Eleventh Edition

NURSING IN TODAY'S WORLD

TRENDS, ISSUES, AND MANAGEMENT

Amy J. Stegen, EdD(c), MSN, RN

Assistant Professor
Weber State University
Ogden, Utah

Holli Sowerby, EdD, MSN, CNE, RN

Assistant Professor
Weber State University
Ogden, Utah

 Wolters Kluwer

Philadelphia · Baltimore · New York · London
Buenos Aires · Hong Kong · Sydney · Tokyo

Vice President and Publisher: Julie K. Stegman
Senior Acquisitions Editor: Christina C. Burns
Director of Product Development: Jennifer K. Forestieri
Development Editors: Dan Reilly, Greg Nicholl
Editorial Coordinator: Tim Rinehart
Marketing Manager: Katie Schlesinger
Editorial Assistant: Kate Campbell
Design Coordinator: Stephen Druding
Art Director: Jennifer Clements
Illustrator: Bot Roda
Production Project Manager: Kim Cox
Manufacturing Coordinator: Karin Duffield
Prepress Vendor: SPi Global

11th Edition

Library of Congress Cataloging-in-Publication Data
Names: Stegen, Amy J., author. | Sowerby, Holli, author. | Preceded by (work): Ellis, Janice Rider. Nursing in todays world.
Title: Nursing in today's world : trends, issues, and management / Amy J. Stegen, Holli Sowerby.
Description: Eleventh edition. | Philadephia : Wolters Kluwer, [2019] | Preceded by Nursing in todays world / Janice Rider Ellis, Celia Love Hartley ; Illustrations by Tomm Scalera. 10th ed. c2012. | Includes bibliographical references and index.
Identifiers: LCCN 2018030664 | ISBN 9781496385000
Subjects: | MESH: Nursing—trends | Nursing Care—trends | Nursing Care—organization & administration | Legislation, Nursing
Classification: LCC RT82 | NLM WY 16.1 | DDC 610.73—dc23 LC record available at https://lccn.loc.gov/2018030664

CCS0818

We would like to dedicate this book to Janice Rider Ellis and Celia Love Hartley, whose hard work and commitment to this textbook made our job easy.

Amy J. Stegen
Holli Sowerby

Barbara Blozen, EdD, MA
Associate Professor
New Jersey City University
Jersey City, New Jersey

Irene Colson Coons, PhD, RN, CNE
Professor and Director of Nursing
College of Southern Nevada
Las Vegas, Nevada

Brenda A. Davis, DNP, MSN, RN, FNP, APRN
Assistant Professor
City Colleges of Chicago – Malcolm X
Chicago, Illinois

Frances C. Gray, DNP, RN, CCM
Assistant Professor
Norfolk State University
Norfolk, Virginia

Jane Hedrick, PhD, RN
Professor
Saint Luke's College
Kansas City, Missouri

Susan Jacob, PhD, RN
Assistant Dean of Quality and Strategic Affairs
University of Tennessee Health Science Center
Memphis, Tennessee

Ginger Meriwether, MSN, BSN
Instructor
Holmes Community College
Grenada, Mississippi

Valerie Pauli, EdD, MSN, RN, ACNS-BC, CNE
Associate Professor
Mercy College of Ohio
Toledo, Ohio

David Peruski, EdD, MSN, BSN
Associate Professor of Nursing
Saginaw Valley State University
Auburn, Mississippi

Boniface Stegman, MSN, BSN
Assistant Professor of Nursing
Maryville University
St. Louis, Missouri

Ana Stoehr, PhD, RN
Assistant Professor
George Mason University
Fairfax, Virginia

Lori Sullivan, DNP, MSNE, BSN
Associate Professor
Finlandia University
Hancock, Missouri

Michael L. Williams, PhD, RN, CCRN, CNE
Associate Professor
Eastern Michigan University
Ypsilanti, Michigan

Nursing in Today's World: Trends, Issues, and Management, 11th edition, focuses on the non-clinical aspects of the professional nursing role. Much of this content is just as critical to practicing safely as is competence in the performance of clinical skills. As nursing steps up to play a major role in the changes brought about by healthcare reform, knowledge of the profession and its place in the healthcare environment has never been more important.

We keep the content of this textbook current by revising and updating each chapter with the latest information on the delivery of care, the structure of the healthcare milieu, roles performed by the variously prepared caregivers, the impact of technology, and the changing financial picture. Additionally, we make every effort to be responsive to suggestions provided by our readers and reviewers. Thus, the 11th edition provides information to help the reader understand the changes that are occurring in healthcare and suggestions for moving from the role of the student into that of a contributing professional in today's healthcare setting. The nursing profession is our focus, and bringing you this content in a concise, readable format is our goal.

ORGANIZATION

This textbook is organized into three major units of study. We provide a flexible approach to instruction, and each chapter is written to stand alone, with frequent cross-referencing throughout. Content may be reordered if so desired. For example, instructors who prefer to skip the historical development of nursing as a profession and move directly to leadership and management are encouraged to adapt the book to match this preference. One possibility is first to present the content in Unit III (Accepting Greater Responsibility for Nursing Practice), which focuses on the nurses' role in working with others in the management of care. Another approach would be to begin with Unit II (Understanding Healthcare in Today's Society) and present information about the healthcare environment, its financing, and its legal and ethical aspects. Similarly, some content areas might be combined or perhaps eliminated if they appear elsewhere in the curriculum of your program.

Unit I: Moving Into the Profession of Nursing

Chapters 1 to 5 focus on nursing itself—its development as a profession, the various educational avenues available to licensure, employment, organizational structures of healthcare environments, and delivery of healthcare.

- **Chapter 1** covers the development of the profession and the challenges to its professional standing, helping prepare students to participate in the nonclinical activities and discussions that are part of nursing.
- The diverse educational paths that prepare graduates for registered nurse licensure are discussed in **Chapter 2**, including the controversy over which form of educational preparation is most appropriate for entry into practice, the implementation of differentiated practice, and whether continuing education should be mandatory or voluntary.

- **Chapter 3** delves into the credentialing of nurses with a discussion of the history of licensing in the United States, explains the process of obtaining and retaining a license, and speculates on the future of licensure in the United States.
- **Chapter 4** discusses current employment opportunities, employer expectations of new graduates, and steps to be taken to realize career goals.
- **Chapter 5** presents information about organizational structures, especially those that provide healthcare, as well as patterns of care delivery and collective bargaining.

Unit II: Understanding Healthcare in Today's Society

This unit includes information on healthcare settings, legal and ethical implications of nursing care, Quality and Safety Education for Nurses (QSEN), and prevention of medication errors.

- **Chapter 6** begins this unit with a description of the various healthcare facilities that provide care to individuals and their families and the evaluation and accreditation of those facilities. Methods and sources of funding for that care and how power is distributed within the system are explained.
- **Chapter 7** deals with the legal responsibilities for practice and includes legal issues common in nursing, malpractice, and the role of the nurse as a witness.
- **Chapter 8** provides a foundation for ethical decision-making, including a broad discussion of ethical issues that affect nursing and nursing practice with a special focus on bioethics.
- Reports released by the Institute of Medicine on errors that have resulted in death or increased hospitalization and cost to clients have highlighted the need for greater safety in the delivery of care. **Chapter 9** presents common errors and the necessary steps to reduce their occurrence.
- **Chapter 10** ends the unit with a discussion of community-based nursing and the nurse's role in that environment. Health promotion and disease prevention are included with a discussion of *Healthy People 2020* and alternative and complementary approaches to healthcare.

Unit III: Accepting Greater Responsibility for Nursing Practice

The book concludes with Unit III, five chapters devoted to the nurses' professional role in the various aspects of healthcare.

- **Chapter 11** provides a basis for understanding leadership and management and the importance of communication in the process of directing the activities of others. Concepts of power, time management, and performance evaluation are also included.
- **Chapter 12** is devoted to management skills: team building, coaching, motivating others, delegating, leading change, and managing conflict.
- It is followed by **Chapter 13** with a discussion of the challenges found in today's workplace: reality shock, burnout, and workplace safety for nurses.
- **Chapter 14** addresses the nurse and the political process and concludes with a description of the various nursing organizations.
- **Chapter 15** looks to the future of nursing, nursing research, and evidence-based practice. Information technology in healthcare is discussed.

FEATURES

Each chapter begins with the following:

- **Learning Outcomes** introduce each chapter and guide learning efforts.
- **Key Terms** used in the chapter discussion are listed to help focus the reader.
- **NEW! Stegen & Sowerby Stories: Part 1** illustrate real-world application of the material presented in each chapter with follow-up discussion questions to further expand understanding. These stories are further explored in **Part 2** at the end of each chapter and online at thePoint®.

Throughout the chapter, students will find special features to help them apply what's learned to real nursing practice:

- **Critical Thinking Activities** engage the reader to envision and apply critical analysis to the topic under discussion.
- **Communication in Action** emphasizes the role of effective communication in every aspect of nursing.
- **NEW! Daily Ethical Dilemmas** in each chapter provide students with the opportunity to apply ethical decision-making to real-life healthcare situations.
- **NEW! Nursing Theory Alerts** highlight a particular nurse theorist in each chapter to introduce students to the many contributions of nursing theory to the practice and profession of nursing.
- **NEW! Evidence-Based Practice** boxes introduced in each chapter highlight how research drives positive practice outcomes.

Every chapter ends with the following, in addition to the References:

- **Stegen & Sowerby Stories**: **Part 2**, the continuation from Part 1 at the beginning of the chapter
- **Want to Know More?** box that lists the additional learning tools found in thePoint®
- **Key Concepts** connect with the Learning Objectives and provide an effective learning tool for content retention.
- **NCLEX-Style Questions** follow each chapter to provide further NCLEX preparation and assess understanding of content.

CARTOON CURRICULUM

The cartoons of *Nursing in Today's World* provide an eye-catching and provocative interpretation of concepts presented in each chapter. We believe that a little humor keeps us healthier and we hope that you, too, will appreciate this hallmark feature that complements the accessible reading style and logical approach of this textbook.

Cartoons in the 11th edition are enhanced by classroom activities and discussion questions, located on thePoint® (see below), that add valuable teaching tools to a favorite component of the book.

TEACHING AND LEARNING RESOURCES

To facilitate mastery of this text's content, a comprehensive teaching and learning package has been developed to assist faculty and students.

Resources for Instructors

Tools to assist you with teaching your course are available upon adoption of this text on thePoint® at http://thePoint.lww.com/Stegen11e.

- A **Test Generator** lets you put together exclusive new tests from a bank containing hundreds of questions to help you in assessing your students' understanding of the material. Test questions link to chapter learning objectives.
- **Open-Book Test** ensures students hone in on core concepts covered in the text.
- A new **Cartoon Curriculum** provides discussion questions as well as cartoon-related activities such as role plays, debates, papers, and projects.
- An **Image Bank** lets you use the photographs and illustrations from this textbook in your PowerPoint slides or as you see fit in your course.
- **PowerPoint Presentations** provide an easy way for you to integrate the textbook with your students' classroom experience, either via slide shows or handouts. Multiple-choice and true/false questions are integrated into the presentations to promote class participation and allow you to use i-clicker technology.
- **Answers and Rationales to Features** include the in-text Critical Thinking Activities and Stegen & Sowerby Stories as well as the accompanying online Cartoon Curriculum and Open Book Test.
- A sample 15-week **Syllabus**.
- Plus **Strategies for Effective Teaching** and **QSEN & BSN Essentials Maps**.

Resources for Students

An exciting set of free resources is available on thePoint® to help students review material and become even more familiar with vital concepts. Students can access all these resources at http://thePoint.lww.com/Stegen11e using the codes printed in the front of their textbooks.

- **NCLEX-Style Review Questions** for each chapter help students review important concepts and practice for the NCLEX.
- **Stegen & Sowerby Stories** include the full unfolding case studies from each chapter as well as questions to help students understand the connection between what they are learning and their careers.
- **Journal Articles** provided for each chapter offer access to current research available in Wolters Kluwer journals.
- **Chapter supplements** provide additional content including history of nursing, state boards, Web site links, and a variety of lists.
- Plus **Learning Objectives** and the **Carrington Professional Guide**.

Acknowledgments

We would like to thank Dan Reilly and Robin Levin Richman for their editorial support through this process, as well as the excellent Wolters Kluwer staff. We are honored to work on a textbook that has such an outstanding history and look forward to continuing its legacy. We both appreciate the support of friends and family, especially our spouses. Without them, we would be unable to make this happen.

Amy J. Stegen

Holli Sowerby

Contents

UNIT ONE

■ Moving Into the Profession of Nursing   1

UNIT   TWO

■ Understanding Healthcare in Today's Society   179

UNIT THREE

■ Accepting Greater Responsibility for Nursing Practice   381

■ Moving Into the Profession of Nursing

You are entering the nursing profession at a time when it is being affected by a number of sociologic issues. As we see in the country at large, there is a graying of the profession with the number of nurses over age 45 increasing. The recession affected retirements and job opportunities. The healthcare environment is rapidly changing, and the forces of healthcare reform may create even more change. The purpose of Unit One is to help you understand nursing as it is today by increasing your perception of the events affecting its development.

Learning about the history and development of the profession can help you to appreciate the heritage of the discipline, understand the events that resulted in nursing offering the opportunities and challenges that it provides today, and interpret the changes occurring now. Chapter 1 begins with a brief history of nursing that describes its growth from early times to an era when preparation for nursing existed as apprentice-type training to a profession that now encompasses doctoral and postdoctoral education. Many believe that nursing is a young profession. Others note that nursing has always existed in some form, while some question whether nursing should be considered a profession at all. This unit considers those debates and addresses the results of the studies that were conducted about nursing and their impact on the development of the profession.

The educational processes by which we prepare nurses continue to experience revision, modification, refinement, and innovation in response to changes that occur in the broader educational environment as well as in the healthcare delivery system. Chapter 2 discusses these as well as the various routes to educational preparation for a nursing career, including a history of the different avenues. You will learn about some of the individuals who made significant contributions to the profession.

Throughout the healthcare system, accreditation of institutions and the licensure and certification of individual professionals serve to safeguard the public. Understanding the various mechanisms by which approval is given helps you to develop your personal career goals and select the organizations where you wish to be employed. As you move into your career as a professional nurse, you will first need to pass examinations that qualify you for a nursing license and may then seek further credentials attesting to your expertise. The various approaches to credentialing are presented in Chapter 3 of this unit.

Once licensed, you will be concerned with finding employment. Chapter 4 focuses on your beginning job search. Information is provided about the competencies needed for the wide variety of opportunities available to nurses today. The various career opportunities in nursing are outlined as well as the expectations of employees. Helpful strategies for seeking that special first job are provided, including writing resumes and composing letters of application and letters following up on interviews.

The final chapter in this unit provides information on the basic structure underlying the healthcare environment, including the mission and/or vision statement, organizational charts, chains of command, and approaches to governance. Also discussed are the forms of nursing care delivery and some major areas of nursing practice in which negotiation occurs, including collective bargaining. Thus, you are moved through the history of the profession into your first role as a practicing professional.

CHAPTER 1

Exploring the Growth of Nursing as a Profession

LEARNING OUTCOMES

After completing this chapter, you should be able to:

1. Discuss the early origins of nursing and factors influencing nursing's development as a profession. Pg 4
2. Describe Florence Nightingale's contribution to nursing and to the growth and improvement of nursing education. Pg 5-8
3. Discuss the development and characteristics of the early nursing schools. Pg 8 – 12
4. Analyze the impact wars and conflicts have had on nursing and nursing education. Pg 12-13
5. Analyze the challenges of defining nursing and formulate your personal definition of nursing. Pg 13-14
6. Identify the major differences between nursing and medicine. Pg 14-15
7. Describe the seven characteristics against which social scientists have evaluated professions, and analyze how these can be applied to nursing. Pg 19
8. Compare and contrast the terms "profession" and "professional" and explain why the issue is of significance to nursing. Pg 20
9. Describe some of the traditions in nursing and explain why the nursing profession has embraced them. Pg 21- 24
10. Discuss the history of the image of nursing in the United States and why it is important for nursing to have a positive image within society. Pg 25-26
11. Analyze areas of nursing about which studies have been conducted and explain why each is important. Pg 27 – 29
12. Explain how a universal language for nursing that includes the North American Nursing Diagnosis Association International (NANDA-I), Nursing Outcomes Classification (NOC), and Nursing Interventions Classification (NIC) systems of nursing classification supports the growth of nursing as a profession globally. Pg 31-33, 34
13. Discuss the ultimate goal of specific documentation systems for nursing and describe how the use of these systems might affect nursing practice. Pg 33

KEY TERMS

Characteristics of a profession
Classification systems
Florence Nightingale
Folk image

International Classification for
  Nursing Practice Project (ICNPP)
Military influence

(continued on page 3)

KEY TERMS *(continued)*

Minimum Data Set for Nursing
   Home Resident Assessment and
   Care Screening (MDS)
North American Nursing Diagnosis
   Association-International
   (NANDA-I)
Nursing Interventions Classification
   (NIC)
Nursing nomenclatures

Nursing Outcomes Classification
   (NOC)
Omaha System
Profession
Professional
Religious image
Servant image
Taxonomy

Stegen & Sowerby Stories: Part 1

Brian is a new nurse and has been working on the medical unit for the last 2 months. Last month, a client died because of a nosocomial infection. The hospital administration and educators have been speaking to staff about reducing nosocomial infection rates and the importance of hand hygiene in that endeavor. Brian notices that Dr. Wells enters his client's room without using hand sanitizer or washing her hands, assesses the client, and then goes to the next client. Brian is aware that this is poor hygiene and against hospital policy. Brian is concerned for his client's safety and those of other clients and wonders how best to address the problem.

Brian is worried that because he is new that he may not be the best person to address the issue. He feels certain that since this is a big problem, others must be watching and they will speak to the doctor, so he chooses to say nothing.

1. What are possible actions that Brian could have taken instead of silence?
2. What could the possible outcomes be of each action?
3. If Brian's client develops an infection as a result of poor hand washing practices, will Brian be held responsible since he was aware of the problem and did nothing?
4. What are Brian's ethical and legal responsibilities as a nurse?

Nursing as a profession is, and will continue to be, responsive to and influenced by the society it serves. Thus, the major activities occurring within the nursing field are also a reflection of what is happening in the society as a whole. Understanding this interrelationship and the progression of nursing as it has developed will help you to evaluate issues arising while you are in practice. Placing the concepts found within this chapter into the broader framework of society may serve to help make the background of nursing more relevant, easier to understand, and more memorable. Throughout the chapter, we mention some of the eras of nursing.

There is no particular date or time period when nursing came into being. While nursing as we know it today may go back less than 150 years, the early origins of nursing, like those of medicine, are intertwined with the ancient civilizations and cultures of the world. With little recorded history, our best speculations regarding the origins of nursing are tied to our knowledge of the varied cultures that existed in the past and to the contributions that these cultures left for future generations.

HISTORY OF HEALTHCARE AND NURSING

Throughout ancient times, suffering and sickness were believed to be caused by evil spirits although the methods and sophistication of care varied greatly from one culture to another. Evil spirits were dealt with by performing incantations or dances, making offerings or sacrifices, and working with medicine men to drive away the demons. Health rules were often part of the religious codes, which gave them authority. A sound theory of disease was absent from most early cultures.

Although ancient cultures developed medicine as a science and a profession, writings about early healthcare make little or no mention of nursing or nurses. One might assume that a family member, particularly the wife or mother, provided the needed care. The possible exceptions to this were the male attendants in early Buddhist hospitals in India and midwives who had an established role in several cultures. It was not until the early Christian period that nursing as we think of it today began to develop.

Nursing has carried forward three heritages from the past that some believe impeded the development of nursing as a profession. They are the folk image of the nurse brought forward from primitive times, the **religious image** of the nurse inherited from the medieval period, and the **servant image** of the nurse created by the Protestant-capitalist ethic from the 16th to 19th century. Whether or not these images hampered progress can be debated, but these concepts of the nurse have certainly had an impact. A summary of these images is provided in Table 1.1.

3 Heritages

Table 1.1 **Nursing Heritages From the Past**

Image of the Nurse	Comments
The **folk image** of the nurse	Primary responsibilities focused on nourishing and nurturing children, caring for older adults, and caring for aging family members. Skills were learned through trial and error and passed from one generation to another. This image presents the nurse as a "caring" person who uses common sense to help the sick individual.
The religious image of the nurse	Groups were organized in conjunction with the establishment of churches in the Christian era with their primary concern focused on care for the sick, the poor, orphans, widows, the aged, slaves, and prisoners. These groups included the deaconesses of the Eastern Christian Church, the Order of Widows and the Order of Virgins, and monastic orders including the Benedictines, which still exist. The first hospitals were also developed at this time, being located close to monasteries. The Crusades (1096–1291) witnessed the founding of military nursing orders, such as the Knights Hospitallers of St. John, the Knights Templars, and the Knights of the Teutonic Order. Nurses in this setting were expected to devote their lives to caring and to exhibit selfless commitment based upon their religious faith.
The servant image of the nurse	The Reformation, which began in Germany in 1517, brought with it a change in the role of women, limiting it to the confines of the home. Duties were those of bearing children and caring for the home. Hospital care was relegated to uncommon women, a group consisting of prisoners, prostitutes, and drunks who had no status in society and were treated as servants who did distasteful tasks. This began what may be called the "Dark Ages" of nursing reflected in Charles Dickens's (1936) description of Sairey Gamp and Betsy Prig in his book *Martin Chuzzlewit*. This image may have greatly influenced the development of nursing as a profession as many capable and desirable persons were unwilling to enter nursing while it had this image.

Table 1.2   **Early Providers of Nursing Care**

Source of Nursing Care	Comments
Sisters of Charity in France and the United States	Founded in Paris in 1633 and receiving help from St. Vincent de Paul, the Sisters of Charity recruited and educated intelligent young women to care for abandoned children as well as provide hospital care. In 1809, the Sisters of Charity established a nursing order in the United States under the direction of Elizabeth Bayley Seton.
Sisters of the Holy Cross in France and the United States	Founded in 1839 in Le Mans, France and in the United States in Bertrand, Michigan in 1844, the Sisters of the Holy Cross provided care to the sick in hospitals and orphanages.
Catholic Religious Orders in Mexico and South America	Following the Reformation, several Roman Catholic religious groups traveled to the Americas. In 1524, the first hospital on the American continent, the Hospital of Immaculate Conception (Hospital de Nuestra Senora O Limpia Concepcion) was built in Mexico City, and mission colleges were founded. The first medical school in America was founded in 1578 at University of Mexico and the second at the University of Lima before 1600.
Ursuline Sisters in Canada	Accompanied Augustinian nuns from France to Quebec, Canada in 1639 to staff the Hotel-Dieu-de Quebec (a hospital that opened that year), and organized the first training of nurses on the North American continent, teaching the native women to care for their families during a smallpox epidemic.
Deaconesses at Kaiserwerth, Germany and Pittsburgh, Pennsylvania	Led by Theodore Fliedner (1800–1864) with the assistance of his first wife, the Christian deaconess movement was revived in Germany in 1836 and a training institute was reestablished. Deaconesses cared for the sick, made visitations, worked in the parish, and taught. In 1849 Pastor Fliedner traveled to the United States to help establish the first Motherhouse of Kaiserwerth in Pittsburgh, Pennsylvania. The Deaconesses managed Pittsburgh Infirmary, which later became Passavant Hospital, the first Protestant hospital in the United States.
Nursing Sisters in England and Ireland	Institute of Nursing Sisters, a secular group, was organized in England by Elizabeth Fry (1780–1845). Sisters of Mercy: A Roman Catholic group formed in 1827 by Catherine McAuley (1787–1841). Irish Sisters of Charity: A Roman Catholic group formed in 1815 by Mary Aikenhead (1787–1857).

During the 17th century, social reform began in Europe. Several nursing groups were organized. These groups gave money, time, and service to the sick and the poor, visiting them in their homes and ministering to their needs. Their activities established many of the early images that were carried forth in nursing, particularly the religious image. Some of these groups and their work are presented in Table 1.2.

THE NIGHTINGALE INFLUENCE

As we look back to the middle of the 19th century, we encounter a world in the throes of an industrial revolution. Factories were built, schools were established, and travel and communication took giant leaps. The telegraph had revolutionized communication, making the happenings on a far-flung battlefield immediately available to the newspaper-reading public. The first rumblings regarding women and their right to vote occurred in England. This is the period in which nursing as a **profession** (an occupation with training and specific qualifications) was born.

During this time, one woman dramatically changed the form and direction of nursing and succeeded in establishing it as a respected field of endeavor. This outstanding woman was **Florence Nightingale (Fig. 1.1).**

Figure 1.1. Florence Nightingale. (From Everett Historical, circa 1880.)

Born May 12, 1820, the second daughter of a wealthy family, she was named after the city in which she was born—Florence, Italy. Because of her family's high social and economic standing, she was cultured, well traveled, and educated. By the age of 17, as the result of tutoring from her father, she had mastered seven languages and mathematics and was extremely well read. This was very unusual for a woman of her time, as she was expected to select a desirable husband from the influential people she met, marry, and assume her place in society. Therefore, further education was deemed unnecessary for her role in life.

Florence Nightingale had other ideas, however. She wanted to become a nurse, but this aspiration was unthinkable to her family because of the terrible conditions of the hospitals at that time and what we now refer to as the "servant image" of nursing. She continued to travel with her family and their friends and, in the course of these travels, met Sidney Herbert and his wife, who were interested in hospital reform. At the time, the public health movement and concerns about hospital reform were growing across England. Inspired, she began collecting information on public health and hospitals and soon became recognized as an important authority on the subject.

Through friends, she learned about Pastor Fliedner's institute at Kaiserwerth where care was provided and nurses were trained. She visited Kaiserwerth briefly in 1850. Because it was a religious institution under the auspices of a Protestant church, her parents would permit her to go there, although she could not go to English hospitals. In 1851, at age 31, she spent 3 months studying at Kaiserwerth.

In 1853, she began working with a committee that supervised an "Establishment for Gentlewomen During Illness." She eventually was appointed superintendent of the establishment, a position she held from August 1853 to October 1854. As her knowledge of hospitals and nursing reform grew, she was consulted by reformers and physicians who were beginning to see the need for trained nurses.

After the Crimean War began in March 1854, war correspondents communicating through the newly developed telegraph wrote about the abominable conditions in which the British Army cared for sick and wounded soldiers. Florence Nightingale, by then a recognized authority on hospital care, wrote to her friend Sir Sidney Herbert, who was then Secretary of War, and offered to take a group of 38 nurses to the Crimea. (At the same time, he had written a letter proposing that she assume direction of all nursing operations at the war front. Their letters crossed in the mail.) Her tireless efforts in the Crimea resulted in greatly reduced mortality rates among the sick and wounded. There is a museum in her honor in the barracks where she worked in what is now part of Istanbul, Turkey.

Public Health measures

When the war ended in 1856, Florence Nightingale returned to England as a national heroine. Her next major project involved working to change the entire approach to health for the British soldier. These activities included constructing hospitals and improving basic hygiene and public health measures for the army. Her focus was on providing cleanliness, wholesome food, fresh air, and separation of people from garbage and sewage both for living environments and for hospital construction (Fig. 1.2). These simple public health measures were revolutionary in the late 1800s.

Throughout her lifetime, Florence Nightingale wrote extensively about hospitals, sanitation, health, and health statistics (creating the first pie chart), and especially about nursing and

Figure 1.2. A focus on cleanliness was a turning point in the history of nursing.

nursing education. Among her most popular books is *Notes on Nursing*, published in 1859. She crusaded for and brought about great reform in nursing education. Her reform of the nursing system and nursing education eventually spread to many nations.

In 1860, she devoted her efforts to the creation of a school of nursing at St. Thomas' Hospital in London, financed by the Nightingale Fund, established to honor her work in the Crimea. The basic principles on which Miss Nightingale established her school included the following:

Basic Principles for School

- Nurses would be trained in teaching hospitals associated with medical schools and organized for that purpose.
- Nurses would be selected carefully and would reside in nurses' houses designed to encourage discipline and form character.
- The school matron would have final authority over the curriculum, living arrangements, and all other aspects of the school.
- The curriculum would include both theoretic material and practical experience.
- Teachers would be paid for their instruction.
- Records would be kept on the students, who would be required to attend lectures, take quizzes, write papers, and keep diaries.

In many other ways, Florence Nightingale advanced nursing as a profession. She believed that nurses should spend their time caring for clients, not cleaning; that nurses must continue learning throughout their lifetime and not become "stagnant"; that nurses should be intelligent and use that intelligence to improve conditions for the client; and that nursing leaders should have social standing. She had a vision of what nursing could and should be. Further discussion of Florence Nightingale's definition of nursing occurs later in this chapter.

Florence Nightingale received many honors from foreign governments, and in 1907, she was recognized by the Queen of England, who awarded her the British Order of Merit. It was the first time it was given to a woman.

Florence Nightingale died in her sleep at the age of 90 on August 13, 1910. The week during which she was born is now honored as International Nurses Week. The enthusiastic student is encouraged to learn more about this fascinating woman in Mark Bostridge's biography *Florence Nightingale: The Making of an Icon (2008)* or by pursuing the topic of Florence Nightingale through the Internet.

THE BEGINNING OF NURSING EDUCATION IN THE UNITED STATES

After the establishment of the Nightingale School in England, nursing programs flourished, and the Nightingale system spread to other countries. In the United States, much of the push for nursing education occurred shortly after the Civil War, during which the lack of trained nurses presented a serious concern.

The Establishment of Early Schools

First System of Instruction

As with many other significant events that have evolved from a variety of influences, it is difficult to pinpoint the first nursing program in the United States. As early as 1798, a pioneer physician, Dr. Valentine Seaman, is said to have initiated the first system of instruction for nurses at New York Hospital. A society was formed in 1839 under Quaker influence, called the Nurse Society of Philadelphia, and a combined Home and School were opened. Historical records show that before 1850, some intermittent preparation was provided to individuals who cared for the sick. A plan of instruction also had been developed for women who would supply maternity service in the home, under the guidance of Dr. Joseph Warrington, who was the obstetric physician for the Philadelphia Dispensary for the Medical Relief of the Poor (Donahue, 2010).

In 1850, a commission of the Massachusetts legislature recommended that institutions be formed to educate nurses. A plan for educating nurses was included in the formation of the *New England Female Medical College*, and a few nurses were educated through this institution. Other hospitals operated training programs, although the course of studies lasted only 6 months. The *Woman's Hospital of Philadelphia*, which operated under the direction of two female physicians, opened a training school in 1861, but it made little progress until it was endowed in 1872. Despite these efforts, the nursing services provided by most hospitals during the 1860s were disorganized and inadequate. In many cases, nursing care was provided by women who had been recruited from among the poor who were sheltered in almshouses or from those who had been arrested for drunkenness or disorderly conduct and who were serving out 10-day sentences. The better hospitals benefited from the work of Catholic sisters or Protestant deaconesses, although most of them also were untrained (Kalisch & Kalisch, 2004, pp. 60–61).

In 1869, responding to the impetus given to nursing during the Civil War, the American Medical Association established a committee to study the issue of training for nurses. The committee, chaired by Dr. Samuel D. Gross (1805–1884), was charged with identifying the best possible method to organize and manage institutions for training nurses. Its report concluded that every large hospital should have a nursing school, emphasized that the union between religious exercises and nursing would be conducive to the welfare of the sick, and recommended that schools be placed under the guardianship of county medical societies (Donahue, 2010).

Formal Programs

The *New England Hospital for Women and Children* is often credited with being the first hospital to establish a formal 1-year program to train nurses in 1872. It operated under the guidance of a female physician, Susan Dimock, who had received her medical education in Europe and had some knowledge of the work of Florence Nightingale. Five probationers started the program on September 1. It was from this school that Melinda Ann (Linda) Richards graduated in 1873, to become America's first trained nurse. This school was also the alma mater for the first black nurse graduate, Mary Eliza Mahoney, in 1879.

Separate Programs

By 1873, three additional schools had opened: the *Bellevue Training School* in New York City, the *Connecticut Training School* in New Haven, and the *Boston Training School*. Typically, these schools did not admit men. In 1888, the *Mills School of Nursing* at Bellevue Hospital opened to train male nurses for client care. Separate schools to educate black nurses also opened; among them were *Spelman Seminary* in Atlanta in 1886, *Hampton Institute* in Virginia and *Providence Hospital* in Chicago in 1891, and *Tuskegee Institute* in Alabama in 1892 (Kalisch & Kalisch, 2004). Table 1.3 identifies some of the early schools.

Similar movements to establish nursing schools occurred in other countries. In 1868, a school was organized in Sydney Hospital, Australia. In Edinburgh, Scotland, a program was started at the Royal Infirmary. The *Mack Training School* in St. Catharines, Toronto, Canada, was started in 1884 (Kalisch & Kalisch, 2004).

Table 1.3   Early North American Training Schools for Nurses*

Date	Name and Place	Comments
1798	New York Hospital—New York	Dr. Valentine Seaman initiated a system of instruction for nurses. His lectures covered the topics of anatomy, physiology, maternal nursing, and care of children.
1839	Philadelphia Dispensary—Philadelphia	Dr. Joseph Warrington provided obstetric training to a group of women who would work with families who would otherwise not receive care. The Nurse Society of Philadelphia grew out of this training.
1861	Bellevue Hospital—New York	Dr. Elizabeth Blackwell converted Bellevue Hospital into a training center for nurses. About 100 women were trained to provide care during the Civil War in an intensive 4-week course.
1861–1862	Woman's Hospital of Philadelphia—Philadelphia	Opened a training school, but it progressed slowly until 1872, when it became endowed—the first endowed school of nursing in America. Organized and conducted by two female physicians.
1862	New England Hospital for Women and Children—Boston	Dr. Marie Zakrzewska, a colleague of Dr. Blackwell's, offered a 6-month program to nurses.
1872	New England Training School—Boston	An expansion of the New England Hospital Program was identified as the first formal school for nurses, directed by Dr. Susan Dimock. The first graduate was Linda Ann Richards. Mary Mahoney, the first black nurse to graduate from a nursing school, also attended this school.
1873—May	Bellevue Training School—New York	First of a trio of schools modeled after the Nightingale model— Lavinia Dock was one of the early graduates.
1873— October	Connecticut Training School— New Haven	Second of the trio of schools started in 1873—introduced first textbook, *New Haven Manual of Nursing*, written by a committee of nurses and physicians.
1873— November	Boston Training School—Boston (attached to Massachusetts General)	Third of the trio—Linda Richards became superintendent of nurses in November 1894. Idea for school initiated by the Woman's Educational Association. Medical staff did not support initiation of the school.
1874	St. Catharine's General and Marine Hospital—Ontario, Canada—later called the Mack Training School	Patterned after the Nightingale schools, this program included instruction in the art of nursing, chemistry, sanitary science, physiology, and anatomy.
1877	Training School of the New York Hospital—New York	Offered an 18-month course to prepare graduates for nursing.
1878	Boston City Hospital Training School—Boston	Required graduates to complete a 2-year program of study.
1884	Toronto General Hospital— Toronto, Canada	Mary Agnes Snively became superintendent of this school, which had early beginnings in 1877.
1884–1885	Farrand Training School for Nurses—Harper Hospital, Detroit	Considered one of the better schools—students had two annual series of lectures, approximately 20 hours totally.
1886	Spelman Seminary—Atlanta	The first separate school to educate black nurses, who were often denied admission to other schools.
1888	Mills School of Nursing at Bellevue Hospital—New York	First school established for male nurses. Prepared them to give general client care.
1889	Johns Hopkins School of Nursing—Baltimore	Program opened under direction of Isabel Hampton Robb. Mary Adelaide Nutting graduated in 1891.
1890	Montreal General—Montreal, Canada	Although wanting a nursing program as early as 1835, hospital conditions would not allow. Nora Gertrude Livingstone established the school in 1890.

*Compiled from Donahue (2010), and Kalisch and Kalisch (2004).

Characteristics of the Early Schools

The life of the nursing student at the turn of the century was not an easy one. The strong militaristic and religious influences over nursing were embodied in the expectations held for nursing students. The nurse in training was expected to yield to her superiors and demonstrate the obedience characteristic of a good soldier with actions governed by the dedication to duty derived from religious devotion (Kalisch & Kalisch, 2004).

The typical nursing student was about 21 years of age, single, and female. The first weeks or months of their education were spent as probationers, or "probies," and their duties, although helping with the operation of the hospital, did little to educate them as nurses. For example, they spent much of their time washing, scrubbing, polishing, folding, stacking, and the like. Rules of conduct were rigid and unforgiving; early superintendents saw it as their responsibility to discipline pupils, ensuring that they possessed good morals and were honest, conscientious, obedient, respectful, loyal, passive, and devoted to duty. Nursing students were expected to be unselfish, thinking not of themselves but of the happiness and well-being of others. This is in keeping with the "religious image" of the nurse.

Initially, nursing education was largely an apprenticeship and resulted in students providing much of the workforce of hospitals. The workday was long and arduous, often starting at 5:30 AM and ending with nursing prayers very late at night, and consisted primarily of work on the hospital wards. The superintendent or her assistants provided instruction. There was no standardization of curriculum and no accreditation. The few lectures that were part of the program were usually given by physicians and scheduled at 8 or 9 PM after a long day of work. A 7-day workweek was the standard, and the help needed on the hospital units took precedence over the education of the young women. Lectures were canceled if students were needed to care for clients.

As schools developed, facilities to house nursing students became necessary. Although some of the early programs provided sleeping quarters in the hospital, nursing students usually were housed in a building next to the hospital, often referred to as the "nurses' dormitory." A "housemother" often controlled the nurses' residence. In religious affiliations, a deaconess or Sister served the same purpose. Housemothers ensured that codes of behavior were adhered to and that curfews were enforced. Violations usually resulted in expulsion from the program or the loss of a part of the uniform, such as a cap or the bib section of an apron. This signified to all that some infraction had occurred. Young women, who were attracted to nursing because of the imagined glamour of wearing a long, crisp, white apron and ministering to sick (though handsome) young men, often became discouraged with the severe duties and routine. The attrition rate was high in the early schools.

From about 1900 to 1920, nursing in Western Europe, Canada, and the United States was beginning to establish itself with the growth of schools, the publication of journals and textbooks, and the formulation of organizations for nursing (see Chapter 15). For both society and nursing, it was an era of great growth. Schools proliferated, as even small hospitals established nursing programs, recognizing the valuable commodity available in students who provided the majority of care given. As early as 1905, early pioneers and advocates for nursing, concerned about the proliferation of schools, championed programs that offered a sound educational foundation and reasonable working hours. During the time Isabel Hampton was principal of the Johns Hopkins Training School (a position she accepted in 1889 and continued until her marriage to Dr. Robb in 1894), she arranged for a regular period of 2 hours of free time during a day that was limited to 12 hours. She would have liked to limit the workday to 8 hours, however. Time was allowed for recreation and for meals.

Although there were some changes in the curriculum—work hours were decreased, the length of study was increased, and the theory component was organized into specific areas of care such as medical, surgical, and obstetric nursing—hospital-based programs remained largely unchanged through the 1940s and 1950s.

Early Textbooks and Journals

First Textbooks + Journals

There were few textbooks before 1900, a factor that complicated the learning process. Many of the lectures presented by physicians were given from notes they had taken while medical students. The first nursing textbook was reportedly the *Hand-book of Nursing for Family and General Use*, written by a committee composed of physicians and nurses associated with the *Connecticut Training School* at New Haven Hospital and published by Lippincott in 1878. Other books followed over the next 2 years. Table 1.4 describes some of the early textbooks.

Nursing journals also appeared toward the end of the 19th century. Five journals for nurses were published before 1901. The first appeared in 1886 and was entitled *The Nightingale*. In 1889, under the direction of Mary E. P. Davis, a company was formed with 550 cash subscriptions, and a new journal called the *American Journal of Nursing* made its debut in October 1900 (Kalisch & Kalisch, 2004, p. 106). The journal continues to be published today.

THE MILITARY INFLUENCE

Wars have had a major impact on nursing and the practice of medicine. The **military influence** is reflected in the innovations in practice made during the heat of battle and in response to the needs of soldiers and veterans that have brought about significant changes. The American Revolution saw the development of dispensaries with the Philadelphia dispensary being the first place to vaccinate against smallpox as preventative medicine. The Civil War saw the invention of ambulances and was instrumental in the development of nursing. The Red Cross was born during the Spanish–American War, and at the end of that war, the Army Nurse Corps was established by legislation in 1901 with the Navy Nurse Corps following in 1908.

Table 1.4   Early Nursing Textbooks*

Year	Author	Title
1878	A committee of physicians and nurses	*Hand-book for Family and General Use*
1885	Clara Weeks Shaw	*A Textbook of Nursing for the Use of Training Schools, Families, and Private Students*
1890	Lavinia Dock	*The Textbook on Materia Medica for Nurses*
1893	Diana Kimber	*The first anatomy book for nurses, Anatomy and Physiology*
1889 (about)	Isabel Hampton	*Nursing: Its Principles and Practices for Hospital and Private Use*
1894 (about)	Isabel Hampton Robb	*Nursing Ethics*

*Compiled from Donahue (2010), and Kalisch and Kalisch (2004).

Figure 1.3. Nurses were widely recruited for service in the military.

More than 30,000 nurses served in World War I after the United States joined the war on April 6, 1917, and those same nurses won the right to vote in 1919 possibly due to the contributions they made during the war **(Fig. 1.3)**. World War II brought about increased status and authority, and flight nursing came into existence. The GI bill came into existence at the end of World War II and made it possible for many nurses to enter bachelor's and master's degree programs after serving with the military.

The Korean and Vietnam wars brought about many developments in triage and surgery with MASH units (Mobile Army Surgical Hospitals) combined with further demand for flight nurses. Nurses have made significant contributions throughout all the wars and conflicts throughout the years and up to the present. Nurses, working with other healthcare professionals, have saved lives, improved medical care, and brought many positive changes throughout our society.

DEVELOPING A DEFINITION FOR NURSING

When you entered the nursing program in which you are now enrolled, what was your perception of nursing as a profession? Has that perception of nursing been changed by the experiences you have had as a nursing student? Some might ask, "Why spend so much time and effort trying to define nursing?"

Over the years, the profession has worked at establishing a definition of nursing; however, nurses themselves cannot agree on a single definition. A major factor that has made it difficult to define nursing is that it is taught as encompassing both <u>theoretic</u> and <u>practical</u> aspects, but it is pursued (and continues to be defined) primarily through practice, until recently a little-studied area. This failure to chart and study our practices and clinical observations has deprived nursing theory of the uniqueness and richness of the knowledge embedded in expert clinical practice. When attempting to define nursing, we often stumble over theoretical concepts and the practical, hands-on application of nursing and how to combine the distinct and unique aspects of both. Despite the challenges, serious efforts were put into defining nursing in the late 1970s and early 1980s.

Early Definitions of Nursing

A nurse is a person who nourishes, fosters, and protects—a person who is prepared to care for the sick, injured, and aged. In this sense, "nurse" is used as a noun and is derived from the Latin *nutrix,* which means "nursing mother." The word nurse also has referred to a woman who suckled a child (usually not her own)—a wet-nurse. Dictionary definitions of nurse include such descriptions as "suckles or nourishes," "to take care of a child or children," and "to bring up; rear." In this way, *nurse* is used as a verb, deriving from the Latin *nutrire*, which means "to suckle and nourish." References to "the nurse" can be found in both the Talmud and in the Old Testament, and appear more similar to the wet-nurse than to someone who cared for the sick.

Over the centuries, the word nurse has evolved to refer to a person who tends to the needs of the sick. <u>Florence Nightingale</u>, in her *Notes on Nursing: What It Is and What It Is Not,* described the nurse's role as one that would "put the client in the best condition for nature to act upon him" (Nightingale, 1954, p. 133), a definition that often is quoted today.

In the past, nurses undoubtedly were more concerned about carrying out their responsibilities than about defining the role of the nurse. Through the years, we have seen the concept of the nurse grow and evolve from the nurse as mother, nourishing and nurturing children, to the nurse without specific reference to gender, with responsibilities encompassing expanded roles and involved in providing vital services to people needing healthcare.

Not surprising, the development of nursing as a profession, the defining of its role and language for society, and the placing of it among other attractive careers have been inextricably tied to the <u>role of women in society</u> at various times in history and to the forces that have had an impact on society. If we are frustrated at what appears to be the slow development of nursing as a profession, we need to remember that it was 1916 when Margaret Sanger opened the first birth control clinic in the United States. And not until 1919, after 40 years of campaigning, were women in the United States granted the right to vote, through the 19th Amendment to the Constitution.

Distinguishing Nursing From Medicine

The formulation of clear and concise definitions of nursing also has been hindered by the lack of an obvious distinction between nursing and medicine. For example, it is not unusual to hear a prospective nursing student say, "I've always been interested in the medical field, so I decided to go into nursing." Something of an interdependence exists between medicine and nursing, and they have somewhat paralleled one another in historic development.

However, anyone who has been involved in the profession of nursing for any period of time will be quick to assure you that distinct differences exist, and more and more the reference is to healthcare rather than to medicine when speaking of the entire field.

The primary differences between nursing and medicine are the purpose and goal of each profession and the education needed to fulfill each role. Further, historically, medicine was perceived as a profession for men and nursing as a profession for women although that situation is much changed today. Finally, the subservient role of the nurse in relationship to the physician in the past—often referred to as the handmaiden of the physician—which has been significant in shaping the definition of nursing can also be dismissed as a stereotype today. In general, medicine is concerned with the diagnosis and treatment (and cure, when possible) of disease. Nursing is concerned with caring for the person from a holistic perspective in a variety of health-related situations. The caring aspects of nursing are well documented in nursing literature (Benner & Wrubel, 1989; Bevis & Watson, 1989; Carper, 1979; Watson, 1979). We think of medicine as being involved with the cure of a client and nursing with the care of that client. The role of the nurse in client care also involves teaching about health and the prevention of illness, as well as caring for the ill individual. It also may encompass case management and is increasingly being practiced outside the walls of hospitals. Nursing takes place in the community and the home, hospice centers, ambulatory care environments, schools and day care centers, and rehabilitation facilities. In all environments, nurses play a key role in promoting higher standards of health.

With advancing technology in the healthcare fields, the diverse areas of specialization within those fields, the different routes to educational preparation for nurses, and the distinct practice settings and roles occupied by the nurse, it is critical that nurses provide clear information for themselves and for the public. To state that you are a registered nurse (RN) says little about what you do. It conveys nothing about where you are employed or your educational background. For example, as an RN, you might be employed in a community hospital or in a long-term care facility, have a role in a critical care unit, have earned additional credentials, be working in advanced practice, or be a nurse educator.

Thus, you can see that the words "nurse" and "nursing" have been applied to a wide variety of healthcare activities, in many different settings, performed by people with a variety of educational backgrounds. The old adage "A nurse is a nurse is a nurse" is out of place in a highly technical healthcare delivery system that struggles to keep "high touch" and "high tech" compatible.

Daily Ethical Dilemma 1.1: The Role of a Nurse

Sue is an RN. One day, her neighbor Judy comes over and asks for some medical advice. Judy was playing with her cat and has a cut on her arm from the cat's claw. She is worried that it's infected and wants Sue to look at it. Sue takes off the bandage and evaluates the wound. Sue tells Judy that it is clearly infected and that she needs Keflex (an antibiotic).

Is Sue acting appropriately as a nurse? What is the role of a nurse versus a physician? What could Sue tell Judy that would be within the scope of a nurse? What are the ethical principles involved? Is this a legal dilemma or an ethical dilemma?

Influences on the Definition of Nursing

A number of factors have influenced the definition of nursing. One might first think of technologic advances that have significantly affected the definition of nursing and the role of the nurse. The acute care hospital provides care to clients who are much more acutely ill with conditions from which they would not have survived 25 years ago. Today, recovery is anticipated after careful evaluation and treatment that can require diagnostic imaging, sophisticated laboratory tests, delicate medical procedures, and specialized critical care utilizing a host of variously prepared healthcare providers. Critical thinking skills are essential to the successful performance of the diverse tasks expected of a nurse. Nurses in many positions have been required to assume ever-greater levels of responsibility. Only recently are nurses beginning to receive the official authority, autonomy, and recognition that should accompany those responsibilities.

Another factor influencing the definition of nursing is the work of nursing theorists. As nursing has grown into a profession, many nursing theorists developed definitions of nursing consistent with their conceptual frameworks. Table 1.5 presents the definitions of some of the theorists.

Table 1.5 Definitions of Nursing by Major Theorists

Theorist	Major Theme	Definition
Florence Nightingale (1954[1860])	Environment/Sanitation	The goal of nursing is to put the client in the best condition for nature to act upon him, primarily by altering the environment.
Hildegard Peplau (1952)	Interpersonal process	Nursing is viewed as an interpersonal process involving interaction between two or more individuals, which has as its common goal assisting the individual who is sick or in need of healthcare.
Faye Abdellah (1960)	Nursing problems	Nursing is a service to individuals, families, and society based on an art and science that molds the attitudes, intellectual competencies, and technical skills of the individual nurse into the desire and ability to help people cope with their healthcare needs, and is focused around 21 nursing problems.
Ernestine Wiedenbach (1964)	Nursing problems model	Nursing is a helping, nurturing, and caring service rendered with compassion, skill, and understanding, in which sensitivity is key to assisting the nurse in identifying problems.
Virginia Henderson (1966)	Development/Needs	Nursing's role is to assist the individual (sick or well) to carry out those activities … he would perform unaided if he had the necessary strength, will, or knowledge.
Myra Levine (1969)	Conservation and adaptation	Nursing means the nurse interposes her/his skill and knowledge into the course of events that affect the client. When influencing adaptation favorably, the nurse is acting in a therapeutic sense. When the nursing intervention cannot alter the course of adaptation, the nurse is acting in a supportive sense.
Ida Orlando Pelletier (1972)	Interpersonal process	Nursing's unique and independent role concerns itself with an individual's need for help in an immediate situation for the purpose of avoiding, relieving, diminishing, or curing that individual's sense of helplessness.
Jean Watson (1979–1988)	Caring	The essence and central unifying focus for nursing practice is caring, a transpersonal value. Nurse behaviors are defined as 10 curative factors. Focuses on the spiritual subjective aspects of both the nurse and the client and the "caring moment" relating to the time when the nurse and client first come together (LeMaire, 2002).

Table 1.5   Definitions of Nursing by Major Theorists (continued)

Theorist	Major Theme	Definition
Dorothy Orem (1980)	Self-care	Nursing is concerned with the individual's need for self-care action, which is the practice of activities that individuals initiate and perform on their own behalf in maintaining health and well-being.
Dorothy E. Johnson (1980)	Systems approach	Nursing is an external regulatory force that acts to preserve the organization and integration of the client's behavior at an optimal level, under those conditions in which the behavior constitutes a threat to physical or social health, or in which illness is found.
Imogene M. King (1981)	Open systems approach	The focus of nursing is the care of human beings resulting in the health of individuals and healthcare for groups, who are viewed as open systems in constant interaction with their environments.
Rosemarie Rizzo Parse (1981)	Man-Living-Health	Nursing is rooted in the human sciences and focuses on man as a living unity and as qualitatively participating in health experiences. Health is viewed as a process.
Betty Neuman (1982)	Systems approach	Nursing responds to individuals, groups, and communities, who are in constant interaction with environmental stressors that create disequilibrium. A critical element is the client's ability to react to stress and factors that assist with reconstitution or adaptation.
Sister Callista Roy (1984)	Adaptation	The goal of nursing is the promotion of adaptive responses (those things that positively influence health) that are affected by the person's ability to respond to stimuli. Nursing involves manipulating stimuli to promote adaptive responses.
Martha E. Rogers (1984)	Science of unitary man	Nursing is an art and science that is humanistic and humanitarian, directed toward the unitary human, and concerned with the nature and direction of human development.
Katharine Y. Kolcaba (1992)	Holistic theory of comfort	The immediate desirable outcome of nursing care is enhanced comfort. This comfort positively correlates with desirable health-seeking behaviors.
Sharon Van Sell and Ioannis Kalofissudis (2010)	A Complexity Integration Nursing Theory	Nursing is an art and a science that can be depicted in mathematical format that shows the relationship among philosophy, science, culture, and the human being in which the socialization of the nurse into nursing is important (Van Sell & Kalofissudis, 2010).

In 1958, Virginia Henderson, a nurse educator, author, and researcher, was asked by the nursing service committee of the International Council of Nurses (ICN) to describe her concept of basic nursing. Hers is still one of the most widely accepted definitions of nursing:

Widely Accepted Definition

> The unique function of the nurse is to assist the individual, sick or well, in the performance of those activities contributing to health or its recovery (or to peaceful death) that he would perform unaided if he had the necessary strength, will or knowledge. And to do this in such a way as to help him gain independence as rapidly as possible (Henderson, 1966, p. 15).

The American Nurses Association (ANA) first defined nursing in its *Social Policy Statement* published in 1980. The definition was significantly expanded in later editions. The third edition of *Nursing's Social Policy Statement: The Essence of the Profession* states,

> Nursing is the protection, promotion, and optimization of health and abilities, prevention of illness and injury, alleviation of suffering through the diagnosis and treatment of human response, and advocacy in the care of individuals, families, communities, and populations (ANA, 2010).

The National Council of State Boards of Nursing has as one of its major responsibilities the management of licensure of nurses throughout the United States. Through the Model Nurse Practice Act, the NCSBN states,

> The Practice of Nursing means assisting clients to attain or maintain optimal health, implementing a strategy of care to accomplish defined goals within the context of a client-centered health care plan, and evaluating responses to nursing care and treatment (NCSBN, Article III, Section 2, 2014).

Perhaps nothing so affects the definition of nursing as its legal definition found in each state's nursing practice act (see Chapter 3). This legal definition is critical because it provides the foundation and guidelines for education, licensure, scope of practice, and, when necessary, the corrective actions against people who violate the practice act.

Legal
Definition
Commonalities
No state adopts the exact wording of any recommended definition, but most states include references to performing services for compensation, the necessity for a specialized knowledge base, the use of the nursing process (although steps may carry different names), and components of nursing practice. Several states include some reference to treating human responses to actual or potential health problems. Most states refer to the execution of the medical regimen, and many include a general statement about additional acts that recognize that nursing practice is evolving and that the nurse's area of responsibility can be expected to broaden.

Defining Nursing for the Future

As the profession grows and responsibilities change, undoubtedly we will continue to refine the definition of nursing. By being responsive to changes, nursing has become more closely aligned with professions such as law, theology, and education, in which changing practices have required greater precision and refinement of definitions of the profession.

Critical Thinking Activity: Nursing Theories
Analyze the definitions of the major nursing theorists. What is similar among them? What is different? What concepts found in those definitions are most closely aligned with your perception of nursing? Develop your own definition of nursing and compare it to those of the theorists and to those of your classmates.

CHARACTERISTICS OF A PROFESSION

The meanings of profession and professionalism as applied to nursing have been a subject of debate for many years. From approximately the 1950s through the 1970s or mid-1980s, nursing periodically was reviewed against the **characteristics of a profession** that had been established in the sociologic literature. Some critics believe that nursing falls short of meeting these criteria. Amid these challenges, nurses have worked to advance the standing of nursing

Table 1.6   How Nursing Meets the Traditional Criteria for a Profession*

Criterion	How Nursing Meets the Criterion
Possession of a Body of Specialized Knowledge	Critics state that nursing borrows from biologic sciences, social sciences, and medical science, and then combines the various skills and concepts. This amalgamation and synthesis may be one of nursing's distinctive qualities. Nursing researchers work to develop an organized body of knowledge unique to nursing along with a specialized language of nursing (discussed later in this chapter). As this body of knowledge expands, this criterion is more nearly met.
Use of Scientific Method to Enlarge the Body of Knowledge	Much work has been done toward systematically gathering and analyzing data, correctly identifying problems, selecting alternates, and evaluating client care. Evidence-based practice and evidence-based education are at the forefront of nursing today (see Chapter 16).
Education Within Institutions of Higher Education	Over time, the settings in which nurses are educated have changed, with most programs under the auspices of colleges or universities. Controversy over the length of nursing programs (associate degree vs. baccalaureate degree) and the technical aspects of client care continues. A few programs continue to be offered by hospitals.
Control of Professional Policy, Professional Activity, and Autonomy	Today, nurses are responsible for planning, implementing, and evaluating the care clients receive and are accountable for that care. Nursing policies and protocols, standards of practice, and evaluative measures and criteria have been developed by nurses (see Chapter 6). In some settings, nurses are eligible for third-party payment. More collaborative relationships are occurring with other healthcare team members, including physicians.
A Code of Ethics	The general standard for the professional behavior of nurses in the United States is the ANA *Code for Nurses,* which is periodically revised. The International Council of Nurses also has developed a code for nurses that sets the standards of ethical practice by nurses throughout the world (see Chapter 8).
Nursing as Lifetime Commitment	Most nurses view themselves as committed to their profession and continue to identify themselves as nurses long after they retire. However, some do leave the profession due to "burnout" and stress. Better educational and clinical pathways encourage continued growth and retention in the profession.
Service to the Public	Although discussion occurs with regard to altruism, remuneration for services, and collective bargaining (see Chapter 5), there is no question that nursing provides a service to the public.

*The criteria identified in this table are developed from criteria set forth by Bixler and Bixler (1945).

through the development of a code of ethics, standards of practice, and peer review. Table 1.6 outlines the seven major criteria for a profession and briefly discusses how nursing is meeting them or falls short of doing so. This set of characteristics corresponds to those being used by the American Association of Colleges of Nursing (AACN) when they refer to "**professional**" nursing as requiring a baccalaureate degree in nursing or higher.

Critical Thinking Activity: Characteristics of the Nursing Profession

In reviewing Table 1.6, select one of the characteristics of a profession that you believe nursing has difficulty meeting. Describe the actions that you believe should occur in the nursing profession that would result in nursing fully meeting that criterion. How would you go about implementing those actions?

Differentiating Between the Terms "Profession" and "Professional"

Nursing involves activities that may be performed by many different caregivers. These people include nursing assistants, practical (vocational) nurses, and RNs prepared for entry into nursing through any of several educational avenues (see Chapter 2). Each of these caregivers contributes to nursing as a profession. To meet the nursing needs of the public, it is essential that caregivers function at various levels of practice. This has led to confusion about the use of the terms profession and professional. Is there a difference between looking at the practice of nursing in its totality and the "professional" practice of nursing?

A Profession as Defined by Legislation

In at least one instance, federal legislation has helped to establish a list of the characteristics of a professional. Public Law 93-360 (Labor Management Relations Act, 1947 [amended, 1959, 1974]), which governs collective bargaining activities, defines the professional employee as follows:

a. Any employee engaged in work (i) predominantly intellectual and varied in character as opposed to routine mental, manual, mechanical, or physical work; (ii) involving the consistent exercise of discretion and judgment in its performance; (iii) of such a character that the output produced or the result accomplished cannot be standardized in relation to a given period of time; (iv) requiring knowledge of an advanced type in a field of science or learning customarily acquired by a prolonged course of specialized intellectual instruction and study in an institution of higher learning or a hospital, as distinguished from a general academic education or from an apprenticeship or from training in the performance of routine mental, manual, or physical processes; or
b. Any employee, who (i) has completed the courses of specialized intellectual instruction and study described in clause (iv) of paragraph (a), and (ii) is performing related work under the supervision of a professional person to qualify himself to become a professional employee as defined in paragraph (a).

Based on this definition, all RNs are considered professionals.

Popular View of a Professional

A popular view of a professional involves the approach a person has to the role that is required. Most professionals approach their activities earnestly, strive for excellence in performance, and demonstrate a sense of ethics and responsibility in relationship to their careers. Such people consider their work a lifelong endeavor rather than a stepping stone to another field of employment. They place a positive value on being termed professional and perceive being termed nonprofessional or technical as an adverse reflection on their status, position, and motivation. Using this definition, we again find that it would apply to all RNs.

Certain people suggest that professionalism has a great deal to do with attitude, dress, conduct, and deportment. The attributes that are considered professional vary according to the personal values and stereotypes of the person doing the evaluation.

Theory Alert *Florence Nightingale*

Florence Nightingale believed that the environment has a direct impact on a client's well-being, which is why she was very concerned with cleanliness and fresh air. Her nursing theory is the Environmental Theory in which the nurse uses the environment to assist the client in his or her recovery. Nightingale believed that a lack of certain environmental factors such as clean water, fresh air, cleanliness, sunlight, and appropriate nutrition would impair a client's recovery. Nightingale recognized the importance of diet and rest in recovery. Monitoring a client's environment to improve recovery remains an important part of nursing care (Petiprin, 2016).

TRADITIONS IN NURSING

Because of its history, nursing has developed many traditions. Some of them are being questioned or eliminated, primarily because they are not practical in today's workplace (eg, the wearing of a nursing cap). It is worthwhile, however, to reflect just a little on the development of these traditions and to discuss their relationship to nursing. Many believe that enduring traditions are important; they keep the reality of today connected to the history of the past.

The Nursing Pin

The nursing pin may date back to the time of the Crusades, when Crusaders marched to Jerusalem to recover the Holy Land. Among the Crusaders were the Knights Hospitallers of St. John of Jerusalem. Their uniform, introduced by a man named Gerard, included a black robe with a white Maltese cross. The Maltese cross became a familiar sight on the battlefields of the Holy Land. Following the capture of Jerusalem in 1099, some of the Crusaders noted the excellent nursing care provided by the Hospital of St. John and decided to join the nursing group. The Maltese cross is an eight-pointed cross formed by four arrowheads joining at their points. The eight points of the cross signified the eight beatitudes that knights were expected to exemplify in their works of charity. When the Knights Templars and the Knights of the Teutonic Order were formed, in 1118 and 1190, respectively, this symbol was carried forward, and later, the Maltese cross became a symbol of many groups who cared for the sick, including the United States Cadet Nurse Corps.

[margin note: Maltese Cross as a symbol]

The actual symbolism of the pin relates to customs established in the 16th century, when the privilege of wearing a coat of arms was limited to noblemen who served their kings with distinction. In time, the privilege was extended to schools and to craft guilds, and the symbols of wisdom, strength, courage, and faith appeared on buttons, badges, and shields. Perhaps it was this spirit that Florence Nightingale attempted to capture when she chose the Maltese cross as a symbol for the badge worn by the graduates of her first nursing school.

As nursing developed as a profession, each school chose a unique pin, awarded on completion of the program, as a public symbol of work well done. Many of the early schools, particularly those associated with hospitals supported by religious groups, incorporated the cross into their pin. The first Nightingale School of Nursing in the United States was at Bellevue Hospital and is credited with developing the first school badge or pin, which was presented to the class of 1880 (Kalisch & Kalisch, 2004, p. 76). The nursing journal *RN* has collected nursing pins from across the United States and has occasionally created a cover display of pins from that collection.

[margin note: Each School has their unique pin]

The Nursing Cap

Inspiration

Purpose

The history of the nursing cap is less certain. Several explanations of the origin of the cap have been suggested. It probably evolved during the period of time when nursing was greatly influenced by religion. It may have originated in the habit worn by the Sisters of Charity of St. Vincent de Paul, who established the first modern school of nursing in Paris in 1864. Another opinion suggests that the cap was influenced by the Institute of Protestant Deaconesses, founded by Pastor Theodor Fliedner at Kaiserwerth in Germany and the institution where Florence Nightingale studied. The white cap of the deaconesses of the early Christian era and the nun's veil of the Middle Ages have been said to be the forerunners of the nursing cap as we know it today (Mangum, 1994). The veil was modified to become a cap and was associated with service to others. We need to remember, also, that in Florence Nightingale's day, every lady wore a cap indoors. If you look at pictures of Queen Victoria, you notice the cap of plain white stiffened muslin framing her face. It was considered proper for women to keep their heads covered; thus, the cap would be viewed as the proper dress for a young woman of the day. The cap worn by students at Kaiserwerth when Florence Nightingale was a student was hood shaped, had a ruffle around the face, and was tied under the chin. A final conjecture is that the cap originally was designed to cover and help to control the long hair that was fashionable in the late 19th century, when short haircuts were not acceptable for women (Kalisch & Kalisch, 2004).

In the United States and Canada, the head covering became smaller and lost its scarf or veil as women's hairstyles changed and hair was worn shorter. (The hair-covering aspect remained a part of the cap in many areas of Europe.) As nursing education programs developed in hospitals, they each created their own cap, as with their nursing pin, to symbolize that particular hospital and nursing school. Some of these caps were rather frilly and were fashioned after the cloth cone through which ether was dropped. Again, as hairstyles changed, the size of the cap also changed, until it became one of individual taste or preference. A capping ceremony was part of the ritual of the nursing student and is discussed later.

Regarding Impracticability

As the role of nurses changed and as high technology became a significant part of the hospital work environment, nurses found that caps were bothersome as they tried to carry out their duties. They were knocked askew by curtains, equipment, and tubing. By the 1980s, many hospitals no longer required the cap as a part of the uniform. Nursing programs responded by dropping the cap as a required article of dress. If students wished to have a cap, it was purchased from a local uniform store and had no particular identification with the program.

The Nursing Uniform

White Uniform

Like the nursing cap, which is actually a part of the early nursing uniform, the requirement for special dress came from the religious and military history of nursing and has always been significant in nursing. This is due to the fact that dress provides a strong nonverbal message about one's image. The nurse attired in a white uniform, at least in the 1950s and 1960s, communicated an impression of confidence, competence, professionalism, authority, role identity, and accountability. As nurses have adopted more casual dress, some of this identity has been lost, and hospital committees, nursing programs, and nurses have spent considerable time discussing appropriate attire.

Early uniforms were long, usually stiffly starched, and had detachable collars and cuffs. A full uniform often included a long cape that would cover the uniform. Kalisch and Kalisch (2004, pp. 75–78) credit the New York Training School for Nurses at Bellevue Hospital with being the first school to adopt a standard uniform for student nurses in 1876. The uniform consisted of a gingham apron worn in the morning and a white apron worn in the afternoon over a dark woolen dress. A well-bred young woman, Euphemia Van Rensselaer, is credited with updating the basic uniform, which students were opposed to wearing. Given 2 days' leave of absence to have a uniform made for herself, she created a tailored uniform consisting of a long gray dress for winter and a calico version for summer, both worn with a white apron and cap. The attractiveness of her appearance resulted in other students accepting the uniform as standard dress. Later, a more easily laundered dress that could be worn throughout the year replaced both dresses.

A regulation uniform became a distinguishing mark of each nursing school by the end of the 19th century. Typically, the uniform consisted of a bodice and skirt of white material, adjustable white cuffs, a stiff white collar, and a white cap. To maintain the feminine hourglass image popular at the time, a tightly laced corset was worn beneath the uniform and ankles were hidden from view. Some suggest that the adoption of a distinctive and attractive uniform played a significant role in developing a professional image for nursing, giving it status, respect, and authority.

By the 1900s, the uniform became more functional, and the hemline was raised. By the mid-1960s, pantsuits became accepted, and nurses in certain settings, particularly psychiatric and pediatric units, challenged the appropriateness of uniforms, especially white uniforms. By 1970, significant changes occurred in uniforms, with the acceptance of styles that were designed to "make the nurse more approachable." In psychiatric settings, "no uniform" became the standard of the day. Today, athletic shoes are acceptable footwear, and scrubs have become the uniform of choice in many institutions. As dress styles have become increasingly casual, many hospitals have been forced to institute dress codes that restrict dangling jewelry, message T-shirts, body piercing, and fake fingernails. With all these changes, often, the nurse is no longer identifiable by dress; only a hospital badge provides information regarding a caregiver's preparation for the role.

Controversy over the appropriate attire for nurses continues. Many hospitals are instituting a dress code with nurses wearing a certain color of uniform so that clients can easily tell who the nurse is. Uniforms remain a complex issue that generates strong feelings from many nurses as nurses want to appear professional while being able to perform their job.

Ceremonies Associated With Nursing Programs

Long-standing traditions embraced by nursing include the ceremonies that mark various points along the educational paths of nursing students. Primary among these are the capping and the pinning ceremonies.

Few schools have capping ceremonies today because most nurses and nursing students no longer wear caps. Traditionally, the cap was awarded to students after they completed a certain part of the program. In hospital schools, it may have been awarded on completion of the probationary period, but more often, it was given after the completion of the first year. Often held in a nearby church, a special ceremony was planned, to which students invited family and others who were interested in their progress. The director of the school, assisted by other school dignitaries and faculty, solemnly placed the cap on the head of each student. Students proudly wore the cap throughout the remainder of the program. Often, a stripe was added to one corner of the cap to signify completion of the second year of study, and a black band was

---

BOX 1.1 THE NIGHTINGALE PLEDGE

I solemnly pledge myself before God and in the presence of this assembly:

To pass my life in purity and to practice my profession faithfully;
I will abstain from whatever is deleterious and mischievous and will not take or
    knowingly administer any harmful drug;
I will do all in my power to maintain and elevate the standard of the profession, and
    will hold in confidence all personal matters committed to my keeping and all family
    affairs coming to my knowledge in the practice of my calling;
With loyalty I will endeavor to aid the physician in his work, and devote myself to the
    welfare of those committed to my care.

Deans, A. G. & Austin, A. L. (1936). *The history of the Farrand Training School for nurses* (p. 58). Detroit, MI: Alumnae Associate of the Farrand Training School for Nurses, as cited in Kalisch and Kalisch (2004).

added at the time of graduation. While very few schools still have a capping ceremony, the tradition of seasoned nurses welcoming new nurses to the profession with a stethoscope or other significant gift continues with the pinning ceremony, as described next.

The second traditional ceremony in nursing, the pinning, was of even greater significance and is continued by many schools today. The pinning heralded the completion of the program. Amid much pomp and circumstance, family and friends gathered to watch as the nursing director or another nurse ceremoniously pinned the school pin on each new graduate. Graduates often recited, in unison, the Nightingale Pledge (Box 1.1) written in 1893 by Lystra E. Gretter, superintendent of Farrand Training School for Nurses at Harper Hospital School in Detroit and a small committee of nurses (Kalisch & Kalisch, 2004). This tradition is often repeated in nursing schools today, although a modified version of the original pledge is often used. Some schools include additional tradition through the "passing of the lamp." A representative of the graduating class hands a lamp (symbolizing the lamp carried by Florence Nightingale) to a representative of the next graduating class, thus reinforcing the concept of the continual caring represented in nursing.

As nursing education moved into institutions of higher education, some of the traditional ceremonies were discontinued. Some argue that the ceremony recognizing program completion in the collegiate environment is the college commencement, and that special celebrations for students of particular areas of study are not appropriate. However, in many large universities, the various disciplines now have separate ceremonies or an additional ceremony for their members. In other cases, the tradition is continued, although there is some tendency for graduates not to purchase a pin.

Critical Thinking Activity: Nursing Traditions
Review the traditions established in nursing. Which is the most meaningful to you, and why? Which is the least meaningful to you, and why? Do you believe traditions should be continued in nursing? Provide a rationale for your answer.

THE IMAGE OF NURSING TODAY

During the late 1970s and early 1980s, much time and energy were invested in studying the image of nursing, with much of this work done by Beatrice and Philip Kalisch, who have written prolifically about the topic. Their writing focuses on segments of an overall study of the image of the nurse in various forms of mass media, including radio, movies, television, newspapers, magazines, and novels. They believe that popular attitudes and assumptions about nurses and what nurses contribute to a client's welfare can greatly influence the future of nursing. It is their contention that since the 1970s, the popular image of the nurse not only has failed to reflect changing professional conditions but also has been based on derogatory stereotypes that have undermined public confidence in and respect for the professional nurse. Nurses should be concerned about negative or incorrect images because such images can influence the attitudes of clients, policy makers, and politicians. Equally important, negative attitudes about nursing may discourage many capable prospective nurses, who will choose another career that offers greater appeal in stature, status, and salary. This issue is of great concern today as we deal with a shortage of nurses.

Negative Image

Although some might argue that nurses have better things to do than to worry about how the nurse is portrayed in the media, a consistently misrepresented image can negatively affect how the public views nurses. Therefore, nurses have responded to television advertisements or programs that portray nurses and nursing in a negative light with letters and telephone calls. Boycotts on the purchase of products that present nurses poorly in advertisements as well as organized written protests have proven to be an effective way to bring about change.

Response to misrepresentation

NURSING'S IMAGE AND THE NURSING SHORTAGE

Throughout the last few decades, nursing has had periods of extreme shortages and times of plenty. Currently the country is experiencing a shortage of nurses that is projected to continue as baby boomers retire, creating more clients and fewer nurses (AACN, 2017). Nursing schools turn away qualified applicants due to a lack of clinical space and insufficient faculty. The problem is complex and likely to continue for at least the next decade (AACN, 2017).

A number of factors are suggested as contributing to the long-term shortfall of RNs. First of all, nurses are getting older. In the United States, the nursing workforce has grown faster than the growth of the U.S. population, but one third of nurses are over the age of 50, with many anticipating retirement within the next decade (HRSA Health Professions, 2013). Another concern centers on the fact that members of the baby boom generation are beginning to enter their senior years, thus increasing the need for nurses in the healthcare system. New nurses often enter nursing as a career change in midlife. They will have fewer years in the profession than will those who entered as young adults.

Nursing Shortage

However, a factor that demands serious consideration relates to the fact that nursing has always been a female-dominated profession. Women today have more educational and occupational alternatives. Many other careers may seem more attractive than nursing in terms of salary, the working conditions, and the prestige given to the role. The percentage of males in nursing has increased from 7.7% in 2000 to 9.1% in 2010 (HRSA Health Professions, 2013), which demonstrates that improvement is still necessary.

Working to Resolve the Issue

The past and future shortage is of such importance that various groups that command respect for their work have decided to study the issue or take action to try to encourage more individuals to choose nursing as a career. The Robert Wood Johnson Foundation and Johnson & Johnson have both funded endeavors to increase the attractiveness of nursing as a career. Across the United States, the National Forum of State Nursing Workforce Centers has been established with 29 states participating. Within each state, the nursing shortage is addressed with efforts made to assure an adequate supply of qualified nurses to meet healthcare needs. This is accomplished by supporting and advancing workforce initiatives, collecting and analyzing data, publishing reports and information, and making recommendations for changes needed to resolve the nurse shortage (NCSBN, 2016).

Limited Spaces

Another factor affecting the nursing supply is the limited number of spaces in nursing programs. Because nursing education is costly and clinical sites are limited, many educational institutions have not been able to increase the size of their programs. As applications increase, further efforts will be needed to increase the number of individuals who can be admitted. Some states have instituted major efforts to increase the available spaces for nursing students.

To provide advice and recommendations to the Secretary of Health and Human Services and Congress on policy matters relating to the nursing work force, the National Advisory Council on Nurse Education and Practice (NACNEP) was established. This group focuses on "support of nursing education and practice which include: enhancement of the composition of the nursing workforce, improvement of the distribution and utilization of nurses to meet the health needs of the Nation, expansion of the knowledge, skills, and capabilities of nurses to enhance the quality of nursing practice, development and dissemination of improved models of organization, financing and delivery of nursing services and promotion of interdisciplinary approaches to the delivery of health services particularly in the context of public health and primary care" (HRSA, n.d.).

Faculty

Serious concern has been voiced by educational institutions and organizations supporting educational efforts, such as the National League for Nursing, regarding the supply of educationally prepared nursing faculty. Again, in conjunction with Johnson & Johnson, scholarships have been made available in some geographic areas to nurses who would like to prepare for faculty positions.

Retention of Nurses

Another aspect of any nursing shortage is the retention of current nurses. Some states have identified that there are a large number of RNs not currently working in the profession. Many experts have pointed to working conditions such as mandatory overtime, heavy workloads, and lack of respect in the workplace as reasons for people leaving. The ANA is focusing on actions that will improve the work environment and thus increase retention as means of addressing the nursing shortage.

Critical Thinking Activity: Nursing Image
Interview five of your friends who are not nurses. What is their image of nursing? What do they understand of the role of the nurse? Do they view nursing positively? What recurrent information is mentioned? What cultural perspectives influence how your friends perceive nursing?

***Communication in Action 1.1:** Affecting Your Image as a Nurse*

Susan Williams and her friend Johanna Ireland were shopping for uniforms to wear. Susan, a new graduate, had asked Johanna to come with her since Johanna had been working as a nurse for a few years now. Susan commented, "I really like these scrubs with the pink bunnies. They are really cute and lighthearted." Johanna replied, "I want something that doesn't make me look like a young girl. I had a client once refuse to take medications from me because they said that I didn't look like a real nurse. I've found that the clients and doctors treat me with more respect when I am dressed more professionally." "Wow, I never thought of that—maybe I should look for something more professional too," replied Susan.

STUDIES FOR AND ABOUT NURSING

Early in the 20th century, the quality of many nursing schools and their graduates was poor; many of Florence Nightingale's admonitions regarding nursing education had been forgotten or ignored. Nurses, doctors, friends, and critics of nursing became concerned that the preparation being offered was inadequate. Before the problem could be corrected, it was necessary to learn more about the programs and how nurses were being used in the employment market. To accomplish this, studies about nursing and nurses were initiated.

As you read about the studies that have been conducted, you will recognize recurring themes with which we continue to grapple today. Our discussion is limited to those studies that looked at the profession as a whole and does not include any of the myriad studies conducted each year, primarily clinical in focus, that form the basis for evidence-based practice and for the expansion of the body of nursing knowledge.

Although the first nursing studies were not begun until the early 1900s, the number of studies since the 1950s has been voluminous. It is impossible to look at any professional nursing publication and not find mention of some new study in progress. Efforts were made to classify and catalog references to these studies and to report them. One of the first was completed by Virginia Henderson, who prepared *A Nursing Studies Index*. In 1952, a group of nurses, under the sponsorship of the Association of Collegiate Schools of Nursing, launched a new journal called *Nursing Research*, which was designed to disseminate information about nursing research.

A single individual often conducted many of the early studies, typically with a particular purpose in mind. Through the years, studies frequently took the form of a report by a special group of individuals, often appointed by a governmental or professional agency. Although by no means inclusive of all studies and reports, Table 1.7 highlights some of the major significant studies of nursing that have provided benchmarks to the profession, identifies the primary investigator/sponsor, and briefly discusses the focus and recommendation(s) associated with each study.

Critical Thinking Activity: Research About Nursing
Identify at least three areas in nursing that you believe need further study, and describe how you would begin to conduct those studies. Whom would you involve and why? How and to whom would you like to see the results and recommendations disseminated?

Table 1.7   Major Studies About Nursing

Date	Name of Study	Primary Investigator/ Sponsor	Focus and Recommendation
1912	*The Educational Status of Nursing*	M. Adelaide Nutting/ U.S. Bureau of Education	What and how students were being taught and conditions under which they were living. Began to establish nursing as a profession.
1923	*Winslow-Goldmark Report on Nursing and Nursing Education in the United States*	Josephine Goldmark/ Rockefeller Foundation	The educational preparation of students including public health nurses, teachers, and supervisors. It pointed out fundamental faults in hospital training schools and resulted in the establishment of the Yale University School of Nursing.
1923	Committee on the Grading of Nursing Schools—a 3-part study	Francis Payne Bolton and contributions of thousands of nurses	Examined supply and demand for nursing services, job analysis of nursing and nurse teaching, and actual grading of nursing schools. Recommended increased training for public health nursing where it noted a demand and lack of preparation.
1923	*(1) Nurses, Clients, and Pocketbooks*	May Ayres Burgess/ statistician	An inquiry into the supply and demand for nurses. Demonstrated that there was an oversupply of nurses.
1934	*(2) An Activity Analysis of Nursing*	Ethel Johns and Blance Pfefferkorn	Looked at the activities that constitute nursing as a basis for improving curricula.
1934	*(3) Nursing Schools Today & Tomorrow*	Ethel Johns	Described the nursing schools of the period and made recommendations about professional schools.
1937	*A Curriculum Guide for Schools of Nursing*—not truly a study of nursing, but often referred to as one because of its far-reaching effects	National League for Nursing Education	A revision of a 1917 publication, it outlined the curricula for a 3-year course, emphasizing sound educational teaching procedures. Followed by many schools of the time.
1948	*Nursing for the Future*	Esther Lucille Brown/ Carnegie Foundation, the Russell Sage Foundation, and the National Nursing Council	Done to determine society's need for nursing. Described inadequacies in nursing schools. Resulted in recommendations that nursing education be placed in universities and colleges and encouraged recruitment of large numbers of men and members of minority groups into nursing schools.
1948	The Ginzberg Report or *A Program for the Nursing Profession*—a report of the discussions of the Committee on the Functions of Nursing	Eli Ginzberg/Columbia University	Reviewed problems centering around the shortage of nurses. Recommended that nursing teams consisting of variously educated nurses be developed.
1950	*Nursing Schools at the Mid-Century*	Margaret Bridgman/ National Committee for the Improvement of Nursing Services— Russell Sage Foundation	Studied the practices of more than 1,000 nursing schools (including organization, costs, curriculum, clinical resources, and student health) and stimulated improvement in baccalaureate schools.
1955	*Patterns of Client Care*	Francis George and Ruth Perkins Kuehn/ University of Pittsburgh	Assessed the amount of nursing service needed by a group of medical/surgical clients and determined how much of that care could be delegated to nursing aides and other nonprofessional people.
1958	*Twenty Thousand Nurses Tell Their Story*	Everett C. Hughes/ANA and American Nurses Foundation	Looked at nurses, what they were doing, their attitudes toward their jobs, and job satisfaction. Formed basis for development of nursing functions, standards, and qualifications.

Table 1.7 Major Studies About Nursing (continued)

Date	Name of Study	Primary Investigator/ Sponsor	Focus and Recommendation
1959	*Community College Education for Nursing*	Mildred Montag/Institute of Research and Service in Nursing Education— Teachers College, Columbia University	Reported the findings of a 5-year study of eight 2-year nursing programs. Led to the establishment of more associate degree programs.
1963	*Toward Quality in Nursing: Needs and Goals*	W. Allen Wallis— Consultant Group on Nursing—a panel of nurses in the health field/U.S. Public Health Service	A report requested by the U.S. Surgeon General to determine funding priorities. Advised on the need for nurses, recruitment concerns, need for nursing research, and improvement of nursing education.
1970	*An Abstract for Action* (a report of the National Commission on Nursing and Nursing Education)	Jerome Lysaught/ANA, ANF, NLN, Mellon and Kellogg Foundations	Looked at current practices and patterns of nursing. Suggested joint practice committees, master planning for nursing education, and funding for nursing education and research.
1979	*The Study of Credentialing in Nursing*	Inez Hinsvark/ANA	A review of credentialing—especially of nursing. Resulted in the appointment of a Task Force. Supported a freestanding credentialing center for nursing.
1983	*National Institute of Medicine Study*	Katherine Bauer/DHHS	Required by the Nursing Training Act of 1979, determined the need for continued outlay of federal money for nursing education. Resulted in 21 specific recommendations. Found that the shortage of nurses of the 1960s and 1970s no longer existed, that federal support of nursing education should focus on graduate study, and that the federal government should discontinue efforts to increase "generalist nurses."
1988	*Secretary's Commission on Nursing*	Lillian Gibbons/DHHS	Responded to serious nursing shortage. Validated the shortage. Recommended increased financial support of education and improved status and working conditions for nurses
1990	*Secretary's Commission on the National Nursing Shortage*	Caroline Burnett/DHHS	Appointed for 1 year to advise on implementation of 1988 report. Had three main foci; recruitment and retention, restructuring of nursing service, and use of nursing personnel and information systems.
1991	*Report of the National Commission of Nursing Implementation Project (NCNIP)*	Vivian De Back/ANA, NLN, AACN, AONE, Kellogg Foundation	Looked at nursing education, practice, management, and research, and developed recommendations for the future of nursing.
1993	*Health Professions Education for the Future*	E.H. O'Neill/Pew Health Professions Commission—Pew Charitable Trusts	Reinforced the belief that the education of health professions was not adequate to meet the health needs of America. Identified competencies for 2005 and emphasized the need for nurse–midwives, nurse practitioners, and the role of nurses in health promotion.
1995	*Reforming Health Care Workforce Regulation*	Pew Health Professions Commission	Had as its mission assisting schools preparing health professionals to understand the changing nature of healthcare, the needs for the future, and how to design and implement the programs preparing these workers. Recommended reform of the licensing process, specifically elimination of exclusive scopes of practice.

DEFINING A LANGUAGE FOR NURSING

Uses

For many, the development of a special language for nursing is an exciting new development. Structured nursing vocabularies allow nurses to use the acquired information to guide evidence-based clinical decisions, manage information in an electronic format, retrieve information for research, and compare clinical outcomes across settings. It also provides a common means of communication (Box 1.2).

The development of nursing languages began as an effort to build a set of terms that would describe the clinical judgments made by nurses that are not in medical language systems. As early as 1909, nurses with a perceptive view of the future recognized that nursing would one day need a language of its own. Ninety years ago, Isabel Hampton Robb wrote the following after attending a meeting of the newly formed ICN:

> While attending a special meeting of the ICN in Paris, I was naturally at once struck by the fact that the methods and the ways of regarding nursing problems were … as foreign to the various delegations as were the actual languages, and the thought occurred to me that … sooner or later we must put ourselves upon a common basis and work out what may be termed a "nursing Esperanto" which would in the course of time give us a universal nursing language (Hampton-Robb, 1909). (Note: Esperanto was a language developed in 1887 with the goal of being a universal language that could be taught as the second language throughout the world, thus enabling improved communication among peoples.)

Defining a language for nursing primarily involves the development and refinement of **nursing nomenclatures** and **classification systems** that communicate information and guide data collection about nursing activities. The term *nursing nomenclature* refers to the words by which we name or describe phenomena in nursing. A *classification* is the systematic arrangement or a structural framework of these phenomena. As we move toward an international network of healthcare, the development of a language unique to nursing is viewed as critical to communication and decision making. Proponents of a specialized language for nursing emphasize the need for objective, science-based information to use in decision making. These data also provide the basis for accountability and the documentation-supporting processes and outcomes of care. The data can be used further to answer research questions

---

BOX 1.2 RATIONALE FOR THE DEVELOPMENT OF A CLASSIFICATION FOR NURSING

- Permits recognition and communication with others by giving a name to the things nurses do
- Provides a uniform legal record of care
- Supports clinical decision making
- Lays the groundwork for nursing research
- Captures the cost of nursing services for billing and accounting purposes
- Generates a structured retrieval database for quality assurance

about nursing and nursing actions. In the age of information technology, uniform, accurate, and automated client care data are required to conduct analyses that will result in improving the quality of care and costing out that care. At present, the language of nursing primarily addresses nursing diagnoses, implementation activities, and nursing outcomes. Some would suggest that the existing systems are not adequate to reflect the entire scope of nursing practice and urge further development; for example, at the present time, none reflects the intensity of nursing practice.

Nursing Terminologies

As nursing struggled to be recognized as a profession, it became clear that a terminology was necessary to standardize charting and enable clear communication and collection of data. There are currently 12 recognized terminology systems that are recognized by the ANA.

Here we discuss the four systems that are currently most popular; these and others that are approved by the ANA are listed in Table 1.8.

NANDA International

The group, originally called the National Group for the Classification of Nursing Diagnosis and then North American Nursing Diagnosis Association (NANDA) and now **NANDA International (NANDA-I),** became a formal organization after its fifth conference in 1982. The Association has two main purposes: to develop a diagnostic classification system (also known as **taxonomy**) and to identify and approve nursing diagnoses. The list of nursing diagnoses (concepts that are given word labels) continues to grow as nurses encounter diagnoses in clinical practice that have not been included and submit these to NANDA-I for consideration. As a student, you have some familiarity with nursing diagnoses from the nursing care plans you develop for client care and in the case studies you discuss in your classes. The following is the definition of a nursing diagnosis accepted by NANDA-I:

> Nursing diagnosis is a clinical judgment about individual, family, or community response to actual or potential health problems/life processes. Nursing diagnoses provide the basis for selection of nursing interventions to achieve outcomes for which the nurse is accountable. These were approved at the 9th conference in 1990 with the latest 2015–2017 addition available on the NANDA.org website.

Nursing Interventions Classifications

Started in 1996 at the University of Iowa, the **Nursing Interventions Classification (NIC)** is a comprehensive, standardized language that describes actions nurses perform in all settings and in all specialties, and includes both physiologic and psychosocial interventions. The interventions are numbered to facilitate computerization and are organized into classes, and *Interventions* the classes are assigned to domains. The domains are functional health, physiologic health, psychosocial health, health knowledge and behavior, perceived health, family health, and community health. Each intervention has been linked with NANDA-I nursing diagnoses and with the **Nursing Outcomes Classification (NOC)** below and with Omaha system problems. Many institutions have adopted NIC as a standardized terminology for use in computerized documentation systems. An overview of NIC is available online (https://nursing.uiowa.edu/center-for-nursing-classification-and-clinical-effectiveness).

Table 1.8   **Major Nursing Classifications Approved by the American Nurses Association**

Title & Web Site	What It Is
NANDA International (formerly North American Nursing Diagnosis) www.nanda.org	Provides taxonomy of nursing diagnoses. Defines a nursing diagnosis as a clinical judgment about an individual, family, or community responses to actual or potential health conditions/life processes. A nursing diagnosis provides the basis for selection of nursing interventions to achieve outcomes for which the nurse is accountable (NANDA-I, 2009).
Nursing Intervention Classification www.nursing.uiowa.edu/center-for-nursing-classification-and-clinical-effectiveness	Provides a comprehensive standardized language, describing treatments that nurses perform in all settings and in all specialties.
Clinical Care Classification (CCC) Version 2.0 (previously Home Healthcare Classification Diagnoses and Interventions) www.sabacare.com	Adapted, revised, and expanded NANDA to include additional home healthcare nursing diagnostic conditions. Now used to assess, document, and classify client/client care across all settings and is being used in Electronic Health Records (Saba, 2004–2008).
The Omaha System www.omahasystem.org/overview.html	A system of client problems, interventions, and client outcomes referred to as the Problem Classification Scheme, the Intervention Scheme, and the Problem Rating Scale for Outcomes (The Omaha System, 2010).
Nursing Outcomes Classification www.nursing.uiowa.edu/cnc	Defines a nursing outcome as a variable concept that represents a client or family caregiver state, behavior, or perception that is measurable along a continuum and responsive to nursing interventions (Moorhead, Johnson, & Mass, 2004).
Nursing Management Minimum Data Set (NMMDS) www.nursing.umn.edu/center/center-nursing-informatics	Provides resources nurse executives need to make informed decisions and manage nursing services delivery and care coordination.
Perioperative Nursing Data Set (PNDS) www.aorn.org/syntegrity/pnds-with-documentation	Standardized language for documenting and evaluating perioperative nursing care (Association of Perioperative Registered Nurses, 2018).
Systematized Nomenclature of Medicine (SNOMED) www.ihtsdo.org/snomed-ct/	Comprehensive system for indexing the entire medical record, including signs and symptoms, diagnoses, and procedures (SNOMED, 2005).
Nursing Minimum Data Set (NMDS) www.cms.hhs.gov/NursingHomeQualityInits/	Identified the four elements of nursing diagnosis, nursing interventions, nursing outcomes, and nursing intensity.
International Classification of Nursing Practice www.icn.ch/icnp.htm	Collaborative project under the auspices of the International Council of Nursing for classifying nursing phenomena (diagnoses, interventions, and outcomes). Includes definitions and provides unifying framework to enable comparison of data internationally.
Alternative Billing Codes Developed by ABC Coding Solutions www.ABCcodes.com	Identifies alternative medicine, nursing, and other integrative healthcare services and related products that facilitate measuring, validating, managing, and reimbursing for care.

Nursing Outcomes Classification

Also developed at the University of Iowa, the NOC was first published in 1997. An out-come is defined as a variable concept representing a client or family caregiver state, behavior, or perception that is measurable along a continuum and responsive to nursing interventions. Project developers believed that stating the outcomes as variable concepts rather than goals would allow the identification of positive or negative changes (or no changes at all) in the client's status. Each outcome has a definition, a list of indicators that assist in evaluation of client status, a rating scale for evaluation, and a suggested target rating. Listed in alphabetical order, the outcomes are grouped into classes and use the same domains as NIC. Both NIC and NOC are continuing in development. An overview of the NOC is available online (https://nursing.uiowa.edu/cncce/nursing-outcomes-classification-overview), and the detailed system is available in print (Moorhead, Johnson, Maas et al., 2013). A presentation of the linkages among NANDA, NIC, and NOC (Bulechek, Butcher, Dochterman, et al., 2013) is a useful tool for those seeking a better understanding of how the three systems can be coordinated.

The Omaha System

The **Omaha System**, another example of classification efforts, is a research-based taxonomy designed to document client care from admission to discharge. It was designed as a three-part, comprehensive yet brief approach to documentation and information management for multidisciplinary healthcare professionals who practice in community settings. It offers terms and codes to classify the client's health-related concerns or problems, the interventions that nurses and other healthcare professionals use, and the client's outcomes (The Omaha System, 2016). Client problems can be identified for individuals, families, and groups. The interventions describe both plans and interventions for specific client concerns. The outcome scales evaluate a client's health-related changes through the use of problem-specific knowledge, behavior, and status ratings. The Omaha System has been recognized by the ANA since 1992 and has been translated into numerous languages. Automation and technology advances and healthcare delivery changes have markedly expanded its use nationally and internationally. Users represent a broad continuum of care with location, size, organization, types of service, and employees becoming increasingly diverse. An overview of the Omaha System is available online (http://omahasystem.org/index.html).

Other Classification Systems

Currently, 12 Data Element Sets and Terminologies are recognized by the ANA (ANA, 2015). All of these are presented in Table 1.8 with a brief description of each and a Web site where more information is provided.

The Minimum Data Set for Nursing Home Resident Assessment and Care Screening

Although not referred to in terms of nursing terminology, the **Minimum Data Set for Nursing Home Resident Assessment and Care Screening (MDS)** bears some mention here.

MDS:
Care for
the Elderly

When the Omnibus Budget Reconciliation Act was passed in 1991, it required assessment of long-term care facility residents. This assessment, done on admission and every 3 months thereafter, must be standardized, comprehensive, accurate, and reproducible. It must be transmitted electronically to data centers in each state. Whenever problems are identified during the assessment, Resident Assessment Protocols (RAPs) must be instituted. The RAPs lists factors that might be associated with the problem, clarifying information to be considered in making a diagnosis and describing the environment that will help reduce the symptoms. Complete documentation of the situation, including nature of the problem, complications, risk factors, referrals, and rationale for action, is required of nurses. The MDS is used as the basis for determining payment to long-term care facilities. The implementation of the MDS nationwide has resulted in a significant collection of data that can be used as a basis for improving the care of the elderly. The MDS 3.0 is developed and was implemented in 2010. An overview and interactive training are available on the Centers for Medicare & Medicaid Services (CMS) Web site (CMS, 2016).

The International Classification for Nursing Practice Project

The **International Classification for Nursing Practice Project (ICNP)** is an effort of the ICN to establish a unified nursing terminology system. It is a compositional terminology for nursing practice that facilitates the development of and the cross-mapping among local terms and existing terminologies (ICN, 2015). In addition, ICNPP is a classification of nursing phenomena, nursing actions, and nursing outcomes.

Importance
of international
classification
System

Although the United States has been involved in the development of classification and information systems for some time, the need for a unified language is now recognized internationally. Because cultural and language differences exist, many of the classification systems currently employed in the United States are not useful in other countries. For example, the concept of self-care reflects the cultural values and norms of American society but may be perceived quite differently in other cultures. In 1989, the ICN was asked to encourage member National Nurses Associations to become involved in developing information and classification systems and nursing data sets that could be used by nurses in all countries to identify and describe nursing. The project began a year later. In 1996, an alpha version of the Classification of Nursing Phenomenon and Nursing Interventions was field tested, and a beta version was launched in June 1999 at ICN's Centennial Conference. The ICNPP Programme has established a formal evaluation and review process to advance the project. ICNP releases a new version approximately every 2 years (ICN, 2015).

Critical Thinking Activity: Nursing Classification System
Analyze the history of the development of a classification and nomenclature specific to nursing. Describe possible future developments, and provide a rationale for your answer. What do you see as major impediments and why? What do you believe will be the long-term benefits and why?

Stegen & Sowerby Stories: Part 2

emember Brian who failed to speak to or report the doctor who was not washing her hand? Brian's client has now developed a nosocomial infection in the surgical site, and the family states that they intend to sue. Can Brian be liable? What is your role in preventing infections and advocating for clients? Read the rest of the story at www.thePoint.com.

Want to Know More?

A variety of resources are available on thePoint° to enhance your learning and understanding of this chapter, such as:

- Full Stegen & Sowerby Stories
- NCLEX-Style Student Review Questions
- Journal Articles
- Case Studies
- Learning Objectives
- Relevant Web sites
- And more...

KEY CONCEPTS

- In its development as a profession, nursing has struggled with its definition, its image, and its role in the healthcare delivery system, due in part to its history and the fact that it has both theoretical and practical aspects. The role of the nurse in the healthcare delivery system has probably never been more important than it is today.
- Florence Nightingale dramatically changed the form and direction of nursing. She set down standards for nursing education and made significant recommendations for changes in how hospitals operated and how nursing was practiced. Many of her recommendations are valid today.
- Early schools of nursing were established shortly after the Civil War with curricula fashioned much like the Nightingale School in England. Early programs were primarily apprenticeships, with long hours during which students provided much of the workforce of the hospital with little time left for study.
- The wars in which the United States have been involved have had a significant impact on nursing. Nurses have always played an important role in the care of the wounded and dying and, over the years, have taken increasingly important roles.
- Nursing is distinct from medicine. Medicine deals with diagnosis and treatment of disease, and nursing is concerned with caring for the person.
- The position nursing occupies as a profession is often judged against sociologically developed characteristics or standards of a profession. Not everyone agrees that nursing meets those standards.

- The standards of a profession typically include seven requirements: (1) possess a well-defined and well-organized body of knowledge, (2) enlarge a systematic body of knowledge and improve education, (3) educate its practitioners in institutions of higher learning, (4) function autonomously in the formulation of policy, (5) develop a code of ethics, (6) attract professionals who will be committed to the profession for a lifetime, and (7) compensate practitioners by providing autonomy, continuous professional development, and economic security.
- Nursing also has struggled with the terms "profession" and "professional." At times, the characteristics of the professional become confused with the formal concept of a profession.
- Nursing as a profession has many traditions, some of which are challenged today, while others are much honored and valued. Among the traditions are the pin, the cap, the uniform, and nursing ceremonies.
- Nursing has struggled with its image. Various groups have waged campaigns to improve the image of nursing and thus make it a more attractive profession. The image of nursing today is viewed as a critical issue because of the nurse shortage. A positive image is needed to attract qualified individuals into the profession.
- Since the beginning of the 20th century, nursing has been a much-studied profession. Early studies dealt with nursing education; later studies dealt with the image of nursing, nurses themselves, and with nursing's role in healthcare delivery.
- As nursing has developed as a profession, more attention has been directed to establishing a unique classification and nomenclature for nursing. Efforts are being made to do this on an international basis.

NCLEX-STYLE PRACTICE QUESTIONS

1. Identify the contributions of ideas from Florence Nightingale to the nursing profession (select all that apply).
   A. Improving basic hygiene
   B. Constructing hospitals
   C. Promoting immunizations
   D. Reforming nursing education

2. What distinguishes nursing from medicine?
   A. Nursing is composed of women
   B. Holistic perspective of caring
   C. Concern with treatment of disease
   D. Dependent on the physician → stereotype

3. What is the purpose of the nursing terminology and classification systems and how do they benefit nursing? (select all that apply).
   A. To classify disease processes in nursing
   B. To compare clinical outcomes across settings
   C. To provide a common means of communication
   D. To manage information in an electronic format

4. Why is the image of nursing important for nurses?

   A. Influences the attitudes of others about nursing

   B. Important to remain fashionable

   C. Influences the type of care provided

   D. Changes how nurses work in the hospital

5. What is the difference between NIC and NOC?

   A. Nursing versus medical

   B. Interventions versus outcomes

   C. Positive versus negative changes

   D. Input versus output data

REFERENCES

Abdellah, F. G. (1960). *Client-centered approaches to nursing.* New York: Macmillan.

American Association of Colleges of Nursing (AACN). (2017). Nursing shortage. *AACN media relations.* Retrieved June 19, 2017 from http://www.aacn.nche.edu/media-relations/fact-sheets/nursing-shortage

American Nurses Association. (2010). *Nursing's social policy statement: The essence of the profession* (3rd ed.). Silver Spring, MD: Author.

American Nurses Association. (2015). *Position statement: Inclusion of recognized terminologies supporting nursing practice within electronic health records and other health information technology solutions.* Retrieved from https://www.nursingworld.org/~490b56/globalassets/docs/ana/inclusion-of-recognized-terminologies-within-ehrs-and-other-health-information-technology-solutions.pdf

Association of Perioperative Registered Nurses. (2018). *Perioperative nursing data set (PNDS) and syntegrity standardized perioperative framework (SPF).* Retrieved from, www.aorn.org/syntegrity/pnds-with-documentation

Benner, P., & Wrubel, J. (1989). *The primacy of caring.* Menlo Park, CA: Addison-Wesley.

Bevis, E. O., & Watson, J. (1989). *Toward a caring curriculum: A new pedagogy for nursing.* New York: National League for Nursing.

Bixler, G. K., & Bixler, R. W. (1945). The professional status of nursing. *American Journal of Nursing, 45*(9), 730.

Bostridge, M. (2008). *Florence Nightingale: The making of an icon.* New York: Farrar, Straus and Giroux.

Bulechek, G., Butcher, H., Dochterman, J., & Wagner, C. (Eds.). (2013). *Nursing interventions classification (NIC)* (6th ed.). St. Louis, MO: Elsevier.

Carper, B. A. (1979). The ethics of caring. *Advances in Nursing Science, 3,* 11–19.

Centers for Medicare & Medicaid Services. (2016). *MDS 3.0 Training.* Retrieved June 12, 2017, from https://www.cms.gov/Medicare/Quality-Initiatives-Patient-Assessment-Instruments/NursingHome QualityInits/NHQIMDS30TrainingMaterials.html

Donahue, M. P. (2010). *Nursing: The finest art* (3rd ed.). St. Louis, MO: CV Mosby.

Hampton-Robb, I. (1909). *Report of the third regular meeting of the International Council of Nurses.* Geneva, Switzerland: ICN.

Henderson, V. (1966). *The nature of a science of nursing.* New York: Macmillan.

Health Resources and Services Administration (HRSA). (2013). *Nursing workforce trends.* Retrieved March 30, 2017, from https://bhw.hrsa.gov/sites/default/files/bhw/nchwa/projections/nursingworkforcetrendsoct2013.pdf

Health Resources and Services Administration (HRSA). (n.d.). *National Advisory Council on Nurse Education and Practice.* Retrieved on March 30, 2017, from https://www.hrsa.gov/advisorycommittees/bhpradvisory/nacnep/

International Council of Nurses. (2015). *Vision, goals & benefits of ICNP*. Retrieved June 19, 2017, from http://www.icn.ch/what-we-do/vision-goals-a-benefits-of-icnpr/

Johnson, D. (1980). The behavioral system model for nursing. In J. P. Riehl & C. Roy (Eds.), *Conceptual models for nursing practice* (2nd ed., pp. 207–216). East Norwalk, CT: Appleton-Century-Crofts.

Kalisch, P. A., & Kalisch, B. J. (2004). *The advance of American nursing* (4th ed.). Philadelphia, PA: Lippincott Williams & Wilkins.

King, I. M. (1981). *A theory for nursing: Systems, concepts, process*. New York: John Wiley & Sons.

Kolcaba, K. Y. (1992). Holistic comfort: Operationalizing the construct as a nurse-sensitive outcome. *Advances in Nursing Science, 1*, 1–10.

Labor Management Relations Act (1947) as amended by Public Laws 86–257 (1959) and 93–360. (1974). *Section 2 [On-line]*. Retrieved September 28, 2005, from https://www.nlrb.gov/who-we-are/our-history/1947-taft-hartley-substantive-provisions

LeMaire, B. (2002). Jean Watson, on her theory of caring. *Nurse Week (Mountain West Edition), 3*(40), 7.

Levine, M. E. (1969). *Introduction to clinical nursing*. Philadelphia, PA: F. A. Davis.

Mangum, S. (1994). Uniforms and caps: Do we need them? In O. L. Strickland & D. J. Fishman (Eds.), *Nursing issues in the 1990s* (pp. 46–66). Albany, NY: Delmar Publishers.

Moorhead, S., Johnson, M., Maas M., Swanson E. (Eds.). (2013). *Nursing outcomes classification* (5th ed.). St. Louis, MO: Elsevier.

NANDA-I. (2009). *Glossary of terms*. Retrieved September 18, 2009, from http://www.nanda.org/DiagnosisDevelopment/DiagnosisSubmission/PreparingYourSubmission/GlossaryofTerms.aspx

National Council of State Boards of Nursing, Inc. (2014). *NCSBN model act*. Retrieved March 14, 2017, from https://www.ncsbn.org/14_Model_Act_0914.pdf

National Council of State Boards of Nursing. (2016). The 2015 national nursing workforce survey. *Journal of Nursing Regulation, 7*(1), S4–S6. Retrieved from www.ncsbn.org/2015ExecutiveSummary.pdf

Neuman, B. (1982). *The Neuman System model: Application to nursing education and practice*. East Norwalk, CT: Appleton-Century-Crofts.

Nightingale, F. (1954). *Notes on nursing: What it is, and what it is not. [An unabridged republication of the first American edition, as published by D. Appleton and Company in 1860]*. New York: Dover Publications.

Omaha System. (2016). Retrieved March 14, 2017, from www.omahasystem.org.overview.html

Orem, D. (1980). *Nursing: Concepts of practice* (2nd ed.). New York: McGraw-Hill.

Orlando, I. J. (1972). *The discipline and teaching of nursing process*. New York: G. P. Putnam's Sons.

Parse, R. R. (1981). *Man-living-health: A theory of nursing*. New York: Wiley.

Peplau, H. E. (1952). *Interpersonal relations in nursing*. New York: G. P. Putnam's Sons.

Petiprin, A. (2016). *Florence Nightingale-Nursing Theorist*. Retrieved from Nursing Theory: http://www.nursing-theory.org/nursing-theorists/Florence-Nightingale.php

Rogers, M. E. (1984). *Science of unitary human beings: A paradigm for nursing*. Paper presented before the International Nurse Theorist Conference, Edmonton, Alberta.

Roy, C. (1984). *Introduction to nursing: An adaptation model* (2nd ed.). Englewood Cliffs, NJ: Prentice-Hall.

Saba, V. (2004–2008). *Clinical care classification system*. Retrieved August 31, 2009, from www.sabacare.com

SNOMED International. (2005). *SNOMED International [On-line]*. Retrieved September 28, 2005, from www.snomed.org/index.html

Van Sell, S. L., & Kalofissudis, I. A. (2010). *The evolving essence of the science of nursing: A complexity integration nursing theory* (2nd ed.). Chania, Crete: The Authors.

Watson, J. (1979). *Nursing the philosophy and science of caring*. Boston, MA: Little, Brown.

Wiedenbach, E. (1964). *Clinical nursing: A helping art*. New York: Springer Publishing Co.

Educational Preparation for Nursing

After completing this chapter, you should be able to:

1. Compare the educational preparation of the nursing assistant, the licensed practical (vocational) nurse (LPN/LVN), and the graduates of the various types of programs preparing registered nurses (RNs), hospital-based programs, associate degree programs, generic baccalaureate programs, and graduate degree entry programs.
2. Explain how other forms of nursing education, including external degree programs, RN baccalaureate programs, master's preparation, doctoral studies, nondegree programs, and articulated programs, serve students and the profession.
3. Discuss some of the innovative approaches to earning a higher degree in nursing.
4. Identify factors that have prompted changes in nursing education, including studies and sociopolitical events, and analyze the effect of each.
5. Analyze the positive and negative effects the American Nurses Association's (ANA's) *Position Paper on Nursing Education* would have had on nursing licensure if adopted nationwide.
6. Critique the major points supporting both mandatory and voluntary continuing education, and explain the mechanisms for documenting and recording continuing education.
7. Analyze the ways in which nursing theories serve to advance the profession.

KEY TERMS

Accreditation
Advanced nursing practice
Articulation
Associate degree education
Baccalaureate degree nursing
  education
Stackable credentials
Competencies
Continuing education unit (CEU)
Diploma programs
Educational mobility
Entry into practice
Evidence-based practice
External degree
Generic program
Grandfather clause

Home health aide
Hospital-based programs
Internships and residencies
Interstate endorsement
Mandatory continuing education
Nursing assistants
Position paper
Practical (vocational) nurse
Scope of practice
Second-degree students
Theorist
Theory
Titling
Unlicensed assistive personnel (UAP)

Voluntary continuing education

Stegen & Sowerby Stories: Part 1

ymeshia has been working full time as a nursing assistant for the past 2 years while going to school to try to become a nurse. Tymeshia has completed all of her general education classes with a 3.5 GPA and was accepted into the nursing program at the community college. Tymeshia has been in the nursing program for exactly 1 month and is beginning to wonder if she made the right choice. It is harder than she expected and her first exam scores are lower than she is used to. Tymeshia meets with her advisor who encourages her to talk to others and assists her in making a study plan. The advisor encourages Tymeshia to wait for another month or two before making a decision. As a nursing student, do you empathize with Tymeshia?

What advice would you give Tymeshia about balancing life and school and how to study?

What can nursing students do to support each other and make the experience better?

Unlike most professions that provide a single route for the educational preparation of its practitioners, nursing offers three major types of educational programs as well as less common ones that prepare graduates to write the National Council Licensure Examination (NCLEX) for registered nursing. These circumstances have resulted in options and opportunities for prospective students, and the multiple-entry points are viewed by some as one of nursing's strengths.

Despite this acknowledged strength, the existence of multiple-entry points has resulted in confusion for both healthcare consumers and employers. Those consumers often find it difficult to understand the various nursing credentials—and probably have little interest in credentials as long as they receive satisfactory care. Employers may have difficulty differentiating among the three major types of RN graduates who, at least initially, enter the work environment performing similar activities. This confusion led to a recommendation from the Pew Commission that nursing distinguishes between the practice responsibilities of the graduates educated in each of the different educational environments (Giordano, 1995). This task has proven difficult at best.

Some nurse educators, charged with the responsibility of graduating a "safe" practitioner, are not entirely clear about how the various educational routes to professional preparation should differ in purpose, structure, and outcome. Certainly, there are basic skills and understandings that all beginning nurses must master to ensure safe client care. Nursing leaders frequently debate aspects of the educational preparation of nurses, such as where it should take place, what content should be included in which programs and to what depth, which tests should measure the various competencies, and which credentials should be awarded.

The three traditional educational avenues that prepare men and women for registered nursing are hospital-based diploma programs, associate degree programs (primarily found at junior and community colleges), and baccalaureate programs (offered at 4-year colleges and universities). It is also possible for students to begin their nursing education in programs that culminate in a master's degree before being eligible to write the state licensing examination for registered nursing.

At least two other groups of caregivers are identified with nursing: the nursing assistant, who may be certified, and the **practical (vocational) nurse,** who is licensed through a separate and different examination from that taken by the RN. We begin with a discussion of those roles.

THE NURSING ASSISTANT

For years, individuals called nursing aides or assistants have provided care to clients in hospitals and long-term care facilities. In the past, these caregivers were hired without formal preparation for their responsibilities and were provided on-the-job training. The use of the nursing aides likely started during World War I and certainly was reinforced during World War II, when approximately 150,000 trained volunteer nursing aides served in wartime hospitals. Nursing aides or assistants have always provided the majority of care in nursing homes. **Nursing assistants** are within a group that is often referred to as **unlicensed assistive personnel (UAP)**.

In 1987, Congress passed the Omnibus Budget Reconciliation Act, which regulates agencies receiving federal funds and includes an amendment regulating the education and certification of nursing assistants who work in nursing homes. The amendment stipulated that by October 1, 1990, all people working as nursing assistants in nursing homes (hospitals and assisted living units were not included) would be required to complete a minimum of 75 hours of theory and practice and pass both a theory and practice examination to be certified. Certification falls under state jurisdiction but is guided by federal regulations. In many states, the hours of preparation required exceed the 75 hours established by federal law. The state agency responsible for certifying and maintaining the list of nursing assistants varies from state to state; most commonly, it is the board of nursing or the state department of health services.

The certified nursing assistant (CNA)—referred to as the nursing assistant or client care assistant in some states—functions under the direction of the RN or the LPN. Each state determines the skills that may be performed by the nursing assistant. Typically, these include basic nursing skills, such as changing bed linens; measuring temperature, pulse, respirations, and blood pressure; bathing clients and helping with personal care; helping clients with eating, walking, and exercise programs; and supporting clients when they are allowed to get out of bed. The preparation of the CNA emphasizes the importance of a safe environment and includes instruction in clients' rights and the use of side rails and restraints. A number of states also require a designated number of hours per year of continuing education.

There are no national regulations governing the educational preparation and **scope of practice** of nursing assistants in areas other than long-term care, although some states have legislation to regulate the practice of those in other settings. Typically, training in hospitals or other agencies occurs under the sponsorship of the employing facility and without formal certification; student backgrounds may vary from less than a high school diploma to advanced degrees. For example, some physicians licensed in foreign countries but who cannot secure licensure in the United States may work as UAPs in healthcare settings.

A number of states have a category of UAP, known as unlicensed medication administration personnel or medication aides. Many of these workers are employed within the primary school system and routinely dispense medications to students; in other instances, these individuals are employed in assisted living and similar facilities. In a few states, CNAs may receive additional instruction and become certified medication aides and are allowed to give medications in a nursing home. The criteria for hospital **accreditation** established by the Joint Commission (formerly the Joint Commission on Accreditation of Healthcare Organizations) now require that hospitals ensure the competence of all employees, including nursing assistants. This has led many hospitals to the practice of hiring only those who were certified as nursing assistants in long-term care facilities and to the development of courses to prepare individuals as nursing assistants for acute care settings. States vary in their requirements for hospital nursing assistants. Many states expect the hospitals to determine what their requirements will be and to then provide their own training.

The **home health aide** is prepared to assist individuals with basic care in their home; thus, a program of instruction includes content related to shopping for groceries, cooking, and doing laundry. Some long-term care nursing assistant programs offer an additional period of training and education for roles as home health aides to those who have completed their nursing assistant program. Other states have a shorter program without a certification examination for home health aides. In some states, there is no standardized certification requirement for those who work in homes.

Training for the various types of nursing assistant occurs in many settings, including high schools, long-term care facilities, hospitals, community colleges, regional occupational programs, and privately operated programs. Some consider this preparation the first rung on the ladder of nursing education, and, in some states, the nursing assistant may be exempt from certain classes required in LPN programs. Some registered nursing programs establish certification as a nursing assistant as an admission requirement.

The employment of UAPs has been of concern to nursing. Some state boards have issued a list of tasks that may be performed by UAPs, and both the ANA and the NCSBN have issued definitions and guidelines for the use of UAPs. More discussion of UAPs in healthcare occurs in Chapter 12.

PRACTICAL NURSE EDUCATION

The practical nurse (titled vocational nurse in Texas and California) is no newcomer to the healthcare delivery system. In the past, the practical nurse was the family friend or community citizen who was called to the home in emergencies. This person, usually self-taught, learned by experience which procedures were effective and which were not. The practical nurse would perform basic care procedures, such as bathing, and also would cook and perform light housekeeping duties for the family, much like the home health aide does today. Although controls on the licensing of practical nurses and the accreditation of their curricula were slower to evolve than those regulating professional nursing, states gradually enacted licensure laws governing practical nursing. By 1945, 19 states and one territory had licensure laws, but licensure of the practical nurse was mandatory in only one state (Kalisch & Kalisch, 2004). Most, if not all, of these people are now retired from nursing practice. By 1955, all states had licensure laws for practical nurses.

It is not clear when formal preparation for practical nursing began. The most widely accepted view is that the first programs were initiated through the YWCA in Brooklyn, New York, around 1892. The school established through the YWCA was known as the Ballard School, after Lucinda Ballard, who provided the funding to operate it. The course of study lasted approximately 3 months, and the students, called "attendants," were trained to care for invalids, the elderly, and children in a home setting.

A YWCA may seem a strange place for a practical nursing program. But YWCAs were an important source of inexpensive housing for many young women who, in the late 1890s and early 1900s, traveled from their homes to large cities in search of new careers and better lives. Because most of these women were untrained and had no marketable skills, the YWCA was a natural site for a school. Box 2.1 outlines some of the significant history in the development of practical nursing.

BOX 2.1 HISTORY OF THE DEVELOPMENT OF PRACTICAL NURSING

1892	YWCA in Brooklyn, New York, establishes a program in practical nursing named after Lucinda Ballard, who provided the funding for it.
1907	Thompson School is founded in Brattleboro, Vermont.
1908	The American Red Cross founds a practical nursing program.
1918	The Household Nursing Association School of Attendant Nursing begins in Boston.
1938	New York becomes the first state to require licensure for the practical nurse.
1941	The Association of Practical Nurse Schools (APNS) is founded.
1942	Membership in the APNS is opened to practical nurses and the name changed to the National Association of Practical Nurse Education and Service (NAPNES). The first planned curriculum for practical nursing is developed.
1945	NAPNES establishes and accredits service for schools of practical nursing; the accrediting portion of this program was discontinued in 1986.
1949	The National Federation of Licensed Practical Nurses (NFLPN) is organized.
1957	Working with the American Nurses Association, NFLPN seeks to clarify the role and function of the practical nurse. The National League for Nursing (NLN) establishes the Council on Practical Nursing.
1966	The Chicago Public School Program becomes the first practical nurse program to be accredited by the NLN.
1979	The NLN publishes a list of competencies of graduates of practical/vocational nursing programs.
1996	The National Council of State Boards of Nursing (NCSBN), working with NAPNES, offers a certification examination for licensed practical nurses in long-term care.

The general curriculum for practical nurses, which typically takes 1 year to complete, varies considerably from state to state and even from school to school. In some states, the education is measured in clock hours instead of credit hours. Most of today's practical nursing education programs stress clinical experience, primarily in structured care settings such as hospitals and long-term care facilities. Basic therapeutic knowledge and introductory content from biologic and behavioral sciences correlate with clinical practice; usually, one third of the time is spent in the classroom and two thirds in clinical practice.

The educational preparation of the practical nurse takes place in a variety of settings. High schools, trade or technical schools, hospitals, junior or community colleges, universities, or independent agencies may offer programs. If the rules and regulations of the state board(s) of nursing allow it, practical nursing and associate nursing degree programs can be incorporated in the community college as part of a career ladder or **stackable credentials** approach to nursing education. These programs sometimes are referred to as one-on-one programs: 1 year of preparation for practical nursing, followed by one more year qualifying the graduate to take the licensure examination for registered nursing. All nursing students in these colleges are grouped together for core courses, including basic nursing content, during the first academic year. At the end of this time, a student has the option of stopping the educational program to seek licensure as a practical nurse or continuing for an additional year to be eligible to write the NCLEX-RN. Many students opt to do both. Graduates of these core programs in practical nursing usually have a broader and more in-depth understanding of the biologic sciences and sometimes the social sciences (also a part of the core curriculum), especially if these are college-level courses that are transferable to a 4-year institution. Because issues related to **educational mobility** and **articulation** between programs (matching courses between one institution and another) have received much attention, these combined programs have become popular.

Graduates of practical nursing programs take the NCLEX-PN; if they pass the exam, they use the title licensed practical nurse (LPN) or, in California and Texas, the title licensed vocational nurse (LVN). Their scope of practice focuses on meeting the healthcare needs of clients in hospitals, long-term care facilities, clinics, and the home. Typically, LPNs or LVNs working in acute and long-term care facilities care for clients whose conditions are considered stable, giving direct client care; observing, recording, and reporting; administering treatments and medications; and assisting in rehabilitation procedures. They also work in clinics and urgent care centers. They receive direction from an RN or a licensed physician.

As with the associate degree and hospital-based diploma programs for RNs, the educational preparation for practical nurses and the future of practical nursing are topics of much discussion. Some advocate two levels of nurses: the practical nurse prepared with an associate degree and the RN prepared with a baccalaureate degree. Others would eliminate practical nursing altogether. In 1987, North Dakota passed legislation that required all candidates taking the licensure examination for practical nursing to have completed an associate degree in practical nursing. In 2003, this requirement was rescinded, and the state moved back to requiring a minimum of 1 year of study for practical nurse licensure and a minimum of 2 years of study for RN licensure.

The nursing shortage has had a major impact on the practice of LPNs/LVNs. In many nursing homes, positions that would have been filled with RNs are being filled with LPNs. The effects of this are not clear, with the concern that in some instances LPNs may be asked to practice beyond the scope for which they were originally prepared. With the "graying" of the United States, and the growing need for nurses in home healthcare and in long-term care facilities, practical nurses will continue to play a significant role in healthcare delivery.

PROGRAMS THAT PREPARE GRADUATES FOR RN LICENSURE

A number of different avenues of education now prepare individuals for licensure as RNs. The most traditional of these are diploma programs, associate degree programs, and baccalaureate programs. Innovative programs that offer generic masters and doctoral educational routes in nursing are also available (to be discussed later in this chapter).

Diploma Education

The earliest type of nursing education in the United States took place in **diploma programs** administered by hospitals, also referred to as **hospital-based programs**. The early development of these schools is synonymous with development of nursing as a whole.

Development of Hospital-Based Diploma Nursing Programs

The first hospital with a nurse training school was the New England Hospital for Women, which accepted five probationers on September 1, 1872 (Kalisch & Kalisch, 2004). The characteristics of these early schools were discussed in detail in Chapter 1.

By the late 1940s and early 1950s, many hospital-based nursing schools had affiliated with nearby colleges and universities; these schools adopted general education requirements, such as anatomy, physiology, sociology, and psychology, as part of the curriculum. During this time, the National League of Nursing Education—later to become two organizations, the National League for Nursing (NLN) and the National League for Nursing Accrediting Commission (NLNAC)—assumed an active role in curriculum guidance and accreditation. NLNAC has since changed its name to the Accreditation Commission for Education in Nursing or ACEN. Nursing programs gained a stronger educational foundation because they were required to align themselves more closely with other types of postsecondary education, that is, education occurring after the completion of high school.

Hospital-Based Programs Today

Thus, diploma schools in operation today have educational programs that meet the criteria necessary for accreditation. They employ qualified faculty who have developed clinical learning experiences that meet the student's learning needs rather than the hospital's service needs (which often took priority in the past). These programs vary in length from 27 to 36 months. Many diploma schools are affiliated with a college or university so that college credit can be awarded formally. Graduates are provided with a foundation in the biologic and social sciences and may have taken some courses in the humanities. There is a strong emphasis in diploma programs on client experiences. The course of study includes experience in nursing management (eg, being in charge of a nursing unit). Graduates work in acute, long-term, and ambulatory healthcare facilities, fulfilling the responsibilities established by the scope of practice for RNs as defined by the state in which they are licensed.

Before the 1970s, diploma schools were a popular avenue to nursing education with over 800 schools in operation. There are fewer than 100 diploma programs left with the majority in the south and Midwest regions of the country (NLN, 2014b). As more nursing education programs were moved to institutions of higher education, many hospital-based schools elected to discontinue their programs. Some merged with a local community college or university that assumed administrative responsibility for managing the nursing program and awarded an associate or baccalaureate degree when graduation requirements were satisfied.

The elimination of hospital-based programs has occurred because hospitals could not sustain the costs of supporting the programs and because students became more attracted to programs located in colleges and universities. Long-standing programs in some areas of the United States (predominately the East) have continued due to financial support from strong endowments and private funding and community traditions that encourage student enrollment.

Associate Degree Nursing Education

The movement toward **associate degree education** began in 1952. Today, associate degree nursing programs prepare more graduates for licensure as RNs than do any of the other programs and comprise over one half of all students enrolled in prelicensure RN programs (NLN, 2014a). Associate degree programs have helped to alleviate the nursing shortages of the 1960s, 1980s, and today.

Development of Associate Degree Education

Four events undoubtedly influenced the beginning of associate degree nursing education. First, these programs followed in the wake of the organization and growth of 2-year community colleges in the United States. Community colleges are located locally, offer the first 2 years of a traditional 4-year college program, offer technical and vocational programs, and make some form of college education accessible to everyone. Second, the cadet nurse program, which was created during World War II, demonstrated that qualified students could be educated adequately in less than the traditional 3 years of the diploma program. Third, the development of associate degree education was influenced by the studies conducted on nursing education in the United States, as discussed in Chapter 1. The final factor influencing the development of associate degree education was the critical national nursing shortage of the 1950s, which occurred because nurses employed during World War II returned home to raise families. It was anticipated that the 2-year program would put graduates into the work market more quickly, thus helping to reduce the shortage of nurses while, at the same time, helping to move nursing education into the overall system of higher education in the United States.

Associate degree in nursing (ADN) programs have the distinction of being the first (and, to date, the only) type of nursing education established on the basis of planned research and experimentation. They were initiated through the Cooperative Research Project in Junior and Community College Education for Nursing at Teachers College, Columbia University. The original 5-year research project, which was directed by Mildred Montag, included seven junior and community colleges and one hospital school, located in six regions of the United States. Students graduating from these programs received an associate degree and were eligible to take the RN licensing examination. ADN programs have expanded from these seven programs in 1952 to more than 1,000 in 2014 (NLN, 2014b).

Characteristics of Associate Degree Education

Accrediting groups ensure that ADN programs are an integral part of the college in which they are housed, that faculty and students have the same rights and privileges as their counterparts in other fields of study, and that the curriculum is sound.

In a typical program, approximately 40% of the credits needed for the associate degree must be fulfilled by general education courses such as English, anatomy, physiology, speech, psychology, and sociology; the rest are to be fulfilled by nursing courses. Clinical learning experiences are carefully selected to correspond with the content delivered in classroom lectures; the preconferences and postconferences help to reinforce the relationship between the two. Some modifications in this structure are occurring, as associate degree educators strive to meet the expectations of employers and the community while remaining true to the concept of associate degree education.

Traditionally, nursing students were a homogeneous group—typically single white women, ranging in age from 18 to 35, who graduated in the upper third of their high school classes. The advent of associate degree education in nursing increased diversity in the students who enroll in nursing programs attracting older students, married women, minorities, men, and students with a wider range of educational experiences and intellectual abilities (Fig. 2.1). People who already possess baccalaureate or higher degrees in other fields sometimes seek admission to an associate degree program, often because it can be completed in a shorter period of time than would be needed to earn another baccalaureate degree. Additionally, community college programs tend to be more geographically accessible than baccalaureate programs in 4-year colleges and universities, which are characteristically located in major urban areas.

Figure 2.1. The public does not always understand nursing credentials.

Challenges to Associate Degree Education

Associate degree education, like other educational programs, has experienced change. With these changes have come some challenges.

The Selective Admission Process

A concern with which educators struggle is the processes used in selecting students for a nursing program. This challenge becomes greater when the number of students seeking admission either increases dramatically or drops significantly, a phenomenon many programs have experienced during the past 15 to 20 years. In response to this problem and in an effort to select students who can realize success in their endeavors, many programs have developed selective admission processes. Although this is common in 4-year schools and colleges, it is a departure from the open-door policy of most community colleges. Some nursing programs use a waiting list, which honors the concept of first come, first served. Other schools use systems similar to a lottery. Also popular are point systems that award numeric scores for courses completed, past work experience, cumulative grade point average, or a combination of all of these, with the students acquiring the greatest number of points being selected for the next class. These factoring systems often require that a student spends at least a year in college to secure a position in the beginning nursing class, resulting in what began as a 2-year program extending to at least 3 years.

Misunderstandings About Associate Degree Education

For many years, associate degree education was poorly understood by employers, the public, and, to some extent, nursing educators in baccalaureate and higher degree programs. Although this route to nursing education is now firmly established as credible preparation for a nursing career, it continues to receive some opposition. The controversy regarding **entry into practice**

> ### *Ethical Dilemma 2.1: Education and Nursing Practice*
>
> Ruth is working with a new nurse, Alex, who has recently moved to Massachusetts from Texas. Ruth is also from Texas and asks where Alex went to school. Ruth does not recognize the name of the school. Ruth notices that Alex does not seem familiar with some of the equipment and does not perform some of the basic skills of nursing correctly. At first, Ruth believes Alex is just nervous and still new, but she is very concerned about Alex's poor skill performance, as this could be detrimental to clients. Ruth looks up the school Alex named and finds that it does not have a nursing program. What should Ruth do?

and the preparation needed for professional nursing (which is discussed later in this chapter) is renewed from time to time. Thus, faculty, graduates, and advocates for associate degree education continue to find themselves clarifying facts such as the actual number of nursing credits and the focus on critical thinking and decision-making, as well as technical skills, and emphasizing the contributions made by graduates of the programs.

Baccalaureate Education

Baccalaureate degree nursing education occurs in a 4-year college or university and is championed by many to provide the minimum educational preparation for professional practice.

Development of Baccalaureate Education in Nursing

The first school of nursing to be established in a university setting was started at the University of Minnesota in 1909 as a quasi-autonomous branch of the university's school of medicine. The program was not very different from the 3-year hospital-based program operating at that time; nothing was required in the way of higher general education, and graduates were prepared for the RN certificate only. Education took place predominantly through apprenticeship, and students provided service to hospitals in exchange for education. However, nursing education did become a part of an academic organization, with 16 colleges and universities developing programs by 1916.

Many of the early programs offering a baccalaureate degree in nursing extended over a 5-year period. This allowed for 3 years of nursing school curriculum similar to that of the hospital-based programs and for an additional 2 years of liberal arts. While the increase in the number of schools was not rapid, in 1924, the Yale School of Nursing became the first to be established as a separate department within a university; Annie W. Goodrich was its dean.

Although the development of baccalaureate education for nurses may not seem like a major step to young people today, remember that it was not until 1920 that the 19th Amendment to the Constitution of the United States granted women the right to vote. Many people considered nursing to be a less than desirable occupation: vocational in its orientation; overshadowed by militaristic, religious, and technical characteristics; and confined to women. Liberal education, scholarship, and knowledge were thought to be incompatible with the female personality and capable of interfering with marriage—for many years, nursing students generally were not allowed to marry (Kalisch & Kalisch, 2004). The nursing curriculum, with its emphasis on the performance of skills rather than on the philosophic and theoretic approaches used in the humanities, was not well accepted by universities. Opposition to collegiate education for nurses also came from physicians, who argued that nurses would be overtrained. Physicians were not certain that a sound knowledge base was as important as the technical skills and manual dexterity that could be acquired with brief training at the bedside and argued that a baccalaureate education would make nursing services too expensive.

Many nursing leaders advocated for baccalaureate education as the minimum educational preparation for supervisory and administrative nursing roles. Baccalaureate education also provides the background needed for addressing the community as a client and incorporating research into practice and the educational base for entry into graduate education in nursing. In 1965, the ANA recommended baccalaureate preparation in nursing as the minimum educational preparation for entry into professional nursing practice, an issue discussed later in this chapter.

Characteristics of Baccalaureate Education

A baccalaureate nursing program is termed a basic or **generic program** when it is a prelicensure program leading to eligibility to take the NCLEX-RN. It includes an upper-division (junior and senior years) nursing major that is built upon 2 years of liberal arts and science courses taken during the freshman and sophomore years. A RN-BSN program is part of a ladder program or stackable credentials and allows the associate prepared nurse to take additional nursing and general education classes in order to obtain a baccalaureate degree in nursing. Some schools have also added programs designed to admit the LPN, who will emerge with a baccalaureate degree in nursing and be eligible for RN licensure. These programs carry different names in different parts of the country, including baccalaureate registered nurse programs, two-on-two programs, and, in the Midwest, capstone programs.

Nine essential components have been identified by the AACN as critical to professional nursing education, which remain current. They include a liberal education; organizational and systems leadership; scholarship for **evidence-based practice (EBP)**; information management and application; healthcare policy, finance, and regulatory environments; interprofessional communication and collaboration; clinical prevention and population health; profession and professional values; and baccalaureate generalist nursing practice (AACN, 2008).

Applicants to such programs must meet the entrance and graduation requirements established by the university and those of the nursing school. The admission requirements usually specify academic preparation at the high school (or preadmission) level, including courses in foreign language and higher-level mathematics and science, and a high cumulative grade point average. Relatively high scores on college admission tests also may be required.

During the freshman and sophomore years, students who pursue a nursing education take humanities, social, life, and physical science courses with college students who are preparing for other majors. The number of required liberal arts and science courses may vary from program to program but usually constitutes about one half the total number of credits specified for graduation—typically 120 semester credits or 180 quarter credits. Students usually begin their study of nursing content during their junior year, thus the term "upper-division major" in nursing. Nursing theory can be taught so that it builds on an understanding of the physical and biologic sciences and liberal arts studied the previous 2 years.

Students in baccalaureate nursing programs learn basic nursing skills. They also learn concepts of health promotion and disease prevention at an individual and population level.

Supervisory and leadership theory and skills are taught, along with an introduction to research. Clinical course work includes experience in community health settings and leadership responsibility. Emphasis is placed on developing skills in critical decision-making, exercising independent nursing judgments that call for broad background knowledge, and working in complex nursing situations in which the outcomes often are not predictable. These call for the application of current evidence into one's practice. Acting as a client advocate, the graduate with a baccalaureate degree in nursing collaborates with other members of the healthcare team in structured and unstructured settings and supervises those with lesser preparation. Baccalaureate graduates often work with groups as well as with individuals. Knowledge and skills in managing information and client care technology are also essential components of baccalaureate education. The roles of the baccalaureate graduate are defined as provider of care, designer/manager/coordinator of care, and member of the profession (AACN, 2008).

Changes in Baccalaureate Education

In recent years, the nature of baccalaureate education has changed. Many baccalaureate nursing programs have taken steps to respond to the need for more RNs prepared for licensure at the baccalaureate level. Innovative methods include the development of accelerated programs and external degree programs. These are discussed in detail later in this chapter. Table 2.1 provides a comparison of these traditional major avenues to RN licensure.

Master's Prelicensure Programs

Our discussion of the various educational programs for registered nursing would be incomplete without mention of the generic master's program. The first generic master's degree in nursing was opened at Yale University in 1974, and other schools soon followed. Students are admitted with a baccalaureate degree in another discipline and are granted a master's degree in nursing after completing an established 2-year program of study that prepares them for RN licensure. Such programs reflect the thinking of some nursing leaders that the minimum preparation for professional nursing should be the master's degree. The programs also provide a higher degree to those people who possess basic baccalaureate preparation in another area of study and are making a career change. With increasing emphasis on the need for a baccalaureate degree for professional practice, this type of program provides a credible opportunity to those with baccalaureate degrees in another area of study. When programs of this type are not available, many students with degrees in other disciplines choose to pursue a 2-year ADN.

Nontraditional Prelicensure Programs

Throughout the years, various adaptations have been made in the traditional ways of educating nurses. These innovative approaches have occurred primarily because of the need to educate more individuals to become nurses, the need to prepare nurses with higher degrees in nursing, shifts in the economy, and the desire among young people to find work that will make a difference while at the same time making a living.

Accelerated Programs

Accelerated programs prepare students at both the baccalaureate and the master's levels. Building on previous learning experiences, they are designed to transition adults with baccalaureate and graduate degrees in other fields into nursing. Baccalaureate programs may be

Table 2.1   Basic Educational Opportunities for Registered Nursing: A Comparison

	Diploma	Associate Degree	Baccalaureate
Location	Is usually conducted by and based in a hospital	Most often conducted in junior or community colleges, occasionally in senior colleges and universities	Located in senior colleges and universities
Length of study	Requires generally 24–30 months but may require 3 academic years	Requires usually 2 academic or sometimes 2 calendar years—with prerequisites completed before nursing courses, up to 3 years	Requires 4 academic years
Requirements for admission	Requires graduation from high school or its equivalent, satisfactory general academic achievement, and successful completion of certain prerequisite courses	Requires that applicants meet entrance requirements of college as well as those of program	Requires that applicants meet entrance requirements of the college or university as well as those of program
Program of learning	Includes courses in theory and practice of nursing and in biologic, physical, and behavioral sciences that may be taken at a local college or university	Combines a balance of nursing courses and college courses in the basic natural and social sciences with courses in general education and the humanities	Combines courses in the liberal arts as well as the behavioral and physical sciences taken in the first 2 years with concentration of courses in the theory and practice of nursing in the junior and senior years
Clinical component	Clinical component completed in large part in the hospital offering the program	Requires as a significant part of the program supervised clinical instruction in hospitals and other community health agencies	Includes courses in community health, leadership, and research as part of the nursing curriculum as well as clinical instruction in a variety of settings
Opportunity for educational advancement	Little or no transferability of courses unless affiliated with a community college or university	Is structured so that some credits may be applied to baccalaureate degree	Provides the basic academic preparation for advancement to higher positions in nursing and to master's degree
Competency on graduation	Graduate is prepared to plan for the care of clients with other members of the healthcare team, to develop and carry out plans for the care of individuals or groups of clients, and to direct selected members of the nursing team. Has an understanding of the hospital climate and the community health resources necessary for the extended care of clients	Graduate is prepared to plan and give direct client care in hospitals, nursing homes, or similar healthcare agencies and to participate with other members of the healthcare team, such as LPNs, nurses' aides, physicians, and other registered nurses, in rendering care to clients	Graduate is prepared to plan and give direct care to individuals and families, whether sick or well, to assume responsibility for directing other members of the healthcare team, and to take on beginning leadership positions. Practices in a variety of settings and emphasizes comprehensive healthcare, including preventive and rehabilitative services, health counseling and education, and care in acute and long-term illnesses. Has necessary education for graduate study toward a master's degree and may move rapidly to specialized leadership positions in nursing as teacher, administrator, clinical specialist, nurse practitioner, and nurse researcher
Licensure	Must successfully complete licensing examination	Must successfully complete licensing examination	Must successfully complete licensing examination

completed in 11 to 18 months including prerequisites, and master's degree programs generally take about 3 years to complete. Accelerated baccalaureate programs make this the fastest route to licensure as an RN (AACN, 2014). Instruction is intense with all courses offered full-time with no breaks between sessions. These fast-track programs have proliferated over the past 15 years with programs available in 43 states plus the District of Columbia and Puerto Rico—more are in the planning stages.

Typical students, referred to as **second-degree students**, are motivated, older, and competitive and have high academic expectations. Admission standards are high, typically requiring a minimum of a 3.0 GPA. Programs are geared to students who have already demonstrated an ability of succeed at a senior college or university. Students receive the same number of clinical hours as the counterparts in the traditional programs (AACN, 2014). More detailed information on accelerated programs can be obtained at http://www.aacn.nche.edu/students/accelerated-nursing-programs.

External Degree Programs

The concept of an **external degree** is not new to education in general. Universities in Australia, the Soviet Union, and England have long recognized independent study validated by examination. The University of London has awarded college degrees earned in this fashion since 1836. The major difference between the external degree and the traditional educational experience is that students awarded an external degree are not required to attend classes or follow any prescribed methods of learning (however, they may choose to take some classes).

Learning is assessed through highly standardized and validated examinations. This approach to education was not developed in the United States until about the mid-1950s and then only in selected areas. New York's Empire State College and the University Without Walls consortium were the first schools in the United States to recognize the value of self-directed learning. Now known as Excelsior University, the New York Regents External Degree Program of the University of the State of New York has become part of this movement.

The nursing program, like other external degree programs in arts, science, and business, uses an assessment approach and is primarily—although not exclusively—designed for those with some experience in nursing. It is philosophically based on principles of adult learning, which advocate flexible and learner-oriented education. Specifically, the responsibility for demonstrating that learning has occurred is placed on the student, and the responsibility for identifying the content to be learned and objectively assessing that this has occurred rests with the faculty. The nursing major is divided into cognitive and performance components. Cognitive learning is documented through nationally standardized and psychometrically valid written examinations. Clinical skills are evaluated through criteria-referenced performance examinations at regional performance assessment centers throughout the country.

There are some limitations on the use of external degree programs. Some states do not accept Excelsior degrees for initial licensure because their laws mandate that the educational process include supervised clinical practice. Some states will admit to the licensure examination for RNs only those external associate degree graduates who were LPNs and therefore have had supervised clinical practice in addition to clinical examinations. Despite objections, alternative and nontraditional avenues to nursing education appeal to the learner, and these programs continue to evolve. Nursing education, like nursing care, should be tailored to fit the consumer's needs.

Communication in Action 2.1: *Addressing Education and Credentials*

Alice Mason, a recent graduate from an associate degree nursing program, was working on a unit with a new baccalaureate graduate. On several occasions, the baccalaureate graduate made comments such as, "I just don't know how you could learn all you need to know in just 2 years." Alice invited her colleague to join her for coffee. She initiated the conversation by saying, "From some of your remarks, I don't believe you understand the scope of associate degree nursing education, and I'd like to explain a bit about it." Calmly, she further explained, "In an associate degree program, we have the same science requirements as in a baccalaureate program in this state. We do take fewer credits in general education, but we are required to take 2 full years of nursing courses, often using the same texts used by programs such as yours. Although sometimes we earn fewer credits in some of those classes. My understanding is that you have spent time studying the community as a client, which I did not, and that you have more time devoted to statistics, nursing research, and leadership. Although I took a nursing management course, I believe it, too, was fewer credits. In order to complete my bachelor's degree, I will need to take the general education courses I do not have, plus 20 semester credits of nursing." She then said, "Tell me more about your program." Her colleague began to share details of her program, and they both felt they more clearly understood one another's education.

SIMILARITIES AMONG TRADITIONAL ENTRY-LEVEL PRELICENSURE PROGRAMS

Currently, there are as many similarities in the various avenues to nursing education as there are differences. These similarities may be grouped into several broad classifications, including academic standards, administrative concerns, and areas relating to students.

Academic Similarities

The most obvious similarity is that all programs must academically prepare graduates to pass the NCLEX for registered nursing in their state at the same minimum standardized score used across the nation. All schools must meet criteria established for state board approval in their respective state.

Administrative Similarities

Adequate financial support is a major concern for many programs because they are relatively expensive to operate. Lower student-to-teacher ratios, expensive laboratories, and limited federal and state funding for nursing education affect the economics of the programs. Another administrative concern focuses on securing appropriate learning experiences. Schools often compete with one another for clinical spaces in hospitals and healthcare facilities. Certain experiences, such as maternal, child, and psychiatric nursing, may be especially difficult to secure. Developing and maintaining curricula that prepare graduates for current practice often present a challenge. Demographic changes, with people living longer, technologic advances—especially in the area of informatics—changes in venues of care, bioethical concerns, and myriad other changes leave faculty struggling to construct and teach state-of-the-art curricula. Not the least of the administrative similarities is the recruitment and retention of qualified faculty, which has become intensified in recent years. More lucrative salaries in other positions and the aging and retirement of the present faculty both affect this concern.

Similarities Relating to Students

Similarities also exist among students. First of all, recruitment and selection is a major task. Although some schools must turn students away (often because they are unable to find faculty or clinical sites), at the same time, schools must be responsive to an increasingly diverse population that may enter school unprepared for college-level studies. This has resulted in the development of selective admission policies that must be scrutinized carefully by school officials and, in some areas, reviewed by the school's attorney for correct legal form and legal ramifications before being accepted by the school's policy-making group.

Programs are caught up in more legal concerns than in the past because applicants and students are seeking their rights as individuals and challenging admission, progression, and dismissal policies. Another legal concern relates to malpractice coverage for students. Some collegiate programs, now removed from the umbrella coverage of the hospital, ask that students purchase malpractice insurance as protection against any lawsuits that might arise as the result of errors committed in the learning process.

There is greater diversity in the student body. Programs are receiving more applications from men, minorities, older adults, and persons who possess degrees in other fields of study. Students with English as a second language present new challenges to nursing faculty in all types of programs. Special courses and other forms of assistance are being developed to enable students with academic challenges to succeed in nursing.

Critical Thinking Activity: Nursing Education in an Ideal World
Imagine that you could restructure nursing education for an ideal world. Where would you begin? How many levels of nursing education would you incorporate into your model? Would each level be terminal or articulated with others? Where would general education fit into your model? How would you see the graduate of each program functioning on the healthcare team? How would you see each level reimbursed for services?

NURSING EDUCATION AT THE GRADUATE LEVEL

The critical need for nurses with additional preparation to work in educational settings, in supervisory roles, as clinical specialists and to fulfill the expanded role of the nurse has resulted in more programs at the graduate level.

Master's Preparation

As indicated in our earlier discussion of master's education in nursing, there are a variety of models. Some less traditional approaches include outreach programs, summers-only programs, RN-to-MSN tracks (that provide a direct route to the master's degree for RNs who have graduated from diploma or associate degree programs), programs taught primarily online, and programs for students with different educational backgrounds (such as RNs with nonjuring baccalaureate degrees or foreign graduates). Some schools offer off-campus classes, at times rotating sites, and some deliver core content by way of television or through other distance learning technology.

Most programs require at least a full year for completion, and many have been expanded to 2 years. Master's programs in nursing are found in senior colleges and universities that have baccalaureate programs in nursing. They have the option of seeking voluntary accreditation from the ACEN, from the National League for Nursing Commission for Nursing Education Accreditation (CNEA), or from the Commission on Collegiate Nursing Education (CCNE).

Master's preparation is recommended for leadership positions in nursing, for clinical specialization, and is generally the minimum preparation required to teach nursing. The AACN has outlined roles for graduates at the various educational levels. Their vision is for a generalist at the baccalaureate level and an advanced generalist at the master's level that includes the clinical nurse leader (CNL) (see Chapter 14). The CNL oversees the care coordination of clients in any healthcare setting and is prepared to serve as a change agent to improve clinical outcomes, save money, and enhance care coordination (AACN, 2016).

Further identified is advanced specialty nursing education with a doctor of nursing practice (DNP) or a research-focused program (PhD, DNS, or DNSc).

Doctoral Studies

The number of requests for admission to doctoral study in nursing has increased greatly since the early 1980s. The impetus for this movement stems from the need for advanced study for academic advancement or tenure in the educational setting and reflects the need in nursing research for the advancement of the profession as a whole.

Before doctorates in nursing were offered, doctoral study in other fields allowed nurses to benefit from postmaster's preparation. A doctorate outside the area of nursing was often the only doctorate available to persons seeking further education; doctorates in nursing are relatively new to the educational milieu, as opposed to such degrees in psychology, sociology, anthropology, or physiology. Certainly, nursing can benefit and has benefited from other disciplines.

Doctoral programs in nursing offer various degrees, such as the doctor of nursing science (DNS), the doctor of science in nursing (DSN), the doctor of nursing education (DEd), and the more traditional doctor of philosophy in nursing (PhD). Nonnursing doctorates are available to nurses, such as the doctor of education (EdD) and the doctor of public health (DPH).

In 2004, the AACN proposed a DNP degree. The DNP is designed for nurses seeking a terminal degree in advanced nursing practice, as opposed to working in research (AACN, 2017). The DNP was developed with the premise that the challenges of today's healthcare demanded a higher level of preparation for advanced practice nurses (APNs) who could design and assess care and provide leadership. Some universities are changing their nurse practitioner programs from master's degree programs to this type of clinical practice doctorates. The difference in the preparation and function of graduates possessing the various degrees is confusing. Typically, the nurse with a doctorate assumes a leadership role in education, often serving as a faculty member or the dean or director of a nursing program. These nurses also may choose to be involved in the research and development of a body of nursing knowledge.

> ### Critical Thinking Activity: Standards for Nurse Practitioners
> If nurse practitioners are to work collaboratively with physicians, and as primary care providers, what type and level of education do you believe they should complete? How would you ensure that this would occur? What standards regarding continuing education should be mandated for those involved in advance practice? Should it be more stringent than that required at the RN level? Defend your position.

OTHER FORMS OF NURSING EDUCATION

A number of factors have fostered the development of other forms of education for nurses. Most of these are seen in the changing role of the nurse in healthcare delivery and the need this creates for more adequate education to meet the requirements of that role. Another contributing aspect is the continuing push to make nursing truly professional and prepare nurses to complete research. A third significant reason for advancing nursing education relates to the need for leadership in nursing administration and education. Thus, RNs seek baccalaureate, masters, and doctoral degrees to support the complex roles into which they move.

Distance Education

Distance education is being used by a variety of universities and other educational entities to make attaining a baccalaureate or master's degree more accessible. This approach focuses on making education available through a variety of distance technologies including online strategies, video broadcasting to distant sites, and courses taught in areas distant from the campus. A wide variety of approaches and methods are used, including courses that are Internet-enabled, Web-based, computer-mediated, online, synchronous, and asynchronous.

Students may participate in clinical learning through a relationship with a mentor or preceptor in a local clinical setting. These clinical experiences follow prescribed procedures leading to specified outcomes and receive academic credit. Part-time study is welcomed. Some programs have brief, intensive times when all students in a cohort gather at the institution for 1 to 2 weeks in order to foster interaction between students and faculty and enhance the educational experience. Students benefit because they can continue to work while attending school and experience reduced travel costs. The RN who wishes to obtain a baccalaureate or higher degree from such an institution may take some courses, such as general education requirements, at a local college, attain credit by examination for some nursing courses, and enroll in still other courses online, with all accepted as credit by the university granting the degree.

Although these programs offer much flexibility to students, they also demand a great deal of discipline on their part. A single course may require as much as 15 to 20 hours of study time per week. A student attempting such a program needs to be an independent learner. Sufficient faculty time also must be provided for students to receive effective feedback regarding their efforts. Library resources are always a concern for distant learners, and colleges need to provide access to appropriate learning resources for distance learners. Mechanisms for evaluating the learning must be developed thoughtfully to ensure the integrity of resulting credentials.

OTHER POSTLICENSURE EDUCATIONAL OPPORTUNITIES

Several opportunities for continued growth and career advancement are available to registered nurses. Some assist the graduate to move into a professional role, some support continued competence, and others are geared to a particular role development but may not culminate in an advanced degree.

Residencies and Structured Orientation for the New Graduate

When nursing education moved from hospital-based diploma programs into higher education, a new problem arose. Employers of the new graduates expected these graduates to function as experienced and qualified professionals on the day after graduation and complained that the graduates were not prepared to assume staff nurse positions within their institutions.

As nursing education moved into institutions of higher education, all clinical time was recognized in credit hours. If students worked on hospital units on weekends, they did so as hospital employees, not as a requirement of their education. As a result, students spend less time in the clinical area. Many graduates of diploma schools in the 1950s would have had as much as 4,000 clock hours of clinical experience, albeit more as apprenticeship and service to the hospital than as a planned learning experience. Graduates of associate and baccalaureate degree programs, with integrated curricula and outcome-based learning experiences, join the work world with clinical learning time of 800 or fewer clock hours. Hospital-based programs also decreased their clinical hours as curricula were reorganized. Students in all programs receive their clinical experience in a variety of settings as opposed to one primary healthcare facility where they become very familiar with policies, procedures, and the physical plant.

All of this results in new graduates needing orientation to the work facility and their new role and time to become proficient in using their newly learned skills. Although few would question the need for **internships and residencies** for new physicians, the need for similar experiences for new nursing graduates has not been readily accepted. New graduates, when unable to live up to expectations placed on them, often become frustrated and discouraged; some opt for less stressful situations, sometimes even outside nursing. Nursing educators, in defending the education provided, cite other professions, such as law and engineering, in which graduates need time to adapt to the world of work.

As a result of efforts to address this concern, orientation programs, internships, and residencies for new graduates have been instituted by hospitals. The programs are intended to ease the transition from the role of student to that of staff by providing the opportunity to increase clinical skills and knowledge as well as self-confidence. These programs can last from several weeks to a year and are designed for graduates of all nursing programs—associate degree, diploma, and baccalaureate. They often include rotations to various units in the hospital, including specialty areas, and they accommodate different shifts. Usually, some formal classwork is associated with the experience, but the majority of the time is spent in direct client care, often under the supervision of a preceptor.

Institutions receive some direct benefits from such programs in addition to securing a better-prepared employee who remains employed. Inadequacies in policies and procedures have been uncovered and, as a result, rewritten. Performance evaluation tools that are more objective in format have emerged. Nursing practice throughout some agencies has become more standardized. Job satisfaction has increased. It is no longer unusual for hospitals to advertise planned orientation and internships as benefits offered to the new graduate seeking employment, a strong recruitment tool in times of nurse shortages.

The major disadvantage voiced by hospitals is the cost of operating such programs. When cost containment is crucial, hospitals may not be eager to deal with these additional costs. Another problem is that some employees who benefit from such programs may resign from their positions soon after completing an internship. This has resulted in many hospitals stipulating a period of required employment following the orientation or internship.

Continuing Education

Continuing education in nursing is defined as a planned learning experience beyond a basic nursing educational program. The learning experiences are designed to promote the development of knowledge, skills, and attitudes for the enhancement of nursing practice, thus improving healthcare to the public (ANA, 1974). Continuing education programs are widely publicized in today's nursing literature. They often are presented just before and during major nursing conventions. Some professional meetings carry continuing education credit. Other continuing education programs exist as extensions of nursing programs at colleges and universities.

Like so many other areas of nursing, continuing education is not new. In an article entitled "Nursing the Sick," written around 1882, Florence Nightingale wrote: "Nursing is, above all, a progressive calling. Year by year nurses have to learn new and improved methods, as medicine and surgery and hygiene improve. Year by year nurses are called upon to do more and better than they have done. It is felt to be impossible to have a public register of nurses that is not a delusion" (Nightingale, as cited in Seymer (1954, p. 349).

The first continuing education courses for nurses probably would be considered postgraduate instruction today. In 1899, Teachers College at Columbia University instituted a course for qualified graduate nurses in hospital economics. Nursing institutes and conferences were first offered to nurses in the 1920s; often, these were given to make up for deficiencies in basic nursing curricula. The first hospital in-service classes or staff development programs were discussed in nursing literature around this time. Today, most hospitals employ someone who is responsible for the staff education program. By 1959, federal funds became available for short-term courses, giving much thrust to continuing education. In 1967, the ANA published Avenues for Continued Learning, its first definitive statement on continuing education; and in 1973, the ANA Council on Continuing Education was established. The Council, which is responsible to the ANA Commission on Education, is concerned about standards of continuing education, accreditation of the programs, transferability of credit from state to state, and development of guidelines for recognition systems within states. In 1974, the first edition of Standards for Continuing Education in Nursing was published by the ANA, and the federal government altered the Nurse Traineeship Act of 1972 to include an option that would provide continuing education as an alternative to placing more students into programs receiving federal capitation dollars.

By the 1970s, most nursing publications had something to say about continuing education for nurses. Practically, all states were organizing or planning to organize some method by which the nurse could receive recognition for continued education. These systems were called continuing education approval and recognition programs, or continuing education recognition programs, and most state systems followed the guidelines and criteria prepared by the ANA.

The **continuing education unit (CEU)** became a rather uniform system of measuring, recording, reporting, accumulating, transferring, and recognizing participation in nonacademic credit offerings. The National Task Force on the Continuing Education Unit, which represented 34 educational groups, developed the definition of a CEU. Although nursing was not one of the groups, the profession has accepted the definition. Ten hours of participation in an organized continuing education experience under responsible sponsorship, with capable direction and qualified instruction, is equal to one CEU. Many states and organizations, however, simply report clock hours of instruction. Following a system for accreditation and approval of continuing education in nursing that was developed and implemented by the ANA in 1975, programs or individuals offering courses for continuing education now receive authority to do so from a recognized body, thereby ensuring quality programs and standardization in their approach.

Today, colleges, universities, hospitals, voluntary agencies, and private proprietary groups all offer continuing education courses to RNs (Fig. 2.2). The cost of this education varies tremendously. Nurses can earn continuing education credits for merely attending meetings and conferences. Attempts to assess whether learning has occurred vary tremendously. Professional journals include sections of programmed instruction that can be completed in the comfort of one's living room. These have an evaluation mechanism. Workshops, institutes, conferences, webinars, short courses, and evening courses abound.

However, some nurses do not feel the need to keep up with these offerings. An issue today is whether continuing education should be mandatory or voluntary. **Mandatory continuing education** affects licensure, meaning that any nurse renewing a license in a state requiring (mandating) continuing education will have to satisfy that requirement. **Voluntary continuing education** is

Figure 2.2. Technology and equipment are changing rapidly so continuing education is essential to stay current with knowledge and skills.

not related to relicensure. Government agencies and state legislatures are exerting pressure on nurses, as they have on physicians, attorneys, dietitians, dentists, pharmacists, and other professionals, to provide evidence of updated knowledge before license renewal.

A position supporting mandatory continuing education raises some questions. How should the learning be measured? Who should accredit the programs? How can quality be ensured? By whom and where should records be retained? Who should bear the cost? What should be the time frame for continuing education? How many hours, courses, and credits should be required? You can contact any state board of nursing for information on specific requirements for that state.

Advanced Practice Preparation

Specialized programs have been developed to help individuals prepare for roles of increased breadth and scope. Programs may be incorporated into the preparation leading to a particular degree, exist as part of a school's continuing education program, or result in certification after examination.

Recent healthcare reform has resulted in an increased emphasis on the role of **advanced nursing practice** in healthcare delivery and more demand for educational programs to prepare these practitioners. An APN is an umbrella term that includes nurse practitioners, clinical nurse specialists, certified nurse–midwives (CNM), and certified registered nurse anesthetists (CRNA).

The RN anesthesia and midwifery programs both award a certificate after completion of a standardized and rigorous course of study lasting from 18 months to 2 years. At one time, admission requirements stipulated RN licensure only; however, a baccalaureate degree in nursing is now required for admission to schools of anesthesia, with a master's degree awarded on completion. The American College of Nurse-Midwives requires a master's degree for completion of a CNM program as of 2010.

Other programs offer nurse practitioner and nursing specialist preparation in areas of nursing practice such as pediatrics, gerontology, family health, genetics, and women's healthcare. In the 1990s, the Pew Commission encouraged growth in the number of master's level nurse practitioner training programs, and many more were developed (de Tornyay, 1996). Programs that prepare nurse practitioners concentrate study in specific areas during a period lasting from several months to a year or more. Requirements for admission vary tremendously. Most programs require a bachelor's degree in some field and a current RN license to enter and award the master's degree on completion. Still others require that the education occur at the postmaster's degree level. The ANCC requires the master's degree for all those seeking initial nurse practitioner certification.

The development of new APN programs has been so great that a complete listing is impossible. A student interested in pursuing such preparation is encouraged to write to the college or university of choice for information about available programs.

Critical Thinking Activity: Continuing Education
Do you believe continuing education should be a mandatory requirement for the renewal of one's license? Why or why not? If your answer is no, how would you ensure competence? If you believe it should be mandatory, what kind of record keeping would you require? Who do you believe should keep the records?

FACTORS THAT BRING ABOUT CHANGES IN NURSING EDUCATION

During the 20th century, society experienced tremendous change. Nursing, as a part of that society, has also experienced enormous change. A number of factors influenced nursing education.

The Brown Report

In 1948, Esther Lucile Brown, who was not a nurse, conducted one of the important early studies of nursing. She was concerned that young women were not choosing nursing as a profession and believed, as a result of her study, that the majority of nursing schools failed to provide a professional education. In *Nursing for the Future*, Brown (1948) recommended that nursing education move away from the system of apprenticeship that predominated at the time (see earlier discussion of hospital-based programs in Chapter 1) and move toward a planned program of education similar to that offered by other professions. She recommended that the schools be operated by universities or colleges, hospitals affiliated with institutions of higher learning, medical colleges, or independently. She also recommended that programs periodically be examined or reviewed and that a list of accredited schools be published and distributed.

The Brown report attracted the attention of many nursing leaders, who shared her concerns about recruiting qualified women into nursing. The study took place shortly after World War II, and nurses who had been involved in the military had a new sense of autonomy and independence that they were not willing to leave behind. Committees were formed to respond to the suggestions put forth in the Brown study, particularly those related to the accreditation of programs. At the same time, the National League for Nursing Education (NLNE), later to become the NLN, recommended that hospital schools of nursing consider transferring control and administration of their programs to educational institutions. The NLNE also urged that federal grants be provided to nursing schools to allow for their improvement.

Development of a National Examination Standard

Along with the push for the improvement of nursing education, licensing authorities were pressured to establish a uniform licensing examination. The development of the State Board Test Pool Examination, which gradually expanded until all states required that same examination, helped all schools to focus on common goals and laid the foundation for **Interstate endorsement** of licenses. The test required to obtain licensure is now known as the NCLEX for registered nursing (or practical nursing for practical nursing program graduates) (see Chapter 3).

National Accreditation of Nursing Programs

By 1952, the NLN had a temporary accreditation program in place and was helping schools to find ways to improve their programs of instruction. Accreditation of all kinds requires that the institution studies its own practices in relationship to standards. Peers, prepared as accreditation visitors, then examine the institution, and a determination is made as to whether the school meets the standards. The accreditation of programs had a noticeable effect on standards of nursing education. As a result of accreditation activities, schools were forced to look at the educational preparation of faculty, the workload of faculty and students, the structure of clinical teaching, withdrawal rates, the self-evaluation of the program, and the state board examination scores. This system of program assessment enhanced the quality of education;

graduation from a nationally accredited school meant added opportunities for advanced education or certain types of employment. Today, accreditation of nursing programs is carried out by the ACEN or CNEA for practical, associate degree, baccalaureate, masters, and clinical doctorate programs in nursing. For baccalaureate, graduate, and residency programs, accreditation is also available through the CCNE (see Chapter 3).

Changes in Nursing Service

While changes were occurring in the education of nurses, nurses in the workplace also experienced significant changes. With the advent of antibiotics, major advances in medical protocols, and medical technology that allowed treatment of very serious conditions but resulted in clients who were in more critical condition, the public received care in hospitals rather than treatment in the home. Births that previously took place at home now occurred in hospitals. Federal funds were allocated for the construction of hospitals. Increased hospitalization drove the need for qualified nurses to a new high. Hospitals were desperate to find nurses to fill needed positions, and nurses represented half of all hospital personnel. Today, RNs constitute the largest healthcare occupation, with over 4 million nurses (The Henry J. Kaiser Family Foundation, 2016).

The role of the nurse changed in response to changes in the workplace. Nursing staff began assuming responsibilities formerly associated with physicians. Unfortunately, they also assumed responsibilities that could have been assumed by housekeeping, dietary, laboratory, and pharmacy departments. Nurses began spending more time managing personnel, delegating responsibilities, and carrying out other administrative duties. Nurses at higher levels in the organization needed higher levels of education (ie, baccalaureate and master's degrees).

The Report of the Surgeon General's Consultant Group

In 1961, the Surgeon General of the United States Public Health Service appointed a group to advise him of the federal government's role in providing adequate nursing services to the country. This group was known as the Surgeon General's Consultant Group on Nursing, and they published their report in 1963.

The report emphasized the need for more nurses and identified the lack of adequate financial resources for nursing education as a major problem. Several other major concerns also were reported. Of critical importance were the reports that too few schools were providing adequate nursing education, that too few college-bound young people were being recruited into the profession, and that more nursing schools were needed in colleges and universities. (By now, you are recognizing this as a recurrent theme regarding nursing.) Educational preparation at the baccalaureate degree level was recommended as the minimum preparation for nurses assuming leadership roles (U.S. Public Health Service, 1963).

The Surgeon General's Consultant Group on Nursing also recommended that federally funded low-cost loans and scholarships be made available to students in both professional and practical nursing programs. It advocated the use of federal funds to construct additional nursing school facilities and to expand educational programs. The Nurse Training Act of 1964 was an outgrowth of these recommendations.

The American Nurses Association Position Paper

In the early 1960s, the educational preparation of nurses became a major concern of the ANA. The ANA believed that the improvement of nursing practice and the profession as a whole

---

BOX 2.2 FOUR MAJOR POSITIONS OF THE ANA POSITION PAPER ON EDUCATIONAL PREPARATION

1. The education of all those who are licensed to practice nursing should take place in institutions of higher education.
2. Minimum preparation for beginning professional nursing practice at the present time should be baccalaureate degree education in nursing.
3. Minimum preparation for beginning technical nursing practice at the present time should be associate degree education in nursing.
4. Education for assistants in the health service occupations should be short, intensive preservice programs in vocational education institutions, rather than on-the-job training programs.

American Nurses Association. (1965). American Nurses Association's first position on education for nursing. *American Journal of Nursing, 65*(12), 106–107.

---

depended on the advancement of nursing education. After studying the issue for 3 years, *A Position Paper on Educational Preparation for Nurse Practitioners and Assistants to Nurses* was published in December 1965. In 2000, the ANA reaffirmed this position (ANA, 2000), which resulted in the entry into practice controversy. The positions of the paper are listed in Box 2.2.

No other single action or position has affected nursing more or has there been any issue that has been more divisive or contentious than the ANA position paper. For 45 years, the profession has been plagued with the issues it brought forth. A basic concern related to the fact that the roles, functions, and responsibilities (**competencies**) of programs offering three different routes to preparation for registered nursing was not clearly differentiated for graduates. All graduates took the same examination and performed similar activities when hired as new graduates in acute care facilities.

Associate degree nursing programs in community colleges and hospital-based diploma programs took serious exception to the paper. To this group, not being considered professional was unacceptable, and they were unwilling to compromise title or licensure. Because of the dissension the position paper created among nursing groups, little immediate action followed although four states—Oregon, Montana, Maine, and North Dakota—were chosen as focus states for early adoption. However, groups slowly began to take action regarding the paper, with many nursing organizations supporting the position, and others adamantly opposed to it and the controversy continues today (Clarke, 2017).

Problems Associated With Changing Educational Requirements for Licensure

Several problems are associated with making any changes in educational requirements for licensure. Four major problems are related to titling, scope of practice, grandfathering, and interstate endorsement.

Titling

One of the most controversial problems associated with changing requirements for licensure involves **Titling**, or the use of titles. The RN title has a long history and is clearly recognizable to the public and to the healthcare community. Currently, graduates of all nursing programs preparing graduates for registered nursing use this title if they pass the NCLEX-RN. If a differentiation were to be made among those with a baccalaureate degree, those with associate degrees, and those prepared in hospital-based programs, which graduates would use the title registered nurse? What alternate titles would be available for graduates from the other programs currently preparing individuals for licensure?

Scope of Practice

Of equal concern is the description and delineation of the scope of practice for the two levels of caregivers. The scope of practice (discussed in Chapter 3) is that section of the Nurse Practice Act that outlines the activities a person with a particular license may legally perform. This would mean the separate testing of each level as it currently exists between the RN and the practical nurse licensure examination. This problem might be of less concern if the nursing profession could agree on an approach to differentiated practice. In some suggestions for two levels of practice, the process of making nursing diagnoses and developing nursing care plans was at times included in the scope of practice of the baccalaureate-prepared nurse only, a position totally unacceptable to associate degree advocates. Again, the diploma graduate was left out of the discussion.

The Grandfather Clause

The application of a **grandfather clause** presents another challenge to nurses. Traditionally, when a state licensure law is enacted, or if a current law is repealed and a new law enacted, a grandfather clause has been a standard feature that allows persons to continue to practice their profession or occupation after new qualifications have been enacted into law. The legal basis for the process is found in the 14th Amendment to the U.S. Constitution, which declares that no state may deprive any person of life, liberty, or property without due process of law. The Supreme Court has ruled that the license to practice is a property right. A grandfather clause is not new to nursing; for example, it was applied when psychiatric nursing became a requirement of all programs. Nurses who were licensed without psychiatric nursing experiences were grandfathered into the new role. In other words, they continued to practice as RNs without taking a formal course in psychiatric nursing and without being required to write a psychiatric examination to maintain their licenses. If nursing began to require a baccalaureate degree for individuals using the RN title, under the provisions of a grandfather clause, all associate graduates licensed before the implementation date for the change would continue to use the title "registered nurse." Those licensed after the change would use whatever new title was established. Although this serves to protect the title of currently licensed nurses, it does not prevent employers from writing job descriptions stipulating a baccalaureate degree as the minimum educational preparation acceptable for a particular position.

Complicating this matter is the fact that some nurses believe a grandfather clause should be conditional. If it were conditional, nurses licensed before the changes in the licensure law would continue to use their current title for a stipulated period of time—for example, 10 years. At the end of that period, if they had not completed the education mandated in the changes (or any other conditions that might have been added), they would have to use the title stipulated in the new law for nurses with their educational preparation. Because of the complexity and the difficulties associated with implementation, it is unlikely that conditional grandfathering will ever become a reality.

Interstate Endorsement

A fourth concern is that of interstate endorsement. Nursing is one of the few professions to have developed a process whereby national examinations with standardized scores are administered in each state or jurisdiction, thus allowing a nurse who has passed the licensing examination in one state to move to another state and seek licensure without the need to retake and pass another examination. (However, with the exception of those states participating in the licensure compact [see Chapter 3], they do need to secure licensure in each state in which they practice.) Because nurses can be highly mobile, this has been a great advantage. As the profession examines multistate licensure, this issue takes on new dimensions.

The Position Paper and Nursing Today

Because the initial thinking and work on the position paper occurred 45 years ago, nursing leaders are raising questions about its relevancy today. The education of nurses has changed greatly with less than 10% of the new graduates coming from diploma programs and greater than 60% completing associate degree programs, many of which have articulation agreements with baccalaureate schools. If one views the position paper as a move to close hospital-based programs and place all nursing in colleges and universities, certainly that goal has been realized. However, two thirds of the graduates still possess less than a baccalaureate education, resulting in the majority of registered nurses being the least educated of all health professionals.

In 2011, a report on *The Future of Nursing* outlined the increased complexity of healthcare and healthcare environments that requires nurses to be more highly educated. The report specified increasing BSN nurses to 80% by 2020 and recommends doubling the number of nurses with a doctorate degree from 1% to 2% (The Institute of Medicine, 2011). Some nursing groups target a specific year for requiring the baccalaureate in nursing as the educational preparation for entry into practice as an RN. It becomes clear that this contentious issue is not one of the past but, rather, is one with which the nurses of tomorrow will continue to grapple.

Critical Thinking Activity: ANA Position on Nursing Education
Take a stand on the ANA position on nursing education. Provide a rationale for the position you have taken. What do you see as outcomes of the position paper? How would your position be implemented in the future? What implications might it have for nursing practice? Do you believe the salaries of nurses educated at different levels and practicing at differentiated levels should differ? Why or why not? If so, how?

FORCES FOR CHANGE IN NURSING EDUCATION

As the nursing profession advances and education remains responsive to the changes that occur, it is imperative that nursing education undergoes modifications. A discussion of some of the most significant challenges follows.

Theory Alert   Isabel Hampton Robb

Isabel Hampton Robb is considered to be one of the original founders of modern nursing theory in America. She graduated from the Bellevue Hospital Training School for Nurses in 1883 and then first worked as a nurse in Rome. Upon returning to the United States, she was the superintendent of nursing at the Cook County nursing school in Chicago, Illinois, and then moved to head John Hopkins School of Nursing in 1889. She wrote Nursing: Its Principles and Practices, Nursing Ethics: For Hospital and Private Use (1900), and Educational Standards of Nurses with Other Addresses on Nursing Subjects (1907).

Robb was important contributor to nursing education, which is her contribution to nursing theory. She developed and implemented a grading system that is still relevant today. She advocated for improving nursing education and reducing long clinical hours. She was one of the founders of the American Journal of Nursing. Through her writings and work, Robb was instrumental in making nursing education what it is today (Petiprin, 2016).

Incorporating Computer Technology in Nursing Education

Nursing education has experienced no transformation more dramatic than the incorporation of computer technology into all aspects of teaching, learning, and healthcare. These changes encompass activities covering everything from entire degrees that can be earned via online courses to separate courses that are taught online to the incorporation of computer technology in the classroom and learning laboratory. In the healthcare setting, computers are used for client records, business functions, and as a support to effective decision-making.

Computer Technology in the Classroom

The computer plays a major role in nursing education and is as essential to the operation of colleges and universities as it is to the operation of hospitals. Additionally, it is an important instructional tool. The computer offers a variety of approaches to instruction that are appealing and helpful to a diverse student population. Classroom teaching is augmented by computer-assisted instruction in the form of interactive and linear video programs, client simulations, drill and practice routines, problem-solving programs, and tutorials, to name a few examples. Faculty also use computers for word processing, literature review, and the development and scoring of tests. Some faculty use computers in the classroom to enhance their lectures and discussions through PowerPoint presentations, response "clickers," and other computer technologies. E-mail and the Internet are also a part of most teaching environments. Some instructional programs are delivered to sites far from the main campus through distance learning modalities using computer technology. At the end of their program of study, all students demonstrate their ability to practice safely on computerized licensing examinations in the form of computerized adaptive testing. In the nursing skills laboratory, mannequins that can blink their eyes, have dilating pupils, breathe, and have a heartbeat and a pulse assist students in the process of learning about heart attacks, diabetic shock, and other emergencies.

Computer literacy among students and faculty is no longer an issue—they possess computer skills. Nursing educators express concern about the initial cost of the equipment and programs needed for this instruction, as well as the increasing cost of keeping both equipment and programs current. For example, the mannequin mentioned above carries a price tag of $215,000. At a time when the budgets of educational institutions are experiencing severe cuts, people responsible for purchasing supplies and equipment increasingly must find creative ways to acquire needed items. Another challenge to faculty is finding time to evaluate the existing software and integrate it into the approved curriculum.

Increasing Community-Based Practice Experiences

Another significant change in nursing practice is the trend toward community-based practice. Most nursing programs, especially hospital-based and associate degree programs, have a history of being strongly oriented toward the hospital as the primary clinical teaching environment. *Community*, as the term was used in nursing education, was associated with public health nursing and was to be found in baccalaureate education only.

Earlier hospital discharge to the home and an increasing emphasis on prevention have created new demands on nursing. Nurses are expected to provide care in clients' homes, the workplace, schools, nursing homes, community health agencies, clinics, shelters, and community gathering places. As the arena in which nursing is practiced begins to shift, nursing educators are challenged to define what part of the nursing curriculum should be taught in a community setting. Often, this requires different clinical teaching strategies and approaches. Some faculty, reticent to shorten any time in acute care facilities, are uncertain how a community experience should be provided and evaluated and about the legal ramifications associated with having students in many different environments and in less controlled situations. Tremendous strides have been taken in developing innovative approaches to community-based nursing; more will follow.

Increasing Emphasis on Research

As the nursing profession continues to grow, one of the areas receiving more emphasis is nursing research. It is difficult to open any nursing journal today without learning more about EBP and nursing decisions (see the following).

Other research, that of nursing **Theorist**, received much attention in the 1980s until the beginning of the 21st century when attention was diverted to EBP. Many curricular patterns responded to the work of nursing theorists. Most approval bodies, state and national, stipulate that a nursing program must have a coherent organizing or conceptual framework around which the program of learning is developed. Some programs have chosen to select the approach of a particular nursing theorist and structure the program of learning around that theorist's work. The program in which you are enrolled may reflect this trend. Perhaps, one of the hospitals to which you are assigned for clinical experience also uses the principles of a nursing theory to structure the delivery of care, although this is less common than using a theory in curriculum development.

A **Theory** is a "scientifically acceptable general principle which governs practice or is proposed to explain observed facts" (Riehl & Roy, 1974, p. 3). Because nursing as a developing profession is seriously involved in research, theories are valuable to use in building a sound body of nursing knowledge. They provide the bases for hypotheses about nursing practice. They make it possible for us to derive a sound rationale for the actions we take. If the theories are testable, they allow us to build our knowledge base and to guide and improve nursing practice.

Today, there are many published nursing theories. In an attempt to structure and organize those theories, various authors have categorized or classified them. Not all are classified similarly. Included are general classifications such as the art and science of humanistic nursing, interpersonal relationships, systems, and energy fields. Other categories include growth and development theories, systems theories, stress adaptation theories, and rhythm theories.

Examples of growth and development theories with which you are probably familiar are those of Maslow, Erikson, Kohlberg, Piaget, and Freud discussed in most basic nursing texts. The theories are so named because they focus on the developing person and arrange this development in stages through which a person must pass to reach a particular level of development. They allow nurses to monitor progress through the stages and evaluate the appropriateness of that progress. These theories are not truly theories of nursing, however, because they were not developed for the purpose of explaining, testing, and changing the practice of nursing. They represent some of the borrowed knowledge around which we build our profession.

Most nursing theories are developed around a combination of concepts. Among these concepts, four approaches usually include those directed to the human person, health and illness, the environment (or society), and nursing.

Nursing theories usually are classified according to the structure or approach around which they are developed. Theories that speak to the art and science of humanistic nursing were among the earliest pure nursing theories developed. Some authors have looked back at the contributions of Florence Nightingale and have included her work in that grouping. Among others are Virginia Henderson and her *Definition of Nursing*, Faye Abdellah and the *Twenty-One Nursing Problems* (which is often cited as one of the early attempts at classification of nursing behaviors), Lydia Hall and her *Core, Care, and Cure* model, and Madeleine Leininger's *Transcultural Care Theory*.

Interpersonal process theories deal with interactions between and among people. Many of these theories were developed during the 1960s. Included in this grouping could be Hildegard Peplau's *Psychodynamic Nursing*, Joyce Travelbee's *Human to Human Relationship*, Ernestine Wiedenbach's *The Helping Art of Clinical Nursing*, and Imogene King's *Dynamic Interacting Systems* model, although the last also could be classified as a systems theory.

Systems theories are so named because they are concerned with the interactions between and among all the factors in a situation. A system usually is viewed as complex and in a state of constant change. It is defined as a whole with interrelated parts and may be a subsystem of a larger system as well as a suprasystem. For example, a person may be viewed as a system composed of cells, tissue, and organs. The person is a subsystem of a family, which in turn is a subsystem of a community. In a systems approach, the person usually is considered as a "total" being, or from a "whole" being viewpoint. Systems theories also provide for input into the system and feedback within the system. The systems approach became popular during the 1970s. Included in this group of theorists are Dorothy Johnson, Sister Callista Roy, and Betty Neuman.

Stress adaptation models are based on concepts that view the person as adjusting or changing (adapting) to avoid situations (stressors) that would result in the disturbance of balance or equilibrium. The adaptation theory helps to explain how balance is maintained and therefore directs nursing actions. One often finds Sister Callista Roy's adaptation model and Betty Neuman's work included in this group, but both also may be considered systems models, as mentioned above.

One of the most recent classifications of theories is by energy fields. These theories, although developed earlier, received growing recognition during the 1980s. Included in this group are the works of Myra Levine, Joyce Fitzpatrick, Margaret Newman, and Martha Rogers.

Humanistic models are also fairly recent. These focus on man's humanness and needs for love, caring, personal meaning, and living in concert with the environment. Theorists noted for developing these theories include Jean Watson, Rosemarie Rizzo Parse, and Margaret Newman.

It is not our purpose to discuss and critique the many approaches to nursing theory. The student who wants to pursue nursing theorists further is encouraged to consult the section on further reading at the end of the chapter or visit enursescribe.com and click on research and theory. Table 2.2 outlines the approaches of several recognized nursing theorists.

Table 2.2   Nursing Theories and Theorists

Theorist	Theory or Model
Lydia Hall	Viewed illness and rehabilitation as learning experiences in which the nurse's role was to guide and teach the client through personal caregiving. Role involves therapeutic use of self (core), the treatment regimen of the healthcare team (cure), and nurturing and intimate bodily care (care).
Dorothy Johnson	A behavioral systems approach that focuses on health viewed as a state of equilibrium that the nurse assists in maintaining or balancing.
Imogene King	A model in which three open systems interact with the environment: personal, individual, and social. Nurse's role is to assist individual to perform daily activities and includes health promotion and maintenance. Involves goal attainment.
Madeleine Leininger	Focused on a caring model that must be practiced interpersonally. Emphasized a transcultural approach.
Myra Levine	Developed around the four concepts of conservation of energy, structural integrity, personal integrity, and social integrity. Supports a holistic approach to nursing based on recognition of the total response of the person to the interaction between the internal and the external environment.
Betty Neuman	A systems model influenced by Gestalt theory, stress, and level of prevention. Employs lines of resistance and lines of defense in creating a healthy being. Nurses are to identify the stressors and assist the individual to respond. Involves primary, secondary, and tertiary prevention.
Dorothea Orem	Recognized as a self-care theory of nursing, supports the concept that each person has a need for the provision and management of self-care actions to achieve "constancy." When the individual is unable to provide these, a self-care deficit exists. The role of the nursing system is to help eliminate the self-care deficit through wholly compensatory, partially compensatory, or supportive–educative actions.
Martha Rogers	Includes complicated approaches to health that involve helicy, resonancy, and complementarity. The holistic individual moves through time and space as part of an expanding universe with potential states of maximum well-being. Nurses act to promote symphonic interaction between man and environment by repatterning the human and environmental fields.
Sister Callista Roy	Identified as an adaptation model that conceives of the individual as being in constant interaction with a changing environment, thus requiring adaptation. Four adaptive modes, or ways in which a person adapts, are identified through (1) physiologic needs, (2) self-concept, (3) role function, and (4) interdependence relations. The nurse's role is to assess a client's adaptive behaviors and the stimuli that may be affecting the person to manipulate the stimuli in such a way as to allow the client to cope or adapt.

> **Critical Thinking Activity: Nursing Theorists**
> Select one nursing theorist. Describe what you find interesting and attractive about that person's nursing theory. Give a rationale for your decision, and describe how using that theory might affect your practice of nursing.

Education That Supports Evidence-Based Practice

The term *evidence-based practice* has a variety of definitions and interpretations. Evolving from evidence-based medicine, it generally refers to the integration of the best evidence available into expert nursing care. It requires that nurses and other healthcare providers have access to the latest research, expert opinion, and understandings of cultural and personal values as a basis for planning and delivering nursing care. EBP is discussed in detail in Chapter 15.

Stegen & Sowerby Stories: Part 2

T ymeshia did not drop out and is now at the end of the first semester of her program. She is getting As and Bs in her classes and is feeling better about her study skills. Tymeshia reduced her work hours and went to a 30-hour per week schedule, instead of 40 hours per week. This gave her the extra study time she needed. Tymeshia is now considering getting married during the next semester and trying to buy a house. As a classmate, what would you advise Tymeshia to consider? Will these choices be compatible with nursing school? How do you set priorities to help you achieve your goals? Read the rest of the story at www.thePoint.com.

Want to Know More?

A variety of resources are available on thePoint® to enhance your learning and understanding of this chapter, such as:

- Full Stegen & Sowerby Stories
- NCLEX-Style Student Review Questions
- Journal Articles
- Case Studies
- Learning Objectives
- Relevant Websites
- And more

KEY CONCEPTS

- Educational programs prepare nursing assistants and LPNs for roles in the healthcare delivery system. As these programs have grown, greater oversight of the programs by approval bodies has occurred. The education of UAP can vary tremendously.

- Three major avenues to preparation for licensure as a registered nurse exist in the United States: the hospital-based diploma, the college-based baccalaureate degree, and the associate degree (usually offered in community colleges). Many similarities exist among these programs. In addition, various nontraditional approaches to nursing education have evolved.
- The nursing shortage of the late 1980s and 1990s, coupled with recommendations or mandates from important groups, has resulted in greater creativity and collaboration in educational approaches. Articulated programs exist in most states created through the pressure of legislation or agreement between schools.
- Master's and doctoral programs that prepare nurses for leadership positions in the profession continue to grow, with more emphasis on the master's degree for advanced practice. The actual degree awarded at the end of doctoral studies varies. A variety of new educational approaches to higher degrees in nursing have evolved.
- One of the most rapidly growing areas is that of advanced practice; this growth was accelerated by healthcare reform. Recommendations from major commissions have urged continued expansion of advanced practice programs and the educational qualifications for such positions.
- Continuing education, whether further education that results in a higher degree or rather in the form of classes, seminars, or workshops that update and increase expertise, is being encouraged by more and more organizations. Staying current in practice is critical to safe client care.
- Nursing education has been influenced by the ANA position on nursing education that advocated the baccalaureate degree as the minimum educational preparation for professional practice. Many nursing educators, particularly those in diploma and associate degree programs, disagreed with this position. This issue may take on new life in the 21st century.
- Many changes are occurring in nursing education. These include more emphasis on articulation and career ladder programs and a shift in educational settings from acute care facilities to community-based experiences.
- No change has affected nursing education as greatly as has the computer age. Entire programs can be completed online. Computer technology has changed the structure of the typical nursing classroom, and instructors prepare graduates who will be able to function in a healthcare environment that makes heavy use of computerized services.
- Nursing theories continue to influence nursing and nursing education. Nursing theories assist us in building a body of nursing knowledge and describing and defining nursing practice.
- The advent of EBP is impacting the curricula of nursing education programs.

NCLEX-STYLE PRACTICE QUESTIONS

1. Which of the following roles is considered an unlicensed assistive personnel?

   A. LPN
   B. RN
   C. CRNA
   D. CNA

2. What is the purpose of continuing education? (select all that apply)
   A. Required for licensure
   B. Promote skill development
   C. Provide networking opportunities
   D. Learn improved practices

3. Why do schools seek accreditation? (select all that apply)
   A. Ensure a minimum level of quality
   B. Allow students' access to federal aide
   C. Promote continuous quality improvement
   D. Ensure students pass NCLEX exam

4. What order would the following stackable credentials be attained in practice?
   A. RN-BSN ____3____
   B. LPN ____1____
   C. ADN ____2____
   D. CRNA ____4____

5. If the position paper from the ANA in 1965 had been adopted, which of the following would be true? (select all that apply)
   A. Nursing assistants would have on-the-job training only.
   B. LPNs would have an associate degree to start.
   C. All RNs would have a minimum of a bachelor degree.
   D. Diploma nurses would have a special status.

REFERENCES

American Association of Colleges of Nursing. (2008). *The essentials of baccalaureate nursing education for professional nursing practice*. Washington, DC: Author.

American Association of Colleges of Nursing. (2014). *Accelerated nursing programs*. Retrieved June 21, 2017, from http://www.aacn.nche.edu/students/accelerated-nursing-programs

American Association of Colleges of Nursing. (2016). *Why hire a certified Clinical Nurse Leader? The CNL bulletin*. Retrieved from http://www.aacn.nche.edu/leading-initiatives/cnl/cnl-certification/pdf/15Fall-Winter-CNL-Bulletin.pdf

American Association of Colleges of Nursing. (2017). *The Doctor of Nursing Practice (DNP)*. Retrieved June 21, 2017, http://www.aacn.nche.edu/media-relations/fact-sheets/dnp

American Nurses Association. (1965). American Nurses Association's first position on education for nursing. *American Journal of Nursing, 65*(12), 106–107.

American Nurses Association. (1974). *Standards for continuing education for nursing*. Kansas City, MO: American Nurses Association.

American Nurses Association. (2000). *ANA reaffirms commitment to BSN for entry into practice-supports new certification program to be offered by ANCC*. Retrieved December 7, 2010, from http://www.nursing-world.org/FunctionalMenuCategories/MediaResources/PressReleases/2000/CommitmenttoBSN.aspx

Brown, E. L. (1948). *Nursing for the future*. New York, NY: Russell Sage Foundation.

Clarke, S. P. (2017). The BSN entry into practice debate. *Nursing Made Incredibly Easy! 15*(1), 6–8. Retrieved from https://doi:10.1097/01.NME.0000508544.59940.19

de Tornyay, R. (1996). Critical challenges for nurse educators. *Journal of Nursing Education, 35*(4), 146–147.

Giordano, B. P. (1996). Pew Heath Professions Commission task force releases policy considerations for reforming health care workforce regulation. *AORN Journal, 63*(2), 343–348. Retrieved from https://doi.org/10.1016/S0001-2092(06)63218-3

Henry J. Kaiser Family Foundation. (2016). *Total number of professionally active nurses.* State Health Facts. Retrieved March 28, 2017, from http://kff.org/other/state-indicator/total-registered-nurses/?currentTimeframe=0&sortModel=%7B%22colId%22:%22Location%22,%22sort%22:%22asc%22%7D

Institute of Medicine-IOM. (2011). *The future of nursing: Focus on education.* Health and Medicine Division. http://www.nationalacademies.org/hmd/Reports/2010/The-Future-of-Nursing-Leading-Change-Advancing-Health/Report-Brief-Education.aspx

Kalisch, P. A., & Kalisch, B. J. (2004). *American nursing: A history* (4th ed.). Philadelphia, PA: Lippincott Williams & Wilkins.

National League for Nursing. (2014a). Proportion of Basic RN Programs, 2014. Annual Survey of Schools of Nursing, Academic Year 2013-2014. http://nln.matrixdev.net/docs/default-source/newsroom/nursing-education-statistics/proportion-of-basic-rn-programs-2014-(pdf).pdf?sfvrsn=0

National League for Nursing. (2014b). *Number of basic RN programs, total and by program type: 2005-2014.* Nursing Education Statistics. http://nln.matrixdev.net/docs/default-source/newsroom/nursing-education-statistics/number-of-basic-rn-programs-total-and-by-program-type-2005-to-2014.pdf?sfvrsn=0

Petiprin, A. (2016). Isabel Hampton Robb. *Nursing Theory.* Retrieved from www.nursing-theory.org

Riehl, J. P., & Roy, S. C. (1974). *Conceptual models for nursing practice.* New York, NY: Appleton-Century-Crofts.

Seymer, L. R. (1954). *Selected writings of Florence Nightingale.* New York, NY: Macmillan.

U.S. Public Health Service. (1963). *Toward quality in nursing: Needs and goals. Report of the Surgeon Generals' Consultant Group on Nursing.* Washington, DC: U.S. Government Printing Office.

CHAPTER 3

Credentials for Healthcare Providers

LEARNING OUTCOMES

After completing this chapter, you should be able to:

1. Define and discuss the concept of credentialing for healthcare professionals.
2. Describe how each of the following types of credentials differs: diploma, certificate, certification, and license.
3. Outline the purposes of accreditation and the general process for seeking accreditation.
4. Identify and analyze the major elements addressed by nursing practice acts.
5. Outline the role of the state boards of nursing or other state regulatory authority.
6. Differentiate between licensure by examination, licensure by endorsement, and mutual recognition of licensure.
7. Discuss personal strategies to avoid violating the provisions of the nursing practice acts and encountering the disciplinary process.
8. Discuss issues in licensure, including ensuring continued competence, multistate licensure, and licensure for graduates of foreign nursing schools.
9. Explain the various uses of certification in nursing.
10. Discuss current trends in credentialing within the healthcare workforce.

KEY TERMS

Accreditation
Administrative law
Advanced practice registered nurse
   (APRN)
Certification
Computerized adaptive testing
   (CAT)
Credentials
Disciplinary action
Enacted (statutory) law
Grandfathering
Home state
Injunctive relief

Licensure by endorsement
Licensure by examination
Mandatory licensure
Mutual recognition of licensure
NCLEX-PN
NCLEX-RN
Nurse Practice Act
Party states
Remote state
Revocation
Rules and regulations
State board of nursing
Telenursing

Stegen & Sowerby Stories: Part 1

A fter working as a CNA in a long-term care center for 2 years, Stephanie was finally finished with nursing school and waiting to take her state board exam. She spoke with the Human Resources Department to see if it would be possible for her to complete the orientation process while she waited to take her exam. The facility was eager to have Stephanie continue as a staff nurse and agreed to the early orientation. Stephanie supposed that she would be working with a licensed nurse as she had while she was in nursing school.

Stephanie attended orientation with other new graduates where she received her name badge identifying her as a nurse and she completed paperwork to have access to pharmacy medications. The facility director gave them a tour of all the areas of the facility and introduced them as new graduate nurses. After a one-week orientation, Stephanie arrived to work where she was assigned to do blood glucose finger sticks, something she had done as a CNA. She was also taught how to do medications, how to avoid medication errors, charting, treatments, and narcotic counts. She had completed these tasks in a previous job at an assisted living facility so she felt comfortable doing them.

1. What problems can you identify in the scenario?
2. Who is responsible for the problems you identified?
3. What are the advantages and disadvantages of early orientation?
4. Which activities were okay for Stephanie to perform and which were not?
5. What action do you think the employer should take?
6. What else may happen?

Credentials provide information regarding qualifications and whether standards have been met. Credentials for organizations or institutions are awarded by bodies (either professional or governmental) that set standards for specific type of organizations (such as hospital or nursing homes). Approval or accreditation from one of these bodies demonstrates to the public that the healthcare organization adheres to accepted standards. Credentials for individuals communicate to others the nature of the person's competence and provide evidence of preparation to perform in a specific capacity. Credentials for individuals include certificates, degrees, and diplomas awarded by educational institutions; legal licenses awarded by a government body; and recognition by a professional organization usually termed **certification**. Those who are engaged in careers in health occupations want to be assured that the standards of practice in their discipline and in healthcare organizations remain high to ensure competence and to protect the public. All these types of credentials are discussed in the following.

APPROVAL AND ACCREDITATION OF INSTITUTIONS AND PROGRAMS

Institutions are approved by government bodies to operate within their state borders. States have varying standards and processes for approval of educational institutions such as technical institutes, colleges, and universities. The approval of most educational institutions is carried out by a state board of education or similar educational authority. States also have approval processes for programs that provide education for licensed health professions. These are most commonly carried out by professional boards.

Accreditation of Educational Institutions

Accreditation is review of the quality of higher education institutions and programs. In the United States, accreditation is a major way that students, families, government officials, and the press know that an institution or program provides a quality education (Council for Higher Education Accreditation [CHEA], 2016). Educational institutions and programs may voluntarily seek this type of accreditation for both their general education and specialized programs.

Organizations that have the authority to offer this type of national or regional accreditation of educational institutions must be approved by the Council for Higher Education Accreditation or the U.S. Department of Education. Some accreditations recognize the entire educational institution, such as the accreditation offered by regional bodies for colleges and universities. In many instances, academic credits, degrees, and certificates are accepted by the public, employers, or other educational institutions only if offered by an accredited educational institution. Although a nonaccredited institution might award a degree, there is no guarantee that the school meets educational standards; therefore, the degree might not be accepted as an adequate evidence of qualifications. Similarly, only course work completed at an accredited institution may be accepted for transfer to another accredited institution. You may have experienced the need for this type of accreditation if you transferred academic credits from one college to another. Accreditation is also necessary for the institution and its students to have access to federal funds (CHEA, 2016). Some academic accreditation is specialized, applying only to a particular program in an institution. Specialized accreditation is voluntary and requires that the specific program meets professional standards for excellence established by a specialized accrediting agency. An educational institution might have general accreditation for its degrees but still not have specialized accreditation. Certain educational organizations are not degree-granting institutions and therefore are not eligible for general accreditation, but they are still eligible for specialized accreditation. This is true of hospital-based diploma schools of nursing.

Government Approval of Nursing Programs

For its graduates to be eligible to take the National Council Licensure Examination (NCLEX) in any state, a nursing program should be approved by a state board of nursing or another designated state government department. In most states, this is called approval, but in a few states, it is called accreditation (a term most commonly associated with a voluntary process described above).

Through the American Nurses Association (ANA), the Council of State Boards of Nursing was created to have a common forum for state boards of nursing. In 1978, the National Council of State Boards of Nursing, Inc. (NCSBN) was formed to replace the ANA Council. NCSBN provides the mechanism for state boards of nursing to collaborate in terms of licensing examinations and other issues of importance to the regulation of nursing practice.

When a new nursing program is to be initiated, it must provide preliminary information to the appropriate state government department while in the planning phase. The nursing program must be approved prior to admitting students to assure prospective students that they will be eligible to become licensed upon graduation. Each state also has a designated time frame to renew its approval of existing nursing programs. This often involves a comprehensive evaluation study, done by the program/school and submitted to the state. Representatives of the state approval authority may visit the program. In some jurisdictions, a school that has received specialized accreditation is exempted from an additional review.

Accreditation of Nursing Education Programs

The specialized accreditation of nursing education programs arose from concerns about the quality of nursing education among nurses. Accreditation helps to strengthen uniform national standards for nursing education. Some employers and educational institutions offering additional education require graduation from a nursing program that has specialized accreditation. In 1893, the American Society of Superintendents of Training Schools for Nurses was established to develop and maintain a universal standard for nursing education. It was renamed the National League for Nursing Education in 1912, and in 1917, it released the first Standard Curriculum for Schools of Nursing. Throughout the first half of the 20th century, the National League for Nursing Education continued to provide guidance for quality in nursing education. In 1952, seven organizations combined into one and became the National League for Nursing (NLN), which assumed responsibility for accrediting nursing education programs. In 1997, in response to the Department of Education's expectations for greater separation of the membership organization (NLN) and the accrediting process, the NLN formed the NLNAC as an independent subsidiary to provide accreditation of nursing programs. Further separation came in 2010 when NLNAC became Accreditation Commission for Education in Nursing (ACEN). ACEN accredits nursing programs at all levels: practical nursing, hospital diploma nursing education, associate degree nursing education, and baccalaureate and higher-degree education programs.

In 1999, the Council on Collegiate Nursing Education (CCNE), a subsidiary of the American Association of Colleges of Nursing, began offering accreditation for baccalaureate and higher-degree nursing programs only. Advanced practice nursing organizations such as the American Association of Nurse Anesthetists provide specialized accreditation for institutions offering advanced practice/nurse practitioner programs (Evidence-Based Practice 3.1).

Evidence-Based Practice 3.1: *Preparing for Accreditation*

Hanna, K., Duvall, J., Turpin, R. L., Pendleton-Romig, K., & Parker, S. (2016). Mastering the journey to continuous compliance: Process improvements for excelling at CCNE accreditation. *SAGE Open*, 6(2). doi:10.1177/2158244016656231

There are many steps in the process of preparing for accreditation. The process requires many hours of data gathering, research, and writing and is often completed by administrators and senior faculty as part of their workload. Accreditation through CCNE is awarded for 10 years with a Continuous Improvement Progress Report (CIPR) due at the 5-year mark.

The authors of this paper were involved in preparation of the 5-year CIPR and the institution developed an effective method of completing this report. The nursing program formed a committee comprised of four full-time faculty members and staff support person. They located a computer software system to assist with managing data and report/review capabilities. With these tools, they were able to more easily gather and maintain the data needed to complete the required reports for CCNE.

The authors reported these findings. By centralizing the data, the required reports were more easily completed. Having a committee helped to distribute the workload at a manageable level. By instituting policies and procedures that would continually gather and maintain data, the nursing program was able to complete the required reporting and was ready for their accreditation visit.

Communication in Action 3.1: *Speaking With an Evaluator of an ADN Program*

Jerry Wilson was a student in an associate degree nursing program. His program was being evaluated for reaccreditation, and an evaluator visited his clinical site. As part of the process, the evaluator interviewed Jerry. The evaluator said, "Please tell me about your objectives for today's clinical experience." Jerry was nervous but pleased to be able to be prepared to respond. "I am working on my neurological assessment skills today," he said. "Although I have performed them in the lab, this is my first opportunity to use those skills with a client and to interpret their meaning in a real-life situation. This assignment is also giving me an opportunity to increase my abilities to communicate with family members as well as the client, because a family member is always with the client." The evaluator then asked, "Would you give me some feedback on the adequacy of this clinical site in providing opportunities for the learning that you need?" Jerry responded, "This unit has provided an exceptionally good learning environment. The nurses are very helpful and supportive. They go out of their way to help us find good learning experiences. I am always able to find clients that will help me meet the course objectives." Jerry's communication was clear, direct, and provided important information to the evaluators.

If Jerry had been less prepared, when the evaluator asked about his goals he might have answered, "I don't really have any goals, just to make it through the day." Another example of a poor response to the question about the adequacy of the clinical site would be, "Well, it is okay and some of the nurses are nice." These responses do not provide the evaluators with any concrete examples of the adequacy of the site or the experience.

Voluntary accreditation is based on a systematic self-study and evaluation by the nursing program itself that focuses on the standards and criteria for accreditation. Peer evaluators from the accrediting organization visit the nursing program; review the self-study; meet with faculty, students, and other interested parties; and provide an independent evaluation. After the site visit, the report and recommendations of the visiting evaluators, along with the self-study document, are submitted to a panel in the organization composed of peer educators. A nursing program may be granted accreditation, granted accreditation with conditions that must be remedied, placed on a warning status for being deficient, or denied accreditation. A program that is accredited meets the national standards of the organization for quality in nursing education. Accreditation exists for limited period of time and must then be renewed.

Accreditation of Continuing Education Programs

The American Nurses Credentialing Center, which is best known for providing certification for individual nursing specialties (discussed later in this chapter), also provides an accreditation mechanism for institutions or organizations that want to be approvers or providers of nursing continuing education programs. State nurses associations and specialty organizations often seek accreditation as *approvers of programs*. These organizations then approve specific continuing education offerings as meeting appropriate standards for content and process. Accreditation as a *provider of a program* assures the nurse consumer that the specific continuing education offering meets appropriate standards.

Many of the states that require continuing education for renewing a nursing license require approval or accreditation by an official group. This ensures that the continuing education is of high quality and will be meaningful for a nurse. Some states operate their own approval systems. When evaluating continuing nursing education offerings, it is important to know whether that class, workshop, or course has been approved and by whom.

CREDENTIALS FOR INDIVIDUALS

Individuals may hold multiple types of credentials. As people progress in their careers, they are likely to attain additional credentials.

Diplomas, Degrees, and Certificates of Completion

A school or business offering instruction awards a diploma or certificate to those who complete a designated program of study. Licensed practical nursing (LPN) programs offer a certificate of completion. Hospital-based programs preparing registered nurses (RNs) offer a diploma. College-based nursing programs offer academic degrees, such as the associate, baccalaureate, or master's degree, which require the fulfillment of certain general education courses and course work specific to a particular career, such as nursing. The value of a diploma or educational certificate or degree is related to the quality of the educational institution or program, as well as to the actual title of the certificate or degree. So, when deciding which institution to attend, check on both the approval of the institution and the specific accreditation of the program.

Licensure

A license is a legal credential, awarded to an individual, to practice a given profession. Most states require licensing only of those who have more direct contact with clients. Physicians, dentists, pharmacists, and nurses are licensed in all states. The licensing of other healthcare workers varies. An individual state or province determines eligibility for licensure and the type of testing required for that profession within that state. Each state develops and enforces its own practice act, which includes the scope of practice for the profession the license represents. We will discuss the nursing practice act later in this chapter.

Certification

For some groups, a standard credential is available in the form of certification provided by a nongovernmental authority, usually a professional organization. Workers with this credential are referred to as *certified* or *registered*. This type of credential should not be confused with a legal license or a simple certificate of completion (nursing is an anomaly in that the term "registered nurse" was adopted early in this century and refers to legal licensure). Certification usually is granted on completion of an education program and the passing of a standardized examination. The program usually has been approved by the professional organization and the organization that administers the examination. Certification does not include a legal scope of practice. Scope of practice will be discussed later in this chapter.

While some professional organizations conduct their own certification, in most instances they have established an independent national affiliated organization whose sole purpose is credentialing. By having an independent organization that focuses all of its efforts on certification, they better ensure objectivity and enhance the confidence of others in the process.

One of the concerns regarding certification is the potential for confusion that exists because regulatory agencies (such as state boards of nursing) and professional associations may use the term *certification* differently and in different contexts. In nursing, certification is used for identifying licensed RNs who have specialized or advanced competence in a specific area of nursing. Certification in nursing will be discussed after the information on basic licensure.

> ### Critical Thinking Activity: Credentials
> Choose an allied health occupation found in a healthcare facility in which you have clinical practice. Investigate the credentials needed for that occupation and how they would be obtained in your state. Analyze a way in which you could work collaboratively with an individual in this health occupation.

NURSING LICENSURE IN THE UNITED STATES

Legal licensure provides a standard mechanism for judging competence and therefore protects the safety of the public **(Fig. 3.1)**. Through the efforts of nurses working collectively, a licensure process was developed and state agencies were established to regulate the practice of nursing.

The History of Licensure in Nursing

Recognizable credentials were not always available for nurses. After schools of nursing became common, a rudimentary means of identifying the qualifications of a caregiver was the certificate of completion issued by the nursing school. This was the first true nursing credential.

Figure 3.1. Licensure: protecting the public from unsafe practices.

However, because the quality of education offered in the nursing schools varied greatly—programs varied in length from 6 weeks to 3 years—it became apparent that a completion certificate was not an adequate guarantee of competence.

The Nurses' Associated Alumnae of the United States and Canada was created in 1896. This organization later evolved into the ANA. One of the major concerns of the association was the establishment of legal licensure for nurses. The ANA campaigned vigorously for the adoption of state licensing laws. Nurses, legislators, and the public had to be educated about the value of licensure for the profession and encouraged to support it. The set of laws regulating the practice of nursing is termed the **Nurse Practice Act**.

The early laws provided for permissive licensure. Permissive licensure is a voluntary system whereby an individual could choose to become licensed to provide evidence of competence, but a license was not required to practice. The requirements for permissive licensure included graduating from a school that satisfied certain standards established in the practice act for that state and passing a comprehensive examination. Only those who had met these standards could use the title RN; others used the title "nurse." Under this system, no one was required to have a license to practice nursing, and variability in standards from one state to another continued.

After permissive licensure laws came into being, nurses' activity regarding licensure became less intense because most individuals graduating from nursing schools sought and received licenses to practice. However, there was still concern that some individuals were practicing nursing without having demonstrated skill and knowledge. The majority of those functioning without licenses were nursing school graduates who had failed the licensing examinations; they were referred to as graduate nurses, rather than RNs. Other nurses who practiced without licenses included individuals who had been educated as nurses in other countries.

To end this situation and provide greater protection to the public, many nurses began to call for **mandatory licensure**. Mandatory nursing licensure requires that all persons who wish to practice nursing meet the established standards for education, pass standardized examinations, and secure a license to practice in the state, province, or territory in which they wish to work.

The first mandatory licensure law took effect in New York in 1947. Today, mandatory licensure is the standard in the United States, Canada, and most other countries. Therefore, if you wish to work as a nurse in any state, territory, province, or other country, you must obtain a license that is valid in that jurisdiction before you begin working (Box 3.1).

Although the terms RN and LPN (or licensed vocational nurse [LVN], as used in Texas and California) were protected in law, the more general term *nurse* has not been protected traditionally. Many individuals describe themselves as nurses, when their roles in healthcare are assistive. Their employers also may refer to them as nurses to support those individuals' status. Thirty-nine states have made *nurse* a protected term. In these states, only RNs or LPNs may use the title nurse. Others, such as certified nurses' aides/assistants and medical assistants, may use only their specific title.

Current Nursing Licensure Laws

"The purpose of a professional license is to protect the public from harm by setting minimal qualifications and competencies for safe entry-level practitioners. Nursing is regulated

---

BOX 3.1 THE HISTORY OF NURSING LICENSURE

1867	Dr. Henry Wentworth Acland first suggested licensure for nurses in England.
1892	American Society of Superintendents of Training Schools for Nurses organized and supported licensure in the United States.
1901	First nursing licensure in the world: New Zealand.
1903	First nursing licensure in the United States: North Carolina, New Jersey, New York, and Virginia (in that order).
1915	ANA drafted its first model nurse practice act.
1919	First nursing licensure in England.
1923	All 48 states had **enacted (statutory)** nursing licensure **laws**.
1935	First mandatory licensure act in the United States: New York (effective 1947).
1946	Ten states had definitions of nursing in the licensing act.
1950	First year the same examination used in all jurisdictions of the United States and its territories: State Board Test Pool Examination.
1965	Twenty-one states had definitions of nursing in the licensing act.
1971	First state to recognize expanded practice in the nursing practice act: Idaho.
1976	First mandatory continuing education for relicensure: California.
1982	Change to nursing process format examination: National Council Licensure Examination for Registered Nurses (NCLEX-RN).
1986	Only state to require baccalaureate degree for initial RN licensure and associate degree for licensed practical nurse licensure: North Dakota (effective 1987 and rescinded in 2003).
1994	Computer-adapted testing initiated nationwide.
1998	Mutual Recognition Nurse Licensure Compact finalized. Utah is the first state to become part of the Compact.
2008	Consensus reached on a model for Advanced Practice RN education and practice.

---

because it is one of the health professions that poses a risk of harm to the public if practiced by someone who is unprepared and/or incompetent" (NCSBN, 2011). The authority for establishing a licensure law lies with the legislature of each jurisdiction. The government agency that has the legal authority to regulate nursing is usually named the board of nursing (although some states use different titles). This body establishes the administrative rules and regulations regarding practice and enforces the provisions of the statute as well as the rules and regulations.

A proposed change in the law enters the legislative process through an elected member of the legislature who has been persuaded that the change is in the best interest of the public. That individual introduces a bill (see thePoint for an overview of how a bill becomes a law). A group, such as the nurses association, wishing to instigate this action may spend months preparing and planning the content for a bill and gaining the support of legislators who might introduce the legislation. With over 4 million professionally active nurses in the United States, nurses, as a group, have to potential to influence the decisions made regarding healthcare.

Rules and Regulations

Each state has its own set of administrative **rules and regulations** to carry out the provisions of laws regulating nursing. These rules are considered **administrative law**. Most states require that public hearings be held regarding proposed rules and regulations, but the board has the authority to make the final decision. The rules and regulations that are accepted by the appropriate board have the force of law unless they are challenged in court and are found not to be in accord with the legislature's intent.

In some states, the Nurse Practice Act is detailed and specifies most of the critical provisions regarding licensure and practice. In other states, the practice act is broad, and the administrative body is given a great deal of power to make decisions through rules and regulations. Both the Nurse Practice Act and state rules and regulations govern nursing in every state.

Nursing Licensure Law Content

In the early 1900s, the ANA, assuming its leadership role in nursing licensure, formulated a model nurse practice act to be used by state associations when planning legislation. The last ANA revision of this model was in 1990 by the ANA Congress for Nursing Practice (ANA, 1990). When the responsibility for overseeing the licensure process shifted to the NCSBN, that group also developed a model nursing practice act. In addition, it wrote the model nursing administrative rules. The NCSBN updated its entire model act and model rules and regulations in 2014 (NCSBN, 2014). Carefully read the Nurse Practice Act for the state in which you will practice. A copy of the Act may be obtained from the state board of nursing (check the NCSBN website, www.ncsbn.org). Many states make these documents available online. In some states, one act includes both practical nursing and registered nursing; other states have separate, but similar, acts. Historically, the role of the nursing assistant was not outlined in nursing laws. As federal legislation mandating classes and certification for nursing assistants in long-term care took effect, some states modified laws and rules and regulations to address the role of the nursing assistant. In other states, regulations governing nursing assistants rest within a different department of the state government.

The following general topics (purpose, definitions and scope of practice, qualifications, titling, license renewal and continuing competence requirements, nursing education programs, grounds for disciplinary action, exceptions, administrative provisions, and grandfathering) usually are covered in state licensure laws for nursing.

Purpose

The purpose of regulating the practice of nursing is twofold: Regulations protect the public and make individual practitioners accountable for their actions. Note that the protection of the status of the licensed individual is not the reason for licensure. With this in mind, you can better understand the inclusion of some other topics in the act.

Definitions and Scope of Practice

All of the significant terms in the act are defined for the purpose of carrying out the law. This is where the legal definition of nursing and the scope of practice are spelled out. The NCSBN has given the following definition:

> Nursing is a scientific process founded on a professional body of knowledge; it is a learned profession based on an understanding of the human condition across the lifespan and the relationship of a client with others and within the environment; and it is an art dedicated to caring for others. The practice of nursing means assisting clients to attain or maintain optimal health, implementing a strategy of care to accomplish defined goals within the context of a client-centered healthcare plan, and evaluating responses to nursing care and treatment. Nursing is a dynamic discipline that is continually evolving to include more sophisticated knowledge, technologies, and client care activities (NCSBN, 2014a).

The document then proceeds to distinguish between RN and LPN practice.

No state adopts the exact wording of any recommended definition. Many states include references to performing services for compensation (which has been deleted from the NCSBN definition), the necessity for a specialized knowledge base, the use of the nursing process or its parts, and components of nursing practice. Most states refer to the execution of the medical regimen, and many include a general statement about additional actions that recognize that nursing practice is evolving and that the nurse's area of responsibility can be expected to broaden.

Definitions of practical nursing are more restrictive and usually state that the individual must function under the direction of an RN or a physician, in areas demanding less judgment and knowledge than is required of the RN. In the NCSBN model act, this is referred to as "a directed scope of nursing practice" (NCSBN, 2014a). Practical nurse standards usually focus on data collection rather than comprehensive assessment, and they specify that the practical nurse contributes to the plan and evaluation of care rather than being accountable for them.

The scope of practice for any profession is directly tied to the legal definition and includes those activities, processes, and skills that are part of that profession. The education of the professional provides the basis for scope of practice and therefore differs for RNs, advanced practice nurses, and LPNs. The scope of practice also differentiates those activities that are nursing actions from those that are a part of other professions.

Because the legal definition of nursing is written in broad terms, it is sometimes difficult to determine whether a specific action is permitted as part of the scope of practice. **Figure 3.2** provides a decision-making process to help you examine whether any action is within your scope of practice as an RN. In some instances, when the issue is very complex, an advisory opinion regarding whether a specific action is within a nursing scope of practice may be sought from the state board of nursing.

Healthcare facilities employ a variety of nursing assistants, mental health technicians, telemetry technicians, nursing assistants, or medication technicians, for example. The preparation and scope of practice for these individuals are a matter of serious concern to the public. Laws regarding educational requirements and legal definitions of scope of practice have been adopted for nursing assistant practice. Through the Omnibus Budget Reconciliation Act of 1987 regulations for long-term care facilities, a nationwide standard was established for the

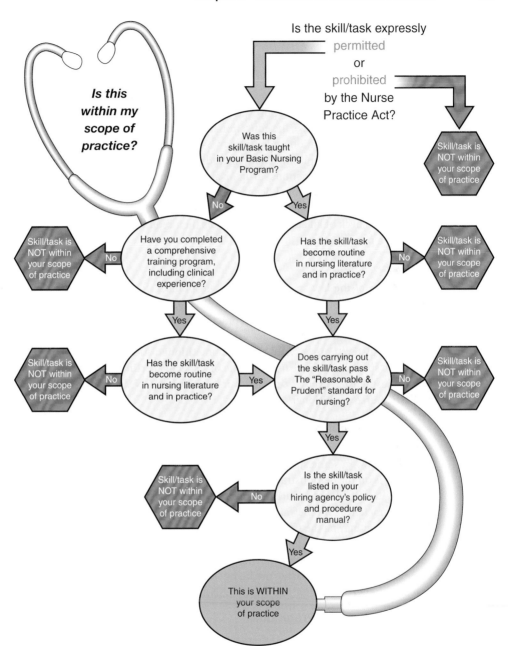

Figure 3.2. Nursing scope of practice: a decision-making model. (Decisioning Model, 2004, with permission of South Dakota Board of Nursing.)

training and certification of nursing assistants employed in these facilities. Each state administers the regulations and is free to raise the standards but may not lower them.

Qualifications for Licensure Applicants

The most common basic requirements for licensure are completion of an application, payment of fees, graduation from an approved educational program, and proficiency in the English language. Some states make the educational requirements more specific—requiring, for example, high school graduation and either an associate or baccalaureate degree, or a diploma in nursing, for the RN applicant. Many include a provision that the applicant report any mental illness, criminal convictions, drug or alcohol dependence, or disciplinary action taken in regard to another professional license that will then be evaluated by the board of nursing in relationship to standards of safety for the public. Most states now require a criminal history background check of all applicants. All states then require completion of a licensing examination with a passing score.

Titling

This section of the law specifies the titles to be used for those who have met the licensure requirements. In some states, only the titles RN and LPN/LVN are regulated. Many states also regulate the use of titles for advanced practice, such as nurse practitioner and nurse–midwife. Titles used in these expanded roles vary from state to state. Some current titles are **advanced practice registered nurse** (APRN), nurse practitioner, and advanced RN practitioner. In some states, the specialized nurse uses the title of a specific certification, such as certified registered nurse anesthetist (CRNA), certified nurse–midwife (CNM), family nurse practitioner, and pediatric nurse practitioner.

License Renewal and Continuing Competence Requirements

The length of time for which a license is valid and any requirements for its renewal are specified in the law. In some states, license renewal requires only the payment of a fee. A growing emphasis is on the demonstration of continued competence for relicensure. In its 2013 survey, the ANA identified that 35 jurisdictions require evidence of continuing education as an indicator of competence for renewal of an RN license (ANA, 2013b). The documentation of continuing education may be the submission of records, or it may be attested to by signing a form with random verification. Requirements vary greatly, with an average of 15 hours of continuing education per year commonly specified. As various states address the issue of continuing competence, additional approaches are being included. Eighteen states reported setting minimum practice hours required for relicensure (ANA, 2013b).

Nursing Education Programs

Some state laws describe the requirements of nursing education programs in only the most general terms, leaving the details up to the board of nursing; in other states, the laws are specific. The law may specify the number of years of education required, which courses or what content must be included, and the approval process for particular programs. If the law is general, then the board sets more specific standards through regulations. Virginia Henderson was a proponent of university level education for nurses. Read more about this nurse theorist in the theory alert.

Theory Alert   Virginia Henderson

Virginia Henderson is often referred to as the modern-day mother of nursing, or the Florence Nightingale of the 20th century. Her work was instrumental in advancing the quality of nursing care and education. She was born in Kansas in 1897 and earned her nursing diploma from the Army School of Nursing at Walter Reed hospital in Washington, D.C. She then went on to receive and bachelor's and master's degree from Teacher's College at Columbia University.

Henderson's theory centers on the nurse temporarily performing for the client those items of care that the client would perform if they were well enough. Key to her theory was the belief that the education and preparation of the nurse and the belief that quality of care was more important than the amount of hours of care. She was a proponent of higher education and felt that nurses should be educated at the university level. Her many writings have been used to organize and improve nursing education programs around the world.

She was very involved in nursing education and nursing research. The Sigma Theta Tau International Honor Society of Nursing electronic library, called the e-Repository, bears her name as a tribute to this forward thinking, education-focused nurse theorist (nursing-theory.org).

Grounds for Disciplinary Action

Disciplinary action refers to all penalties that may be imposed against an individual who has violated provisions of a licensing law. The Nurse Practice Act for a state identifies the basis for disciplinary action, and the board is empowered to prosecute those who violate the law. Disciplinary actions may include fines, reprimands, restrictions on practice (such as working only under supervision), suspension of a license for a specified period, or **revocation** (removal) of a license. The board may be authorized to ask a court to halt a specific practice that it believes is contrary to the law until a full hearing can be held. This is called **injunctive relief**. This term refers to the court order called an injunction that requires an individual or organization to stop a particular activity. The board also may immediately suspend a license, pending investigation, if the situation holds a serious threat to the public.

Disciplinary action can only be taken based on criteria stated in the law **(Fig. 3.3)**. Most courts have supported revocation of a license only when the offense was related in some way to practice issues that affected public safety. Thus, most modern nurse practice or disciplinary acts contain specific concerns such as the following:

- Fraud or deceit in obtaining a license
- Criminal conviction

Figure 3.3. Disciplinary action refers to all penalties that may be imposed against an individual who has violated provisions of a licensing law.

- Unethical conduct
- Drug diversion
- Unsafe or unprofessional practice (including practicing while chemically impaired)
- Practicing outside the scope of practice

Another problem faced by disciplinary boards is the misuse of social media the NCSBN states, "The use of social media and other electronic communication is expanding exponentially. While social media is an exciting and valuable tool to nurses when used wisely, it can pose risks when used inappropriately. NCSBN has developed social media guidelines for nurses, along with a number of resources to help disseminate best practices" (NCSBN, 2017) (see **Fig. 3.4**). Some states also have clauses that call for license revocation for individuals who default on government-sponsored education loans or on agreements regarding service in return for scholarship aid.

Exceptions

Certain provisions may allow those who are not licensed to act as nurses in specific situations. The primary exception is usually for those performing as a student enrolled in a nursing program. Those who care for family members or friends without pay are also exempted from license regulations. Those who practice nursing in a federal agency, such as a military hospital, are exempted from seeking a license in the state where they are stationed as long as they maintain a current license in another state. Some states are adopting exceptions for self-directed care by the disabled. In these situations, a paid care provider may perform certain care that is usually considered nursing when directed to do so by the mentally competent, physically

Figure 3.4. Nurses have a responsibility to maintain client confidentiality and to use social media appropriately.

disabled client. This includes administering medications in the home and carrying out specific care procedures, such as catheterization.

Administrative Provisions

Each law requires administrative specifications detailing when the law will become effective and when a previous act will no longer be in force. Although the Nurse Practice Act itself usually does not specify the fees to be charged for obtaining or renewing a license, general authority for setting fees is provided.

All states charge a fee for processing an application for licensure, for taking the licensing examination (which is paid to the company that prepares and scores an examination), and for license renewal. For specific information about current fees, contact your state board of nursing or visit its website.

Grandfathering

When a new law is written, it usually contains a statement specifying that anyone currently holding a license may continue to hold that license if and when requirements for the license change. This is termed **grandfathering**. Without this provision, the enactment of a new law would require individuals who are currently licensed to reapply and to show that they meet the new standards.

However, not all changes in the law are grandfathered. When new requirements are instituted that the legislature believes are important for the safety of the public, all currently licensed individuals may be required to meet the new standards within a given time period. A good example is the requirement for continuing education for relicensure. When this requirement was added, all applicants had to meet the requirement by a specific date.

Sunset Laws and Nurse Practice Acts

Most laws remain in effect until the legislature votes to rescind or replace them. Because this has resulted in archaic laws remaining in effect for many years, some states have passed what are known as "sunset laws." Sunset laws provide that any regulatory act, such as the Nurse Practice Act, will automatically be rescinded after a predetermined length of time if not reauthorized. Nurses must identify when "sun-setting" will occur and work in advance to sustain the current law or make changes. The advantage of sunset laws is that they guarantee that the legislature will review and evaluate agencies and programs.

Advanced Practice Registered Nurses

Advanced practice registered nurses (APRNs) include nurse practitioners, nurse anesthetists, nurse–midwives, and, in some states, clinical nurse specialists (CNSs). Licensure requirements for advanced practice vary from state to state. Most, but not all, require the master's or doctoral degree in nursing. Gradually, states are moving toward the master's degree as the minimum standard. None of the states administers a state licensing examination for advanced practice nursing.

Certification for advanced practice forms the basis of legal approval of APRN qualifications. The certification may be from the American Nurse Credentialing Center (ANCC) or a nursing specialty organization. A collaboration of more than 40 organizations have been working to create uniformity in advanced nursing practice (ANCC, 2017). The document

Consensus Model for APRN Regulation: Licensure, Accreditation, Certification & Education (NCSBN, 2008) provides the basis for this move toward greater symmetry in licensing and scope of practice.

The consensus model includes recommended titles. All are termed APRN with one of four roles: CRNA, CNM, certified nurse practitioner, or CNS. Education for all of these roles would be in an accredited master's or doctoral degree program or in a postgraduate certificate program. These programs would have to meet broad-based expectations that include pathophysiology, pharmacology, and physical assessment as well as significant clinical practice. Certification by an appropriate organization that includes both review of education and a rigorous examination would be required. APRNs would be licensed as independent practitioners without requirements for collaboration or supervision (NCSBN, 2008). A plan for an APRN compact for multistate licensing has been developed but not yet implemented.

Advanced practice nurses have the skills and abilities to help meet the needs of the millions of individuals expected to enter the system through the healthcare reform process. State regulations that do not allow APRNs to practice within the full scope of their abilities create a barrier to their being able to make this contribution. The most current Institute of Medicine (IOM) report *The Future of Nursing: Leading Change, Advancing Health 2010* recognizes the contributions of APRNs and the work that still needs to be done to ensure their full utilization to meet the healthcare needs of the public.

The Role of the State Board of Nursing

The **state board of nursing** (or its equivalent) is the administrative department of the government legally empowered to carry out the provisions of the Nurse Practice Act. Each state board must operate within the framework of its own state law regarding the practice of nursing, but all cooperate through the NCSBN. For example, state boards acting together through the NCSBN contract with the company that prepares the licensing examinations for RNs and practical nurses that are used throughout the United States. They also cooperate with other organizations, such as the ANA, the NLN, and the NLNAC, in some matters, but maintain the separation that is required of a group whose focus is protection of the public through effective licensure of nurses.

The board of nursing typically performs the following functions:

- Establishes standards for licensure
- Examines and licenses applicants
- Provides for interstate endorsement
- Renews licenses, grants temporary licenses, and provides for inactive status for those already licensed who request it
- Enforces disciplinary codes
- Provides rules for revocation of license
- Regulates specialty practice
- Establishes standards and curricula for nursing programs
- Approves nursing education programs

Some or most of these duties may be performed by a centralized state agency acting in that capacity for all licensed occupations. When a centralized agency has the majority of the responsibility, the board of nursing may act in an advisory capacity in regard to issues.

Board membership, the procedures for appointment and removal, and the qualifications of board members are determined by the Nurse Practice Act. The governor of the state usually appoints the members of the board. The law specifies the occupational background of the candidates; nominations may be made by nurses' organizations and other interested parties. North Carolina is the only state in which the RN members of the state board are elected by the RNs in the state.

Most states have a single board for RNs and LPNs. Each state board has a paid staff that usually is headed by an RN with advanced education who is employed as the executive director of the state board of nursing. The executive director is responsible for administering the work of the board, for seeing that rules and regulations are followed, and for working with the NCSBN and other state boards.

OBTAINING A NURSING LICENSE

There are two procedures for obtaining a nursing license. The first is used for obtaining an initial license and is termed **licensure by examination**. The second is for obtaining a license when the nurse is already licensed in another jurisdiction and is called **licensure by endorsement**. In both instances, the applicant for licensure must meet all provisions of the law (such as educational preparation, language proficiency, and legal residency status) in the state where he or she seeks licensure. In the initial licensure process, the applicant must take and pass the NCLEX. When seeking licensure by endorsement, the applicant is not required to take another examination—the licensing examination results from the initial state are accepted as proof of minimum safe practice—but other requirements must be met.

Licensure by Examination

The establishment of a licensing examination was an important part of early efforts to achieve a professional standard for the RN. When each state adopted a licensing law, it also established a mechanism for examining license applicants. A major achievement in the history of nursing licensure was the formation of the Bureau of State Boards of Nurse Examiners, which eventually led to the use of an identical examination in all states in 1950. The original examination, called the State Board Test Pool Examination, was prepared by the testing department of the NLN, under a contract with the state boards. Although each state initially determined its own passing score, eventually all states adopted a common passing score. The current examination, called the **NCLEX-RN** for registered nursing and the **NCLEX-PN** for practical nursing, is used in all states and territories of the United States. Beginning in October 2002, Pearson Professional Testing of Minnesota was granted the contract for preparing and administering all NCLEX exams.

Content of the Examination

The NCSBN supports a study called the RN Practice Analysis every 3 years. This is used to guide the development of test questions. There is a similar cycle for studying PN practice. These studies identify nursing behaviors critical to maintaining a safe and effective standard of care. In all of these studies, newly licensed, practicing RNs or PNs are studied to determine both the frequency and the importance of various behaviors. These studies are reflected in the 2017 NCLEX-RN Test Plan (NCSBN, 2016a) and the 2017 NCLEX-PN Test Plan (NCSBN, 2016b).

Table 3.1   2016 Test Plan for NCLEX-RN

Client Needs Categories/Subcategories	Percentage of Items
Safe Effective Care Environment	
Management of care	17–23
Safety and infection control	9–15
Health Promotion and Maintenance	6–12
Psychosocial Integrity	6–12
Physiological Integrity	
Basic care and comfort	6–12
Pharmacologic and parenteral therapies	12–18
Reduction of risk potential	9–15
Physiological adaptation	11–17

Source: National Council of State Boards of Nursing, Inc. (NCSBN), 2015.

The test plans are available for downloading without charge from the NCSBN website. The NCLEX-RN questions are organized into client needs and the integrated process. The four client need categories (safe effective care environment, health promotion and maintenance, psychosocial integrity, and physiological integrity) and their subcategories form the basis of the exam (Table 3.1). There are five integrated processes: (1) nursing process, (2) caring, (3) communication and documentation, (4) teaching/learning, and (5) culture and spirituality. The nursing process is further divided into five steps: (1) assessment, (2) analysis, (3) planning, (4) implementation, and (5) evaluation. These client need categories and the integrated processes form a matrix in which each question tests both an integrated process and one category or subcategory of client need.

The NCLEX-PN exam (the licensure exam for LPNs/LVNs) has a similar construction pattern. A PN Job Analysis study is conducted, and then the test plan is developed. The most recent PN Job Analysis was completed in 2015; the newest test plan for the PN was approved in 2016 and implemented in April 2017. A practical nurse is expected to assume a more dependent role in assessment; therefore, that step is titled data collection. Analysis is not part of the test plan. Whereas the RN examination includes management of care, the PN examination focuses on coordination of care. Even when topics are the same, the level of judgment expected of the PN differs from that expected of the RN. The newest test recognizes that many LPNs are employed in long-term care settings, with clients older than 65 years of age; therefore, it focuses on the older population (NCSBN, 2016b).

Preparing and Administering the Examination

Preparing questions for the examination is a complex process. Nursing educators and RNs who work with new graduates are brought together to write exam questions based on the test plan. Content experts who are also nurses currently working with new graduates review all questions. Another panel of individuals reviews the questions for bias. Each question then is verified for accuracy by using current nursing references; test-construction experts also review the structure of all of the questions. The final versions of all questions are tested by inclusion in a nongraded part of the license examinations being given to new graduates; the questions are evaluated for their level of difficulty and appropriate use as part of a future scored examination.

In addition to assuming responsibility for test preparation, the testing service administers the computerized tests through contracted testing centers, scores the examinations, and reports scores to the state boards. The testing service is authorized to sell statistical information related to the examinations to the states and to individual schools. The entire testing process is explained in the candidate booklet (NCSBN, 2017), which is also available online at the testing website www.vue.com/nclex. An overview is presented as follows.

Computerized Adaptive Testing

All NCLEX (both RN and PN) exams are administered through **computerized adaptive testing** (CAT). CAT consists of a bank of examination questions administered through a computerized system. It was first field tested in 1990 and then across the country in 1993 and finally adopted for all testing beginning in April 1994.

In this computerized test, the multiple-choice questions are delivered on a computer screen. The computer contains a large bank of questions, and different individuals may be presented with different questions. The computer program evaluates each response and then selects an appropriate question to present next, choosing a slightly harder question if the previous question was answered correctly or an easier question if the response was incorrect. The computer program ensures that all essential aspects of the test matrix plan are part of every examination. The development of questions and the design of the computer program ensure that all tests are equivalent, even when they are not identical. On the NCLEX-RN, the minimum number of questions that might be administered is 75 and the maximum is 265. The maximum length of time for the examination is 6 hours, but a candidate performing either especially well or very poorly might complete the exam in just 1 hour. Optional breaks are offered at 2 hours and again at 3.5 hours, others may be taken at the discretion of the applicant. Testing ends when the scoring analysis clearly indicates a pass or fail, the maximum number of questions has been answered, or the maximum time has been completed.

Each candidate for licensure makes an individual appointment at a testing site. Security at the center is tightly monitored using photo identification, a fingerprint, and a palm vein scan. The computers are located in a quiet room without distractions. No test study materials are allowed at the testing center and no food or drink is allowed in the test environment. An erasable note board is provided for notes or calculations. An optional on-screen calculator is provided.

The multiple-choice questions in the examination typically are based on situations that require a nursing response. They are designed to test judgment and decision-making, not simply knowledge of facts. Setting priorities, delegating, and communicating with the health team are aspects of that judgment. In addition to multiple-choice questions, there are several alternative question types that involve computation, short answer, identifying items on the screen, or multiple answers. These are described in the NLCEX-RN Candidate Bulletin (2017). A tutorial on how to use the computer, including the on-screen calculator, along with some practice questions is provided to ensure that the individual understands the process.

Scoring the Examination

The computer calculates the score as the applicant answers questions. As soon as the statistical computation provides a prediction with 95% certainty of pass or fail, the test is terminated. If the computerized score has not provided a 95% certainty of pass or fail by the end of the examination (because either time is up or the maximum number of questions are answered), the system identifies whether the estimate of ability is above the standard even if it does not meet the 95% certainty standard. If it meets or is above that standard, the person passes.

Although the computer immediately determines pass or fail (upon the completion of the examination), the individual is not notified of the result at that time. The scoring information is communicated to the testing service, which then notifies the appropriate board. The board of nursing then notifies the individual whether he or she passed or failed. Every 3 years, the NCSBN considers the appropriateness of the passing standards for both the PN and RN examinations and may modify them.

Preparing for the NCLEX Exam

Individuals must determine how best to prepare for the licensure examination based on their background and preferred study style. A review of the knowledge basic to nursing is important for most individuals. This may be done using course notes and texts. Those who become anxious in testing situations may want to focus on exercises to decrease anxiety during the examination. Those who find the process of test taking difficult can gain greater self-confidence by practicing test-taking techniques. This can be done through printed tests in books or computerized test preparation programs.

For both the NCLEX-RN and the NCLEX-PN, many commercial study aids are available. To prepare applicants to take the examination, the NCLEX Candidate Bulletin (NCSBN, 2017) explains the examination, how it is written, and the scoring system, and provides sample questions to familiarize applicants with the way the test is written. Many companies also prepare NCLEX-RN and NCLEX-PN review books, sample examination questions, audiotapes, and computerized practice examinations that are used to prepare for the licensing examinations. Manuals that outline standard nursing practice relative to many different healthcare problems may be useful for reviewing nursing content. Live and videotaped review courses, produced both by individual schools of nursing and by commercial publishers, are available to those who want assistance with preparation. During your preparation, remember that the goal is to solidify your knowledge and skills and to develop your critical thinking and problem-solving skills. Memorizing answers to test questions presented in study books will not help you with the problem solving in regard to the unique questions presented in the actual examination.

Critical Thinking Activity: Multistate Licensure
A student about to graduate from an RN program in New York plans to live and practice nursing in New Jersey. What options are available to her to become licensed? Investigate the steps she should take to ensure that she may legally practice nursing in New Jersey as soon after graduation as possible.

Licensure by Endorsement

The process of obtaining a nursing license in a new state (while already licensed in another state) is called licensure by endorsement. In licensure by endorsement, each case is considered independently, based on the rules and regulations of the state to which one is applying for licensure. However, due to the uniformity of licensing laws throughout most of the United States and its territories, nurses have enjoyed easy mobility between geographic areas.

Because the same licensure examination and passing standards are used nationwide, no state requires that the examination be retaken. Basic educational and legal requirements of the individual state where a license is sought must be met. Sometimes a nurse moving to a new state must meet the current criteria for new licensure. In other states, a nurse must fulfill only the requirements that were in effect at the time of the original licensure. A state may require a nurse to meet other criteria, such as those for continuing education, before granting licensure by endorsement. In all cases, appropriate paperwork must be completed, necessary fees paid, and a license obtained before a nurse may begin employment. A temporary license, which allows the applicant for licensure by endorsement to be employed while credentials are being verified and processed, is available in some states. If a nurse wishes to maintain licensure in more than one state, this may be done by paying the renewal fees and meeting other requirements for continued licensure, such as continuing education, in each state in which a license is maintained. Some nurses hold licenses in several states to be able to work as a traveling nurse or to choose work in different locations. Nurses working close to state lines may need more than one license to be employed by an agency that operates in more than one state. This might also be true of a nursing education program that has clinical sites in two adjacent states or a home care agency with clients in two states.

Mutual Recognition of Licensure

The process of mutual recognition of licensure in nursing has been established through the NCSBN based on a multistate agreement called the Nurse Licensure Compact. **Mutual recognition of licensure** involves an individual receiving an RN license in the state where he or she resides (the **home state**) and being legally permitted to practice in additional states without obtaining additional licenses for those states. This is sometimes referred to as "multistate licensure." Those states that have entered into the NCSBN Nurse Licensure Compact have all passed legislation adopting the terms of the Compact into their licensure laws (NCSBN, 2015). At the time of this writing, 25 states have entered the compact agreement. For the most current information on states participating, go to the NCSBN website and link to Nursing Licensure Compact.

Processes Involved in Mutual Recognition

All of the states that have signed the compact are referred to as **party states**. An individual maintains only one license, the license granted in the home state in which he or she resides and has a registered nursing license, but is legally permitted to practice in any party state. When renewing a license, the individual renews in the home state. The individual nurse cannot hold a license in two party states at the same time. When an individual changes residence to a new party state, he or she applies for a new home state license based on residency. Individuals who wish to practice in a nonparty state still need to apply for a license in the nonparty state before practicing nursing.

The individual nurse must comply with the state laws regulating nursing practice in the state in which the client is located. Any party state where nursing care occurs, whether the home state or the **remote state** (a party state other than the nurse's home state), may institute disciplinary action based on appropriate procedures. The home state is notified of the action being taken in the remote state through a coordinated information data bank system called NURSYS. When a remote state institutes disciplinary action, it may revoke a nurse's privilege to practice in that state only. Only the home state may revoke the license itself. If an individual has been assigned to some type of alternative program (such as drug treatment and monitoring) as part of the disciplinary process by any party state, the conditions of the disciplinary process must prohibit the individual from practicing in other states in the compact until the problem is resolved.

NURSYS was completed in 2000. This data bank contains licensure and disciplinary information from approximately 49 states that have chosen to use the system (NCSBN, 2017). NURSYS provides online access to this computerized data bank for member state boards of nursing. It also provides an effective mechanism for individuals to have their records sent from one state to another when seeking endorsement.

As you can see, the RN who is licensed in a Nurse Licensure Compact state who chooses to work outside the home state must follow the directives contained in the compact and become familiar with the nursing practice act in any state in which clients are located. The state board of any state participating in the compact will provide complete information on the specific requirements to be met.

A separate APRN compact has also been developed and passed as model law in 2015. States participating in APRN compact will have to meet the expectations for education and licensure requirements found in the Consensus Model for APRN Regulation (NCSBN, 2008).

Reasons Nurses Seek Mutual Recognition of Licenses

Under standard licensing laws, the nurse who practices in more than one state must hold multiple nursing licenses. This is both costly and complex. As the healthcare system grows more diverse, it is not uncommon for a healthcare-providing organization to operate across state boundaries.

Telenursing includes the use of telecommunications technology (e.g., telephone, fax, computers, teleconferencing, interactive television, and video phone) to provide nursing services to individuals and groups. A telenurse in one state may care for a client in a distant state, NCSBN states that the nurse should be licensed in the state where the client resides (NCSBN, 2014b). Another area of concern is the nurse who works for an agency that serves clients across state borders. This nurse needs to visit clients in more than one state. The nursing case manager may follow clients in several states. All of these situations create a demand for a simpler licensing system for working in multiple states.

Concerns Regarding Mutual Recognition of Licenses

Not all nurses have supported mutual recognition of licenses. The ANA has identified that nurses who have differing requirements for relicensure could be practicing side by side; for example, one home state requires continuing education and another does not. Some state attorneys general have given opinions that it would be unconstitutional in their state to allow another state to control the requirements for practice. Issues of privacy regarding the data stored in the NURSYS system are another area of concern. The mutual recognition of licenses system may save money for the nurse who practices in multiple states because only one license would be purchased. However, if fewer nurses are licensed in the state, but the same number practice in the state, one would expect that disciplinary costs would remain even. The cost of licenses for all nurses, therefore, would have to rise to ensure adequate funds to support disciplinary costs. A major concern is the disciplinary process. Although the board of nursing can investigate nursing practices and enforce its own standards in the state, it cannot change the licensure status of the person whose licensure originates in a different state; this fact is troubling to some boards of nursing. They are concerned that this does not allow them to protect the public adequately. A person disciplined in a remote state will still possess what would appear to be a valid home state license, but perhaps would not be able to practice legally in the remote state. For the individual nurse, the differences in licensure regulations could result in the same behavior being the cause of disciplinary action in one state but not in others; however, if the license were removed by the home state, then it would be invalid in all states (ANA, 2013a, 2013b, 2013c).

The future not only holds many exciting possibilities for nursing but also poses many potential pitfalls. This is a complex issue, because state licensing agencies are charged with protecting the public and have legitimate concerns regarding such areas as disciplinary action.

REVOCATION OR LIMITATION OF A LICENSE

The procedure for revoking a license includes a fact-finding process and a hearing, which functions in many ways like a court proceeding. The state board or a specially designated hearing board is responsible for conducting the hearing and making a decision. The board may provide a license with conditions, suspend a license until certain conditions are met, or revoke a license completely. For example, a nurse faced with charges of chemical dependency might be directed to enter a treatment program, to refuse employment involving direct responsibility for clients who need controlled substances or access to drugs, and to be monitored for compliance. If these conditions are met, the individual may be allowed to work in a restricted environment and then be reinstated to full rights and privileges of licensure when treatment is completed. The board's decision may be appealed in a court of law in most states. If a board of nursing finds that the individual's actions constitute a felony, the board is obligated to report that to the criminal authorities for prosecution.

Daily Ethical Dilemma 3.1: *Substance Abuse*

RNs Mary and Ann are friends and were working together for the day. Mary had a headache that was getting worse and she asked Ann if she had any medication for a headache. Ann stated that she had some in a brown bottle in her purse, in her locker. Mary retrieved two white pills from the brown bottle in Ann's purse that looked like the Tylenol she had taken for headaches before. After taking the medication, Mary began to have trouble focusing and she was unable to keep up with her client care and charting.

1. What do you suspect has happened?
2. Identify the potential problems in this scenario.
3. Her supervisor questioned her unusual behavior and Mary denied using any mood altering medication. She was required to provide a urine screen and sent home pending investigation. Her urine was positive for hydrocodone for which she did not have a prescription.
4. What action do you think the employer will take?
5. Who is at fault here, Mary or Ann?

Retrieved March 23, 2017 from http://kbn.ky.gov/conprotect/Pages/casestudies.aspx

The individual being investigated for any violation of the Nurse Practice Act should have an attorney who is knowledgeable about professional disciplinary issues from the time of notification of the complaint. Some nurses fail to take this important action: they may have the mistaken impression that only those guilty of misconduct need an attorney; they may believe that if they made an error they deserve punishment; or they may worry about the cost of an attorney. Just as in a criminal proceeding, the law is complex and a knowledgeable attorney provides direction and support throughout a disciplinary process. Penalties may vary greatly and the naïve nurse may not realize that extenuating circumstances or negotiations may change penalties. Although attorney costs are substantial, a license to practice nursing is extremely valuable to the individual nurse. Some malpractice insurance policies include payment for attorney fees in the case of disciplinary action (see Chapter 7). The state nurses association or the local chapter of the National Association of Nurse Attorneys can often provide referrals of attorneys who are familiar with the disciplinary process.

As a licensed professional, be aware that you are responsible to your clients and to the state in which you practice. You can act to protect your license through maintaining current knowledge and appropriate standards of practice. Also, understand and abide by the scope of practice as described in your individual nursing practice act. If you take a position in a new state, it is your responsibility to become informed about that state's Nurse Practice Act. Evidence-Based Practice 3.2 discusses current research regarding the misuse of social media that can be a problem for RNs and for nursing students before licensure.

LICENSURE OF GRADUATES OF FOREIGN NURSING SCHOOLS

Many nurses from other countries have immigrated to the United States and sought licensure to be able to work in their new home. Some nurses have come to the United States for additional education and need a license to engage in clinical practice associated with that education. Still others are attracted by the higher salaries and better living conditions for nurses in the United States. During the nursing shortage of the early 1980s, and again in the nursing shortage in the first part of this century, employers in the United States actively recruited foreign nurses, sometimes providing support for travel and relocation expenses.

Evidence-Based Practice 3.2: Social Media Use By Nurses

Westrick, S. J. (2016). Nursing students' use of electronic and social media: Law, ethics, and e-professionalism. *Nursing Education Perspectives (National League For Nursing), 37*(1), 16–22. doi:10.5480/14-1358

There is an increasing problem with the misuse of social media by nursing students. The misuse of social media can lead to expulsion from nursing programs and legal action against schools of nursing and nursing faculty. It is important to be aware of what constitutes a breach of client confidentiality and to prevent such occurrences.

This article analyses several legal cases where breach of confidentiality occurred resulting in legal action. Students are routinely cautioned about client privacy and the use of social media. Nursing programs are adding social media policies in student handbooks, and these policies should specify the consequences for the violation of the social media policy.

Several concerns have been expressed regarding the recruitment of foreign-educated nurses to the United States. In many of the countries from which nurses immigrate to the United States, shortages exist. Thus, the United States depletes other countries of an important health resource. Some nurses in the United States believe that overseas recruitment replaces the need to address workplace problems that contribute to the shortage. Nurses educated in other countries may lack understanding of the US healthcare system and the expectations for scope of practice. Further, they may lack English language proficiency.

For the foreign-educated nurse, there are two requirements that must be met in order to work in the United States. The first of these is a visa that permits employment, either a visa granted to a permanent immigrant or one granted to a temporary worker. The employer is required to verify the individual's eligibility for employment in the United States. When the visa is contingent upon employment, the foreign-educated nurse may feel constrained from changing employers if circumstances differ from what was promised during recruitment.

The second requirement is that the foreign-educated nurse must obtain a state license to practice nursing. To obtain a license, all graduates of foreign nursing schools who want to practice nursing in the United States must provide verification to the state licensing authority that their nursing education meets state requirements and they must take the appropriate NCLEX exam. In the past, institutions would sometimes hire foreign nurses into lower paying positions until they obtained a license. When many did not pass the examination, the nurses felt exploited by the system.

CGFNS International

The U.S. Department of Labor, the Department of Health and Human Services (HHS), the Immigration and Naturalization Service (INS), the ANA, and the NLN are all concerned about the safety of the public and about the well-being of the foreign-educated nurse. To address these problems, these organizations and government agencies collaborated in the development of an independent organization originally called the Commission on Graduates of Foreign Nursing Schools (CGFNS—pronounced "cog-fens") and now titled CGFNS International (Fig. 3.5).

While some nurses who come to the United States possess regular immigrant visas, the majority come on special-preference visas. Special immigration regulations allow a foreign nurse to obtain a special-preference visa from the INS or a work permit from the U.S. Labor Department because of the need for nurses. To obtain this special-preference visa, an individual nurse must obtain a visa certificate from an HHS-approved agency, such as CGFNS. The Department of Homeland Security ruled in July 2005 that nurses from Mexico and Canada, who were formerly exempted from this requirement under NAFTA, were subject to this same requirement for a certificate.

The CGFNS service *VisaScreen* provides a certificate enabling an individual to apply for a visa. A VisaScreen includes (1) a review of the foreign nurse's education, (2) evaluation of all current and previous licenses to practice, (3) assessment of English language proficiency, and (4) completion of either the CGFNS Assessment of General Nursing Knowledge Examination or the NCLEX-RN. The CGFNS Assessment is offered around the world for individuals to take before emigrating. Because many foreign-educated nurses still come to the United States without having taken the CGFNS examination, it is also offered in selected cities in the United States. When these requirements have been completed satisfactorily, a certificate is issued that can be presented to the immigration service to obtain a special-preference visa (CGFNS, 2016).

Figure 3.5. The Commission on Graduates of Foreign Nursing Schools, now CGFNS International is concerned about the safety of the public and about the well-being of the foreign-educated nurse. This figure illustrates the global communication and international messaging concept.

International Centre on Nurse Migration

The International Centre on Nurse Migration is a project of the CGFNS and the International Council of Nurses (ICN). The goals of the Centre relate to both effective client care and the well-being of nurse migrants. To achieve its goals, the Centre works on policies worldwide that affect nurse migration, collects and reports data on nurse migration, and serves as a resource for those working with regulations regarding nurse migration (International Centre on Nurse Migration, 2016). Because there is a worldwide shortage of nurses and a wide disparity of wages and recognition between developing and developed countries, nurse migration will continue to be an important international issue.

NURSING LICENSURE AROUND THE WORLD

Nursing education and nursing licensure differ greatly throughout the world. Additionally, practice patterns and expectations of nursing behaviors may differ between countries. In Australia, nursing education has been moved into university settings, and future applicants for licensure in that country are required to have a university education. In Italy, nursing education is now consolidated under broad, multisite programs administered by university nursing departments. The European Union is moving toward a system that allows freer movement of professionals between its nations. The nations of Eastern Europe have faced many drastic changes in their healthcare systems as they changed internally and formed different relationships with the West. Nursing education was restricted during Soviet domination, and many nurses had limited nursing educational opportunities, with basic nursing education sometimes occurring at the high school level. Nursing in those countries is moving toward contemporary expectations.

Individuals who are interested in international nursing need to consider both their language proficiency and their educational backgrounds. Organizations actively working in the international health field, such as the World Health Organization and medical relief organizations, usually will provide information on opportunities and licensure requirements in various countries. The ICN in Geneva can provide addresses of appropriate government authorities to contact regarding licensure in other countries. During times of emergency, such as the tsunami in the Indian Ocean, countries may welcome nurses as part of relief groups without requiring licensure in that country. Additionally, there are opportunities for short-term healthcare work in developing countries through charitable agencies and international missions.

CERTIFICATION IN NURSING

As mentioned earlier, certification in nursing is primarily a professional, not legal, credential, and it focuses on knowledge and skills related to a particular area of practice. The definition of certification adopted by the Interdivisional Council on Certification of the ANA (1978) states, "Certification is the documented validation of specific qualifications demonstrated by the individual RN in the provision of professional nursing care in a defined area of practice." Certification is available from many professional nursing and healthcare organizations.

American Nurses Credentialing Center Certification

In 1988, the ANA established the ANCC, which assumed all of the ANA credentialing activities. The ANA invited all other organizations providing credentialing for nurses to join; some joined, but many retained their individual programs.

ANCC certification is a method of recognizing nurses who have special expertise. Applicants must demonstrate current practice and knowledge beyond that required for licensure as an RN. After submitting evidence of completing all requirements, a nurse may take the national examination for a specific certification. Certification is granted for a period of 5 years, after which a nurse may renew the certification by submitting new evidence of current practice and ability.

The master's degree currently forms the basis of the requirement for certification as a CNS, a nurse practitioner, or other advanced practice roles but is moving toward the use of the doctor of nursing practice. For specialty certifications, there are requirements for continuing education and hours of practice in the area of specialization. All certifications require passing an examination. See Box 3.2 for a list of ANCC certifications available.

BOX 3.2 NURSING CERTIFICATION AVAILABLE THROUGH THE AMERICAN NURSES' CREDENTIALING CENTER

Nurse Practitioners
Acute Care Nurse Practitioner
Adult Nurse Practitioner
Adult Psychiatric & Mental Health NP
Diabetes Management—Advanced
Emergency NP
Family NP
Family Psych & Mental Health NP
Gerontologic NP
Adult-Gerontology Acute Care NP
Adult-Gerontology Primary Care NP
Pediatric NP
School NP

Clinical Nurse Specialists
Adult Health CNS
Adult-Gerontology CNS
Adult Psychiatric & Mental Health CNS
Child/Adolescent Psych & Mental Health CNS
CNS Core Exam
Diabetes Management—Advanced
Gerontologic CNS
Home Health CNS
Pediatric CNS
Public/Community Health CNS

Other Advanced-Level Specialties
Ambulatory Care Nursing

Cardiac Rehabilitation Nursing
Cardiac–Vascular Nurse
Certified Vascular Nurse
College Health Nursing
Community Health Nursing
Diabetes Management—Advanced
Faith Community Nursing
Forensic Nursing—Advanced
General Nursing Practice
Genetics Nursing—Advanced
Gerontologic Nursing
Homeostasis Nursing
Home Health Nursing
Informatics Nursing
Maternal–Child Nursing
Medical–Surgical Nursing
Nurse Executive
Nurse Executive—Advanced
Nursing Case Management
Nursing Professional Development
Pain Management Nursing
Pediatric Nursing
Perinatal Nursing
Psychiatric–Mental Health Nursing
Public Health Nursing—Advanced
Rheumatology Nursing
School Nursing

Detailed information on requirements and credentialing process available from ANCC at www.nursecredentialing.org/.

Other Nursing Certifications Available

In 1991, eight national nursing certification programs joined to establish the American Board of Nursing Specialties; now called the Accreditation Board for Specialty Nursing. Since that time, a number of other nursing organizations that provide certification have joined this organization. The goals of this board are to ensure quality in specialty nursing, improve the public's perception of specialty nurses, and provide specialty nurses who bring a consistent standard of education and experience to their practice. This was major breakthrough in the entire certification process for nursing. This board established a peer review process for certification organizations that provides evaluation and recognition of the certification granted.

> **Critical Thinking Activity: Certification Requirements for an RN**
> An RN with 5 years of general medical–surgical acute care experience is interested in obtaining certification in medical–surgical nursing. Research the requirements for such certification and outline what she will need to do to be eligible to be certified as a medical–surgical nurse.

Certification for Licensed Practical Nurses

Certification for LPNs/LVNs is available for those practicing in long-term care. The National Association of Practical Nurse Education and Service determined that many LPNs have responsible positions in long-term care and that recognition of their abilities through certification would be appropriate. They contracted with the NCSBN to develop and administer a certification examination. Those taking this examination use the title certified in long-term care (CLTC).

THE FUTURE OF CREDENTIALING IN HEALTHCARE

Because credentialing in nursing involves so many aspects of education, licensure, and certification, it has confused the public, nurses, and other healthcare professionals. The ideal credential clearly communicates qualifications and competence; therefore, it is important for nursing to have a credentialing system that can be understood by others. Current changes are moving nursing closer to an effective credentialing system.

Institutional Control of Credentials

Many new healthcare occupations related to new procedures and processes in medical care are being developed as new technology develops. Those who believe the state should take positive action to protect the public continue to exert pressure to license additional healthcare providers. Those who oppose credentialing of additional individual groups of healthcare workers believe that modern-day employers are able to assess workers and to differentiate among them on the basis of competence. Some who oppose credentialing of individual health occupations believe that licensing the institution that hires the employees would be an adequate safeguard for the public.

Another approach to credentialing in healthcare is certifying specific competencies rather than an entire field of practice. Those advocating this approach believe that it would facilitate the development of individuals with a broad range of competencies suited to a particular setting. For example, in a rural area, one individual might be certified as competent to perform certain basic x-ray examinations (such as for simple fractures), basic laboratory studies (such as complete blood count and urinalysis), and some basic client care procedures (such as bathing, toileting, feeding, and positioning). Because more complex procedures are sent to a larger center and there is no need for a full-time person in any of these positions, basic care would be made available in a convenient and low-cost manner. Certification of specific competencies by the employing agency is sometimes referred to as site-based examination and site-based certification. One concern about this method of certifying competencies is its focus on technical skills, without adequately recognizing the knowledge base needed for decision-making and judgment. Other concerns are the complexity of keeping track of the many specific competencies and the difficulty with job mobility when competencies are not standardized.

Institute of Medicine Recommendations and the Future of Approval/Accreditation

In the IOM report *The Future of Nursing: Leading change, Advancing Health* (2010), the study committee concluded that "no single profession, working alone, can meet the complex needs of clients and communities. Nurses should continue to develop skills and competencies in leadership and innovation and collaborate with other professionals in healthcare delivery and health system redesign" (IOM, 2010). Since then, progress toward promoting higher education for RNs has happened along with changes to the scope of practice for APRNs. "The progress report asked state action coalitions to be broader in stakeholder engagement and to include as many interprofessional partners as possible" (IOM, 2015). Another previous recommendation was that those with responsibility for oversight of the various health professions (approval and accreditation bodies) meet to develop specific core competencies that relate to the following:

- Delivering client-centered care
- Working as part of interdisciplinary teams
- Practicing evidence-based healthcare
- Focus on quality improvement
- Using information technology

These have been incorporated into accreditation criteria for nursing education and healthcare delivery agencies. As nursing grows and moves forward, the dual expectations of state approval and national accreditation create a substantial workload and cost for the individual nursing program. The IOM report recommended that both licensing bodies and specialty certification bodies require health professionals to demonstrate in some way their continued competence in the previously determined core competencies. Again, this has become an accepted practice for most licensing and certification bodies.

Stegen & Sowerby Stories: Part 2

Remember Stephanie, the CNA waiting to take her state board exam for nursing? A couple weeks after she started working, she was called in to see the director regarding her working without a license. Read the rest of the story at www.thePoint.com.

Want to Know More?

A variety of resources are available on thePoint® to enhance your learning and understanding of this chapter, such as:

- Full Stegen & Sowerby Stories
- NCLEX-Style Student Review Questions
- Journal Articles
- Case Studies
- Learning Objectives
- Relevant Websites
- And more...

KEY CONCEPTS

- Credentials are written proof of qualifications and may include diplomas awarded by educational programs, certification, or registration by professional groups, and legal licenses awarded by governmental agencies.
- Permissive licensure allows for those meeting certain standards voluntarily to be licensed, whereas mandatory licensure requires that all individuals who wish to practice in the field be licensed to practice.
- Nursing leaders began efforts to obtain legal licensure in 1896. The first permissive licensure law was passed in 1903 by North Carolina, and the first mandatory licensure law was passed in New York in 1947.
- Legal rules governing nursing practice are found in the licensure law passed by a legislative body. Further provisions governing nursing are found in the rules and regulations established by the administrative agency in which the legislation vests authority.
- The state nursing practice acts usually contain a definition of nursing and address qualifications for licensure applicants, use of titles, renewal and continuing competence requirements, grandfathering, financial concerns, nursing education programs, disciplinary action, violations and penalties, administrative provisions, and expanded nursing roles.
- The state boards of nursing (or their equivalent) are the administrative agencies that have the authority to carry out the provisions of the Nurse Practice Act.
- A license to practice nursing must be obtained from the state or province in which you wish to work, except in the case of states that belong to the Multistate Compact. An initial license is termed licensure by examination, and subsequent licenses may be obtained in other jurisdictions through licensure by endorsement.
- Advanced practice nurses are regulated by each state. Most require professional certification in an advanced practice nursing specialty to be licensed in that role.
- Mutual recognition of licensure involves a compact between certain states that allows nurses who are licensed in one of those states to work freely among all the compact states belonging to the Multistate Compact without the need for obtaining additional licenses.
- The NCLEX-RN is administered through a computerized plan that covers the four integrated processes, nursing process, communication and documentation, caring, and teaching/learning, and four areas of client needs and that identifies competence for entry-level safe nursing care.
- Graduates of foreign nursing schools must have their credentials reviewed and may be required to take the CGFNS examination, which reviews nursing content and a test for English language ability, before being admitted to take the NCLEX exam.
- A license may be revoked by the state board of nursing, a designated disciplinary board, or a court of law based on specific reasons stated in the Nurse Practice Act.
- Certification provides evidence of specialized clinical knowledge and ability beyond the basic level. Certification as a nurse practitioner may be used as a basis for legal approval for the advanced registered nurse practitioner role.
- Concerns about the future of healthcare worker credentialing include issues of public accountability and continued competence.

- The IOM report on the future of nursing reiterated a series of recommendations, several of which focus on developing a set of core competencies that could be used for both education and ongoing professional regulation.
- The NCSBN has endorsed the core competencies identified by the IOM and encourages movement toward recommendations of the Future of Nursing report as part of approval and accreditation decisions.

NCLEX-STYLE PRACTICE QUESTIONS

1. After moving to a new state and securing a position as an RN at a large hospital, where would you find your scope of practice?

   A. The human resources department of the facility
   B. The office of the Chief Nursing Officer (CNO) of the hospital
   C. Online through the National Council of State Boards of Nursing (NCSBN)
   D. Through the new state board of nursing in the nurse practice act

2. As a new nurse, you have heard about the Nurse Licensure Compact. What is the relationship between the member states?

   A. The nurse can work in any state as long as she has a compact license.
   B. The nurse can have as many licenses as she wishes as long as they are all compact states.
   C. The nurse can hold a license in the state where she lives and work in another state as long as they are both part of the compact.
   D. The nurse must have a license for each state that she works in that is a member of a compact state

3. Several education programs prepare students for NCLEX-RN. Identify the types of RN education programs. (Select all that apply)

   A. Diploma nursing education
   B. Associate degree nursing education
   C. Baccalaureate degree nursing education
   D. Correspondence degree nursing education

4. Identify what is meant by licensure by endorsement.

   A. The nurse receives a letter from the program endorsing them for licensure
   B. The nurse signs her license when it arrives, endorsing licensure
   C. The nurse has already licensed in another state and pays a fee to license in another state
   D. The nurse takes the licensing exam for a second time which is called endorsement

REFERENCES

American Nurses Association. (1980). *Nursing: A social policy statement*. Kansas City, MO: American Journal of Nursing Co.

American Nurses Association. (2013a). *Title "Nurse" protection*. Kansas City, MO: Author. Retrieved February 22, 2017, from http://www.nursingworld.org/MainMenuCategories/Policy-Advocacy/State/Legislative-Agenda-Reports/State-TitleNurse/Title-Nurse-Summary-Language.html

American Nurses Association. (2013b). *States which require continuing education for RN licensure.* Kansas City, MO: Author. Retrieved February 22, 2017, from http://www.nursingworld.org/ MainMenuCategories/Policy-Advocacy/State/Legislative-Agenda-Reports/NursingEducation/ NursingEducationAdvancement/RN-CE-LicensureChart.pdf

American Nurses Association. (2013c). *Nursing licensure portability.* Kansas City, MO: Author. Retrieved February 22, 2017, from www.nursingworld.org/MainMenuCategories/Policy-Advocacy/Positions-and-Resolutions/Issue-Briefs/Nursing-Licensure-Portability.pdf

American Nurses Association, Congress for Nursing Practice. (1990). *Suggested state legislation: Nursing Practice Act, Disciplinary Diversion Act; Prescriptive Authority Act.* Kansas City, MO: Author.

American Nurses Credentialing Center. (2017). *APRN factsheet.* Silver Spring, MD: American Nurses Credentialing Center. Retrieved February 22, 2017, from http://www.nursecredentialing.org/ certification/aprncorner/aprn-factsheet

CGFNS-International. (2016). *Overview.* Retrieved February 27, 2017, from http://www.cgfns.org/ services/visascreen/

Council for Higher Education (CHEA). (2016). *Information about accreditation.* Washington, DC: Council for Higher Education Accreditation.

Institute of Medicine. (2010). *The future of nursing: Leading change, advancing health.* Washington, DC: National Academies Press.

Institute of Medicine. (2015). *Assessing progress on the IOM report the future of nursing.* Washington, DC: National Academies Press.

International Centre on Nurse Migration. (2016). *Mission, vision, and goals.* New York: Author. Retrieved March 23, 2017, from www.intlnursemigration.org

National Council of State Boards of Nursing. (2008). *Consensus model for APRN regulation: Licensure, accreditation, certification & education.* Retrieved March 23, 2017, from https://www.ncsbn.org/ Consensus_Model_for_APRN_Regulation_July_2008.pdf

National Council of State Boards of Nursing. (2011). *What you need to know about nursing licensure and boards of nursing.* Chicago, IL: Author. Retrieved May 11, 2018, from https://www.ncsbn.org/Nursing_ Licensure.pdf

National Council of State Boards of Nursing. (2014a). *Model nursing act and rules.* Chicago, IL: Author. Retrieved March 23, 2017, from https://www.ncsbn.org/3867.htm

National Council of State Boards of Nursing. (2014b). *State based licensure and telehealth.* Chicago, IL: Author. Retrieved February 22, 2017, from https://www.ncsbn.org/federal.htm

National Council of State Boards of Nursing. (2016a). *2017 NCLEX-RN test plan.* Chicago, IL: Author. Retrieved February 22, 2017, from https://www.ncsbn.org/8628.htm

National Council of State Boards of Nursing. (2016b). *2017 NCLEX-PN test plan.* Chicago, IL: Author. Retrieved February 22, 2017, from https://www.ncsbn.org/9812.htm

National Council of State Boards of Nursing. (2017). Chicago, IL: Author. Retrieved February 22, 2017, from https://www.nursys.com/LQC/LQCJurisdictions.aspx

National Council of State Boards of Nursing. (2017). *Professional boundaries.* Chicago, IL: Author. Retrieved May 11, 2018, from https://www.ncsbn.org/professional-boundaries.htm#3502

CHAPTER 4

Making Professional Goals a Reality

LEARNING OUTCOMES

After completing this chapter, you should be able to:

1. Describe the various employment opportunities available to nurses today and discuss the educational requirements of each.
2. Describe the competencies needed by the new graduate as outlined by the job analysis study that is the basis for the National Council Licensure Examination (NCLEX).
3. Analyze the eight common expectations employers have of new graduates explaining why each is important and relate them to your own background and education.
4. Develop a list of your personal short- and long-term career goals.
5. Prepare a personal résumé and sample letters of application, follow-up, and resignation.
6. Describe aspects to consider when preparing for an interview.
7. Formulate possible responses to an employment interview.

KEY TERMS

Application letter/cover letter	Proficiency
Competency	Résumé
Long-term goals	Short-term goals

Stegen & Sowerby Stories: Part 1

After working at your first RN job for 6 months, you are asked to be part of the hiring committee that will interview and hire RNs for two open positions. Having vacancies on your unit means that everyone is working extra shifts and it is important that the positions be filled quickly. There are a dozen applicants. The top six are identified and interviews are scheduled. There will be four people from the committee at each interview.

Interviews go well and the committee has determined the top two candidates that are equally qualified. When discussing the two candidates, at a meeting of the hiring committee, your supervisor feels that you should not hire one of the candidates because she alluded to the fact that she has diabetes and people with diabetes get sick a lot. She feels the candidate will be unreliable and unable to do her share of the work on the unit.

1. How do you feel about your supervisor's suggestion?
2. What are the ethical implications?
3. Are there any legal implications?
4. What are your personal feelings?
5. Do you agree with your supervisor?

When you graduate, one of your first goals will be to obtain employment as a registered nurse (RN). You probably look forward to practicing in the nursing role you have spent so long attaining. Although some new graduates have worked as unlicensed assistive staff or practical (vocational) nurses during their education, for others their only contact with healthcare settings may have been as students rather than as employees. You may not have experienced all of the many settings in which RNs are employed. You may have questions regarding employer expectations and your own role as an RN.

Planning a nursing career can be complex and finding that first job may be a challenge. In this chapter, we try to assist you as you survey the RN job market and plan for a successful approach to obtaining that important first position.

EMPLOYMENT OPPORTUNITIES TODAY

In 2008, the sudden economic recession affected healthcare institutions as well as every other part of society. Positions for new graduate RNs decreased. This was due in part to the effects of the economic recession—people without insurance put off all care; elective procedures were avoided, causing hospital census to drop; nurses who could retire continued working; and nurses who had been employed part-time accepted full-time positions. Orientation programs for new graduates are costly and if experienced nurses could be hired that was the preference.

According to the U.S. Bureau of Labor Statistics (2018), the long-term outlook for all nursing positions is excellent with 439,300 new jobs created between 2014 and 2024. This represents an increase of 16%, much greater than the average for all occupations. While the predicted shortage of nurses did not develop as predicted, there are still many parts of the country that are experiencing a lack of qualified nurses. Evidence-Based Practice 4.1 gives a good overview of the current issue.

Evidence-Based Practice 4.1: *The RN Workforce*

Clarke, S. P. (2016). RN workforce update: Current and long-range forecast. *Nursing Management, 47*(11), 20–25.

In the early 2000s, huge shortages in qualified RNs were predicted. Because of these predictions, many nursing programs expanded and applicants to these expanded programs were abundant. As the years passed, the predicted shortages have not materialized to the extent predicted. While there are still specific areas of the country where there are not enough RNs to fill vacancies, in general, the supply and demand are well balanced, and new graduates are finding jobs within a few months after graduation and in some areas may even have a job waiting before graduation.

Healthcare is a major sector of the economy and will continue to bring better than average employment prospects. There will be areas of the country that will experience significant shortages in the next decade. Nurses willing to relocate could find good career opportunities in those areas of the country.

In planning a job search, flexibility will be key. You may find it most productive to consider a range of positions you would like or to examine whether your most desired position would best be obtained by starting in a different position and moving to the desired position after becoming more experienced. You might consider changing your geographical location; some areas have a greater need for RNs than do others.

While just 61% of nursing jobs are located in hospitals (U.S. Bureau of Labor Statistics, 2018), most new graduates choose to begin their careers in structured healthcare settings where planned orientations and mentoring provide support for the novice in making the adjustment to the RN role. In its trend studies, the National Council of State Boards of Nursing (NCSBN) has identified changes over time in the work environments, employment characteristics, and job activities of newly licensed nurses. The most recent publication includes the data from the 2014 survey (NCSBN, 2015a). Of those responding, over 72% worked in hospital settings. Fifteen percent worked in long-term care and 10% worked in community-based or ambulatory care settings. This study showed that 18.7% of new graduates were employed in critical care and 27.7% were in medical–surgical units.

When reporting the types of clients for whom they care, newly licensed nurses most frequently identified acutely ill clients as the population for whom they cared with 50% including this population. 30.2% indicated they cared for clients older than 85 years, and 52.8% indicated caring for those aged 18 to 64. Much lower percentages indicated they care for children. Of those working a regular shift, 43.8% reported working day shift and 31.4% on the night shift. Rotating shifts are less common than a straight shift assignment with 12.5% reporting that they work rotating shifts (NCSBN, 2015a).

The number of positions for RNs in many settings other than those involved in providing direct client care has grown. Healthcare-oriented businesses, such as insurance companies and medical equipment supply companies, have found that it is often easier to teach nurses about business than to teach business people about healthcare. As a result, nurses are being employed in what some individuals see as nonnursing positions. Others argue that these, too, should be considered nursing positions, because the expertise that makes the individual successful is nursing expertise. Although experienced nurses usually hold these positions, moving into such positions may be a part of a career plan of the new graduate.

The number of men in nursing, which remained relatively small for many years, is beginning to grow as society reassesses its attitude toward labeling jobs as women's or men's work. In 2011, the number of men in nursing was estimated at 9.6%—up from 6.6% in 2008 (U.S. Census Bureau, 2013). Men have been attracted by the career opportunities and the improving economic picture offered by a career in nursing. The economic position of the nurse has improved for several reasons. One reason is the extension of laws governing fair labor practices to non-profit institutions and the advent of collective bargaining (see Chapter 5). Another major reason was the nursing shortage that occurred in the 1980s. The demand for nurses rose faster than the supply; employers began increasing salaries and benefits to attract nurses. This trend was especially notable in urban communities. Nurses comprise one of the largest segments of the US workforce and are among the highest paid with RN salaries averaging $67,490 per year (U.S. Bureau of Labor Statistics, 2018).

All these factors bring you, as a new graduate, into a world of uncertainty, but one also filled with opportunity and promise. We encourage you to look forward to the positive contribution that you can make to clients and to nursing practice.

> **Critical Thinking Activity: RN Employment**
> View several online job board for your location. Count the advertisements for RNs. How many employers are represented? Think of all the different healthcare agencies in the community. Do the ads represent most of them, some of them, or only a few of the potential employers of nurses? Of those listed, how many specify background or experience beyond that which a new graduate would have? How many specify the shift or work schedule? If wages are noted, what is the range of wages quoted? Reflect on your own expectations for employment after graduation. How do your expectations compare with what you find in these advertisements?

COMPETENCIES OF THE NEW GRADUATE

Recently, you may have heard the term *competency* used a great deal, especially as it applied to you as a student. **Competency**, as used here, refers to the ability of the person to effectively and safely perform specified nursing actions, including the application of critical thinking skills. Some have differentiated competency, which is an entry-level expectation, and proficiency, which is expected of the experienced nurse (Fig. 4.1).

Competencies Identified by Nursing Organizations

A number of nursing organizations have developed statements regarding the competencies expected of the new graduate. Chief among these organizations is the NCSBN.

Figure 4.1. New graduates are expected to know both their own abilities and when to seek appropriate help.

National Council of State Boards of Nursing Competencies

The most definitive statements on the competencies needed by the newly licensed practical nurse (PN) and the RN have been developed by the NCSBN based on its job analysis studies, which serve as the basis for the NCLEX-RN and NCLEX-PN.

In these studies, frequency and importance of activities reported by a stratified random sample of newly licensed, entry-level nurses were examined. Both the frequency of the nursing activities and their importance were studied. Importance was scaled from 1 (not important) to 5 (critically important) and was in regard to the maintenance of client safety and/or threat of complications or distress (NCSBN, 2015a). The last published RN study was completed in 2015; the results of that study supported changes to the current test plan for 2016 (NCSBN, 2015b). The most recent PN study was completed in 2015 (NCSBN, 2016a) with a new test plan initiated in 2017 (NCSBN, 2016b).

In addition to looking at activities for all new graduates in general, the study also looked at activities in relationship to the care setting. Physiologic and psychosocial integrity were supported by many individual nursing actions. Some, such as assessing vital signs, seemed almost universal. Others, such as monitoring for side effects of radiation therapy, were needed in a minority of settings. Allowing clients to talk about their concerns and assisting them to communicate effectively were almost universal activities.

When recent graduates were surveyed regarding important postgraduate competencies, they were provided with a list of activities and asked to rank the amount of time spent on each category (NCSBN, 2015a). The categories, in order of time spent, were

- Management of care
- Safety and infection control
- Health promotion and maintenance
- Psychosocial integrity
- Basic care and comfort
- Pharmacologic and parenteral therapies
- Reduction of risk potential
- Physiologic adaptation

National League for Nursing Competencies

In addition to the NCSBN, other organizations have explored the issue of competencies of new nursing graduates. The various educational councils that were previously a part of the NLN structure developed statements regarding competencies of new graduates during the late 1970s through the 1980s. All educational councils were eliminated in restructuring of the NLN. In 2010, after a great deal of study and work, the NLN developed a comprehensive statement of the expected outcomes and competencies of each level of nursing education from practical/vocational through the research doctorate in nursing. This research was updated in 2012 and is used to guide programs in building curricula (NLN, 2012).

Competencies Expressed by Other Groups

In 1998, the American Association of Colleges of Nursing (AACN) developed a document titled, *Essentials of Baccalaureate Education for Professional Nursing Practice*, which was last updated in 2008 (AACN, 2008). This document identifies essentials for education that are aimed at developing the competencies needed. Additionally, some states have developed statements of competencies for graduates of the nursing programs in those states. This has often been part of a process to improve articulation between programs at different levels.

Employers' Expectations Regarding Competencies

Employers often ask for further clarification of competence. Does competence mean that the new graduate can function independently, or will some supervision still be needed? Further complicating the picture is the confusion surrounding competencies of the graduates of the three types of nursing education programs that prepare individuals for RN licensure (see Chapter 2). Although statements by several organizations have distinguished among levels of functioning, many employers do not differentiate expectations.

What is expected of the new graduate varies across healthcare agencies and geographic areas. The acuity of the client care load and the types of services offered by an agency also may affect expectations. The Joint Commission has a criterion requiring that accredited institutions monitor and ensure the competence of their staff. This requires that an institution identify expected competencies for staff and then design an assessment method. As institutions move to comply with this standard, most direct their initial efforts toward technical skills because these are more easily identified and assessed. Other competencies are more difficult to assess. Patricia Benner, a prominent nurse theorist, explains that RNs go through several stages as they progress in their chosen career. Read more about her Novice to Expert theory in the Theory Alert that follows.

Theory Alert   *Patricia Benner*

Patricia Benner mapped the stages of a nurse's expertise. She earned her bachelor's degree in nursing in 1964. Since earning her PhD from the University of California at Berkley in 1982, she has been teaching and researching at the University of California at San Francisco, where she is currently a professor emerita.

Benner's developed the theory known as *Novice to Expert*. She identifies five levels of experience in nursing: novice, advanced beginner, competent, proficient, and expert. Nurses move through these stages as they progress in their chosen specialty area. If they change areas, they will begin again at a lower level of experience. This theory recognizes that the nurse with the highest pay or most prestigious title may not be the expert nurse.

Experience gained before licensure, working in healthcare, can be very beneficial to the newly graduated RN. However, the licensure exam confirms that the new graduate is prepared to begin his or her nursing career as a novice
(Source: www.nursing-theory.org.)

Some general patterns of expectations can be seen:

1. **Possess the necessary theoretic background for safe client care and for decision-making.** The new graduate must know when an emergency or complication occurs and secure medical help for the client. Many employers believe that new graduates today are very competent in their theoretic foundations for practice.

2. **Use the nursing process in a systematic way.** This includes assessment, analysis, planning, intervention, and evaluation. As noted previously, a large percentage of the new graduates' time is spent in activities they would describe as using the steps of the nursing process. New graduates should be able to develop plans of care and follow plans that have been developed by the agency.

3. **Recognize own abilities and limitations.** To provide safe care, the nurse must identify when a situation requires greater expertise or knowledge and when assistance is needed. Employers may be able to assist if nurses ask for help and direction but cannot accept the risk to clients created by nurses who do not know or accept their own limitations.

4. **Use communication skills effectively with clients and coworkers.** In every setting, there are clients and families who are anxious, depressed, suffering loss, angry, or experiencing other emotional distress. The nurse is expected to respond appropriately to these individuals and to facilitate their coping and adaptation. Effective communication skills are essential to the functioning of the entire interdisciplinary healthcare team. Often, the nurse is expected to help coordinate the work of others, and this cannot be done without effective communication skills.

5. **Work effectively with assistive personnel, delegating and supervising nursing care tasks in an appropriate manner.** In most settings, assistive personnel are a part of the nursing team. The RN, and in some instances the PN, is expected to identify which nursing activities can be delegated and do so in a way that contributes to appropriate client care outcomes.

6. **Provide accurate and complete documentation.** Employers generally recognize that the new graduate must be given time to learn the documentation system used in the facility. However, the new graduate is expected to recognize the need for recording data. It is anticipated that the nurse will keep accurate, grammatically correct, and legible written records and complete electronic records that provide the necessary legal documentation of care.

7. **Possess proficiency in the basic technical nursing skills.** This is an area in which a wide variety of expectations may be present. In most settings, **proficiency** in the basic skills required to support activities of daily living is expected. In some settings, nurses will carry out these tasks, whereas in others they will direct or teach others, such as nursing assistants or family members, to do them. The settings in which nurses practice are wide-ranging, and the technical skills needed in one setting may not be required in another.

8. **Possess basic skills in information technology.** Nurses of today must be able to learn and navigate the computer system in use in a particular facility, manage e-mail communication, seek information resources to support evidence-based care, and use electronic medical records.

In addition to these professional responsibilities performed as a nurse, employers also speak of their concern for worker-related competencies they want to see in all healthcare workers. These include the following:

1. **Demonstrate a commitment to a work ethic.** This means that the employee will take the responsibility of the job seriously and will be on time, take only the allowed coffee and lunch breaks, and will not take sick days unless truly ill. It also means that the new graduate recognizes that nurses are needed 24 hours a day, 365 days a year, and that this may require sacrifices of personal convenience, including working evening shifts or on holidays.

2. **Function with acceptable speed.** This is another area in which expectations differ greatly. Generally, an orientation period is planned—although, with the pressures on healthcare agencies, this often has been shortened considerably. An acceptable speed of function is reflected by the ability to carry out a typical RN assignment within a shift.

PERSONAL CAREER GOALS

In caring for clients, you are involved in the process of goal setting. Many nurses recognize the value of this in client care but never transfer the concept to their personal lives. Nursing as a profession offers many career options. Without carefully setting goals, your professional growth may be impeded. As well as the information here, you may want to explore the websites listed on *thePoint* that relate to personal goal setting.

Focusing Your Goals

You may want to focus on a broad area of clinical competency, such as pediatric nursing, or on a more restricted area, such as neonatal care. Clinical areas available for concentrated effort become more varied as healthcare becomes more complex. Most of these areas offer certification to individuals who possess the expertise and pass the examinations. Many individuals focus their careers on particular client populations without ever seeking formal certification in that field. However, there may be advantages in terms of salary and recognition to holding specialty certification.

Opportunities for additional education and certification in most clinical specialties are available for any experienced RN, although some require that the individual have a bachelor's or master's degree in nursing. Some specialty positions are in advanced practice, such as the woman's healthcare specialist, the family nurse practitioner, and the pediatric nurse practitioner. These advanced practice specialties require a master's degree for certification. Although some educational programs preparing advanced practice nurses require the bachelor's degree in nursing for entry, many will accept an individual with an ADN combined with a bachelor's degree in another field.

Another approach may be to focus your goals on the setting in which care is delivered, such as acute, long-term, or community care. As healthcare needs expand, these separate realms of care delivery all demand more specialized knowledge. Even within the individual area of focus, differences are present. For example, within the community are ambulatory care settings, public health nursing agencies, occupational health nursing departments, and day care facilities.

Another way of focusing your goals is according to functional categories. Although nurses are initially thought of as direct care providers, they also are needed in many other positions. For example, there is need for those who would move into supervisory and administrative capacities, those who teach, and those who conduct nursing research. Additional education supports the ability to advance into these fields. Nursing also lends itself to writing, community service, and even political involvement.

You may decide to set your goals in relation to all three areas identified above; you might identify a clinical area, care setting, and functional category.

Setting Your Goals

The first step in setting personal career goals is a thorough self-assessment. Determine how your abilities and competencies correspond to your own expectations and to those of employers. Other factors to explore are your likes and dislikes and the situations or types of work you particularly enjoyed as a student. Consider the area in which you were most successful. Were there areas in which you or your instructor felt that you were an above-average student? Consider your health and personal characteristics in relation to types of work. Do you have physical restrictions? Do you prefer working independently or with others? Do you prefer a work environment that is relatively predictable, or do you thrive in situations that change frequently? Another factor to consider is your own geographic mobility: would you be willing to move or travel as part of a job?

As you plan ahead, examine the many options offered by nursing. What types of jobs and opportunities are open to you? What education and personal abilities are needed in these areas? Does the education you have meet the educational requirements? Are avenues for additional education available to you? All of these considerations are important as you plan for the future. Career goals need to be both short and long term. They will help you to plan your future constructively. This does not mean that goals are static. Just as client goals must be realistic, personal, and flexible, so must your own goals.

Short-term goals encompass what you want to accomplish this month and this year. What do you want to do and what do you want to be in the immediate future? For example, you might decide that your short-term goal is to have 2 years of solid experience in a busy metropolitan hospital.

Long-term goals represent where you want to be in your profession 5 or more years from now. A long-term goal may be to work in a small, remote community in which you will have the opportunity to function autonomously.

Although both long- and short-term goals may be revised as your life evolves, they guide you in making day-to-day decisions more effectively. In today's world of rapid healthcare change, you may need to keep your goals somewhat broad and flexible. Be ready to consider alternative goals and a variety of pathways to one goal. These approaches will be of value as you enter a system in transition **(Fig. 4.2)**.

Figure 4.2. Clearly visualizing goals helps you to achieve them.

> **Critical Thinking Activity: Professional Goals**
> Write out your short- and long-term professional goals and a brief plan on how you can achieve these goals. Think critically about the obstacles you will need to overcome to reach these goals. How will you deal with the obstacles?

Maintaining and Enhancing Your Competence

Included in your goal setting should be an approach to maintaining and enhancing your competence. Every nurse has an obligation to society to maintain competence and continue practicing high-quality, safe care. Most state boards of nursing have identified a mechanism for identifying continued competence for ongoing practice. Some of the most common ways are through work as an RN, through reflective practice, through continuing education, and through self-directed study.

Practicing as an RN keeps you up-to-date and provides you the opportunity to learn new technology, to see new procedures, and to care for complex clients requiring critical thinking and decision-making skills. Most employers provide in-service education regarding policies and procedures to enhance your competence. Maintaining and enhancing competence through practice requires that you focus your critical thinking on your own development as a nurse. You may develop the habit of reflective practice for this purpose. In reflective practice, you take the time to debrief after incidents and go back over the situation identifying what went well and what needed improvement. This may be done in a group or independently. Reflective practice is often enhanced by keeping a journal in which you write down your reflections (being sure to eliminate any personally identifiable health information regarding clients). Thus, you move your own practice forward improving your own competence. You may set goals for your own learning and professional development.

Continuing education may occur through workshops, conferences, and completing online classes. Computer instruction programs and examinations related to journal articles may be completed on your own time frame. Self-directed study may involve subscribing to and reading journals, participating in a journal club, or researching Web information. Some nurses may want to advance through specialty or higher education. Any of these avenues may be appropriate, depending on the circumstances. As a new graduate, you may be hired at a facility that has a new nurse residency program. These programs are highly effective and help the new graduate gain confidence, which is helpful to transition to practice smoothly. For more inform about gaining professional confidence as a new graduate, see Evidence-Based Practic

MAKING GOALS REALITY

Philosophic questions regarding goals must be resolved by practical appro
new graduate, your first goal simply may be to get a job in nursing. Ke
not applying only for an entry-level job. If you have identified a spe
you wish to work, a specific employer you prefer, or a long-ter
from one position to another, then you need to do those thin
preferred position, not just any position. Additionally, wh
also may be making an impression that will affect later r
opportunities. Those who interview you for an entry-lev
future job assignments. The impression you make initially w

Evidence-Based Practice 4.2: Gaining Professional Confidence as a New Graduate

Ortiz, J. (2016). New graduate nurses' experiences about lack of professional confidence. *Nurse Education in Practice, 19,* 19–24. doi:10.1016/j.nepr.2016.04.001

Professional confidence is something that new graduates lack. This confidence develops over time, and many recent graduates felt that the mentoring or preceptor relationships were key to the development of professional confidence. As new graduates added to their experience, both positive and negative aspects were identified by the participants in this research study.

It was determined that new graduates must experience both positive and negative circumstances to develop the professional confidence that is essential to successful transition into the nursing profession. Some of the negative circumstances were identified as *communication is huge, making mistakes,* and *disconnect between school and practice.* Positive circumstances were labeled *independence, relationship building, positive feedback is important,* and *gaining experience.*

Having a mentor that supports the new graduate through both the positive and negative circumstances is essential for successful transition to the nurse role. The process of gaining professional confidence is dynamic with the new RN feeling both positive and negative emotions about performance of the nursing duties. With good mentorship, professional confidence is increased.

Figure 4.3. Making goals reality.

Whatever the situation, you are more likely to realize your goals if you are prepared to present yourself in the best possible way to a prospective employer. Many of you have held different jobs in the community as students and as adults. You may be familiar with and competent in the job search process. Others have never applied for the kind of job that could be considered the beginning of a career. Employers and prospective employees may hold different expectations in such a situation.

Identifying Potential Employers

To begin your job search effectively, you need to identify potential employers. You might begin your review with those more familiar to you, such as those where you have had clinical experiences during your education, and gradually move outward in an ever-widening circle to identify others. You might network with instructors, colleagues, and fellow graduates for opportunities. If you worked as an employee in a healthcare setting before graduation, you may be given preference in hiring at that institution. This is one reason for seeking healthcare employment during your nursing education process.

Job fairs for healthcare employers are becoming more common. Each employer participating sets up a booth or table to provide information on job openings in its agency. An individual looking for employment may explore a variety of employers, learning about job openings, benefits, and opportunities in a brief time without the difficulty of searching out each employer. The employer may see many potential employees in a focused period. Thus, job fairs benefit both employers and potential employees. Job fairs may be held in the community, attracting experienced healthcare workers as well as students and new graduates. Some colleges arrange job fairs on campus. Nursing programs or nursing student clubs also may arrange job fairs. When attending a job fair, prepare and dress as if you going to an interview (see below). Prospective employers begin to form their impression of you at the job fair.

A prominent source of potential jobs is the Internet. Many government job openings are posted online. An online search may reveal the names of nursing employers in your area as well as those at other locations of interest to you. Using a search engine, look for "employment opportunities," "jobs," or "careers" combined with the term "nursing." Some online service providers have additional support services for a job search that might include career guidance (for a fee) or sample documents such as résumés and letters of application.

Major nursing journals have sections in the back pages devoted to advertisements. Some of these advertise nursing positions. Sometimes, an entire issue is devoted to a specific geographic area. This provides the ability to do a quick overview of possible employers. Your nursing program may receive advertising magazines that are designed to present job opportunities for new graduates. These magazines provide a few articles about relevant job search topics, such as interviewing, as well as advertisements from healthcare agencies. These advertisements present information on the agency itself and how to make contact for an application.

Another source of potential jobs is the classified section of the local newspaper. There you may find jobs in small facilities, as well as general recruitment announcements from larger facilities. However, just because an agency fails to advertise does not mean it will not be hiring any employees. Advertising is expensive and may not result in the desired outcome. Therefore, some healthcare agencies do not advertise and rely on those who independently seek them out as potential employers.

In areas of the country where jobs are very scarce for new graduates, unpaid nursing internships have been developed. These provide job experience to enhance the new graduate's skills and abilities and increase the potential for hiring.

Letter of Application

Writing a letter of **application** is an excellent way to approach many prospective employers (Box 4.1). This letter is often termed a **cover letter** because it is sent with your résumé. You can present yourself positively through a well-written letter. Some question the value of

BOX 4.1 LETTER OF APPLICATION

Maribeth Wilson
3428 1st Ave. N.
Seattle, WA 98103
(206) 274-5978
E-mail: maribethw@email.com
May 20, 2010

Joyce Montgall, R.N.
Nurse Recruiter
Seattle General Medical Center
321 Heath Blvd.
Seattle, WA 98101

Dear Ms. Montgall:

Enclosed please find a copy of my résumé, along with my application to Seattle General Medical Center's New Graduate Residency Program. I will graduate from Shoreline Community College' associate degree nursing program on June 8, 2011. I expect to acquire my registered nurse license by the end of July. I am extremely interested in a medical-surgical nursing position within your upcoming residency program.

I believe that I would bring many strengths to a new graduate position. I have worked here at Seattle General as a nursing assistant for the past year, and my experience has given me an excellent foundation in understanding the philosophy and mission of the Medical Center. During this time I have been assigned to several different units, including 4 West and 4 Center, where new graduate positions are available. The nurses at Seattle General have been generous in their mentoring and have helped me to increase my understanding of the clients' conditions. They have been supportive as I developed increased problem-solving and decision-making skills. I am familiar with the documentation system and the policies of the institution.

Within my nursing student educational experience, I have had the privilege of working in a wide variety of healthcare institutions throughout the city. From these experiences I would bring an understanding of the community standards of care as well as a unique appreciation of the position of Seattle General in the healthcare community.

I hope that I will be selected for an interview and look forward to hearing from you. My phone number, e-mail address, and home address are at the top of this letter. I am available most afternoons. If I do not hear from you within the next 2 weeks, I will contact your office to ascertain the status of my application.

Sincerely,

Maribeth Wilson

the cover letter; however, employment experts support the use of cover letters saying that an effective cover letter forges a connection with the employer and can set you apart from other applicants. The cover letter should package your résumé so that it will get more than just a glance. It provides the opportunity for you to reveal a bit of your personality and connects your experience to the position's requirements.

Before you write your letter, make sure you have information about the prospective employer. What kind of facility is this? What types of clients does it serve, and what special services does it offer? It makes a poor impression to write to a prospective employer stating that your goal is to work in pediatrics when that facility does not provide any pediatric services. Many agencies maintain a website with information regarding their mission, goals, and services. You might also obtain this information by calling the human resources department of the facility or by contacting a public information office. In a small agency, you may simply speak with a receptionist or secretary. If you call for information, be honest and straightforward in explaining that you are considering applying for employment and would like information about the agency before making that decision. The letter is sent to the nurse recruiter (if the agency has one) or to the human resources department along with your résumé. If you are not sure to whom to address your letter, check the agency's website or ask when you call to inquire about the agency itself.

Another part of your advance planning is identifying how you will focus your letter on your special qualifications and what you want to highlight. Focus on the skills or accomplishments related to the position you want. Your letter should be no more than one page in length, but should present all essential information. Introduce yourself and your purpose for writing in the first paragraph so that the reader immediately understands why you are writing. You may want to state briefly your reasons for applying for a position with this particular employer. The more specific the reasons, the better the impression you are likely to make.

Use the body of the letter to briefly highlight your qualifications for the position. This should not be a simple recitation of what is in your résumé, but should either present the information in a slightly different light or add pertinent detail that is not in the résumé. If you are responding to an advertisement, touch on each of the qualifications listed in the advertisement. You might include personal qualities that would make you an effective employee in the position, such as interest in learning and skill in teamwork. Relate your skills and abilities to the needs of this particular agency. If your healthcare experience is limited, point out skills you have gained from other jobs that would be useful in nursing. These might be interpersonal skills, management skills, or adaptability.

In the final paragraph, make a summary statement indicating why you want to work for this employer and ask for an appointment for an interview. Be sure to indicate the times you are available and how and where you can be contacted if the employer so wishes. It also is wise to indicate that you will contact the person to whom the letter is addressed to request an appointment. This allows you to maintain some initiative in the process. Thank the person for considering your application, and close.

Another point to remember is that the letter's appearance and its content both represent you. You will be judged on spelling, grammar, clarity, and neatness, in addition to content. Be cautious about relying on the spell-checking function on your computer. An incorrect word may pass the spell-check but be clearly seen as an error by the careful reader. Your letter of application should be written in standard business format on plain white or off-white business paper. Make it brief and clear. Ask a friend or family member to check your first draft if you have any questions about its correctness.

> **Critical Thinking Activity: Job Search and Application for Work**
> Identify an area of the country and type of nursing position that interests you. Using the various Internet resources, learn about job availability, salaries, and working conditions for at least three employers in that area. Determine which of the three would be of most interest to you and write a letter of application (cover letter) specific to that position.

Preparing an Effective Résumé

A **résumé** is a brief overview of your qualifications for a position. Its purpose is to present you in the most positive light to be considered for the position in which you are interested and to provide the employer with a way to identify quickly whether you have the basic qualifications for a position. Résumés are used primarily to screen applicants for interviewing; therefore, you will want to make a good impression that will result in an interview. You will want to include your résumé with your initial letter. In addition, have copies of your résumé to take with you to any interview or appointment. You may want to leave a copy of your résumé with a unit manager at the end of an interview because your original résumé may be retained in the human resources office. Résumés may be posted online through job search sites. If posting online, check on the privacy policies of the site. Use care in what you place in an online résumé for your own safety.

Appearance of Your Résumé

The appearance of your résumé is important because it initially presents your image to the prospective employer. You want its appearance to reflect a competent, professional image. It is not necessary to have a professionally produced résumé. Nursing employers, when asked, have indicated that it neither adds to nor detracts from their impression to read a résumé that has been produced by some professional printing method. The important point is that it be a somewhat formal, standard, informative document that is neat and without errors.

Your résumé should be on standard-sized (8.5″ × 11″), white or off-white, good-quality paper so that it is easy to handle, file, and read. A résumé that is individually printed (or reproduced well enough so that it appears to be) usually will be received more positively than an obvious photocopy. You will find it valuable to create a résumé and save it in a way you will be able to revise it easily. You will need to be able to tailor it to an individual job situation. In addition to the capabilities of standard word processing software (which usually include résumé templates), there are inexpensive software programs especially designed to facilitate the production of a well-organized and formatted résumé.

To achieve legibility, use sufficient margins (usually 1″), spacing, indentation, bullets, and even line separators to separate different sections and topics. You might want to underline or italicize related items or bold print or highlight important items to draw swift attention. A résumé looks better when the content is evenly balanced on a page. Dense paragraphs do not attract the reader, but lists and topics do. Use capital letters, bold font, and underlining to draw the reader's eye to what you want that individual to notice first, but be careful not to overdo this approach. When an employer is reviewing many such documents, anything that facilitates review and makes you stand out is an advantage. Often, the use of bullets helps to break up the tedium of words. Ask individuals you trust to review the appearance of your résumé and offer feedback.

If your résumé will be viewed online, consider how that will affect the appearance. Special fonts or nonstandard résumé programs may not transfer effectively into the online environment. A job site will provide directions for a posted résumé. If your résumé is sent as an attachment to an e-mail, then it should be composed in a common word processing program such as Microsoft Word or in rich text format (.rtf). You might check with the receiving human resources department as to its preference for format.

Traditionally, applicants have been advised to keep résumés to one page if possible although an online résumé may be longer than one page. To develop a one-page résumé, consider how you might most effectively present employment history. However, more important in today' market is that the information supports your candidacy for the position you are seeking and thus may be more than a single page.

Content of Your Résumé

The content of your résumé is critical. When you are beginning the preparation of a résumé, first list the information that you want to include in some way. Making such a list before beginning the process of actually formatting a résumé helps you to take an organized approach and not forget to include important information. If you will be submitting a résumé online, this process should include identifying specific key words that you want to include within the résumé. Often, employers search online résumés using key words that pertain to the type of position they have available or specific skills and abilities that are needed in the position. If your résumé does not contain these key words, it will not be identified as relevant to the employer.

A standard résumé always begins with your name, address, and telephone number (including area code). If you will be moving, indicate the date the move will be effective and provide an alternate method of contacting you after that date. You may use the address of a permanently settled relative or friend. Employers are not permitted to ask about age, race, religion, marital status, sexual orientation, and dependents, and you should not include this information. An e-mail address is helpful to employers. However, if your e-mail address is an informal phrase, or could be viewed as unprofessional, plan to set up a separate e-mail address for business use. Use a simple derivation from your name that creates a professional impression. One final comment regarding content: be certain that it is accurate. It should be assumed that you will be checked on what you say in your résumé so truthfulness is always the best bet.

Objective

Many résumés include a personal goal or objective. This is helpful to a recruiter or human resources department that considers many different occupations within the agency. The objective immediately alerts the reader to the type of position being sought. This may include both a short-term goal such as "employment as a beginning registered nurse" and a long-term goal such as "with eventual move to employment in coronary care." You may wish to write an objective that is tailored to a specific employer or job announcement. When you are more experienced, you may want to make your objective more specific to a particular department or role (see Box 4.3 later for an example).

Some career advisors today are suggesting a statement of what you can provide for the employer is more effective than an objective that focuses on your own goals. It should show the employer how they can benefit from hiring you, how you can make a contribution. This statement should focus on what you can do rather than on what you want. This must be done very succinctly so as to quickly catch the attention of the individual reading the résumé. The remainder of the résumé should reinforce this first impression (see Box 4.4 later for an example).

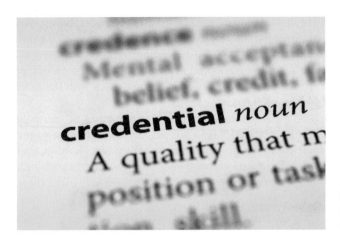

Figure 4.4. A résumé includes information regarding your licensure and other credentials.

Credentials

Include information regarding your licensure and other credentials **(Fig. 4.4)**. Indicate the date your license will be effective and whether you have a temporary permit to work as a nurse. Your nursing license or permit number should be listed after you have received it. If you do not have a license at the time you are preparing your résumé, you may choose to include information about when you expect to have your license in your letter of application.

Education

Educational background should form a separate section and cover your nursing education and any specialized courses or postgraduate work you have completed. It is appropriate to note any college-level work. Do not include high school information. In each group of information, list the most recent items first.

Employment History

Work experience is of critical importance, and you should provide a meaningful employment history. If using a traditional format, for each job you held include employer, address (city and state are sufficient), dates employed, position, and duties. List the most recent employer first and follow with the remaining information in reverse chronologic order. The prospective employer will be especially interested in a previous nursing assistant position or any other position that demonstrates your knowledge of or experience in some area of healthcare or the assumption of responsibility. Other positions also may be important if you are clearly able to identify skills used in those settings that are transferable to nursing.

If you have had only one or two part-time jobs during your educational program, it would be appropriate to include them in detail. However, if during your educational program you held 15 part-time jobs, for example, it is appropriate to list only significant ones that offered valuable experience. If you do not have paid work experience, you could list any internship hours that pertain to the type of employment you are seeking.

Focus on accomplishments and use active verbs to describe skills. These give life to your résumé and create interest in the reader. See the accompanying box for a list of active verbs you might use in describing your skills and abilities (Box 4.2). If you were part of a team that accomplished a significant project or task, you might indicate that. However, be careful

BOX 4.2 POWER VERBS FOR RÉSUMÉS

- Use of verbs without subjects will be more concise and space conserving.
- Use of active, not passive, voice, such as "advanced to" rather than "was promoted to," "earned" rather than "was given," indicates a person who does things rather than receives them.
- Use of "-ed" or "-ing" as verb endings can both be effective.

Accompanied	Directed	Inspired	Processed
Achieved	Discovered	Installed	Procured
Acquired	Displayed	Instructed	Produced
Activated	Doubled	Insured	Progressed
Administered	Earned	Integrated	Promoted
Advanced to	Educated	Intensified	Prompted
Advised	Employed	Interviewed	Proposed
Analyzed	Enacted	Invented	Proved
Arranged	Encouraged	Led	Provided
Assembled	Engineered	Located	Reconciled
Assessed	Established	Maintained	Reduced
Assisted	Evaluated	Managed	Regulated
Balanced	Executed	Marketed	Related
Budgeted	Exhibited	Mastered	Reorganized
Clarified	Expanded	Mediated	Reported
Composed	Facilitated	Motivated	Represented
Conceived	Financed	Negotiated	Researched
Concluded	Formalized	Nominated	Satisfied
Conducted	Formed	Obtained	Secured
Constructed	Formulated	Officiated	Served
Consulted	Founded	Operated	Simplified
Controlled	Generated	Ordered	Solved
Converted	Governed	Organized	Structured
Coordinated	Graduated	Originated	Succeeded
Counseled	Headed	Overcame	Supervised
Created	Identified	Participated	Trained
Decided	Implemented	Perceived	Transferred
Delegated	Improved	Perfected	Transformed
Demonstrated	Improvised	Performed	Unified
Designed	Increased	Piloted	Verified
Detailed	Induced	Pioneered	Won
Determined	Influenced	Placed	Wrote
Developed	Informed	Planned	
Devised	Initiated	Prepared	
Diagnosed	Innovated	Presided	

not to take personal credit for team accomplishments. If you are responding to a specific job announcement, be sure that your résumé reflects the education and skills that are noted.

In a position-focused résumé, you can emphasize the responsibilities you had within each position. See Box 4.3 for an example of a position-focused résumé. You might also highlight

---

BOX 4.3 POSITION-FOCUSED RÉSUMÉ OF A RECENT GRADUATE

Sarah Mitchell
5714 31st Ave. N.
Seattle, WA 98117
(206) 555-0000
E-mail: sarahmit@email.com

Objective
A beginning Registered Nurse position that will provide the opportunity for professional development and advancement toward critical care nursing.
Overall qualifications: Possesses a positive, energetic approach to working collaboratively with others, solving problems, and providing evidence-based, client-centered nursing care.

Experience

2009–present   Seattle General Medical Center   Seattle, WA

Client Care Technician, Medical-Surgical Units

• Provide basic care and ADLs with attention to psychosocial needs for acutely ill medical-surgical clients.
• Assist RN with procedures and carry out delegated duties.
• Work collaboratively with nursing team, assuring prompt response to client needs.
• Effectively manage time to support seven clients on evening shift.
• Document care on computerized system, maintaining accuracy, and confidentiality.

2007–2009   Health Choice Urgent Care Center   Seattle, WA

Nursing Technician, Urgent Care Clinic

• Interviewed clients, took vital signs, initiated documentation, and prioritized care for urgently ill and injured adults and children.
• Under RN supervision, performed assessments, dressing changes, ECGs, nebulizer treatments, and hospital admission processes.
• Attended to psychosocial needs of family and others accompanying a sick or injured individual.

2005–2007 First United Bank Lynnwood, WA.

Bank Teller

• Maintained excellent customer service by following detailed bank policies and procedures.
• Incorporated information from employee training classes into job skills to assure up-to-date function.

Education

2008–2011   Shoreline Community College   Seattle, WA

AAS Nursing, to be Awarded June 2011

specific experiences in an area that especially relates to the position for which you are applying. For example, you might have had a senior leadership practicum on an orthopedic unit—this would be particularly relevant to an application for a nursing position in orthopedics. If you had a practicum in the facility or agency to which you are applying, indicate this in some way. Your familiarity with its policies and procedures will be a valuable asset. If you attended any special workshops, include those in a separate section. Information included in this part of the résumé can be used to demonstrate your ability to meet deadlines, produce good work, and relate to people in ambiguous situations. Use numbers when possible to describe achievements. For example, if you previously worked evenings in a long-term care facility as an LPN, you might state, "Supervised five nursing assistants" or "Administered all medications to 30 clients per shift." Be sure to include language proficiency if you are fluent in more than English. Computer literacy is essential for electronic charting; you might indicate the charting systems you are familiar with if you have used several.

You may choose a more skill-focused résumé and not include details of all your previous positions separately. For individuals who are older and have an extensive employment history, a résumé providing types of positions with a focus on related skills rather than a chronologic list of employers is often the most effective. List a position such as LPN and include responsibilities and skills for all employers followed by a simple list of employers. This keeps the résumé from becoming repetitive as the same information is presented for each employer. See Box 4.4 for an example of a skill-focused employment section.

Additional Experience

Volunteer or community work and awards and honors form two sections when you have these experiences. Choose the items you list under volunteer and community work carefully. Employers are interested in skills you would bring to the job that require decision-making and the exercise of good judgment (both in volunteer work and in past work experience). In some instances, you may want to list briefly the skills or abilities gained, targeting the particular skills you think are important to the position for which you are applying. For example, you might use your volunteer experience to demonstrate past success in the skill of organization, managing or coordinating people and events, and effectively delegating responsibilities.

List awards, honors, and professional associations (such as the National Student Nurses' Association) that would demonstrate your competence, professional involvement, or leadership ability. This provides an opportunity to show responsibility in directing the activities of others, public speaking, and, perhaps, motivating people. You may omit this section if you feel that you have nothing pertinent to enter.

References

References are typed on a separate page and given to the prospective employer or copied onto an application form, if they are requested. Be selective in choosing the people you list as references. Consider people who know you, would be able to speak positively of you to a future employer, and would have credibility with the employer. Seek the person's permission before giving his or her name as a reference.

A primary reference should be an instructor from your basic educational program. This person would be able to affirm your ability in the nursing field. Some agencies request two instructor references, so be prepared for that. Another reference should be someone who has employed you and who can describe your work habits and effectiveness as an employee.

BOX 4.4 SKILL-FOCUSED RÉSUMÉ OF A RECENT GRADUATE

Joseph M. Sanchez
1298 Avenida Diaz
La Quinta, CA 92252
(619) 524-4321

Objective
An opportunity to provide excellent, customer-focused care using evidence-based practice and contributing to Main Medical Center's status as the premier hospital in the tristate region.

Skills/Accomplishments
- Work effectively in a multicultural environment.
- Communication skills: Earned award for communicating in a positive, supportive way with coworkers, clients, and families.
- Bilingual Spanish/English: Developed Spanish language instructions to assist clients.
- Collaborative/cooperative worker: Volunteered to work multiple shifts/floating positions in order to allow colleagues to meet important family needs.
- Excellent critical thinking and problem solving: Identified cost saving approaches to work processes.

Education
College of the Desert, Palm Desert, CA
Management practicum, Desert Health Center 5-West: Working with RN preceptor, demonstrated RN level skills in managing care of a module of five acutely ill clients. Delegated care appropriately to nursing assistant. Facilitated interdisciplinary communication.
Associate in Science in Nursing, June 2011

Experience
Manor Care Center, Palm Desert, CA
Nursing Assistant, Certified: 2005–Present
- Maintained function and dignity of dependent elderly adults by providing direct care, strong interpersonal relationships, and effective collaboration with nursing and allied health.
- Earned promotion to position of mentor for new hires and team leader for a group of nursing assistants. Facilitated team performance to accomplish assigned responsibilities.
Northrup Corporation, Los Angeles, CA
Machinist: 1995–2005
- Performed precision skills with accuracy and attention to detail.
- Followed precise written protocols and procedures to ensure quality.
- Led a team in a program of total quality management within our department.

Awards
- College of the Desert Merit Scholar 2010
- Golden Acorn Award for Leadership in Parent Involvement, Cactus Valley Elementary School PTA, La Quinta, CA

If you have had any healthcare work experience, this would be the best work reference. Also, look at the position in which you assumed the most responsibility. This should be reasonably recent (within the past 10 years). Again, some employers ask for two work references.

If the agency indicates the type of references they want, supply the names of references that comply with the agency' request. When types of references are not specified, include professional or work-related references only. Include full names with titles (if any), addresses, and telephone numbers, so that the employer will be able to contact the references easily.

Employers express differences of opinion about the value of a standardized letter of reference addressed "To Whom It May Concern." Some employers may consider this a useful initial presentation of your qualifications. Other employers want the reference to address the specific position needs or the qualifications outlined on a reference form. If you do obtain this type of general reference letter, be sure to preserve the original carefully (perhaps in a clear, plastic page protector) to show to a potential employer; you then would provide a good-quality photocopy for the employer to place in your file. Even when an employer accepts this as an initial reference, your references are usually be contacted as well.

> **Critical Thinking Activity: Cover Letter**
> Create an effective résumé that presents you as a positive addition to a nursing staff. Create an application/cover letter for a specific nursing position you have learned about in a search of possible employers.

Completing an Application

Whether the application is online or completed in a print format, there are similarities. First, be sure that you fill in all the information requested. Do not simply write on the application form "see résumé" or leave the sections blank. Information often will be entered into a database, and the employer wants it in a standardized format. The failure to follow directions accurately is a poor reflection on your skills and abilities. If the application must be completed onsite, bring all needed information with you, including information about references and names, addresses, and dates for past employers. If it is an online application, you may need to complete it at one time and then submit it. Sometimes, it is beneficial to print out the online form to be certain you have the information before starting it on the computer.

Successful Interviewing

The interview should be a two-way conversation in which you will gain as well as give information. Typically, employers have three major concerns for which they seek answers in the interview: they want to know whether you have the required knowledge and skills to do the job, whether you possess an attitude toward the job and the organization that is compatible with what they are seeking, and whether your personality and style will fit with the image the organization wishes to put forth. They are going to be interested in what you can do for them and, at this point, are often more interested in what you can do than in your opinions. They may be especially interested in your problem-solving and critical thinking skills. When planning for an employment interview, consider your appearance, your attitude and approach, and what the content of the interview will be.

Learning About Your Potential Employer

Once you know that you have gained an interview with a potential employer, learn as much about that specific position and the organization as you can. This can be done a number of ways. Review information you received when you were searching for organizations to which you would apply. Look again at information on its website if one exists. Be sure you have information regarding the organization's mission statement and other public pronouncements. Look especially for information on the various types of healthcare service the institution provides. If possible, contact current employees. Check local newspapers for information regarding the facility.

Preparing Your Questions for the Interviewer

Think through the situation before going to the interview and outline information that you want to obtain and questions that you want answered. It is helpful to write out your questions so that they are clearly stated, and so that you do not forget items while in the tense atmosphere that often exists in an interview situation; for example, "How and when will I learn of your decision?"

Time spent reflecting on your personal views in advance will be valuable for the interview. Remember that an interview is a chance to sell yourself to an employer, a chance to present yourself as a valuable addition to their nursing staff, and an opportunity to determine how you will fit into that work setting. A question such as "Please tell me about the educational opportunities that would be available to me" indicates an interest in learning.

Dressing for the Interview

The minute you walk in the door, people start making assumptions about you. How you dress plays a significant role in this aspect of job seeking. You need to make a conscious decision about the impression you want to create through your attire. Your personal appearance and demeanor may make a significant difference in whether you are offered a position.

Consider what you would like the interviewer's response to be and choose your attire with that in mind. This means that what you wear when applying for one type of job might be different when applying for another type of job. And you don't always know who you will be talking with—someone fairly conservative or someone with an informal approach. Being neat and well-groomed is always essential. In most instances, such as applying for a position at a hospital, you would wear businesslike clothing, such as dress pants or skirt and shirt or blouse or sweater, or a suit or dress. If you were applying for a position in a walk-in healthcare clinic that offered services to persons who are uncomfortable in a traditional environment, it might be appropriate to wear more casual clothing, such as khaki trousers and a polo shirt with a collar. Never appear at a job site wearing leisure or sports clothing such as attire with a bare midriff, shorts, athletic attire, body piercing jewelry other than the earlobe, pants with holes in the legs, or flip-flops. Avoid the use of strong cologne or perfume. Most interviewers indicate that being more businesslike in dress is never a mistake, while being too casual is a frequent mistake. In all instances, your hair should be clean and neatly styled. Do not chew gum while in the interview. If you smoke, avoid smoking immediately before the interview so that the odor of smoke is not apparent on your clothes or person.

Today, many people have tattoos and piercings. They can be limiting when seeking a job. It is advisable to remove jewelry from obvious pierced locations other than earrings (which should not be elaborate) and to wear clothing that covers tattoos. Jewelry should be conservative and limited in amount. You want the attention to be on what you have to say rather than focused on the jewelry you are wearing.

Things to Take With You

Take several copies of your résumé with you to the interview. You may want to refer to it or you may find it appropriate to leave a copy with someone. In addition, be prepared with the names, addresses, and telephone numbers of all references, as well as your Social Security card and photo identification. If you should be offered a position, you will need these last two items to complete employment forms. If you have received your nursing license, take that with you, or in states with a paperless system, have your license number. Take along a black pen to fill out any forms and a notepad with your questions listed and a place to make personal notes of important information obtained during the interview. You might want to purchase a special job interview hard-backed folder that will hold materials in a pocket on one side, has a notepad on the other, has a place for a pen, and will be a surface upon which you can write. You do not want to infringe on an interviewer's space by using that person's desk to take notes. Having all the information and supplies you need with you can increase your self-confidence if you have forms to fill out or if questions about statements on your résumé arise during the interview.

Arriving at the Interview

Plan to arrive at an interview early. This gives you time to check your appearance and focus your thoughts. If you carry a cell phone, turn it off before the interview. Having it ring in the middle of the interview is disrespectful to the interviewer.

Your manner during the interview is important also. It has been said that a first impression is made in the initial 10 seconds of contact. Although the employer expects an applicant to be nervous, he or she will be interested in whether your nervousness makes you unable to respond appropriately. Follow common rules of courtesy. Greet your interviewer with a smile and firm handshake and establish eye contact and maintain it throughout the interview. Making and maintaining eye contact communicates confidence and honesty—two important characteristics employers value. Wait to be asked to sit down before you take a chair. Do not put anything of yours on the interviewer's desk other than your résumé. Avoid any distracting mannerisms, such as chewing gum or fussing with your hair, face, or clothes. Nervousness often causes people to fidget, bounce their feet, or drum their fingers; be careful to avoid these behaviors. Sit up straight, as slouching communicates a message of disinterest. Be serious when appropriate, but do not forget to smile and be pleasant. The interviewer is also thinking of your impact on clients, visitors, and other staff members.

Anticipating Interview Questions

When you prepare your responses, try to anticipate possible questions from the interviewer. To do this, you must know the role of the person conducting the interview; for example, your first interview might be with a human resources department employee, not a nursing department representative. If you are successful at this stage, you might be recommended for an interview in the nursing department. Each might ask different types of questions.

Role-playing an interview situation with a friend or relative may help you to feel more confident in your responses. Another technique is to visualize the interview situation in your mind and mentally rehearse responses to questions.

An interview usually covers a wide variety of subjects. The interviewer may direct the flow of topics or may encourage you to bring up the ones that concern you during the process. Some interviewers focus on asking questions about your past experiences and your future plans. Others focus their questions on specific accomplishments and problems encountered in your past nursing experiences. Presenting hypothetical problems for you to consider and asking you to provide appropriate nursing responses are common. You may find it helpful to use your nursing process approach to any situation presented. Specifically state, "I would need to begin by assessing …." Talk about clearly identifying the problem (analysis of data) and planning for action. Don't neglect to indicate that you would evaluate the effectiveness of your actions. See Box 4.5 for a list of questions you might reflect on as you prepare.

In most instances, be sure to answer questions that are asked, rather than skirting them. However, if the interviewer asks a question that is illegal or inappropriate, such as a question regarding age or marital status, you might want to redirect the question to address what appears to be the concern of the interviewer. For example, in response to a question about your age, you might say, "Perhaps you believe that I appear to be young and inexperienced. I want to assure you that I have demonstrated my maturity and responsibility both in my nursing education and in my position with [name of employer]." In response to a question about marital status or children, you could reply, "Perhaps you are concerned about how long I plan to stay in my first position? I want to assure you that whatever my personal situation, professionally, I am looking for a position in an organization where I can be a long-term employee and plan for advancement within the organization." Avoid simple yes or no answers, but try to describe or explain to give a more complete picture of yourself.

Some interviews are conducted by a group of interviewers. This might include a person from nursing administration, a unit manager, and a staff development nurse. For an applicant to sit across the table from three to five individuals can be intimidating. You will need to look around the group, being sure to make eye contact with each individual. Make sure that you understand the role of each person present. You might actually write down individual names and roles on your notepad. This would allow you to direct a question to a specific individual or to use an individual's name when replying to a question. If you use a name, be sure to address them formally as "Mr.," "Ms." (if marital status of a woman is not known), "Miss," or "Mrs." rather than by first name. If they want you to use another form of address, they will let you know. While replying to the person who asks the question, glance at others as you make your point. Be sure that you do not ignore any individual, even if one of the interviewers does not seem to ask questions or to be as active in the process as the others. Interviews of this type are often longer than interviews with one person.

Some interviewers are less skilled than others; in these situations, the questions may seem less focused and vaguer. You may sometimes feel at a loss as to exactly what is being asked. Before proceeding, seek clarification, but be careful that your manner of asking for clarification does not offend the interviewer. In this situation, you may have to take the initiative to be sure that you have an opportunity to present your strengths and skills. Don't hesitate to elaborate on questions to more effectively present yourself.

BOX 4.5 POTENTIAL INTERVIEW QUESTIONS

Philosophy
- What is your philosophy of nursing?
- Is there a nursing theorist that you use as a basis for your nursing practice?
- What do you believe is the most central concept to support excellence in nursing?

Personal Goals and Planning
- Where do you see yourself in 1 year? 5 years? 10 years?
- Have you developed any professional goals? If so, would you share those with me?
- Why do you want to work here?
- What plans do you have for continuing education in nursing?
- What do you see as your weakest area in nursing?
- What do you see as your strengths in nursing?

Your Experiences
- What experience in your nursing education did you find the most rewarding? Why?
- What experience in your nursing education did you like the least? Why?
- In what kind of settings did you have an opportunity to work as a nursing student?
- What other job experiences have you had? What skill did you develop there that will be useful in nursing?

Problem Solving
- Identify a problem in client care that you encountered as a student and explain how you solved that problem.
- Describe a difficult client with whom you worked. Include why you found that client difficult and how you managed the situation.
- Identify a situation in which you were involved in a conflict and describe how you handled that situation. If you had to do it over again, what would you do differently?
- Explain how you would use the nursing process in client care.
- A problem may be presented to you for your solution. Plan ahead to approach it in a systematic manner.

Technical Skills
- What technical nursing skills do you feel comfortable performing?
- What skills will you require assistance with?
- What do you do when you encounter a technical skill you have not performed before?

The Employment Setting
- In what type of unit do you wish to work?
- Why do you want to work here?
- Why do you think we should hire you for this position?

Communication in Action 4.1: Clarifying Questions in an Interview

Cheryl Layton, a new graduate, interviewed for a nursing position. She found that she did not understand many of the interviewer's questions and decided to use clarifying questions and statements throughout the interview. When there was a rather unclear question about communicating with others, she asked, "Would you give me an example of the type of situation you were thinking about?" Another clarifying approach she used was to state clearly what she perceived to be the central question before continuing: "Let me be sure I understand. You would like me to identify a situation in which I believe I responded effectively to a problem. Is that correct?" Still another clarifying response she used was, "If I understand correctly, your unit will be switching to computerized charting, and you are interested in my experience with computerized documentation. Is that right?" In this way, she indicated interest and attention to accuracy but did not challenge or offend the interviewer.

Almost all interviews provide an opportunity for the interviewee to ask questions before the interview is terminated. You should prepare for this and prepare two or three questions in advance. Make sure your questions are appropriate for the interviewer. In the human resources department, you might ask about the overall mission and philosophy of the organization, its organizational structure, and how authority and accountability are determined. You might also ask, "Do you have any questions about my résumé? Are there other details I can provide?" With a nursing interviewer, demonstrate that you are concerned about how nursing care is given and by whom, where responsibility and authority for nursing care decisions lie, the philosophy underlying care, the availability of continuing education, and where you would be expected to fit into the facility's overall picture. For example, you might ask, "Can you outline for me the responsibilities of this position?" or "What type of individuals do well in this type of position?"

Then, be sure to cover such topics as hours, schedules, pay scales, and benefits. Recognize that the replies to these questions may be quite general when you have not yet been offered a specific position. Before you leave, be sure to ask when you can expect to know the results of your interview and how you can follow up. State clearly that you are interested in the position and hope to be hired (if that is true). An important reason for not getting a position is the failure to clearly state that you want to work there.

If you are unfamiliar with the interview process, you might benefit from reading books on the topic. Reading several different books will give you a variety of viewpoints and might provide you with strategies that are comfortable for you.

Communication in Action 4.2: *Replying Professionally to an Interview*

Rosa Quintana had been interviewing for a position in a new graduate residency program in which she would really like to be a participant. The interviewer said, "Well that concludes my questions, do you have any questions for me?" Rosa responded, "I prepared some questions before I came. Some of those were already answered. However, I would like to hear more about the shared governance system you briefly mentioned on your website. Exactly what types of issues are addressed through shared governance and how might I, as a newly hired new graduate, participate in shared governance?" In this reply, Rosa demonstrated her preplanning and organization as well as her understanding of organizational function. After hearing the response to this question, Rosa then said, "Thank you so much for that information. It confirms that I would really like to work here. I do hope to be chosen to enter this new graduate residency. What are the next steps I can take to learn about my status in the selection process?"

Telephone and Online Interviews

Because interviews are costly to an employer, telephone and online interviews may be conducted and an in-person interview only scheduled for individuals in whom the organization is interested in employing. Do not mistake these telephone or online interviews for unimportant or casual conversations. Plan for them in the same way that you would for an in-person interview. Prepare and have all your materials at hand. You will want to be professional and businesslike in this context also. The one advantage is that you may not need to worry about your appearance if there is no video link.

Interviewing Errors

Several errors can occur during an interview that almost certainly will result in the position being offered to someone else. The first relates to making a negative comment about a former employer. If asked why you left a position identified on your résumé, be careful not to use this as a time to vent your frustrations about the employer or the employment situation. You may be labeled a troublemaker.

Bringing your personal problems to the interview may create a negative response. You may be asked why you would like this position. This is no time to talk about the economic necessity of having the job to repay your student loans, make your car payment, or even meet the monthly rent. Instead, focus on professional issues related to this employer.

Taking a friend or relative with you to the interview gives the impression that you are not an independent thinker. If you take children, they will be a distraction. Some interviewers will refuse to have children in the office. Arrange with a friend who also has children to exchange babysitting time or make other plans.

Do not take over the interview. Let the interviewer lead the interview. It is important to know when to talk and when to listen. When answering questions, be brief and concise; don't ramble. Also, watch your nonverbal responses.

Follow-Up Strategies

After your interview, write a brief thank-you letter to the person who interviewed you. If a group interviewed you, direct the letter to the person who seemed to be in charge. In that letter, thank the individual for the time and attention to your questions and concerns. Restate any agreement you feel was reached. For example, write, "I understand that I am to call your office next week to learn whether I have been scheduled for an interview with the birth center unit manager." Close your letter with a positive comment about the organization. Even if you are not offered a job or do not choose to work at that facility, you are leaving a positive impression. You can never tell when that will be important to you in the future (Box 4.6).

BOX 4.6 INTERVIEW FOLLOW-UP LETTER

Maribeth Wilson
3428 lst Ave. N.
Seattle, WA 98103
(206) 274-5978
E-mail: maribethw@email.com
June 9, 2010

Joyce Montgall, R.N.
Nurse Recruiter
Seattle General Medical Center
321 Heath Blvd.
Seattle, WA 98101

Dear Ms. Montgall:

I want to thank you for meeting with me today to discuss your new nursing graduate residency program at Seattle General. I am particularly interested in the medical-surgical positions available on 4 West and 4 Center, although I am certainly willing to consider another unit.

I am confident that my educational background, clinical experience, and commitment to excellent client care make me an ideal match with Seattle General. In addition, I feel very "at home" in the Seattle General environment, having worked there as a nursing assistant for the last year.

Again, I hope that you will consider me for one of the medical-surgical positions in the July 1 new graduate program. I am available to meet with any of the unit managers, which I understand is the next step in your hiring process. I can be contacted at the above telephone number or by e-mail. I do have an answering machine and would promptly return your call if I were not there to receive it. If I have not heard from you within 2 weeks, I will check with your office regarding the status of my application.

Thank you again for your time and consideration.

Sincerely,

Maribeth Wilson

If you did not obtain an interview, you should continue to contact the potential employer at intervals to learn of other job opportunities and to indicate that you still seek a position. When a new position opens, employers do not necessarily go back through previous employment files. They are more likely to interview a person who appears to be currently searching for a position than one who was searching several months previously. They will assume that you have found desirable employment.

Do not let this letter be your last contact with that potential employer. Call back as agreed. Even if you do not get a position at this time, ask if your application will be kept on file because you are still interested in employment with that particular agency. You might then continue to call back every month or so to find out if any other positions are available.

Setting up your own record-keeping system often enhances managing a job search. Maintain a record of when you contacted an agency, in what manner (letter or telephone call), interviews—including the interviewer's name and the content of the interview—and dates and times of any follow-up letters or calls. Have a place to record your own notes or impressions. This will enable you to keep track of details when you manage an extensive job search. By keeping this type of record, you will not forget to call an agency to recheck on job availability or mistakenly send an inquiry letter and résumé twice to the same agency.

Resignation

When you decide to leave a nursing position, it is important that you provide the employer with an appropriate amount of time to seek a replacement. The more responsible your position, the more time the employer will need. For a staff nursing position, strive to provide a month's notice, unless an urgent matter requires that less notice be given. Notice of resignation should be in a letter that is directed to the manager of your department. Copies should be sent to other supervisory people, such as the chief nursing officer.

The letter of resignation is important in concluding your relationship with the employer on a cordial and positive basis. The feelings left behind when you resign may influence letters of recommendation and future opportunities for employment with that agency. Give a reason for your resignation and the exact date when it will be effective. If you have accrued vacation or holiday time and want to take the time off or be paid for it, clearly state that. Comment about positive factors in the employment setting and acknowledge those who have provided special support or assistance in your growth (Box 4.7).

If you are resigning because of problems in the work setting, such as inadequate staffing, which may result in client harm, it is wiser to address those in person, separate from your letter of resignation, and in a manner that will not affect future recommendations. See Daily Ethical Dilemma 4.1 for an example of this type of situation. However you address problems, do so in a clear, factual, unemotional way. Avoid attacking anyone personally and do not make broad, sweeping negative comments. Remember that the nursing community is not large and a career path may bring you back to this agency or may bring these individuals to a place where you work. Try always to leave with appropriate professional relationships intact.

BOX 4.7 LETTER OF RESIGNATION

1546 Avenida Escuela
Palm Desert, CA 76321
February 14, 2011

Marvin Short, R.N., Unit Manager
Transitional Care Unit
Desert Hospital
509 Desert Highway
Palm Desert, CA 76320

Dear Marvin:

It is with mixed feelings that I am submitting my resignation to be effective March 23. I will be moving to Oregon and returning to school full time beginning spring quarter.

My 2 years here at Desert Hospital has been an excellent foundation for my future career. The nurses were supportive of me as a new graduate and have always encouraged me to think of my career as a lifetime opportunity for growth.

The last day I plan to work will be at the end of this pay period. My understanding is that my unused vacation and holiday pay will be included in my final paycheck.

Thank you again for all of your help.

Sincerely,

John Webster, R.N.
cc: Maria Gonzales, Vice President for Client Care Services

Daily Ethical Dilemma 4.1: *Staffing Shortfall*

A 61-year-old woman was admitted to the hospital through the emergency department. She came in for what she thought was a bad cold and was subsequently diagnosed with pneumonia. Shortly after her arrival on the medical floor, she became feverish and short of breath. Her family called out for help, but there was no one at the nurse's station. The client eventually stopped breathing. After successful resuscitation, she was unable to walk, talk, or care for herself due to lack of oxygen.

- Where do you think the nurses were?
- What mistakes, if any, do you think were made?

When this incident happened, there were only 3 RNs on duty for a client load of 41. There should have been 5 RNs and 2 LPNs. Furthermore, examination of hospital records showed that the hospital staffing standards were below standard for 51 out of the 59 days prior to this incident.

- Do you think there is cause for legal action?
- Who do you think is at fault?

Retrieved March 26, 2017, from https://www.americannursetoday.com/ethics-case-study-poor-staffing-results-in-brain-damaged-client-2/

Stegen & Sowerby Stories: Part 2

R emember that hiring committee that was tasked with filling two vacant positions? After a lengthy discussion, the hiring committee decided to offer the positions to the two candidates who had been identified as the most qualified. One of these candidates was the nurse with diabetes. Read the rest of the story at www.thePoint.com.

Want to Know More?

A variety of resources are available on thePoint® to enhance your learning and understanding of this chapter, such as:

- Full Stegen & Sowerby Stories
- NCLEX-Style Student Review Questions
- Journal Articles
- Case Studies
- Learning Objectives
- Relevant Websites
- And more...

KEY CONCEPTS

- Developing a successful career pathway involves setting personal short- and long-term goals and developing a plan for maintaining and enhancing your own competence.
- Throughout the history of nursing, employment patterns have changed, moving from a focus on the home and the community in the first part of this century to a focus on acute care institutions.
- Competencies expected of the newly licensed RN can be categorized by frequency and by importance.
- Employers have expectations in eight basic areas: theoretic knowledge for safe practice and decision-making, ability to use the nursing process, self-awareness, communication skills, understanding the importance of documentation, commitment to a work ethic, proficiency in specified technical skills, computer literacy, and speed of functioning.
- To obtain a nursing position, you will need to identify potential employers, develop a professional résumé, write appropriate letters to employers, and interview effectively using both in-person and online strategies.
- Successful interviewing involves learning about the organization, dressing appropriately, arriving a bit early, being self-confident, maintaining eye contact throughout the interview, and remaining attentive.
- To make the best impression, interview questions should be answered directly and clearly. The use of clarifying statements and questions may help to assure that you are providing needed data, while specific details rather than generalities in your response often are

received more favorably. Approaching problem-solving questions using the nursing process provides a pattern for effective response.

- Following up after the interview has been completed includes sending a note of thanks to the key decision-makers, and checking back to learn of decisions about the position, and maintaining contact with the institution if not selected if you still would like to be considered for a position there.
- When resigning from a position, communicating your plans to the head of the department with a sufficient time interval to allow the organization to find a replacement to fill your position leaves a professional impression and may result in a more positive reference.

NCLEX-STYLE PRACTICE QUESTIONS

1. You are leaving your current RN position to relocate with your spouse. What information should you include in your resignation letter?

   A. A thank you for the opportunity to work at the facility, information regarding your grievances during the time you have worked there, and your intended last day
   B. A thank you for the opportunity to work at the facility, the names of unsafe nurses that you have concerns about, and your intended last day of work
   C. That you are relocating with your spouse, a thank you for the opportunity to work at the facility, and your last intended day of work
   D. That you are relocating with your spouse, your last intended day of work, and suggestions to improve client care that you have observed are needed

2. In preparing your résumé, which elements would you choose to emphasize?

   A. Objective, credentials, education, and employment history
   B. Career goals and trajectory, references, and mission statement
   C. Mission statement, education, and references
   D. Objective, education, and career goals

3. You have submitted a job application and been called to schedule an interview. When planning for an interview, what should you consider to improve your chances of being hired? (Select all that apply)

   A. Questions about evening and weekend differentials
   B. Attention to professional dress and grooming
   C. Presenting a positive attitude and approach
   D. Check the location so you can arrive on time

REFERENCES

American Association of Colleges of Nursing. (2008). *The essentials of baccalaureate nursing education for professional nursing practice*. Washington, DC: Author.

National Council of State Boards of Nursing. (2015a). *The 2014 RN practice analysis: Linking the NCLEX-RN® examination to practice* (Research Brief Vol. 62). Chicago, IL: Author. Retrieved March 1, 2017, from https://www.ncsbn.org/15_RN_Practice_Analysis_Vol62_web.pdf

National Council of State Boards of Nursing. (2015b). *2016 NCLEX-RN test plan*. Chicago, IL: Author. Retrieved March 1, 2017, from https://www.ncsbn.org/RN_Test_Plan_2016_Final.pdf

National Council of State Boards of Nursing. (2016a). *The 2015 LPN practice analysis: Linking the NCLEX-PN® examination to practice*. Chicago, IL: Author. Retrieved March 1, 2017, from https://www.ncsbn.org/16_2015LPN_Practice_Analysis_vol67.pdf

National Council of State Boards of Nursing. (2016b). *2017 NCLEX-PN test plan*. Chicago, IL: Author. Retrieved March 1, 2017, from https://www.ncsbn.org/2017_PN_TestPlan.pdf

National League for Nursing. (2012). *Outcomes and competencies for graduates of practical/vocational, diploma, associate degree, baccalaureate, master's, practice doctorate, and research doctorate programs in nursing*. Atlanta, GA: Author.

U.S. Bureau of Labor Statistics. (2018). *Occupational outlook handbook*. Retrieved May 14, 2018, from https://www.bls.gov/ooh/healthcare/registered-nurses.htm

U.S. Census Bureau. (2013). *Male nurses becoming more common place, census bureau reports*. Retrieved May 14, 2018, from https://www.census.gov/newsroom/press-releases/2013/cb13-32.html

The World of Healthcare Employment

After completing this chapter, you should be able to:

1. Discuss the purpose of organizational mission and vision statements and statements of philosophy and analyze how these differ.
2. Discuss the concept of organizational structure and explore the relationships among organizational charts, chains of command, and channels of communication within the structure of organizations.
3. Delineate the characteristics of shared governance, and explain the advantages of a shared governance approach.
4. Discuss the development of the Magnet Recognition Program for hospitals and list the characteristics required to achieve this status.
5. Describe various patterns of nursing care delivery, and identify the major characteristics of each and a situation in which each would be employed appropriately.
6. Compare and contrast the characteristics of a grievance with those of a complaint.
7. Analyze the processes through which resolution is achieved in collective bargaining issues.
8. Discuss the history of collective bargaining as it applies to nursing.
9. Identify at least four professional concerns that should be addressed in a contract for nurses.
10. Discuss the concerns nurses have regarding membership in a collective bargaining group and the reasons for each of these concerns.
11. Outline the advantages and disadvantages of having the state nurses association serve as a bargaining agent for nurses.

Accountability
Agency shop
Arbitration/arbitrator
Authority
Bargain in good faith
Binding arbitration
Bureaucracy
Case management
Case method

Centralized/decentralized/matrix
Chain of command
Channels of communication
Clinical ladders
Collective bargaining
Concession bargaining
Contract
Cross-training
Deadlocked

(continued on page 143)

KEY TERMS   *(continued)*

Functional method	Procedure
Grievance/grievance process	Protocols
Impasse	Ratified
Interest-based bargaining	Reinstatement privilege
Lockout	Shared governance
Mediation/mediator	Span of control—broad, narrow
Mission statement	Standards of care
Modular care	Statements of philosophy
National Labor Relations Board	Strike/strike breaking
(NLRB)	Structure
Negotiate/negotiation	Team nursing
Organizational chart	Total patient care
Organizational hierarchy	Unfair labor practice
Partnership models	Union
Policy	Vision
Primary care	

Stegen and Sowerby Stories: Part 1

The number of clients a nurse is assigned to care for, referred to as a staffing ratio, has long been a source of topic for conversation between managers and staff. With union help, nurses in New York were among the first to develop staffing guidelines with both managers and staff nurses present for the negotiation. Nurses complained that client acuity was not being considered in the current staffing structure, and managers argued that other factors such as no-shows and float nurses who did not want higher acuity work contributed to the problem. Discussions took place several times a month over approximately 4 months, and a professional facilitator was present to keep the discussion moving in the right direction and to be sure everyone adhered to the agenda and rules laid out for the discussion. Jeri, a nurse on the medical/surgical unit, complained of the rising acuity level of the clients, the increasing number of ventilated clients, and an increase in clients requiring the services of an interpreter that makes it difficult to care for clients. The hospital chief nursing officer stated that this situation exists on all the floors and asked what could be done to manage current staffing. (Source: http://www.restructassoc.com/case_newyork.htm)

1. Do you support the concept of nurses becoming members of unions? Why or why not?
2. Do you believe that all employees should be required to pay membership fees if a facility has a union?
3. What staffing ratio problems have you seen at your job or in clinical rotations?
4. List the advantages and disadvantages of union membership.

As you seek employment as a professional nurse, you will most likely find an initial job in a healthcare organization. Organizations—formally constituted groups of people who have identified tasks and who work together to achieve a specific purpose defined by the organization—are the backbone of the American economy. We believe you will move from student to staff nurse more easily and function more effectively in any organization if you have some understanding of the structure and makeup of organizations. By gaining an understanding of the makeup of organizations, you will be best equipped to participate effectively in the activities of the workplace. This also will help you anticipate some of the difficulties that may occur and, thus, handle them with greater ease.

This chapter begins with a brief discussion of the structure of organizations and some of the most common conditions of employment and then presents the most common avenues, including unions, through which employees participate in workplace decisions. Because we can only touch on these topics, you are encouraged to gain greater depth in this area by reading books devoted to this topic.

UNDERSTANDING ORGANIZATIONS

All organizations have structure and purpose. **Structure** refers to the way in which a group is formed, its chains of command, lines of communication, and processes by which decisions are made (Fig. 5.1). These comprise the formal working relationships and serve to identify who is accountable and responsible for the various jobs within the organization. The purpose

Figure 5.1. The structure of an organization.

identifies the goals of the organization—what it intends to accomplish. In other words, the structure outlines how individuals work together to reach the purpose.

Mission Statement and Philosophy

The purpose of an organization is often expressed in the form of a **mission statement**, which outlines what the organization plans to accomplish, including its goals and function. Sometimes, mission statements incorporate **statements of philosophy** (beliefs) and goals or objectives into a single statement; other times, the philosophy and goals are addressed in a statement separate from the mission statement. The mission of an organization may be combined with a **vision**, which is a broad conceptual view of what the organization desires to be and do. The mission statement is the responsibility of the board of directors or board of trustees. Input may be gathered from many sources, and drafts are developed by top management with final approval by the board. Box 5.1 provides an example of a typical mission and vision statement for a hospital.

Mission and vision statements serve as a standard against which an organization's performance can be evaluated. A large research hospital might incorporate into its mission statement obligations for research, teaching, and the care of clients with complex problems. A smaller community hospital may reflect a goal of meeting the healthcare needs of citizens of the community in its mission statement. The hospital's ability to meet these goals would be reviewed as part of the overall evaluation of the organization.

Critical Thinking Activity: Mission Statement

Based on your perception of the needs of the community in which you live, write a mission statement for a hospital in your community. How did you arrive at the decision to offer the services you outlined? What facts support this decision? What services did you not include? Examine your response for personal biases.

BOX 5.1 TYPICAL HOSPITAL MISSION STATEMENT

Mission, Vision, Values, and Strategic Goals for Mercy Valley Hospital

Mission: To provide services resulting in the improved health of all individuals we serve.

Vision: To make available high-quality, high-tech, and high-touch healthcare to residents of the community.

Values:

- Client centered
- Caring, compassion, and consideration
- Cooperation and collaboration
- Ongoing development and improvement
- Leadership
- Best care provider
- Best employer
- Best partner

Organizational Structure

A central goal of most organizations is to seek an organizational structure that is efficient while providing maximum cost-effectiveness. The structure of an organization outlines the formal working relationships and identifies who is accountable and responsible for the various jobs required within the organization. The structure determines the manner and extent to which roles, power, and responsibilities are delegated, controlled, and coordinated and how communication occurs between levels of management (BusinessDictionary.com, 2017). Size, age, services, technical components, and environment influence the structure of an organization.

The concept of organizational structure is credited to a German social scientist, Max Weber, who is known as the father of organizational theory. He highly valued **bureaucracy**—the administration of institutions through departments or subdivisions managed by sets of officials who followed an inflexible routine with clear lines of authority (see Theory Alert). Historically, hospitals have functioned in the bureaucratic mode, which also dominated both government and corporate life throughout the 20th century.

Theory Alert   *Max Weber*

Max Weber was born in Germany in 1864. He was a sociologist by training, and he theorized that administrative structure is based on rational–legal authority and areas of responsibility are clearly specified. Subordinates follow rules of superiors; clearly defined rules govern decisions. His theory states that rules are stable and can be learned.

Employment at an organization is viewed as a career, and a full-time employee looks forward to a lifelong career. Weber viewed this system as reliable and clear and the most stable system for both subordinates and superiors. The system is based on discipline. (Source: https://www.business.com/articles/management-theory-of-max-weber/)

To continue operation, an organization must make enough money to meet its expenses and to improve and develop; some also seek to provide a profit return to investors. This is as true in healthcare as it is in retail businesses. As the values and priorities of our society change and as new technology becomes available, healthcare organizations also must make adaptations in their structure and function. Today, our healthcare system is experiencing tremendous transformation (see Chapter 6).

Types of Structure

The power to make decisions is a key factor in the structure and function of any organization. Organizations may be described as having a **centralized** (or tall) or a **decentralized** (or flat) structure. When the structure is centralized, the authority to make decisions is vested in a few individuals in the top layer of management. For example, in the client services area of a hospital, major decisions may be made by the vice president of client care and two or three associates **(Fig. 5.2)**.

Conversely, when the decision-making involves a number of individuals and individual employees are responsible for making decisions in areas in which they have expertise, the organization is said to operate in a decentralized manner. Currently, many organizations are

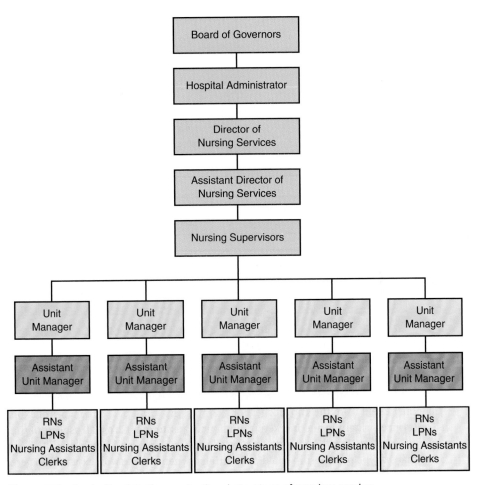

Figure 5.2. Centralized (tall) organizational structure of nursing service.

going through a process of restructuring to embrace a transformational approach to decision-making that places the responsibility for finding solutions to problems at the site where the activity occurs. Decentralized structures have the advantage of simplified communication patterns, which flow easily and directly from lower levels to higher levels. Later in this chapter, we discuss the concept of shared governance, which embraces a decentralized structure and function **(Fig. 5.3)**.

Another type of organizational structure, the **matrix** structure, may be either flat or tall and also may be referred to as cross-functional. The unique characteristic of the matrix structure is that a second structure overlies the first, creating two directions for lines of authority, accountability, and communication. An organization will have an underlying structure (either tall or flat) that is a functional structure over which is imposed a project structure. In short, the individuals in the functional structure perform the duties of operating and maintaining the organization, and the individuals in the project structure oversee the application of various projects or special responsibilities. The relationship that exists among individuals in the

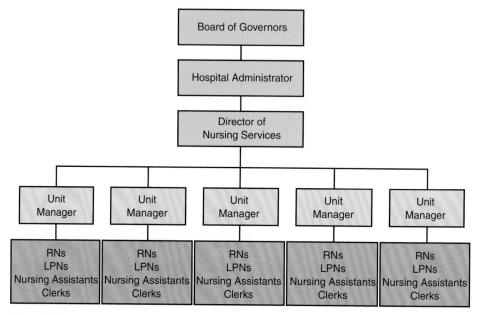

Figure 5.3. Decentralized (flat) organizational structure of nursing service.

project structure is outside the regular chain of command of the underlying structure. We typically see the matrix structure in large, multifaceted organizations. Individuals with special expertise or authority in an area serve as resource persons for several departments, all of which can benefit from the knowledge. For example, in **Figure 5.4**, three types of expertise (financial services, planning and marketing, and quality assurance) cross all aspects of this large hospital corporation, which include acute care, long-term care, and home care. Another example of a matrix-type relationship could be illustrated when a nurse with expertise in gerontologic nursing provides assistance, advice, and information to employees in each branch of this hospital organization.

ORGANIZATIONAL RELATIONSHIPS

When examining organizational function, it is important that you identify relationships among people and departments and realize where the authority and accountability are placed within that organization. When one has **authority**, it means that the individual has the power or the right to take action, give directions or commands, and make final decisions. **Accountability** refers to being obliged to answer for one's actions and sometimes, as when certain tasks are delegated, for the actions of others. A synonym frequently used for accountability is responsibility. We discuss both authority and accountability in more detail in the section on shared governance.

Most organizations have several ways of expressing and defining the relationship of one worker to another. Organizational charts, chains of command, channels of communication, job descriptions, and policies and procedures provide different views of organizational relationships.

Figure 5.4. Matrix organizational structure of nursing service.

Organizational Chart

The structure of any large group comprises both a formal and an informal organization. The formal organization can be seen on an organizational chart. The **organizational chart** is a graphic, pictorial means of portraying roles and patterns of interaction among parts of a system. It identifies formal chains of command, communication channels, and the authority for decision-making.

The organizational chart typically is represented on the page by boxes stacked in a pyramid formation. The greatest authority exists at the top of the chart (often a single box), and authority declines as you move toward the base (many boxes). Persons occupying jobs at the top of the organizational chart are considered administrators, executives, or management, and individuals with jobs closer to the base are considered employees or staff members. Located between these two levels is an area known as middle management, comprising those who coordinate and control activities of specified groups of workers.

The organizational chart may take one of several forms, reflecting the type of administration operating within that organization. One term used to describe these forms is **span of control**, which refers to the number of employees supervised by a manager. A **narrow** span of control exists when a manager has responsibility for only three to five subordinates. If, however, the organization operates with a **broad span** of control, it places authority and responsibility for decision-making in the hands of fewer individuals, with each manager supervising a large number of employees. The larger the number of individuals to be supervised, the more difficult it is to control each worker through direct observation. If two organizations of equal size were to exist—one with a narrow span of control and the other with a broad span of control—the organization choosing to implement a narrow span of control would have more managers. One limitation of the organizational chart is the difficulty in keeping it current. Positions and people change frequently, and each change requires updating the chart.

In most groups, we find an informal organization, sometimes called the "grapevine," that represents informal or social relationships. The informal organization is not depicted on an organizational chart or formally acknowledged in any specific manner, but it can often have a profound effect on how an organization functions.

This informal structure has its own leaders and communication channels. It is responsible for much of the socialization that occurs among employees of the organization and creates a sense of belonging. There may be unwritten and informal rules and expectations regarding performance, dress, communications, and other factors that affect group operation.

Chain of Command

All organizations have a chain of command. The **chain of command** represents the path of authority and accountability from individuals at the top of the organization to those at the base of the organization. It is often referred to as the **organizational hierarchy**. Thus, in hospitals, we typically find that the nursing administrator gives directions to and evaluates the performance of the assistant administrator, who, in turn, gives directions to and evaluates the performance of the nursing unit manager, and so forth. When we look at this process from the base of the organization to the top, we often use the phrase "reports to"—indicating that the unit manager is accountable to the assistant administrator and the assistant administrator is accountable to the nursing administrator. Similarly, we find the registered nurse (RN) giving directions to and overseeing the activities of the practical (vocational) nurse and the nursing assistant. The length of the chain of command varies depending on the size of the organization and whether that organization is centralized or decentralized.

Some individuals are represented as having accountability to those above them but also hold some accountability to other departments. These represent collaborative rather than authoritarian relationships. For example, a clinical nurse specialist in wound care might hold some accountability to nurses on all units, but she has no authority to compel them to consult with her or follow her suggestions.

Almost without exception, the salaries commanded by persons at the top of the organizational hierarchy are greater than those of persons close to the base. Accordingly, the experience, educational requirements, hours worked, and responsibilities are usually greater for persons with positions near the top of the organizational chart.

Channels of Communication

Channels of communication are, as the name implies, the patterns through which messages are delivered within an organization. The channels of communication usually reflect the chain of command; they run up and down the organizational chart, moving from one level of responsibility and authority to the next. Thus, the nurse manager communicates concerns and information to the assistant administrator, who either has the authority and responsibility to deal with the problem or relays the concern to the nursing administrator. The nursing assistant reports her concerns to the staff nurse, who either has the authority to deal with the issue or reports it to the head nurse or clinical manager. Some types of communication move along to individuals in parallel positions.

For nurse managers to report a concern directly to administrators rather than to assistant administrators to whom they report is referred to as *looping* the system. It is generally considered improper and inappropriate to skip or bypass any level in the communication system. For example, if a staff nurse disagrees with a pharmacy technician who delivers medications to the unit and takes this problem directly to the nursing supervisor without first discussing it with the unit manager, this individual is looping the system. You can see how this would put the unit manager at a distinct disadvantage, should the supervisor ask about the incident. Proper channels of communication should be followed while keeping in mind the responsibility to protect the client. See the following Daily Ethical Dilemma for an illustration of the following communication channels.

Daily Ethical Dilemma 5.1: Communication Chain of Command

While caring for a 5-day-old infant in the neonatal intensive care unit (NICU), a nurse noted that the infant was developing a yeast infection. The attending MD told the resident to order a medication, flucytosine, which is commonly abbreviated 5FC. The resident accidentally wrote the order of 5FU, a chemotherapy agent.

The medication was given twice before a new night-shift nurse noted that the medication did not seem to be indicated for the infant. She called the pharmacy to question the medication and also the resident. The resident insisted that the attending MD had ordered the medication and demanded that it be given. The nurse then gave the 5FU to the infant. The next morning, the infant died.

- Review the five rights of medication administration. Which of those five rights could have helped the nurse to protect her client?
- How did the nurse follow or not follow the chain of command?
- What might the nurse have said to the resident to address her concerns regarding the medication?
- What recourse did the nurse have when the resident demanded she give the medication?

Smalls, H. T. (2009). Nursing liability and chain of command. *Neonatal Network, 28*(6), 401–402.

Communication in Action 5.1: *Missing Supplies*

Mary had been working on a medical unit of a community hospital for 4 months. Over that period of time, she noted that one of the nursing assistants, Jane, often left with towels, washcloths, and other unit supplies in her backpack. Mary approached Jane as they were leaving one afternoon and said, "I've noticed that you often carry home towels and other unit supplies." Jane quickly replied, "Oh, these ones are becoming ragged and should not be used anymore." Further observation suggested that Jane continued to remove unit items. Mary decided she needed to report this to her unit manager. Talking with the manager in private, Mary explained, "On several occasions within the past 3 months I have noticed Jane leaving the hospital with unit supplies in her backpack. I asked her about it 2 weeks ago and she stated that the supplies were worn and should not be used with clients. I thought you should know about this." The unit manager thanked Mary and said, "I'll look into it."

Not all communications follow the formal pathways. New approaches to leadership and management have encouraged communication outside those lines if the result is accomplishing a desired action more efficiently. The informal structure of the organization mentioned earlier also functions outside the formal pathways, often communicating messages much more rapidly than within the formal structure.

Job Descriptions

Job descriptions form another important aspect of any organization. Job descriptions are written statements, usually found in policy manuals, that specify the duties and functions of the various jobs within the organization and the scope of authority, responsibility, and accountability involved in each position. Job descriptions should explain the role of each individual working for the company or organization, from the chief executive officer to the housekeeper.

Sometimes job descriptions are very detailed; other times they are more broadly stated. If broadly stated, policy and procedure manuals may help to specify a task or responsibility. Job descriptions provide the foundation for performance standards for each position and should provide the basis for evaluation. Job descriptions also may include competencies expected of employees and can provide the basis for competency-based orientation. Increasingly in today's healthcare environment, more care is delegated by the RN to those with lesser educational preparation; therefore, it is critical that job descriptions provide sufficient description of the competencies of various workers, so that the document can be used to guide delegation activities (see Chapter 12 for more information on delegation).

Job descriptions also are important when cross-training is used in the organization. **Cross-training** requires that a person hired to perform functions of one position in the healthcare team be trained in the skills needed to perform those of another position. For example, a respiratory therapist might learn to perform basic client care skills and, when not needed for respiratory therapy treatments, be available to answer call lights and respond to client needs. Cross-training is viewed by some administrators as a method by which costs can be reduced by having an individual able to do more than one set of tasks within the organization. It can help manage peak times and provide for greater flexibility in scheduling. It also may be viewed as a method of job enrichment, giving an employee more control or more responsibility. Some persons enjoy the challenge of learning new skills and excel in the stimulation; others prefer to stay in the area they have chosen and know well.

Cross-training of nurses between different specialties has become common, and many nurses welcome the employment flexibility this provides. It also allows nurses to move with greater comfort from one area of the hospital to another when client census surges or drops in an area. Some nurses express concern over their ability to maintain a high level of expertise in multiple areas. As you enter into your first nursing position, check with your state board of nursing to learn what position your practice act has taken regarding cross-training.

Job descriptions also may describe **clinical ladders**. A clinical ladder differentiates and defines the skills and performance expected of nurses in terms of advancing levels. Typically, three or four levels of performance are defined, with each higher level having greater responsibility and authority than the previous one. A new graduate usually enters the system as a clinical nurse I (or similar title) and moves to clinical nurse II and then to clinical nurse III as that individual becomes more proficient. Salary increases typically accompany movement from one level to another, and the responsibility the individual is expected to assume also increases.

Sometimes additional formal education or continuing education is required for advancement. Through this process, the nurse is supported and encouraged to develop greater clinical expertise. The clinical ladder also serves as a mechanism for recognizing and rewarding nurses who wish to remain in direct care positions rather than seek administrative positions.

Policies, Protocols, Procedures, and Standards of Care

A **policy** may be defined as a designated plan or course of action to be taken in a specific situation. In organizations, the governing board holds the responsibility and authority for ensuring that appropriate policies are adopted and followed. The governing board usually delegates the development of policies to the chief administrative officer who usually delegates the responsibility for the development of policies for a specific department to individuals or groups in the department who will be most affected by the policy. The policy once developed is returned to the governing board for review, possible revision, and adoption **(Fig. 5.5)**.

Figure 5.5. Policies, protocols, procedures, and standards of care.

Written copies of all policies may be available in each department, or a current copy should be available online in the institution's computer network. Online policy manuals ensure that all departments refer to the most current policy and that the information is always available. Depending on the area in which you are employed, you will find varying reasons for referring to the policy manual in your role as a new employee. As you might anticipate, the need for special policies related to occurrences in an emergency department, a delivery room, or a critical care unit is greater than in a general medical or surgical unit in a hospital. When you are confronted with a new nonclinical problem to solve, always check your policy manual to see if it offers guidance; if you do not find help there, ask your manager.

Special unit policies are sometimes termed **protocols**. A protocol is a detailed "plan for carrying out a scientific study or a client's treatment regimen" (Dictionary.com, 2017). For example, the protocol for dealing with a client seen in the emergency department suffering from a dog bite determines the wound assessment instrument to be used, a reference to the procedure to be used for wound care, when tetanus immunization would be included in care, discharge criteria, and teaching needed. Protocols are usually available online so that any unit confronted by an unusual situation has access to the protocol even when it is not commonly used.

Procedure manuals are usually available online and contain the written instructions describing the accepted method for satisfactorily performing a particular nursing activity (**procedure**), often describing it in a number of steps. Each unit or department should have access to a procedure manual. In the manual, you might find a procedure for changing the dressing on a central intravenous line, administering chemotherapy agents, and doing many other procedures, such as catheterizations.

Institutions are giving nurses more responsibility for developing institutional policies, protocols, and procedures and serving as representatives to various committees that monitor, review, and update these policies, protocols, and procedures. As hospitals move to broader spans of control and to greater involvement of all employees in decision-making, participation in policy formation is becoming more common. The nature of a policy and the breadth of its scope will determine whether it needs further review within the organization.

Standards of care are authoritative statements that describe a common or acceptable level of client care or performance. In 1973, the American Nurses Association (ANA) first formulated general standards and guidelines for nursing practice, which were revised in 1991, in 2004, and again in 2015. Additionally, standards for more than 20 areas of specialty practice have been developed. They apply across the nation, are broad and general in nature, and have the purpose of establishing the best practice and eliminating as much variation as possible. Similarly, state practice acts contain language describing the standard of practice that applies to all nurses licensed in that state.

Each agency also may develop standards of care for clients with selected healthcare problems. These may take the form of standard nursing care plans or documents termed "care pathways," *critical pathways*, or *clinical pathways*. These are intended to serve as guides to direct the healthcare team in daily care. The individual standard organizes and sequences the care and describes the care required for a client at specific times in the treatment. It involves a multidisciplinary approach and identifies both the care activities and the outcomes for each 24-hour period of hospitalization. These specific standards of care become the basis for evaluation of care, quality improvement within the organization, and cost analysis.

SHARED GOVERNANCE

In the realm of administrative structure, one of the more important changes in healthcare delivery has been the move to a pattern of shared governance within healthcare agencies. Governance establishes how the power and authority for decision-making is structured within an organization.

Shared Governance Model

Shared governance may be viewed as a system in which nurses have organizational autonomy as reflected in control over their practice and have input into decision relating to client care. It is a professional practice model in which both the nursing staff and the nursing management are involved in decision-making, as opposed to the administrative decision area being controlled by the management. Fundamental to the successful implementation of shared governance is the belief that staff nurses at every level within the organization should govern their practice and be involved in decisions that affect that practice. It involves the concepts of equalitarianism, collegiality, and shared professional accountability. Thus, shared governance is more than a structure—it is also a way of thinking.

Effect of Shared Governance on the Roles of the Manager and Staff Nurse

In a shared governance model, the traditional role of the manager as one who hires, evaluates, promotes, and fires becomes a thing of the past. The nurse manager's role is changed to becoming one of facilitator, integrator, and coordinator of the processes that support the work of the staff nurses who have been empowered to control their own practice. They need to participate in professional development sessions that increase nurses' understanding of the decision-making process, team building, group dynamics, leadership and budgeting, and how to participate in and conduct meetings. Managers must learn to share authority over key areas such as scheduling. Many managers have found their new and changing role difficult to accept. The implementation of a shared governance structure requires that staff nurses understand that it is their right and professional obligation to participate in how decisions are made about nursing practice (Joseph & Bogue, 2016).

Pros and Cons of a Shared Governance Model

Strong advocates for the empowerment, autonomy, and professional development of staff nurses encourage the implementation of shared governance. Because shared governance models were introduced to improve nurses' work environments, satisfaction, and retention (Joseph & Bogue, 2016), their popularity has grown. Nurses engaged in evidence-based practice (see Chapter 15) believe the environment that most facilitates and nurtures critical thinking and autonomous decision-making is that of shared governance in which engagement and participation are encouraged.

The Magnet hospital designation, which is awarded through the American Nurses Credentialing Center (ANCC), recognizes that shared governance is beneficial to nurses and involves activities such as accountability for decision-making and establishing committee structures, research projects, and control over practice. Research is ongoing, but shared governance is widely described as empowering and the means for empowerment for direct care nurses (Joseph & Bogue, 2016).

> **Critical Thinking Activity: Shared Governance**
> Research the term *shared governance.* Analyze the information you locate, and make a list of the advantages and disadvantages you see in this form of governance. What steps would you take to implement a shared governance model at a healthcare facility that did not have one?

MAGNET HOSPITALS

Along with the concept of shared governance, the hospital workplace has witnessed the development of the Magnet hospital concept. A Magnet hospital is described as one where nursing delivers excellent client outcomes, where nurses have a high level of job satisfaction, and where there is a low staff nurse turnover rate and appropriate grievance resolution (Stimpfel, Sloane, McHugh, et al., 2016). In the early 1980s, the American Academy of Nursing recognized that acute care facilities, in particular, were having difficulty attracting and retaining RNs. They appointed a task force on hospital nursing practice to examine the situation. The task force determined that it was necessary to research the various factors involved in creating environments that would attract and retain professional nursing staff (McClure, 2005). Nurse researchers, sponsored by the ANA, conducted "reputational" studies to identify successful hospitals, and a body of literature was developed from these studies.

Initially, 41 hospitals were selected as Magnet hospitals. Gold standards were then identified. In 1991, the American Nurses Credentialing Center (ANCC) established a program through which hospitals could apply to be designated Magnet hospitals. Today, more than 448 healthcare organizations in the United States have been awarded Magnet designation for excellence in nursing practice (ANCC Magnet Recognition Program, 2017).

As the study of hospitals continued, characteristics emerged that resulted in the hospitals being considered a good place to work. In the initial study conducted by Kramer and Schmalenberg (2005), 14 forces of magnetism were identified. Over time, some of these became outdated; for others, the operational definition changed. These forces were narrowed down to 10 items staff nurses identified as important enabling them to give quality client care and eventually down to 8 (Box 5.2). Note that many of the forces of magnetism relate to characteristics

---

BOX 5.2   EIGHT ESSENTIALS OF MAGNETISM

- Support for education
- Clinically competent coworkers
- Autonomous nursing practice
- Positive RN–MD relationships
- Supportive nurse manager
- Control over nursing practice
- Adequate staffing
- Culture that values concern for the client as paramount

Data from Kramer, M., & Schmalenberg, C. E. (2005). Best quality client care: A historical perspective on Magnet hospitals. *Nursing Administration, 29*(3), 275–287.

of hospitals discussed earlier in this chapter (ie, flat, decentralized organizational structures, shared governance, and nurse autonomy). Magnet hospitals have been identified as having strong leadership, offering educational resources to employees, providing a work environment in which nurses can grow and challenge themselves, and allowing nurses to be involved in problem solving. A strong aspect of Magnet hospitals is a decrease in the turnover of staff, a factor that speaks to employee satisfaction.

Although Magnet recognition was initiated by nurses and is carried out through the ANCC, the Magnet effort involves all departments and disciplines within the institution. Excellent client care is an interdisciplinary process, and participants in the process of gaining Magnet recognition experience feelings of pride and satisfaction.

PATTERNS OF NURSING CARE DELIVERY

The nursing department of any healthcare institution carries major responsibility for the quality of nursing care delivered. Throughout the years, the structure of the delivery of care has taken many forms, with the particular pattern of care in common use changing about every 20 years. Among the factors influencing the delivery pattern selected in each era were the types of clients served, the type of care provided, the cost of the care, the structure of the hospital, and the number and education level of potential employees. Perhaps a wider variety of patterns of care are being used today than at any other time in nursing's history. In the following table, the typical implementation of several patterns of care delivery is described (Table 5.1, **Fig. 5.6**). However, remember that you might find a particular pattern of care practiced a little differently in different settings.

Table 5.1   Patterns of Nursing Care Delivery

Method	Key Factors
Case Method	• First system used for the delivery of nursing care in the United States (around the beginning of the 20th century) • The nurse works with one client (or case) only and was expected to meet all of that client's needs • The nurse often lived in the client's home and was expected to assume other household duties, such as cooking for the client and family and light housekeeping, when not busy with the client • Chief disadvantage was that nurses worked long hours and were poorly paid • Vestiges of its structure can be seen in today's home health nursing; however, the role of the RN in home healthcare is typically one of assessment, planning, skilled intervention, supervision of care provided by a home health aide, and evaluation of the client's progress
Functional Method	• Emerged during the Great Depression of the 1930s and allowed for the care of greater numbers of clients in hospitals and for the use of advancing technology • A head nurse assigned nursing tasks to various persons employed on the unit—one nurse might take all temperatures and another would do all dressings, while yet another administered all medications • Although economical and efficient, this system of care delivery had the disadvantage of fragmenting care—no single individual was responsible for the planning of care • Nursing care came to be viewed as a list of procedures and tasks • May be used in long-term care facilities or subacute units, largely because of the educational preparation of the care providers

(Continued)

Table 5.1   Patterns of Nursing Care Delivery (continued)

Method	Key Factors
Team Nursing	• Introduced in the early 1950s, with the promise that it would result in more client-centered care • Teams composed of variously educated care providers, for example, two nurse aides, an orderly, an LPN, and an experienced RN as the team leader • Team leader makes assignments, has overall responsibility for the care of clients, typically administers all medications, and gives report • Important part of this form of nursing is the team conference, during which members of the team meet to communicate about the needs of the clients and to plan care • Team nursing has again become a prevalent method of care delivery
Total Client Care	• During the late 1970s and early 1980s, many hospitals returned to total client care in which an RN or LPN was assigned to all the care needs of a group of four to six clients • This approach to care is costly because an individual with less training could satisfactorily complete many of the tasks performed by the RN at a lesser cost • This method requires higher RN staffing, and higher RN staffing is associated with less hospital-related mortality, failure to rescue, cardiac arrest, hospital-acquired pneumonia, and other adverse effects, as well as shorter stays
Primary Care	• Became popular in the 1980s, one nurse was assigned the responsibility for the care of each client from client admission to client's discharge • An associate nurse worked with the same client on other shifts and on the primary nurse's day off • Benefits of this method include the continuity of care for the client and job satisfaction for the nurses • Under this system, every nurse was a primary nurse for a few clients and an associate nurse for others • Concern was the level of expertise and commitment required of all nurses and the fact that nurses who work autonomously with clients soon forget how to delegate responsibilities
Modular Care	• Modular care gained popularity in the mid-1980s • Client care units were divided into modules, and the same team of care providers consistently was assigned to a particular module • Modular nursing looks a lot like team nursing • Advantages: continuity of care, involving the RN in planning and coordinating care, more efficient communication because of the geographic closeness of the unit • Disadvantages: increased costs of stocking each unit and the fact that many hospitals do not lend themselves architecturally to a modular staffing
Partnership Models	• Client care is provided to a group of clients by an RN and an LPN or unlicensed nursing assistant • May also be referred to as "care pairs" • Difficulty of maintaining consistent partnerships among staff creates a major disadvantage
Case Management	• Not a system of care delivery; however, involves nurses in the role of managing client care • System in which the healthcare services are controlled and monitored carefully to ensure that policies are followed and costs are minimized • Case manager typically follows the client from the diagnostic phase through hospitalization, rehabilitation, and back to home

Figure 5.6. Team conference, planning, and communication are critical elements of team nursing.

Critical Thinking Activity: Nursing Care Delivery
Compare the various patterns of nursing care delivery with the pattern being used in a facility where you currently receive clinical experience. Analyze the pattern in current use and evaluate whether another pattern of care delivery would be more or less effective. Provide a rationale for your answer.

WORKPLACE ACTIVITIES THAT INVOLVE NEGOTIATION

Negotiation involves the exchange of ideas and values for the purpose of reaching a mutual decision regarding a particular situation. While it occurs on a day-to-day basis as we work with others, it often is also a part of the mediation process. The following section of this chapter discusses some of the major activities in healthcare environments when negotiation occurs.

Grievance Process

A **grievance** is a circumstance or action believed to be in violation of a contract (or of policies of an institution if a contract is not in place). The **grievance process** represents an established and orderly method to be used in the adjustment of grievances between parties. In this sense, it represents a problem-solving mechanism.

Grievances usually are related to interpretations of a contract or policies and procedures. They may occur as a result of a misunderstanding or difference of opinion about the contract or its language or as a result of direct violations of policies or of the contract. Although either the management or an employee can file grievances, in most instances, it is an employee who initiates the case.

The grievance process spells out in writing a series of steps to be taken to resolve the area of dissension and a timeline for accomplishing those steps. If a contract exists, the steps to be used in mediating grievances are usually included in that document. If there is no formal contract, internal policies exist that outline grievance procedures. Perhaps you are aware of grievance processes from your student handbook, where the processes in place in an educational program are shared with students.

Initially, the employee and the immediate supervisor attempt to resolve the disagreement through an informal talk. If no resolution occurs, the discussion moves to the steps of the grievance process, involving others within the organization. The steps include providing notifications and responses in writing, adhering to strict timelines for action, and eventually involving people at higher levels within the organization (eg, representatives from the bargaining unit, a grievance chairperson, the human resources director, and administrative representatives). Perhaps the services of an arbitrator will be needed toward the end of the dispute. Failure of either side to comply with the timelines that are in effect regarding its own actions or responses ends the process. If an arbitrator is involved, that person's decision is usually binding.

It is important to differentiate between complaints and grievances. Employees may have complaints that are not violations of the contract. For example, Nurse A may object that she was required to float from the postpartum unit to the nursery; she had been oriented to the nursery but preferred to work in the postpartum unit. Nurse B was required to float from a medical unit to a surgical unit to which she had not been oriented. If the contract in this hospital stipulates that no one would be floated to a unit to which he or she had not been oriented, Nurse A had a complaint, whereas Nurse B had a grievance.

The absence of grievances, once thought to be an indication of an effective, well-managed organization, may not be the best indicator of the organization's health. It is entirely possible that problems are not being addressed. By the same token, a high number of grievances may indicate problems within the organization. These problems also may relate to the language of the contract or the education of the employee regarding the conditions of employment. Another barometer of the health of an organization is the level at which the grievances are resolved. It is most desirable to settle most grievances at the informal level, without the involvement of an arbitrator.

Although most grievances are settled short of arbitration, they are still time and energy consuming. Grievances can best be avoided if everyone has a good understanding of the terms of employment and if sound personnel policies are developed and applied consistently and equitably. A part of the orientation of new employees to an organization should be spent reviewing and explaining these features. Open discussions between the employees and management to review mutual concerns and share information help reduce the number of grievances. Mutual respect is a critical element in any organization.

Critical Thinking Activity: Grievances

What are the reasons that grievance processes should be spelled out? How would you determine whether an issue is a grievance or a complaint? What resources are available to you as you search for the answer?

Collective Bargaining

Collective bargaining consists of a set of procedures by which employee representatives (typically a union) and employer representatives negotiate to obtain a signed agreement (**contract**) that spells out wages, hours, and conditions of employment that are acceptable to both. A keyword in this definition is negotiate. The goal of negotiations is to obtain a signed agreement, which is a legal contract that spells out in writing the decisions that are reached.

Because of nursing's long history as a profession of dedication, altruism, and service, collective bargaining initially was a controversial issue within nursing. Some saw this process as detracting from the professional role of the nurse and ethically improper.

Today, however, nurses are vitally concerned about contracts, services, third-party payers, comparable worth, clients' rights and safety, shared governance, staffing ratios, and a host of issues that can be discussed at the bargaining table. Nurses believe that people who choose nursing as a career should have the opportunity to have some voice in client care assignments, length of the workday and workweek, fringe benefits, and wages, without losing face with the public at large, members of the medical profession, or other colleagues. Additionally, at a time when nurses are campaigning for a safer practice environment free of mandatory overtime and other work issues, collective bargaining takes on a new countenance—an avenue by which to address these and other work concerns and gain control over practice.

History of Collective Bargaining

Interest in the rights of workers began to gain attention in the United States as early as the 1850s. The highlights of the history of collective bargaining are presented in Table 5.2.

Understanding the Basic Concepts of Collective Bargaining

Intelligent and effective bargaining begins with an awareness of the process itself. The information that follows is designed to provide a better understanding of the terms and processes involved in bargaining collectively to achieve an agreed-upon contract.

Table 5.2 History of Collective Bargaining

Event	Date	Effect(s)
Horace Greeley writes articles in *New York Tribune* columns regarding collective bargaining	1850	Impetus and interest generated in the issue of workers' rights
National Industrial Recovery Act	1933	Nation required to accept a 35–40-hour workweek and 30–40 cents per hour minimum wage and prohibited child labor
NLRA (Wagner Act)	1935	Gave workers protection in their efforts to form unions and organize for better working conditions Created the NLRB
Taft–Hartley Act (Labor Management Relations Act)	1947	Excluded nonprofit hospitals from the legal obligation of bargaining with employees
Taft–Hartley Act amended	1974	Provided economic security programs for those employed in nonprofit hospitals, thus requiring hospitals to bargain with nurses for better salaries and working conditions Required a 10-day written notice of intent to picket or strike

Bargaining and Negotiating

To **negotiate** means to bargain or confer with another party or parties to reach an agreement. It implies that there will be a discussion of the terms of the agreement and suggests that there will be give and take—that neither party will obtain all items asked for in the contract. Ideally, negotiations would proceed in a somewhat philosophic vein, moving toward reasonable compromises that would allow each side to achieve many of the conditions it requested, but this does not always occur. What is assured is that there will be change. Kurt Lewin developed the Change Theory, which has three phases, all of which are evident in collective bargaining. See the Theory Alert below for more information.

Theory Alert   *Kurt Lewin*

Kurt Lewin is considered to be the father of social psychology. He was born in Germany in 1890. He served in the German army during World War I. He was injured and returned home to Berlin where he completed his PhD. He immigrated to the United States in 1933.

Lewin developed the Change Theory, a nursing model that proposes there are three components to change: driving forces, restraining forces, and equilibrium. These components refer to the situational factors that either cause change, resist change, or seek to maintain the status quo. Lewin labels three distinct stages of change: unfreezing, movement, and refreezing.

For change to take place, people must be willing to let go of the old way of thinking or doing; this is *unfreezing*. The progression to the change is the *movement* phase, and to prevent sliding back to the old way of doing things, *refreezing* need to take place. All of these steps are evident in the adoption of successful collective bargaining agreements.
(Source: www.nursing-theory.org)

A typical bargaining session has three phases. The early sessions include a formal exchange of proposals, during which each side may ask for more than it knows it can expect to receive and emphasizes its commitment to certain issues. The second phase gives the most attention to secondary issues. The third phase occurs as the deadline approaches, and primary issues are discussed realistically.

Several forms of bargaining have evolved. **Interest-based bargaining** represents a nontraditional style of bargaining in which the parties:

• Focus on interests or what each side wants rather than proposals
• Agree on the criteria of acceptability that will be used to evaluate alternatives
• Generate several alternatives that are consistent with their interests
• Apply the agreed-upon acceptability criteria to the alternatives so generated in order to arrive at mutually acceptable contract provisions

Much of the success of the technique depends on mutual trust, openness, and a willingness to share information. But even where these are lacking, the technique, with its focus on interests and on developing alternatives, tends to make the parties more flexible and open to alternative solutions and thus increases the likelihood of agreement (Labor-Management Relations Glossary, n.d.).

Another variation sometimes seen is concession bargaining. **Concession bargaining** is a process in which there is an explicit exchange of reduced labor costs for improvements in job security. This occurs with increasing frequency. An example would be a shift in emphasis from one that asks for increases in salary to one that focuses on eliminating the practice of calling nurses and telling them not to report for work because the census has dropped (on such days, the nurses do not receive salary). These are issues of concern to nurses today.

Unions and Collective Action

A **union** is a legally authorized organization that has been empowered by its members to negotiate and enforce a contract. Therefore, in order to engage in collective bargaining, employees must choose a union that will represent them. This usually is done through an election. The major areas in which a union may bargain are the wages, hours, and working conditions of its members.

When a branch or part of a professional association assumes the role and responsibility of a union, as often occurs in nursing, the negotiating group may be known as a collective action division, although it is legally considered a union. A professional organization works under the same legal constraints as any other union. It provides legal counsel and representatives to assist with negotiations, may lobby on behalf of issues, or may participate in other activities that would further the economic welfare of nurses (Evidence-Based Practice 5.1). It oversees the development of the contract, monitors adherence to the contract, and represents employees in any grievance process.

Contracts

The conclusion of the bargaining process should result in a signed contract that converts to writing the agreements that have been reached. A contract is "an agreement between two or more parties, especially one that is written and enforceable by law" (www.freedictionary.com). This signed contract is enforceable under law and cannot be changed by either party acting unilaterally.

Some would suggest that the contract is the most important product of the collective bargaining process because it is a legal agreement on all issues that have been discussed.

Evidence-Based Practice 5.1: Comparing Wages for Union and Nonunion Nurses

Coombs, C. K., Newman, R. J., Cebula, R. J., & White, M. L. (2015). The bargaining power of health care unions and union wage premiums for registered nurses. *Journal of Labor Research*, *36*(4), 442–461. doi:http://dx.doi.org/10.1007/s12122-015-9214-z

The National Sample Survey of Registered Nurses included a question regarding union status for the first time in 2008. The study then used the data gathered to compare wages for union and nonunion nurses. It also compared various work environments.

A wage advantage for union workers was evident across work environments, with a larger advantage apparent in private sector employment. It also appeared that even nonunion workers benefitted as the bargaining power and lobbying efforts of the union seemed to improve wages for both groups of workers.

It provides the foundation for further activities. Unlike the policies of an agency, which can be changed by the management alone, the agreement of both management and employees is required for any change to be made in a contract. The contract remains in effect until breached or terminated. Most negotiated contracts define the period of time—usually 2 or 3 years—during which the established conditions are effective.

Before being put into effect, a contract must be **ratified**. This means that the members of the bargaining group must accept the terms of the contract. This is usually done by a vote of the membership. Factors to be considered in a contract will be discussed later in this chapter.

Rules Governing Labor Relations

When two parties agree to begin the negotiation process, it is understood that both will **bargain in good faith**. Bargaining in good faith means that the parties will meet at regular times to discuss (with the intent to resolve) any differences over wages, hours, and other employment conditions. Failure to carry out these activities could lead to an unfair labor practice.

An **unfair labor practice** is any action that interferes with the rights of employees or employers as described in the amended NLRA. It is not possible to discuss all of these in detail; however, some examples follow. An employer must not interfere with the employee's right to form a union or other organized bargaining group, join the group, or participate in the group's activities. The employer may not attempt to control a group, once organized, or to discriminate against its members regarding hiring or tenure. Most importantly, the employer must bargain collectively and in good faith with representatives of the employees.

Likewise, labor organizations have constraints placed on their activities. They, too, must bargain in good faith. They must not restrain or coerce employees in selecting a bargaining group to bargain collectively. They may not pressure an employer to discriminate against employees who do not belong to the labor organization.

One of the issues brought up in negotiations that usually results in a dispute is that of agency shop. When an **agency shop** clause is in effect, all employees in the unit pay dues or fees to the union to defray the costs of providing representation. There are several variations in provisions related to an agency shop. If, because of religious or philosophic beliefs, employees are unwilling to pay dues to the bargaining group, provisions may be made to pay the same sum to a nonprofit group, such as a charity or foundation. In some instances, those who are already members of the union are required to remain members for the life of the contract, although no one is required to become a member. In some states, laws referred to as "right to work laws" forbid the establishment of an agency shop. If you seek employment in an agency where nurses bargain collectively, it would be wise to explore the options available to you.

Settling Labor Disputes

When labor disputes arise, several actions can be taken to help resolve the differences. Initially, of course, the parties continue to negotiate and may agree to extend the negotiation period if progress in settling differences is being made. When the two parties negotiating cannot come to an agreement on an issue, they are considered to be at **impasse** or deadlocked on the issue.

Mediation and Arbitration

Perhaps the most commonly used method of seeking agreement between parties when negotiating has not been successful is through mediation and arbitration. A **mediator** is a third person who may join the bargainers to assist the parties in reconciling differences and arriving at a peaceful agreement. Although the mediator may join the parties at any point in the negotiations, due to the cost of mediation, most negotiations proceed until things are at an impasse. **Mediation** involves finding compromises, and the mediator assists with this. He or she must gain the respect of both parties and must remain neutral to the issues presented.

An **arbitrator** is technically defined as a person chosen by the agreement of both parties to decide a dispute between them. The primary difference between a mediator and an arbitrator is that the mediator assists the parties in reaching their own decision, whereas the arbitrator has the authority to actually make the decision for the parties if necessary. However, the terms mediator and arbitrator and mediation and arbitration often are used interchangeably; in fact, a mediator may also serve as an arbitrator **(Fig. 5.7)**.

Arbitration may take several forms. It may be mediation–arbitration, in which a third person joins the parties in the negotiation process and helps establish priorities. If an agreement is

Figure 5.7. The arbitrator's decision may not really please either side.

not reached by a specified date, or if it appears that the issue is **deadlocked**, with neither party willing to compromise, the mediator then assumes the role of an arbitrator and makes a decision based on the information gained in the role of mediator.

Another form of arbitration is called **binding arbitration**. This means that both parties are obligated to abide by the decision of the arbitrator. Some people see this as the least desirable alternative in settling disputes because it may result in a decision that is not satisfactory to either side but one by which both must abide. Binding arbitration has the advantage of resolving deadlocked issues without a strike. It also encourages both parties, knowing that the arbitrator's decision may not please either side, to reach a compromise on their own.

One criticism of any type of arbitration is the expense involved. Arbitrators must be paid for their services. Arbitration is also criticized because it undermines voluntary collective bargaining and allows parties to avoid unpleasant confrontation with their own difficulties by shifting that responsibility to a public authority. However, it is useful in preventing the disruption of services.

Lockouts and Strikes

When the negotiation process breaks down, lockouts and strikes are likely to occur. A **lockout** occurs when an employer refuses to allow the employees to work. It is done to force employees to agree to the terms offered by the employer. The employer may close a place of business, or the employer may choose to remain open, discharge the workers, and use replacement workers. One can see how undesirable this would be in the healthcare system, but it has occurred in rare instances.

A **strike** occurs when workers refuse to continue to work until certain demands are met, thus imposing economic hardship and pressure on the employer. When the negotiation process breaks down, employees may use the strike to emphasize the need to improve their working conditions, salaries, and benefits. The most recent strikes by nurses, however, have been over issues related to client care rather than those related to the economic status of the nurses. Striking places a serious economic hardship on employees and therefore is not undertaken lightly. Sometimes a strike is used to gain public attention to the labor dispute and to create public pressure for a settlement. This is only successful if the public agrees with the position of the striking workers.

At one time, nursing strikes were viewed by some as unprofessional and detrimental to the health of the community and, as indicated in Table 5.3, were forbidden by ANA policy until 1968. When strikes occurred, they drew major media attention, and it was feared that they would damage the image of nurses and nursing.

Some nurses view with great concern the issue of whether nurses should participate in strikes if negotiations break down. These nurses believe that the withholding of services from clients is unethical and unprofessional and, therefore, personally unacceptable. Others view the strike as a final method for bringing attention to the needs of the nurse as a citizen. Fortunately, as bargaining groups representing nurses become more knowledgeable and skilled in the process, strikes occur less frequently. Disagreements at the bargaining table are more commonly resolved through mediation and arbitration, much to the relief of many professionals.

Strikes in nursing are undertaken only with advance notice, to enable clients to be transferred to another facility and to make other plans for care of individuals in the community.

Typically, arrangements are made with another hospital to admit clients during the strike, and all elective procedures are canceled. The striking nurses may also agree to provide staffing to critical care, labor and delivery, and emergency departments of the facility in which the strike occurs. Often, the notification that nurses intend to strike on a certain date is a sufficient incentive to move negotiations to the point of settlement.

In spite of efforts to avoid them, strikes do occur in nursing. When this happens, it is often an unpleasant experience for all. Those who choose to cross picket lines may be subjected to harassment and verbal abuse by their colleagues. Those striking for better working conditions and client safety may feel betrayed by nurses who make the strike less effective. Nurses may feel pitted against one another as well as against the management (National Nurse, 2016).

Reinstatement Privilege

A **reinstatement privilege** is a guarantee offered to striking employees that they will be rehired after the strike as positions become available, provided that they have not engaged in any unfair labor practices during the strike and provided that the strike itself is lawful. The hospital may replace a striking nurse during the strike. If strikers agree unconditionally to return to work, the employer is not required to rehire a striking nurse at that time. However, recall lists are developed, and if the nurse cannot find regular and equivalent employment, he or she is privileged to recall and preference on jobs before new employees may be given employment. Nurses may lose their reinstatement privileges because of misconduct during a lawful strike. For example, strikers may not physically block other nurses and personnel from entering or leaving a hospital during a strike. Strikers may not threaten nonstriking employees and may not attack management representatives. These types of activities usually do not occur during strikes conducted by nurses but are not outside the realm of possibility.

What to Look for in a Contract

The negotiation process should ultimately conclude in the development of a written contract that is signed by both union and management representatives.

A contract must meet certain specified criteria to be legally binding. It must result from mutually agreed-upon items arrived at through a "meeting of minds." Something of value must be given for a reciprocal promise, that is, professional duties for an agreed-upon sum. Contracts can be enforceable whether written or oral but are easier to work with when written. Written contracts are also considered formal contracts. Although each agreement will differ, most contracts have a fairly general format. Box 5.3 includes items included in that format.

Issues Negotiated in Contracts

Many have come to believe that the collective action of nurses provides one of the best avenues for achieving professional goals and exercising control over nursing practice. Provision 6 of the ANA Code (2015) states, "The nurse, through individual and collective effort, establishes, maintains, and improves the ethical environment of the work setting and conditions of employment that are conducive to safe, quality healthcare." As nurses are called on to assume greater responsibility for complicated decisions and control over practice, collective bargaining through a professional organization may provide the means to implement the concept of collective action. Today, the terms and conditions of employment have taken on a prominence over wages and hours in contract negotiations.

BOX 5.3 ITEMS TYPICALLY INCLUDED IN CONTRACTS

- A preamble stating the objectives of each party
- A statement recognizing the official bargaining groups
- A section dealing with financial remuneration, including wages and salaries, overtime rates, holiday pay, and shift differentials
- A section dealing with nonfinancial rewards, that is, fringe benefits such as retirement programs, types of insurance available, free parking, and other services provided by the employer
- A section dealing with seniority in respect to promotions, transfers, work schedules, and layoffs
- A section establishing guidelines for disciplinary problems
- A section describing grievance procedures
- A section that may explicitly state codes of conduct or professional standards

---

The ANA (2015) has developed the Nurses' Bill of Rights, which is useful in identifying the important elements of the work environment.

1. Nurses have the right to practice in a manner that fulfills their obligations to society and to those who receive nursing care.
2. Nurses have the right to practice in environments that allow them to act in accordance with professional standards and legally authorized scopes of practice.
3. Nurses have the right to a work environment that supports and facilitates ethical practice, in accordance with the Code of Ethics for Nurses with Interpretive Statements.
4. Nurses have the right to freely and openly advocate for themselves and their clients, without fear of retribution.
5. Nurses have the right to fair compensation for their work, consistent with their knowledge, experience, and professional responsibilities.
6. Nurses have the right to a work environment that is safe for themselves and for their clients.
7. Nurses have the right to negotiate the conditions of their employment, either as individuals or collectively, in all practice settings.

The manner in which the bargaining is conducted greatly influences how it will be perceived. Nurses as a group need to develop the skills necessary to communicate to the public the importance of their role in healthcare delivery. They must be able to handle conflicts and work toward resolution while maintaining integrity and dignity. Nurses need to become enlightened and informed, and they need more than a superficial understanding of the process of collective bargaining. It is important that, as a new graduate, you know whether there is a contract in effect in the institution in which you seek employment or in the community in which you plan to work. You should also be knowledgeable about the terms of the existing contract so that you might best fulfill your obligations and recognize and benefit from the provisions to which you are entitled. The organization to which you are applying for employment can provide you with a copy of the current contract. Contact the state nurses' association for information regarding the organization that represents nurses in a particular hospital or facility. They can also provide a copy of any contracts that have been negotiated for which they represented the nurses.

Critical Thinking Activity: Contracts
As a new employee in a hospital, how will you find out whether there is a contract? To whom will you ask? How will you obtain a copy of the contract? What will you do if the contract includes language that you do not understand? What would you do if you were in total disagreement with some of the stipulations of the contract?

Issues Related to Collective Bargaining and Nursing

Four major issues of collective bargaining affect the nursing profession: the fact that some nurses see collective bargaining as unprofessional, the matter of which bargaining group will represent nursing when nurses participate in collective bargaining, the question of whether to join a union when one exists, and the issue of the role of the supervisor. These issues may take on greater or lesser importance depending on the area of the country involved, the length of time the nurses in that area have been participating in collective bargaining, and the group chosen to represent the nurses at the bargaining table. Additionally, as a staff nurse, you may, at some time, have to make a decision regarding whether to strike. In making this decision, you want to be well grounded in the issues at hand and knowledgeable about the arrangements that have been made for the continuance of services in emergency situations and in special hospital areas, such as labor and delivery.

Collective Action and Professionalism

In addition to the historic view of nursing as an all-serving, altruistic calling with strong religious influences, another factor that has hampered the strong development of unionization in nursing is the socialization of women and the fact that nursing is primarily a woman's profession. Although more men now enter nursing, currently fewer than 10% of the RNs in the United States are male. Early social beliefs that a woman's role should be submissive, supportive, and obedient were extremely compatible with the expectations that our society placed on nurses. The paternalism that has existed in the healthcare delivery system has also made the process of collective bargaining for nurses a slow one. The combination of the role of women and the role of the nurse under earlier paternalistic practices was once described by a nursing author as the nurse caring for the "hospital family," looking out for the needs of all (from client to physician), and being responsible for keeping everyone happy (Ashley, 1976). The tendency to see the physician as the father figure in the healthcare system, the nurse as the corresponding mother figure, and the clients as the children has done little to promote the autonomy of nursing as a profession.

Today, we see nurses involved in collective bargaining in greater numbers than ever before. Several of the factors responsible for this change include:

- Legislated changes that allowed nurses to bargain collectively
- The rising cost of healthcare that resulted in the examination of all factors, including salaries that contributed to the cost
- Issues in the delivery of care such as client–nurse ratios, workplace safety, and overtime that lent themselves to negotiation
- A new generation of nurses who approach the world of employment with different goals and attitudes than did the previous generations

Representation for Nurses

As collective bargaining has become accepted for nurses, the number of groups that seek to represent them at the bargaining table has constantly increased, with many groups now bargaining for nurses. Representation is determined by elections that are supervised by the NLRB. To become the certified collective bargaining representative of a group of employees, the organization seeking that role must receive 50% of the votes cast, plus one.

Activity of the ANA

When nurses first began to organize, the ANA, through the state nurses associations, was the sole bargaining representative; this group still represents more nurses than all other organizations combined. See Table 5.3 for a summary of the activities of ANA in relationship to collective bargaining and workplace advocacy. (For more information on ANA activities related to collective bargaining, see thePoint˚.)

Some would contend that it is not realistic for one group to work with the professionalism aspect of nursing as well as with the issues of wages, benefits, and working conditions. This has encouraged other organizations to compete for the right to represent nurses. As a result, a large number of nurses are represented by the American Federation of Teachers, the Teamsters Union, the National Union of Hospital and Health Care Employees, the Federation of Nurses and Health Professionals, United Food and Commercial Workers, or the Service Employees

Table 5.3 ANA Activities Related to Collective Bargaining and Workplace Advocacy

Year	Activity
1931	Developed within its organization a legislative policy addressing general welfare concerns of its members.
1945	Appointed a committee to study employment conditions.
1946	Established the ANA Economic Security Program as an outcome of the 1945 study. State nurses associations encouraged to act as exclusive bargaining agents for their memberships.
1947	Collective bargaining between nurses and hospital administrations implemented in several states with negotiated contracts in effect.
1949	ANA is certified as a labor organization.
1950	No-strike policy adopted officially by ANA due to the concern for the image of nursing.
1967	ANA identified as the bargaining agent for nurses in Veterans Administration hospitals.
1968	No-strike policy rescinded.
1991	ANA embarked on a Workplace Advocacy Initiative to improve the work environment of nurses.
1999	UAN established as an autonomous arm of ANA to carry out collective bargaining for nurses at the national level and to coordinate the work of state collective bargaining units.
2000	Commission on Workplace Advocacy established to address the needs of individual nurses in the workplace not represented by collective bargaining.
2003	The Center for American Nurses established as an outgrowth of the Commission on Workplace Advocacy. Created a new membership category for Associate Organization Members and addresses challenges and opportunities individual nonunion nurses face in their practice environments.
2009	NNU formed as a *superunion* by three founding organizations, UAN, Massachusetts Nurses Association, and CNA/NNOC.

International Union (SEIU). In some instances, as with the SEIU, the organization represents other workers employed in the organization. The SEIU organizes what are called "wall-to-wall" unions, in which all employees of all categories from housekeeping and maintenance to nurses and pharmacists belong to one bargaining unit. This may be favored by hospital administration, which often expresses frustration with the number of groups with whom negotiations must be carried out. However, when the SEIU is bargaining for all employees, it has the distinct disadvantage of diluting the ability of nurses to include professional issues in the negotiation process.

Nurses face a difficult decision when choosing which group can represent them best. In the past years, this decision has occupied perhaps more time and effort on the part of nurses than has the actual bargaining. Some contend that only RNs should bargain for RNs because nurses face different issues than other workers. Many believe that only nurses can effectively negotiate such items. These people contend that hospital administrations, fearing the power of labor unions, will bargain more constructively and positively with nurses themselves.

The state nurses association serves as a collective bargaining agent in many states. To do this, they must organize in such as way that the collective bargaining is separated in terms of finances and control from the other activities of the organization. Those who are members but not part of a collective bargaining unit pay lesser dues than those who are part of a collective bargaining unit. Only those who are part of bargaining units have a vote regarding collective bargaining issues.

Some nurses prefer two organizations—one to represent issues related to professionalism and another to negotiate salaries. This does require dues to two organizations. Although the dues for the state nurses association are reduced considerably if it does not serve as the bargaining agent for an individual's workplace, there remains an added cost when belonging to two organizations. Because of this, many who are represented by another union do not join their nurses association.

Critical Thinking Activity: Collective Bargaining

If the collective bargaining agent in the hospital in which you worked was other than the state nurses association, would you belong to both organizations? What factors would you use to support your decision? Why are these factors important to you?

Decision to Join or Not to Join

Once nurses have gained an understanding of collective bargaining and have developed a personal philosophy about the professional role of the nurse, they are ready to make a decision regarding membership in the bargaining unit.

In working with students who are soon to embark on professional careers, we find that it is easier for them to decide whether to bargain collectively than it is to decide to part with the money that is required for membership. Many nurses want better working conditions and higher salaries but are all too willing to let someone else fund these endeavors and work to achieve them.

It is in response to these concerns that many agency shop clauses have been added to contracts. Those who are members and are active in the negotiation process believe it is inappropriate for some to benefit from the labors of the bargaining process without having contributed, at least financially, to the effort. The presence of agency shop clauses may serve as either an asset or a deterrent to recruitment, depending on the applicant's viewpoint.

Communication in Action 5.2: *Seeking Information Regarding a Union*

Will Jones had just begun working at the medical center. He was given a copy of the contract for RNs during his orientation. He was also given the name of a union representative on his unit. During his first week there, he approached the representative and said, "Hi Carol, I was told you are the union representative for our unit. Do you have some time to talk with me? I would like to understand more about the process here." She replied, "Sure—let's plan to go down to the cafeteria at 11:30—first lunch. Does that work for you?" He said, "That is when I was scheduled for lunch too. Just so you know, I don't really know anything about the union, what its goals are, the issues here, or anything. I hope you can help me get that kind of information." Will had set the stage to become a knowledgeable participant in the bargaining process.

Collective Bargaining and the Role of a Supervisor

The question of whether nurses are considered supervisors because they direct the care of others first surfaced in 1994, when a nursing home argued before the Supreme Court that the LPNs in its employment were supervisors, directing the work of others, and, therefore, were not protected by the NLRA. The Supreme Court, in a 5 to 4 decision, ruled in favor of the nursing home ("Striking at bargaining," 1994).

This issue was again addressed in February 1996, when the NLRB ended nearly 2 years of deliberation by ruling that charge nurses at Alaska's Providence Medical Center could not be called supervisors simply because the role requires some direction of other workers. The board stated that the essence of the nurse's role was judgment and went on to explain that the authority that arises from professional knowledge is distinct from the authority of a front-line manager ("NLRB to the Supreme Court," 1996). The fact that the nurses did not have the authority to hire, evaluate, and terminate others was important in the court's decision. In another case in 2013, RNs employed as charge nurses in a nursing home were considered to be supervisors as they exercised sufficient, independent judgment when issuing discipline (Rosen, 2013). The issue continues to occur with surprising frequency, often with contradictory results.

Changes in the Number of Bargaining Units

Within hospitals, there are many different positions and job titles, ranging from professional staff through office staff to those responsible for hospital maintenance. In nursing alone, there are groups of RNs, LPNs, and nursing assistants. As these groups have been granted authority to organize into bargaining units, concern has been expressed about the number of unions with which any hospital administration must bargain at any given time. Some fairly elaborate estimates have been made regarding the amount of time demanded by the collective bargaining process.

When the NLRA was first passed in 1974, the NLRB specified that seven employee bargaining units would exist within the healthcare industry (Wilson, Hamilton, & Murphy, 1990, p. 37): RNs, physicians, other professional employees, technical employees, business office employees, clerical employees, and skilled maintenance employees. In 1984, the NLRB determined that bargaining units would be decided on a case-by-case basis. This resulted in reducing the number of bargaining units to three: all professionals, all nonprofessionals, and guards.

In 1989, the NLRB proposed a new rule that resulted in the establishment of eight collective bargaining units. At this time, it was also determined that the rule would apply to hospitals of all sizes. In response, the American Hospital Association (AHA) sought and obtained a permanent injunction against the rule. Subsequently, all-RN units were legally approved. In April 1991, the U.S. Supreme Court upheld the NLRB in its authority to define bargaining units for healthcare workers in acute care hospitals and allowed for all-RN bargaining units ("Supreme Court Okays," 1991). As might be expected, the AHA and the ANA occupied opposite points of view regarding this issue. The NLRB continues to represent the rights of worker. "The **National Labor Relations Board** is an independent federal agency that protects the rights of private sector employees to join together, with or without a union, to improve their wages and working conditions" (NLRB, n.d.).

Changing Trends With Regard to Collective Bargaining

At one time, economic concerns and working conditions may have been the principal motivators for collective action. However, by the mid-1980s, subtle, and at times not so subtle, changes occurred throughout the United States regarding collective bargaining, unionism, and labor–management relations.

Some working in the area of contract management have reported a shift from the adversarial relationship that historically had existed between the employee and the employer (which focused on salaries, work hours, and the like) to one that placed greater emphasis on the quality of work life. These items, such as staffing ratios and assistive personnel, can make the work environment safer for employees and clients. See Evidence-Based Practice 5.2 for more information.

Evidence-Based Practice 5.2: Nurse Unions and Client Outcomes

Dube, A., Kaplan, E., & Thompson, O. (2016). Nurse unions and client outcomes. *ILR Review*, 69(4), 803–833. doi:10.1177/0019793916644251

In this article, the authors compared data from hospitals with unions against hospitals without unions. They were evaluating the information gathered to determine what, if any, effect, unionization had on client outcomes. The information gathered revealed some significant differences.

The authors found that hospitals with unions had better client outcomes on 12 out of 13 areas that were significantly impacted by nursing care. It was also found that unionization often occurred at hospitals that were experiencing a decline in quality as measured by client outcome. The changes ranged from 15% to nearly 60% improvements in unionized facilities. One factor that probably relates to this is staffing ratios that are always a topic of much discussion.

Thrust of Collective Bargaining in Nursing

The focus of collective bargaining issues changed during the 1990s. As nurses have become more comfortable and knowledgeable about the bargaining process, their energies have been directed toward many issues. Originally focusing on wages and benefits, today, the major concerns of nurses also include staffing patterns, involvement in decisions affecting client care, cross-training, the use of unlicensed assistive personnel, workplace safety and the rights of employees to know the hazards with a work environment, comparable worth, and discriminatory practices against employees (both male and female). This shift in emphasis reflects the general acceptance of the process of collective bargaining by nurses and the fact that significant headway has been made through this process regarding basic issues.

Elimination of Unions and Strike Breaking

A trend seen in healthcare institutions during the 1980s, and persisting in some areas today, is an effort toward eliminating unions. Although technically illegal when referring to methods used to eliminate an existing union, the movement has been expanded to include a wide range of legal activities that slow down collective bargaining or prevent a union from forming or functioning effectively. Pressured by rapidly escalating healthcare costs and influenced by the changing attitudes toward work, hospital administrators have hired consultants and law firms to assist and advise in discouraging and impeding organizational activities.

Another closely related approach involves mutual cooperation between the management and the union without undermining the legitimate roles and rights of either. The union encourages wholehearted employee participation by its members while exercising flexibility on issues. With this approach, the union should have input into the managerial decision-making process through representation on committees at every level of the organization. Unions should be expected to be cooperative with management but not be co-opted. Management must be fair with the union, neither seeking to destroy the union nor meekly acquiescing to every union demand.

Strike breaking refers to efforts directed at causing employees on strike to cease the strike without having reached an agreement. In an effort to break a strike, employers hire temporary nurses at very high wages plus living stipends to entice them to come to work. Some temporary agencies specialize in providing nurses to work when the regular employees of the institution are on strike.

Impact of Shared Governance on Collective Bargaining

Although the greater involvement of staff nurses in healthcare agency decision-making may have a significant impact on the collective bargaining process, the number of nurses represented by collective bargaining is increasing. When both collective bargaining and shared governance are present, there is a separation of those issues that are the purview of the union and those issues that can be decided within the shared governance structure. If there is a union, it has the responsibility and authority to negotiate those things that fall under wages, benefits, and working conditions, such as the use of agency nurses, workload, and policies regarding floating from one unit to another. The shared governance committees work with clinical standards. Each nurse has greater accountability for participation in decision-making outside of the bargaining process and for implementing decisions that have been made.

Looking to the Future

As with many of the issues with which nursing wrestles, there are no easy answers to the matter of collective bargaining. Some view it as an absolute necessity; others find it unethical.

Stegen and Sowerby Stories: Part 2

emember the New York nurses and managers that met to discuss staffing ratios with assistance of a facilitator? They continued to meet about twice monthly for 4 months to discuss factors that impact staffing and work toward a mutually agreed upon staffing ratio. There were many differing opinions expressed during those meetings. Read the rest of the story at www.thePoint.com.

Want to Know More?

A variety of resources are available on thePoint® to enhance your learning and understanding of this chapter, such as:

- Full Stegen and Sowerby Stories
- NCLEX-Style Student Review Questions
- Journal Articles
- Case Studies
- Learning Objectives
- Relevant Websites
- And more...

KEY CONCEPTS

- Mission statements provide information about critical elements of the organization. They explicitly outline the purpose of the organization and may also contain the philosophy and the vision or goals of the group. These statements serve as a benchmark against which an organization's performance may be evaluated.
- Organizations may be structured in a number of ways. Some are tall and centralized, where the authority to make decisions is vested in a few individuals. Others are flat and decentralized, with a number of individuals involved in decision-making. Some have a matrix of functional roles.
- All organizations have chains of command, channels of communication, and spans of control that describe lines of authority and accountability. These can be depicted in organizational charts, which represent the formal organization and are a pictorial means of portraying roles and patterns of interaction among parts of a system.
- Written job descriptions outline the roles and responsibilities for all employees and are a necessary and vital part of any organization.
- Policies, protocols, and procedures guide the activities of the employees as they carry out their responsibilities.

- Shared governance, a form of practice model that involves decision-making in which both nursing staff and management participate, results in a decentralized organization and often results in greater job satisfaction for nurses because they have more control over their practice.
- In the late 1980s, studies were conducted to determine what factors resulted in hospitals attracting and retaining RNs. Characteristics of these hospitals were identified, and the awarding of Magnet status to hospitals that achieve these goals has resulted. The process is carried out under the auspices of the ANCC.
- Patterns of nursing care delivery have varied over the years and include the case method, the functional method, team nursing, total client care, modular care, and primary nursing.
- Case management provides an approach to the delivery of all client care services (not just nursing) over an entire hospital stay or even throughout an entire healthcare concern. Nurses are involved in case management and may serve as case managers.
- Many workplace matters require negotiation. Major issues among these are grievances, collective bargaining contracts, and workplace safety issues.
- A grievance is an alleged violation of the provisions of the contract or institutional policies. Should a grievance arise, all steps must be followed as outlined in order for the grievance to be addressed effectively. Nurses need to distinguish between issues that are grievances and those that are simply complaints.
- Approaches to collective bargaining vary and include the historic adversarial approach, interest-based bargaining, and concession bargaining.
- Interest-based bargaining attempts to problem solve differences between labor and industry. Nurses can play a powerful leadership role in the process.
- The collective bargaining process culminates in a contract that places in writing the decisions reached at the bargaining table. Key aspects of a contract are the wages and benefits, issues of seniority and layoffs, grievance procedures, termination procedures, and working conditions (including professional involvement).
- One of the issues surrounding nurses and collective bargaining is related to which group should do the bargaining for nurses. Many believe this process is best conducted by a professional nursing organization; others believe they are served best by an organization that has collective bargaining as its only focus.
- Since 1974, nurses have bargained collectively for salaries, working conditions, and benefits. Collective bargaining may also negotiate for nurses' participation in committees focused on improving client care and client care standards and other issues of concern to nurses including staffing patterns, mandatory overtime, use of temporary nurses, workplace safety, and discriminatory practices.
- Trends regarding the collective bargaining process include constructive adversarialism, union busting, strike breaking, and changes in the number of bargaining units.

NCLEX-STYLE PRACTICE QUESTIONS

1. Which elements should be included in a contract for nurses? (select all that apply)

   A. Financial remuneration
   B. Grievance procedures
   C. Assign unit scrub color
   D. Fringe benefits

2. What is Magnet status?

   A. An award given to hospitals for attracting the most clients in a location
   B. An award that recognizes the attraction between good employers and good nurses
   C. An award designed to measure the strength and quality of nursing at a facility
   D. The way a facility determines if nurses are qualified to work in critical care areas

3. "We strive to provide the kind of care we would want our closest loved ones to receive" is an example of what?

   A. Mediation agreement
   B. Mission statement
   C. Magnet philosophy
   D. Organizational structure

4. Which of the following statements describes mediation?

   A. Mediation is a process using an impartial third party (the mediator) who meets with the employer and employee to resolve disputes.
   B. Mediation is a final decision-making process in which the mediator makes a final decision to resolve an employer–employee dispute.
   C. Mediation is a process to determine who is right and who is wrong in a dispute between employees and employers.
   D. Mediation is a stress-reducing exercise thought to help all members of the medical team relieve stress and promote better quality of life.

REFERENCES

American Nurses Association. (2015). *Code of ethics for nurses with interpretive statements*. Washington, DC: American Nurses Publishing.

ANCC Magnet Recognition Program. (2017). Retrieved March 15, 2018, from https://www.nursingworld.org/organizational-programs/magnet/

Aroostook RNs strike for staffing and investment in nurses. (2016). *National Nurse, 112*(3), 10.

Ashley, J. A. (1976). *Hospitals, paternalism and the role of the nurse*. New York: Teachers' College Press.

Dictionary.com. (2017). *Protocol*. Retrieved March 4, 2017, from http://dictionary.reference.com/browse/protocol

Joseph, M. L., & Bogue, R. J. (2016). A theory-based approach to nursing shared governance. *Nursing Outlook, 64*(4), 339–351. doi:10.1016/j.outlook.2016.01.004

Kramer, M., & Schmalenberg, C. E. (2005). Best quality client care: A historical perspective on Magnet hospitals. *Nursing Administration, 29*(3), 275–287.

Labor-Management Relations Glossary. (n.d.). Retrieved March 7, 2017, from http://www.opm.gov/lmr/html/flexible.htm

McClure, M. L. (2005). Magnet hospitals: Insights and issues. *Nursing Administration, 29*(3), 198–201.

National Labor Relations Board. (n.d.). Retrieved March 7, 2017, from https://www.nlrb.gov/

NLRB to the Supreme Court: Labor law protects nurses. (1996). *American Journal of Nursing, 96*(4), 67, 72.

Rosen, P. B. (2013). *Registered nurses, serving as charge nurses, were supervisors under NLRA, federal appeals court rules*. Retrieved March 7, 2017, from http://www.jacksonlewis.com/resources-publication/registered-nurses-serving-charge-nurses-were-supervisors-under-nlra-federal-appeals-court-rules

Stimpfel, A. W., Sloane, D. M., McHugh, M. D., & Aiken, L. H. (2016). Hospitals known for nursing excellence associated with better hospital experience for clients. *Health Services Research, 51*(3), 1120–1134. doi:10.1111/1475-6773.12357

Striking at bargaining rights, court says RNs are supervisors. (1994). *American Journal of Nursing, 94*(7), 67, 70–71.

Supreme Court Okays all-RN unit. (1991, June). *American Nurse, 33*(3), 1.

Wilson, C. N., Hamilton, C. L., & Murphy, E (1990). Union dynamics in nursing. *Journal of Nursing Administration, 20*(2), 35–39.

■ Understanding Healthcare in Today's Society

T his unit provides you with a basic overview of the healthcare delivery system in the United States. Chapter 6 begins with the part of the system with which you are probably most familiar—those settings that employ nurses—and then expands to include some of those that are lesser known and understood. After gaining an understanding of the various players in the system, you should find it easier to analyze specific issues, such as access, finance, power, and control, which are also addressed.

A well-grounded understanding of the legal and ethical dimensions of practice provides the foundation for professional nursing. Chapter 7 initiates a discussion of the legal ramifications of practice. Concrete examples provide help in understanding specific legal issues of importance to consumers and healthcare providers. The chapter concludes with the role of the nurse as a witness.

Ethical and bioethical issues associated with healthcare constantly challenge us as professionals and as members of society. Each technologic advance brings additional questions and concerns to our attention. Chapter 8 explores these issues and their ramifications for nursing practice. A discussion of major questions posed by ethical and bioethical issues provides an understanding of the basis for ethical decision-making and the factors that significantly affect it and outlines a framework for ethical decision-making. Some of the specific problems you will encounter as you move into a professional role are explored in the hope that considering them before you become directly involved will help you to address them more comfortably.

Chapter 9, Safety Concerns in Healthcare, is devoted to issues related to safe client care. Beginning with findings from the Institute of Medicine study conducted in 1999, the content expands to include a review of actions taken by other national organizations to increase client safety. Areas of major concern are identified with discussion of strategies and tools to eliminate errors. The chapter concludes with a discussion of major areas in which nurses play a critical role in the prevention of adverse events.

The unit concludes with Chapter 10 and a discussion of nursing's role in the community. Wherever their individual practice settings, nurses have an impact on the health of their communities. Moving toward the goals of *Healthy People 2020* will require a commitment from all those in the system. Included in this chapter is a discussion on complementary and alternative healthcare and how that affects the health of both individuals and communities.

CHAPTER 6

Understanding the Healthcare Environment and Its Financing

Stegen & Sowerby Stories: Part 1

M olly is a 52-year-old woman with a history of alcohol abuse. She also suffers from posttraumatic stress disorder and has a history of depression. She was hospitalized for a major depressive episode, and spent 5 weeks in therapy as an inpatient. On discharge, she had almost weekly follow-up appointments with a psychiatrist for 3 months. Her provider was a resident in his last year of training. In June at her final appointment with her psychiatrist, he let her know that his residency was ending and that she would be seeing a new provider.

Because the incoming residents were not in the computer system, they were unable to schedule a follow-up appointment and requested that the client call after July 1st to schedule an appointment. The client did not call, and the incoming resident realized this after approximately 1 month. The new resident's schedule was already booked out through August, so the client was not seen until September. This represented a gap of about 3 months in her care.

- What concerns do you have regarding the mental health of this client?
- What could have been done to better meet the needs of the client?
- What are some possible solutions to the scheduling issues?

Healthcare is an exciting and rewarding field but also a challenging one due to the issues that surround it. The entire healthcare system reverberates with change. The roles of nurses in this system constantly develop and expand. You can function more effectively within this system if you understand the various healthcare agencies and their services, the roles that nurses perform in those agencies, and the colleagues with whom you work. We will begin with an overview of healthcare agencies and then discuss the financing of healthcare.

CLASSIFICATION OF HEALTHCARE AGENCIES

The healthcare industry is so large, diverse, and complex that it is difficult to understand. Generally, agencies providing care are classified according to length of stay, ownership, or type of service. These classifications are somewhat arbitrary, and any agency may be placed in more than one classification. With the systemic changes that are occurring, one large entity may exist that includes multiple lengths of stay, types of service, and ownership patterns. Understanding these categories is useful because they are used to plan for services, to describe institutions, and to allocate funding and reimbursement. Your understanding also can be used to guide clients and families through what sometimes seems a maze of confusion in the healthcare system **(Fig. 6.1)**.

Classification According to Length of Stay

One way of classifying inpatient agencies is according to the average *length of stay*, or how long clients remain in the facility. Ambulatory care, short stay, traditional acute care, and long-term care are terms that reflect the average length of stay in a facility. Table 6.1 outlines the various definitions of care according to the length of stay.

Figure 6.1. The many pieces of the healthcare puzzle in the United States.

Classification According to Ownership

The second method of classifying healthcare agencies is according to ownership. Agencies may be classified as governmental (public), proprietary (private profit making), sole proprietorship, or non-profit. Table 6.2 provides information about the various types of ownership. An important consideration is that all healthcare agencies, regardless of their ownership, need to have income sufficient to meet the costs of the care provided as well as to maintain and upgrade the equipment and physical facilities that support that care. No agency can continue to exist if it is not adequately funded.

Classification According to Type of Care

Healthcare agencies may also be classified according to *type of care* provided. Many agencies provide more than one type of care. The type of care is based on the acuity, which is the

Table 6.1 Healthcare Institutions Classified by Length of Stay

Length of Stay	Description
In-and-out care	Contact with client is measured in minutes vs. hours. Typical examples are office visits, emergency department visits, and therapy sessions.
Short stay	Provides care to clients who suffer from acute conditions or require treatments that require <24 hours of care and monitoring. Diagnostic tests or minimally invasive surgery are examples.
Acute care	Traditionally occurs in hospitals where clients stay >24 hours but <30 days. Stays are shortened since the advent of managed care and DRGs.
Long-term care	Provides care to residents for the remainder of their lives; care also includes services to clients with limited recovery needs, functional losses, chronic disease, mental illness, or major rehabilitation, which may range from 30 to 90 days.

Table 6.2   Healthcare Institutions Classified by Ownership

Ownership	Description
Government	Local, county, state, or federal (includes military and veterans facilities).
Nonprofit organization	Religious and philanthropic groups and community organizations.
Proprietary corporation	Stockholders own shares and the agency is managed for the benefit of stockholders.
Sole proprietorship	Individual person/family owns and operates the agency.

seriousness of the illness and the rate of change that is occurring. Higher acuity signifies that the illness is more serious and/or changing more rapidly and will demand a greater intensity of services. Other types of care are available to those whose need for services differs. Table 6.3 provides an overview of the different types of care.

Table 6.3   Healthcare Institutions Classified by Type of Care

Type of Care	Description
Acute care	Illness needing immediate hospitalization and provision of diagnostic tests, treatments, and/or monitoring that require the continuous availability of skilled nursing care. Goals are recovery from illness or injury and restoration to previous level of function.
Long-term acute care	Illness that has stabilized but still needs the ongoing provision of highly skilled care, such as ventilator support or care for major unhealed wounds. Goals are correction of the underlying problem and eventual move to a less skilled level of care.
Subacute care	Care provided after initial recovery from an acute illness needing inpatient care. Skilled care is needed but on a less frequent and intense basis. Goals are to restore function for discharge to home. It is usually provided in a separate unit in an acute care hospital.
Skilled nursing care	Care provided after initial recovery from an acute illness needing inpatient care or following subacute care. Skilled care is still needed, but on a less frequent and intense basis. Goals are to restore function for discharge to home. It is usually provided in a nursing home.
Custodial care	Care is needed because of functional deficits in the ADLs rather than due to the illness itself. Care may be provided in an assisted-living setting, an adult family home (board and care home), or a nursing home. The goals of care are maintenance of functioning and maximum wellness in the face of disability.
Hospice care	Care provided for the terminally ill in the last 6 months before expected death. Care may be provided in the home or an inpatient hospice. Goals are patient autonomy and relief of symptoms while supporting the patient toward a peaceful death and the family and others in their mourning processes.
Ambulatory care	Care for the person who can come to the healthcare agency, receive needed healthcare, and then be discharged to home. It may be a clinic or office. It may also be in hospital departments that provide skilled care for 24 hours or less. Goals are focused on treating a health problem and returning the person to an independent living situation.
Home care	Care providers visit the home to provide some types of care, teach the client and family how to manage care in the home, and evaluate response to treatment. The goal is effective client and family self-care.

> **Critical Thinking Activity: Healthcare Setting**
> Recall the last time that you needed healthcare. Categorize the place where you received care in regard to length of stay, ownership, and type of care provided. Describe those characteristics of the care setting that formed the basis for your decisions regarding classification.

UNDERSTANDING TODAY'S HOSPITAL

The modern hospital is often viewed as the hub or center of the healthcare delivery system and as central to the healthcare of a community, although more care is moving into community settings and the emphasis is on avoiding and limiting hospitalization. A primary characteristic of hospital care is its focus on the current problem, rapid assessment, stabilization or treatment, and then discharge.

In addition to supplying healthcare to clients, hospitals also provide education to a wide variety of healthcare workers and to the community. In many cases, they also serve as centers for research and research dissemination. Hospitals use their status and position in healthcare to enter into cooperative agreements and alliances with healthcare providers, insurance companies, and even other hospitals.

The Development of Hospitals in the United States

The history of hospitals in the United States can be traced back to the mid-1700s, when most cities built almshouses, also called poorhouses. Almshouses provided food and shelter for the homeless poor and served as homes for the aged, disabled, mentally ill, and orphaned. *Pest houses* also were built at this time to isolate people with contagious diseases, especially those diseases contracted aboard a ship. These facilities housed people suffering from cholera, smallpox, typhus, and yellow fever, and the more common communicable diseases such as scarlet fever. Pest houses opened and closed as needed.

Neither almshouses nor pest houses were institutions from which most individuals would want to seek or receive care. They were crowded and unsanitary, with insufficient heat and ventilation. Cross infection was common, and mortality was high. Those with financial means were cared for in their homes.

The first hospital, founded in what was to become the United States, was started in Philadelphia in 1751, at the urging of Benjamin Franklin. Franklin believed that the public had a duty to provide care to the poor, friendless, sick, and insane. A bill passed that year authorizing the establishment of the Pennsylvania Hospital (**Fig. 6.2**, U.S. History.org, 2017). The New York Hospital in New York City was established in 1773, primarily to prevent the spread of infectious diseases brought by sailors and immigrants. Massachusetts General Hospital in Boston opened its doors in 1816 and New Haven Hospital in Connecticut in 1826.

The early hospitals cared for people with acute illnesses and injuries but did not admit the mentally ill. Separate hospitals were established for this purpose. The first such facility was established as a department of the Pennsylvania Hospital in 1752. The second was founded in Williamsburg, Virginia, in 1773; the third, known as Friends Hospital (established by the Quakers), was located near Philadelphia in 1813. By 1840, eight hospitals to treat the mentally

Figure 6.2. Pennsylvania Hospital, the first hospital in the United States, was started in 1751 in Philadelphia.

ill had been established (National Institutes of Health, 2015). The cruel and inhumane treatment of patients in the early mental hospitals is legendary. Dorothea Dix campaigned vigorously for and brought about much reform in the area of mental health treatment. Although never educated as a nurse (she was a schoolteacher), Dix volunteered as a nurse during the Civil War and is included in the American Nurses Association Nursing Hall of Fame because of her significant contributions to the profession.

Factors Affecting the Development of Hospitals

Six major forces can be cited as influencing the growth of hospitals throughout the United States: (1) advances in medical science, (2) the development of medical technology, (3) changes in medical education, (4) growth of the health insurance industry, (5) greater involvement of the government, and (6) the emergence of professional nursing. Each played a unique role in the continued development of hospitals and patient care.

Advances in Medical Science

By the end of the colonial period, two medical schools had been established in the United States. Before that time, physicians learned their skills through an apprenticeship with a practicing physician. As medicine became more of a science, advances occurred. One of the most significant was the discovery of anesthesia and the rapid progress in surgery that followed. The germ theory also did much to improve the practice of medicine because it inspired the development of agents or techniques that would sterilize or serve as antiseptics and provided a rationale for cleanliness. The growth of hospitals in the United States was a direct result of such progress, which made hospitals safer and more desirable. The discovery of sulfa in the mid-1930s and antibiotics in the mid-1940s heralded even greater changes.

The Development of Medical Technology

The development of specialized medical technology was a natural successor to the advances in medical science. The first hospital laboratory opened in 1889, and x-rays were used in diagnosis in 1896. The electrocardiogram was invented in 1903 and the electroencephalogram in 1929 (Encyclopedia.com, 2016). Since those early days, new technology has continued to expand.

Changes in Medical Education

Advances in medical education also had a significant impact on the development of hospitals. *The Flexner Report*, a study of medical education that was completed in 1910, led to changes in the structure and content of curricula in medical schools. It also expanded the role of hospitals to include education and research and resulted in internships and residencies for medical students.

Growth of the Health Insurance Industry

The growth of the health insurance industry is another factor responsible for the development of hospitals. Although there were some antecedents, most sources indicate that the first hospital insurance plan was initiated at Baylor University Hospital in 1929 to serve the needs of schoolteachers in Dallas, Texas. Their approach formed the model for Blue Cross plans around the country. As health insurance grew more widespread, individuals could more often afford hospital care.

Greater Involvement of the Government

In early times, the government was involved in healthcare delivery primarily at a local level, building almshouses and facilities for the insane. The federal government built public health hospitals for seamen and military hospitals for members of the armed services. By 1935, the government was providing grants-in-aid to assist in the establishment of public health and other programs to furnish health assistance to citizens. The Hospital Survey and Construction Act of 1946 (also called the Hill-Burton Act) resulted in the construction of many hospitals and other health facilities. **Medicare** (the federal health plan for those on Social Security and their dependents) and **Medicaid** (state health plans for certain low-income individuals paid through a combination of state and federal funds) were established in 1965. The passage of the Patient Protection and Affordable Health Care Act of 2010 (healthcare reform) was another major step in the federal government's attempt to assure healthcare for all legal residents of the United States (see Chapter 14 for an overview of this legislation).

The Emergence of Professional Nursing

Another force that significantly influenced the growth of hospitals was the development of professional nursing. In 1892, Congress passed a bill acknowledging the contribution of and granting pensions to the nurses of the Civil War. This was the beginning of a great increase in the number of nursing schools and the beginning of the moving of care from the home to the hospital or clinic (Weatherford, n.d.). Professional nursing education resulted in considerate, skilled patient care that made hospitals acceptable to all people, not just the poor. The role of the nurse and nursing influences the healthcare delivery system more today than ever before.

Hospital Services for Clients and Families

The two terms used frequently to describe today's modern hospital services are *inpatient care* and *outpatient care*. Individuals are termed inpatients when they have been admitted for the purpose of staying 24 hours or longer. The outpatient comes to the hospital for services, but is expected to stay less than 24 hours.

Inpatient units comprise what most people think of when they use the designation *acute care hospital* (see Table 6.1). Nurses work in all of these service departments, coordinating the nursing care for individual clients, managing the care environment, delegating and supervising care provided by others, and providing direct skilled care.

In addition to these usual acute care units, hospitals have developed transitional care and rehabilitation units that provide long-term care services, often closing some units and converting them to areas offering these other types of care. A transitional care or rehabilitation unit allows a hospital to discharge an individual from acute, inpatient care in a timely fashion because the next level of services is guaranteed to be available. Reimbursement for the transitional or rehabilitation care is based on long-term care guidelines, and the care must meet long-term care standards for skilled nursing care. Outpatient care, also termed *ambulatory care*, is care that is provided for a period of time expected to be less than 24 hours. The outpatient goes through an admission process, has a procedure performed or care delivered, is determined to be ready for home care, and is discharged. Many diagnostic and treatment procedures, surgeries, and emergency health needs are treated as outpatient care. The distinction between the categories of inpatient and outpatient is important in regard to both billing and discharge to a nursing home. Both Medicare and Medicaid are billed differently for outpatient care than for inpatient care. Medicare payments for nursing home care after hospitalization require that the person be admitted as an inpatient with a minimum 3-day hospital stay. When these conditions are not met, Medicare payment is denied for a nursing home stay even if it meets the standards for recovery and return to home. Clients and their families may not understand this distinction and how it affects the bills they receive and their eligibility for some types of reimbursement. Nurses must understand that different rules may apply and refer clients and families to appropriate resources for accurate information as they help clients to plan for needed care after discharge.

Hospitals may also be referred to by the mix of traditional inpatient services that are offered (Table 6.4). Not every hospital offers each of the services mentioned earlier, but more are becoming part of a corporate entity that provides all services. The terms most commonly used to describe the mix of services are the *general* or *community* hospital, the *tertiary care* hospital, and the *specialty* hospital.

Hospitals may offer other services that are not directed solely at client care. Day procedures and early discharge for inpatient care may present travel difficulties for individuals who live a long distance from a major care center. To facilitate care for these clients and their families, some hospitals have developed hotel-like services, often termed *hospitality units*, where the client scheduled for day surgery may plan to arrive the day before and stay overnight. A family member may also stay in the unit during the individual's hospitalization. After discharge, both the client and the family member may stay one or more days before traveling home. The cost of staying in a hospitality unit is not covered by insurance, but it is much more

Table 6.4   Hospitals Classified by Mix of Services

Type	Services
General or community hospital	Medical, surgical, obstetric, emergency, and diagnostic, plus laboratory services.
Tertiary care hospital	Referral centers for clients with complex or unusual health problems such as level 1 trauma, major burns, bone marrow transplant, and research-based oncology, in addition to standard care.
	Part of a large medical center associated with a university. Serves a wide geographic area
Specialty hospital	Offers only a particular type of care (ie, psychiatric, pediatric).

convenient than staying in a hotel and typically the cost is less than in a hotel. Additionally, if an emergency occurs, the client in a hospitality unit has care immediately available.

Hospitals as Educational Institutions

The education of healthcare providers is an important function of many hospitals. Although the number of hospital-based schools of nursing offering diplomas has decreased steadily, some are well supported and expect to continue operation. There are also hospital-based programs for respiratory therapy, dietetics, medical laboratory technology, and other health-related professions.

Many hospitals serve as clinical laboratory sites for individuals who enrolled in colleges and universities that provide education for healthcare professionals. These individuals include students in nursing, laboratory sciences, nutrition, pharmacy, radiology and imaging, and other disciplines as well as medicine.

Graduate medical education includes residency programs for physicians preparing for independent practice. Residents receive a salary from the hospital and are responsible for providing services in return. Residents augment the services of primary physicians, who are often referred to as the attending or staff physicians. Residents often provide the majority of medical services for individuals who are part of the medically underserved in a community, consulting with the staff physician in charge as needed. Part of the funding for graduate medical education comes from the money made available through Medicare.

THE LONG-TERM CARE FACILITY

Long-term care refers to any of the different care settings that involve coordination of the entire multidisciplinary team to provide counseling, nursing care, rehabilitation, nutritional support, social services, and sometimes special education programs over months to years. Managing a positive living environment is as important as managing health problems for long-term care residents. Long-term care facilities include nursing homes, assisted-living centers, adult care homes (also called board and care homes), chronic disease hospitals, psychiatric hospitals, and group homes for those with developmental disabilities or chronic mental health problems. The majority of long-term care facilities are nursing homes that care primarily for older adults.

Nursing Homes

The nursing home is the care facility most often associated with long-term care. Although nursing homes suffer from negative images of the past, they do offer a far different environment than they did many years ago. Nursing homes in the United States provide care and a positive living environment for individuals who have the greatest number of deficits in activities of daily living (ADLs). ADLs include dressing, bathing, eating, toileting, and ambulating. Just as the acute care hospital, the nursing home is expanding services beyond those traditionally associated with nursing home care. A nursing home that provides skilled care in nursing, physical therapy, and speech therapy is termed a **skilled nursing facility** (SNF).

History of the Nursing Home

Like acute care facilities, the nursing home had a rather harsh beginning. In the 19th century, almshouses sheltered the destitute elderly. These facilities attracted a strange mixture of residents, including those who needed asylum and detention, as well as the poor, the chronically disabled, and the mentally ill. According to the moral perspective that prevailed at the time, poverty and disability were viewed as indications of an undisciplined and wasteful life. A person who was housed in a county poorhouse often had no financial resources and no family to provide care and assistance and endured a certain social stigma. In time, these almshouses became the community dumping grounds for all of society's cast offs. As the United States grew as a society, various groups became concerned about the conditions that existed in the almshouses. Eventually, people were separated according to their condition, and the mentally and chronically ill were reassigned to different institutions. An increasing number of churches and fraternal organizations started homes to care for their elderly members. As a result of the Social Security Act of 1935, private (for-profit or proprietary) nursing homes emerged during that decade.

In the postwar period, the Hill-Burton Act of 1946, which supported hospital construction, was expanded to include voluntary (nonprofit) nursing homes, and some states also developed grant programs. Since 1950, government funding for nursing home care has increased steadily. Governmental regulation of nursing homes has become increasingly involved and complex.

In the 1950s and 1960s, the deinstitutionalization movement, which saw large numbers of the older population with dementia discharged from mental hospitals, also affected nursing homes. Nursing homes began to assume the role of providing specialized care for older adults. By the 1960s, this role was well established, but the nursing home industry was plagued by constant reports of substandard and negligent care and, in some instances, charges of absolute abuse of clients and misuse or embezzlement of their funds. This resulted in even greater scrutiny and regulation by the government.

Today, *nursing home* is a broad term that encompasses nearly 16,000 facilities ranging from special units in acute community hospitals to those that are a part of the campus of continuing care retirement centers (Centers for Disease Control and Prevention [CDC], 2014). The facilities are licensed by the state in which they operate, and each state has its own definitions and requirements; however, 87.6% are certified for payment by Medicare and/or Medicaid (CDC, 2014), and thus are subject to federal standards. The major reason for admission to a nursing home is functional dependence in terms of basic ADLs and cognitive impairment rather than medical diagnosis.

The Nursing Home Resident

Although most older adults live in community settings, many will spend their last years in a nursing home. Sixty-nine percent of the residents are women, reflecting the longer life span of women and the greater likelihood that a woman's spouse will precede her in death. The most recent data available from the National Nursing Home Survey (NNHS) indicate that over 96% are dependent in at least one ADL and more than half of all residents are dependent in all five ADLs. Typically, nursing home residents range in age from 65 to older than 100, with 41.6% aged 85 and older (CDC, 2014).

The number of individuals requiring nursing home care is expected to steadily increase, based on the increasing number of the elderly. According to the 2010 census, the number of people aged 80 to 84 increased by 16% from the 2000 census, those 90 to 94 increased by 30%, and those over 100 increased by 6% (U.S. Census Bureau, 2011). The percentage of the population that is over 65 has been steadily increasing and in now at 15.1% (U.S. Census Bureau, 2011).

Health Services in Nursing Homes

The majority of residents in nursing homes remain there because of major deficits in self-care abilities and the need for ongoing care that is custodial in focus rather than treatment oriented. Maintenance of function, independence, autonomy, and rehabilitation are all goals for nursing home residents. Residents are concerned with the living environment and the healthcare environment.

Units designed for the cognitively impaired are free of restraints and barriers to mobility. Facility design and alarm systems prevent residents from wandering away. These units provide special approaches to care delivery that decrease stress and reduce the potential for hostile, angry outbursts. Caregivers are trained in responding appropriately to the special challenges of working with the cognitively impaired.

Some nursing homes have entire wings devoted to individuals receiving posthospital convalescent care where the major goal is rehabilitation and return to independent living. These individuals are admitted with a specific planned stay of 14 to 30 days. During this time, the individual is aided in restoring functional abilities and planning for self or family care. Activities might include physical therapy for the person with a hip replacement or speech therapy after a stroke.

Funding Nursing Home Care

The cost of nursing home care is a concern for many. The annual cost of nursing home care in a semiprivate room ranges from $54,024 in Texas to $291,996 in Alaska, with a national average of $82,128 (Genworth, 2016). Medicare pays for only a limited number of days for individuals who meet specific criteria regarding hospitalization and who need skilled care or rehabilitation rather than custodial care. Some individuals have long-term care insurance that will pay part of their costs. An increasing number of individuals are purchasing policies, which are available through a number of organizations. Personal financial resources are frequently exhausted by a prolonged nursing home stay. State-administered public assistance in the form of programs such as Medicaid pays for nursing home care when an individual's personal financial resources have fallen below a certain state-determined level. Payment for an individual resident may come from multiple sources with insurance paying a sum, personal resources (such as savings, Social Security, and/or pension) paying a portion, and Medicaid paying for the remainder. As the number of older adults requiring nursing home care continues to rise, these costs create a serious budget concern in most states.

Regulation of Nursing Home Care

Nursing homes are among the most regulated of all healthcare facilities. Because the federal government pays for some of the care, federal regulations affect nursing homes across the country. Starting primarily with the Federal Budget Act of 1987, government regulations mandate specific assessment tools; planning processes; standards of care, including the use of restraints and psychoactive medications; documentation systems used; and evaluation tools. Data are collected according to a standardized **minimum data set** (MDS). State regulations may place additional requirements on nursing homes. Nursing homes are visited by a survey team that is responsible for ensuring adherence to regulatory standards. The results of nursing home surveys are public documents and must be displayed in each facility in a place accessible to the public and to residents who wish to review them. Nursing home survey results may be seen on the Medicare Web site at www.medicare.gov/Nhcompare/Home.asp.

Critical Thinking Activity: Nursing Homes
Use the Web site www.medicare.gov/Nhcompare/Home.asp to investigate a nursing home in your community. Find out its average length of stay, the types of services it offers, and its type of ownership. Analyze the quality of care provided as represented through the nursing home survey. Compare this facility with two other nursing homes in your geographic area.

Assisted-Living Facilities

The assisted-living facility provides care for those needing help with some ADLs. In an assisted-living arrangement, the resident can maintain maximum independence and use a shared decision-making model to decide when additional help or support is needed. Husbands and wives may reside together and may often bring their own furniture and belongings to create a home-like atmosphere. Those who are able seek the less costly and more independent and flexible living found here. Assisted-living facilities have been much less regulated than nursing homes. Increasing regulation is expected. The Joint Commission provides a voluntary accrediting process for assisted-living centers.

Care in Assisted-Living Facilities

In an assisted-living facility, all instrumental ADLs such as shopping, cleaning, meal preparation, and laundry are provided. A resident is expected to have some mobility (although it may require a walker or a cane) and to eat in a dining room except when the person is temporarily ill. Residents also are expected to manage their own medication and health needs, although they may be assisted with remembering to take medications. Assistance is provided with bathing, dressing, and other personal care as needed. Most care is provided by unlicensed assistive personnel. Licensed nurses may be employed in a supervisory capacity and may plan for care. One area of controversy is the level of assistance with medications and health needs that can be provided by unlicensed, unregulated personnel. Some states are authorizing delegation to appropriately trained assistive personnel of selected nursing tasks, such as giving oral medications, for residents of assisted living.

For some individuals, the transitions from independent living to assisted living and from assisted living to nursing home care are smooth ones, thus avoiding the transition or relocation stress that affects their well-being. This is particularly true when multiple levels of care are available in the same retirement living setting. (See the discussion of continuing care retirement communities that follows.) For others, this change triggers serious stress and is one of the reasons for pressure to allow residents to remain in assisted-living settings even when very incapacitated.

Board and care homes, sometimes termed *adult family homes*, that provide assisted living and some services similar to nursing homes are licensed in some states. These individual residences usually house six or fewer adults needing care and assistance. Originally planned as care in private homes that would be operated by the owner or resident, many now are commercial operations with a paid staff. The costs are usually less than for a nursing home. One concern is the difficulty of regulating these small residences where there are no professional caregivers.

Funding Assisted Living

Assisted living is not supported with Medicare funds and therefore does not have to meet the stringent regulatory standards of federal legislation. Public assistance, in the form of Medicaid, or other programs, may provide some support for assisted living when the alternative would be expensive nursing home care for which the state would be responsible; however, this is not true in all jurisdictions. Most assisted living is paid for by the individual or family.

Retirement Communities

Retirement communities, which continue to grow, may be self-contained towns, retirement villages, retirement subdivisions, retirement residences, or continuing care retirement communities. The basic retirement complex is designed to provide the environment for self-care and may support independence longer than would a regular house or apartment. Home care services are provided to those in retirement communities in the same way that they are provided to those in regular homes or apartments.

Continuing care retirement communities provide a variety of levels of independent and dependent living and care to residents based on each resident's needs. Most residents enter the community to reside in a retirement apartment or home and then move within the community to an assisted-living section and from there to a convalescent or nursing home center if that becomes necessary. The nursing theorist Sister Callista Roy's adaptation model is very applicable to these communities. (See the Theory Alert that follows.) Services such as occupational therapy, physical therapy, and dental care also may be available as home care or for those in the convalescent center. The aim is for people to reside in the setting that provides maximum autonomy and independence while ensuring that needs are met. A major limiting factor is the cost of such communities to the individual residents.

Theory Alert   *Sister Callista Roy the Adaptation Model*

Sister Callista Roy was born in 1939 in Los Angeles, California. She earned her Bachelor's degree in nursing in 1963. Later, she earned a Master's degree in pediatric nursing and also a Master's and Doctoral degree in Sociology.

Roy's theory, called the Adaptation Model of Nursing, is a holistic theory looking at all aspects of a client. She identified four modes of adaptation: physiologic, self-concept, role function, and interdependence. The emphasis of role function is the adaptation to different roles throughout a person's lifetime. As roles change and physical ability changes, people make adaptations. Sometimes, those adaptations are good and healthy, and other times, Roy calls them *maladaptations* and proposes that the nurse's role is to assist in correcting maladaptive behavior.

(Source: www.nursing-theory.org)

Rehabilitation Centers

Rehabilitation centers typically focus on a specific healthcare problem; for example, there are centers for those with spinal cord injuries and other centers focusing on head injuries or cerebral vascular accidents. Although many of these agencies prefer nurses who have taken advanced courses in rehabilitation nursing, many employ nurses with different backgrounds, such as those who have worked in a nursing home focused on rehabilitation principles.

Other Long-Term Care Facilities

Some of the other long-term care facilities available are the group homes for the developmentally disabled and for those with chronic psychiatric illnesses. These smaller residences, most with 12 or fewer residents, strive to create a home-like atmosphere in which individuals can function at their highest capacity. They are often hampered by the lack of stable funding and the difficulty of hiring qualified care providers because of the low wages typically offered.

AMBULATORY CARE SETTINGS

Ambulatory care has long been provided in offices, clinics, and the day-procedure units of hospitals. Some ambulatory care is provided in settings where people work and go to school. Providing care where people routinely spend their days rather than requiring them to go to a different site for healthcare often results in a more effective use of healthcare services. Some ambulatory care settings rely heavily on the skills of registered nurses (RNs) to provide assessment and teaching, while others focus on medical care provided by physicians, nurse practitioners (NPs), and physician assistants (PAs), with medical assistants (MAs) for routine tasks.

Healthcare Provider Offices

One of the major changes in healthcare has been the decrease in the number of solo practice offices and the growth of group and organizational practices. Many medical practices are owned by health systems that also own hospitals. Within a private-physician practice setting, there may be several general practice physicians and many specialists. Advanced practice nurses (APNs) and PAs also are working in many of these group practice settings. Other RNs in these settings may have responsibility for triage, assessment, teaching, and providing direct care. Nursing roles in ambulatory care are expanding as the need for the cost-effective use of physician time is modifying practice patterns.

Walk-In Clinics

Walk-in clinics treat clients with emergent conditions that do not require the high-technology resources of the emergency room. Walk-in clinics may be referred to as immediate care facilities, urgent care centers, or emergent care centers and are usually open during extended hours that include evenings and weekends, in addition to the traditional Monday through Friday office hours. Walk-in clinics have grown in popularity as people find it increasingly difficult to gain access to traditional healthcare settings because of their personal time constraints.

Many walk-in clinics have gradually added services such as sports physical examinations for school-age children, pelvic examinations and Pap tests for women, and routine immunizations. Some are beginning to act as primary care providers, advertising the willingness of staff doctors to become family doctors. Walk-in clinics have relatively small nursing staffs, often employing only one RN during a shift; therefore, each nurse must have a wide variety of skills and be able to function with a high degree of autonomy. Some settings do not use RNs in direct care; they are hired in these settings only to supervise MAs and other clinic staff members and may oversee more than one facility. Licensed practical nurses (LPNs) may be employed in ambulatory care to collect data, carry out specific treatments, and give medications.

COMMUNITY AGENCIES

Agencies providing care in the community include public health agencies, home care agencies, and hospice care.

Public Health Agencies

Public health departments are operated as agencies of the government. In general, the focus of health departments has been on broad community issues, communicable diseases, and infant and child health. Public health nurses originally did a great deal of individual family visiting, but today, fewer funds are available for visits. As a result, public health nurses now focus on individuals who are at high risk and whose health affects the entire community, such as those with tuberculosis. Public health nurses responsible for community health issues are required to have a baccalaureate degree in nursing; however, some agencies operate a variety of clinics (such as immunization clinics) in which RNs with an associate degree or diploma provide teaching and direct care services.

Home Care Agencies

Home care agencies, such as the traditional visiting nurse services and the proprietary home healthcare companies, provide a broad spectrum of care that may include nursing care, personal care assistance, minor housekeeping, physical therapy, occupational therapy, speech/language therapy, and respiratory therapy for individuals in their homes. Teaching family and caregivers is a large part of the home care professional's responsibility. The focus of home care agencies is broad. It ranges from providing short-term visits for clients who need assistance after a hospital stay or acute illness to assisting clients who will need ongoing home care for years, such as those requiring dialysis or ventilator support in the home. People with these conditions may require nursing care for 8- to 12-hour shifts in the home or episodic visits that last from 15 to 60 minutes.

Hospice Care

The goal of hospice care is to assist the terminally ill individual to maintain the highest possible quality of life until death. Hospice care may be provided in the home with care providers visiting as needed. Some hospices provide services to individuals living in assisted-living or nursing home settings. There are inpatient hospice units for those who do not have a family and friends to act as home caregivers or for whom this would be too great a task. Multidisciplinary teams may include physicians, nurses, clergy, occupational and physical therapists, home health aides, social workers, and volunteers who work with both the hospice patient and the family or other caregivers. Nurses provide special skills in symptom management for physical problems, such as pain, nausea, anorexia, and constipation and psychosocial support for end-of-life events and issues. Nurses are usually responsible for the management and coordination of hospice care.

Community Mental Health Centers

Community mental health centers were established to allow individuals with psychiatric problems to remain in their communities. Services may include individual counseling and therapy, group or family counseling, medication management, evaluation, and referral. For those who must be hospitalized, the community mental health center provides follow-up care that facilitates early discharge. These centers usually employ a variety of mental healthcare workers including psychiatrists, clinical psychologists, social workers, marriage and family counselors, psychiatric nurses, and community workers.

Many psychiatric care providers hoped that psychiatric clients who remained in their communities on an outpatient basis, with family and community ties intact, would have more successful treatment outcomes. Another hoped-for advantage of community mental health centers was that people would seek help more readily when it was available in the community. Unfortunately, community mental health centers have not been funded adequately to meet the many and varied needs of individuals with mental health problems. Mentally ill clients often are eligible for care only when they become acutely ill and not for care that can maintain their health. Some people are not eligible for help because of the complex rules and regulations governing funding. Others do not continue with prescribed treatment and experience a relapse; legal constraints do not allow involuntary treatment. Although recognition of the rights of the mentally ill has been important, there also is a concern that society expects mentally ill people to make rational decisions about their own best interests when, in fact, they are not mentally capable of understanding the consequences of their actions. The entire area of community mental health has many challenges.

Adult Day Centers

Adult day centers provide care for adults who cannot safely be alone throughout the day. Transported daily to the center by a family member or a van operated by the center, clients receive a variety of social and health services that enable them to continue to live in their own home or a family member's home. Various maintenance and rehabilitative services usually are available, including exercise classes, medication education and supervision, recreational activities, mental healthcare, and an opportunity to interact with other people. Some centers provide "drop-in" or intermittent services for clients who need only one aspect of the program. Other centers provide care each day for clients who need continuing supervision while family members are at work or school. The nursing role in these settings may vary considerably. Some settings have advanced practice RNs (APRNs) who plan care and work with families. Others have RNs who provide medication supervision, assessment for ongoing health problems, and who may lead groups in reminiscence, reality orientation, or validation therapy. LPNs may be hired to give medications and carry out specific treatments.

Ambulatory Care Dialysis Centers

A dialysis center provides an environment where the individual can go two to three times a week for dialysis. Nurses in dialysis centers must have high-level skills, because clients with renal failure who need in-center dialysis usually have the most complex problems and coexisting illnesses. Both LPNs and RNs may be employed in these centers.

COLLEAGUES IN HEALTHCARE

Hundreds of types of healthcare workers have been identified in the United States, each of which meets the needs of our society in some way. It is not within the scope of this book to discuss each of these occupations individually. Table 6.5 provides a list of the more common healthcare occupations and a web reference for information regarding education and credentialing. The discussion below focuses on some of the issues related to the healthcare professions.

Roles of Healthcare Workers

Although the major health occupations provide academic education with legal licensure and a defined scope of practice, many of the allied healthcare providers have much less defined roles, which creates concerns about how education or training is provided and how the role is regulated. For some, regulations and requirements may differ from state to state. National organizations that provide accreditation for allied health educational programs serve to provide standardization of some occupations.

Even within professions, increasing specialization has sometimes created conflict over expertise and territory (Fig. 6.3). Pressure from insurers has mandated a decreased use of specialty physicians and mandated that more care be delivered by family practice physicians. In some states, clinical psychologists may obtain authority to prescribe medications, a treatment modality formerly limited to physicians and certain APRNs. This eliminates the need for referral to another mental healthcare provider solely for the prescription of medications to treat psychiatric conditions. When nurse anesthetists can be reimbursed independently, more facilities hire those nurse specialists, which decrease the demand for anesthesiologists. Those with greater education argue that the client loses when the provider has a lesser background. The education, regulation, and use of all healthcare workers will continue to be an issue in the coming years.

Access to Primary Healthcare

The healthcare provider contacted initially by clients who seek healthcare is considered a **primary care provider** (PCP), who furnishes entry into the healthcare system. Today, the federal

Table 6.5 Common Health Occupations and Certification Organizations*

Dentistry	
American Dental Association (www.ada.org)	Doctor of dental surgery (DDS) dentist Registered dental hygienist (RDH) Dental assistant
Diagnostic Imaging Technology	
American Society of Radiologic Technicians (www.asrt.org) Society of Diagnostic Medical Sonography (www.sdms.org) Nuclear Medicine Technology Certification Board (NMTCB) (www.mntcb.org)	Radiologic technologist Sonography technologist Nuclear medicine technologist
Nutrition	
American Dietetic Association (www.eatright.org)	Registered dietitian Dietetic technician registered
Occupational Therapy	
American Occupational Therapy Association (www.aota.org/)	Occupational therapist registered Occupational therapy assistant
Optometry/Vision Care	
American Optometric Association (www.aoanet.org)	Doctor of optometry Certified paraoptometric (CPO)-certified paraoptometric assistant (CPOA) Certified paraoptometric technician (CPOT)
Pharmacy	
American Pharmacists Association (www.aphanet.org)	Registered pharmacist Pharmacy assistant
Physical Therapy	
American Physical Therapy Association (www.apta.org)	Registered physical therapist (PT) Physical therapist assistant (PTA)
Physician	
American Medical Association (www.ama-assn.org/) American Osteopathic Association (www.osteopathic.org)	Medical doctor (MD) Doctor of osteopathic (DO) medicine
Podiatry	
American Podiatric Medicine Association (www.apma.org)	Doctor of podiatric medicine (DPM)
Respiratory Therapy	
American Association for Respiratory Care (www.aarc.org/)	Respiratory therapist (RT)
Speech, Language, and Hearing Therapy	
American Speech, Language, and Hearing Association (www.asha.org)	Speech/language pathologist (CCC-SLP) Speech/language pathology assistant (SLPA) Audiologist (CCC-A)

*Organization Web sites provide an overview of the profession and educational requirements.

government considers family practice specialists, pediatricians, internal medicine specialists, obstetricians, PAs, and NPs to be PCPs. The PCP is the mainstay of basic care for most individuals.

All states require licensure of physicians, NPs, and other providers who are authorized to treat illness and prescribe drugs. The cornerstone of many managed healthcare plans is an emphasis on the primary healthcare provider as the gatekeeper for the system. The primary

Figure 6.3. Overlapping roles and unclear boundaries can lead to conflict.

provider implements health maintenance activities that prevent the need for more expensive care as well as provides care for common health problems. Because fewer physicians are choosing primary care fields of practice, the availability of adequate numbers of PCPs has been identified as a concern with the expansion of health plans in the United States through healthcare reform. NPs and PAs may fill this gap.

Lack of **access** to primary care has been one of the healthcare problems for individuals without health insurance, the unemployed, those residing in rural areas and in economically disadvantaged areas in large cities, and those on welfare programs. Often it has resulted in delaying care until the problem is more complex and requires greater resources to resolve. In urban areas, the lack of access to primary care has often resulted in the inappropriate use of emergency room services for routine illnesses.

Interdisciplinary Teamwork

As the healthcare system grows more complex, it is clear that it is impossible for one individual, educated for a specific role, to manage all aspects of care. This has led to an increasing emphasis on collaborative work that will provide the benefits available through the expertise of different professions. Multidisciplinary teamwork has always been part of hospice care—physicians, nurses, social workers, therapists, home health aides, and pastoral staff all bring their unique insights into the client's care. The current regulations for long-term care require that there be interdisciplinary collaboration in planning for resident care.

Healthcare Worker Supply

According to the Bureau of Labor statistics, the long-term expectation is that the employment market for nurses will grow 16% between 2014 and 2024, which is much faster than average

(BLS, 2015). The challenge will be to sustain the nursing workforce and nursing school enrollments in the coming years. If these falter, the future supply will be in serious jeopardy.

Nurses are not the only healthcare workers in short supply. There are predicted shortages in almost all areas of healthcare over the next 15 years. As the population ages and more people enter the system due to the expansion of healthcare insurance coverage, the shortages are likely to persist.

PAYING FOR HEALTHCARE

Throughout the world, the concern over healthcare has everyone's attention. In most of the industrialized world, healthcare is seen as a right, or an **entitlement**, of every citizen. Based on this right, healthcare in most industrialized countries is operated by government systems that provide universal healthcare coverage. In some countries such as Sweden and the Netherlands, there is strong centralization of financing and control. In other countries such as Canada and Germany, systems are controlled regionally through provincial authority. These governmental systems are successful in accomplishing overall health outcomes such as low maternal–infant mortality, high immunization rates, and reduction of preventable deaths. The problems found in these systems are related to the high cost of providing healthcare and subsequent attempts to control those costs. The delay before receiving care may be long, and some care, especially care that is very costly such as dialysis, may be limited. Because of these situations, private medical care that is paid for by individuals also may be available to those with sufficient income.

In developing nations, healthcare may be limited or almost nonexistent. Some care may be paid for by the government and some by private means, but there are not enough individual or institutional providers to meet the needs of the population. The available resources may not meet the standards that those in more affluent countries have come to expect. Hospitals may lack adequate safe water and sanitation. Ordinary supplies such as dressing materials and sterile needles may be unavailable. Drugs may be in short supply, and diagnostic and laboratory testing may be nonexistent. Healthcare outcomes in these countries tend to be poor, especially regarding infant and child mortality. The World Health Organization is most active in these developing nations, trying to improve health outcomes through immunization, sanitation, and other public health programs.

In the United States, there has been no mechanism to build a coordinated healthcare system. Much of the complexity found in the U.S. healthcare system relates to the variety of mechanisms for funding and controlling healthcare. Although the United States has ready access to the most sophisticated medical technology and expertise, deficiencies are seen in some of the key measures of population health.

As noted earlier, in 2010, the U.S. Congress passed the Patient Protection and Affordable Care Act commonly referred to as the Healthcare Reform. This act set up a process through which the United States would move toward healthcare coverage for all by requiring everyone to be enrolled in some type of health plan. The various health plans described below will continue to exist, but enrollment will change. The provisions of this act go into effect over a period of years beginning in 2010. Changes mandated by this act will be identified as part of the discussion that follows. As political power changes, laws may change, so you will need to watch legislative developments carefully to learn what provisions are in place.

Financing Healthcare for Individuals

Currently, there are many different approaches to financing healthcare for individuals in the United States. Personal payment, charitable care, insurance plans, health maintenance organizations (HMOs), and a variety of government programs are all forms of healthcare financing. Agencies such as insurance companies and government programs that pay providers for health services provided to individuals are termed **third-party payers**. Increasingly, decisions about an individual's healthcare are made by a combination of the client–consumer, the provider, and the payer, rather than by any one of them alone.

Under healthcare reform, these options will remain. Individuals will have access to one or more health plan options through employers, subsidies for low-income individuals, expansion of the rules for Medicaid, and the use of insurance pools for high-risk individuals. All are currently mandated to participate by 2019.

Personal Payment

Today, most individuals still pay for healthcare but often in indirect ways that make them less aware of the specific costs. Health insurance premiums may be deducted from a paycheck, or an employer may pay premiums directly, considering them part of employee compensation. Most health insurance plans require the subscriber to pay a deductible (a portion of the bill), which may be computed for each service or may be an aggregate for the year. The size of the deductible that is the individual's responsibility is increasing in many insurance plans, giving people greater incentive to use services wisely. The ACA continues to allow co-pays and deductibles to be part of insurance plans, but it does limit the co-pays for those on Medicare.

Charitable Care

Charitable care has played a significant role in the history of healthcare. The earliest hospitals were religious institutions that provided healthcare as a form of ministry and as a charitable service. Some large charitable groups, such as the Shriners Hospitals for Children, still provide a great deal of care for people who are unable to pay. Although these hospitals do collect insurance and payment from those who can afford care, they also raise money for the purpose of providing high-level care to children in need.

Hospitals constructed with the use of Hill-Burton funds made available in 1946 accepted an obligation to provide some charitable care in their communities. As these obligations expired, concern about what was happening in emergency care led to legislation that requires hospitals to provide emergency care regardless of an individual's ability to pay.

Historically, some money for charitable care was raised through donations. As insurance became more widespread, hospitals often supported charitable care by charging paying clients more than the cost of their care and using the excess income to offset the costs of charitable care. However, as negotiations for lower healthcare costs for managed care continue and regulations have limited Medicare reimbursement, hospitals are experiencing a decreased ability to provide charitable care without severe financial difficulties.

Individual physicians also have provided forms of charitable care. Only rarely did people directly ask physicians for charitable care; rather, the physician sometimes did not pursue the payment of a bill that could not be paid by a family. Physicians and other care providers also have provided charitable care by volunteering their time at free clinics.

To meet the needs of society, free clinics have been established throughout the country and now number more than 1,200. The National Association of Free Clinics (NAFC), founded in 2001, serves as an advocate for the issues and concerns of free clinics, their volunteer and paid staff, and their clients. Free clinics are becoming PCPs for those without other access to care (NAFC, 2016).

Charitable care is expected to continue to be a part of financing of healthcare. There will always be some individuals who fall outside of the system due to immigration status or other such issues. Additionally, individuals with very high healthcare costs may continue to need help with the deductibles and co-pays that can mount during a prolonged or high-cost illness.

Health Insurance Plans

Starting in the 1930s, insurance companies gradually began to pay a larger share of medical fees. The basic framework of insurance coverage is that of shared risk of having high-cost healthcare needs. Individuals pay for coverage whether or not they incur healthcare costs; when an insured individual requires healthcare, the insurance pays for that care. Thus, the individual has a stable healthcare cost without the risk of incurring costs that are difficult to meet from ordinary income, and the insurance company stays financially solvent because more money is coming in than is going out.

Historically, health insurance was for hospital care and related services only. Outpatient visits, immunizations, costs of drugs, and other such benefits were not covered by insurance policies. One disadvantage of this system was that consumers had no incentive to reduce their use of services; they paid the same regardless of their needs or use of the system. People sought to have care delivered on an inpatient basis to obtain reimbursement. Another disadvantage was that individuals often neglected preventive healthcare that had to be paid for out of pocket. Health insurance policies now cover many preventive services, outpatient costs, and some prescription costs.

At the heart of the process of setting insurance rates and specifying coverage are identifying what will be covered, determining the risk (probability) of health services being needed for different groups of individuals, and projecting the costs of care. It has been found that the more heterogeneous the group, the more likely that the average cost for those in the plan will mirror the population average, thereby keeping insurance costs reasonable for all. Limitations on coverage that eliminate individuals with high probability of needing services (such as the older adult diabetic) protect insurance companies from the risk of excessive costs. When high-risk individuals are excluded from insurance, it lessens the cost for low-risk subscribers within the plan, but leaves those who are most in need of assistance without the benefit of insurance.

Most insurance companies are private profit-making companies owned by stockholders. They provide service to policyholders in return for insurance payments and create profit for stockholders in the company. Nonprofit insurance companies are established within different legal regulations from profit-making companies. They are owned collectively by those who hold insurance policies. All profits from the company are theoretically used to enhance benefits or to decrease the cost of the insurance. Additionally, the nonprofit companies have certain advantages in terms of taxes. The *Blues* (Blue Cross and Blue Shield companies) originally were established as not-for-profit organizations.

Legal regulations place restrictions on the rate setting, investments, and general management of nonprofit companies that do not apply to private profit-making companies. This has limited their ability to grow in size and compete for some types of business. In some areas of the country, Blue Cross and Blue Shield companies have asked regulatory authorities for permission to convert from nonprofit to profit-making status and to sell stock in the company (and have changed their names in the process). In some states, courts have required that these corporations provide remuneration to their communities in return for this change in status. In other states, these changes have occurred without public input. In still others, the change was blocked.

One of the major controversies in the 2010 healthcare reform act was the requirement that all individuals be covered by an insurance company plan unless they were enrolled in a government plan such as Medicaid, Veterans' Administration (VA), or Medicare. This mandate provided private companies with a very large source of new subscribers.

As the cost of healthcare has increased, insurance premiums have increased greatly. An additional public concern has been that health insurance has been unobtainable for individuals with existing health problems and often economically beyond the means of those who are not insured as part of an employee group. The new law requires access to insurance for all individuals with preexisting illnesses through high-risk pools. Subsidies have been enacted for those who meet low-income standards, and Medicaid requirements are being changed. Young adults up through the age of 26 have access to insurance through their parents' insurance.

Although insurance companies originally focused on paying for healthcare, they now are involved in establishing standards for care, evaluating care, and negotiating charges. They are active participants in all areas of healthcare and, because of the economic power they wield, have great influence. Insurance companies determine whom they will pay and what procedures they will reimburse. Thus, insurance companies can and do limit healthcare choices.

All insurance plans have written rules regarding notification, acceptable providers, and precisely when and how reimbursement will occur. Sometimes, these rules result in a denial of payment. Many people have expressed concern about the process of reviewing and denying insurance claims. Realistically, the foremost goal of most health insurance plans is to return a profit to investors. Providing good healthcare to an individual is a means to that end and not the focus of effort.

Federal legislation, the Health Insurance Portability and Accountability Act (HIPAA), was passed in 1996. Title 1 of the Act focuses on measures that assist in maintaining healthcare insurance coverage for those who change or lose their jobs (see http://aspe.hhs.gov/admn-simp/pl104191.htm, for the full text of the act). The Centers for Medicare & Medicaid Services (CMS) provide consumer information regarding the protections provided by this federal legislation to allow people to maintain coverage when they change jobs. This legislation also has provided tax incentives for those purchasing long-term care insurance. The HIPAA legislation had additional provisions regarding the privacy of client health records, which will be discussed in Chapter 8.

Managed Care Organizations

Managed care refers to any system for "a system of healthcare (as by an HMO or PPO) that controls costs by placing limits on physicians' fees and by restricting the patient's choice of physicians" (Merriam-Webster, 2017). The concept of managed care has broadened since its beginning, and now it includes many types of health plans.

A managed care plan may be controlled by the payer (eg, an insurance company), include both payers and providers, or be a business entity that serves only as a go-between. HMOs (discussed later) have always acted as managed care systems. Many of the current health plans referred to as HMOs are in reality managed care systems that do not focus on health maintenance.

In some cases, a group of primary healthcare providers, termed an **independent practice association**, may contract with a managed care organization to provide services for a preset fee per individual in the program. Managed care organizations also may directly provide healthcare and therefore employ many healthcare workers, including nurses. In some managed care organizations, clients have a choice of care providers; in others, they do not. Managed care plans that allow an individual the option of going outside of the plan for services that the plan does not or will not provide are called **point-of-service plans**. Usually, the subscriber is eligible for some reimbursement of costs for these outside services, but by a greatly reduced amount.

In a managed care system, someone, usually the primary physician, is assigned to the role of gatekeeper. This person monitors and restricts the use of services by the client. The physician sees the client first and then determines whether referral or diagnostic services are needed. In some managed care systems, the primary physician has decision-making authority. However, in many managed care systems, the actual gatekeeper is a plan manager, who must be consulted regarding the use of services. A written request may be required before the client receives permission for a referral. This may result in delay or denial of needed care and is one source of consumer dissatisfaction with managed care plans.

Managed care usually requires that care be authorized or approved for payment before it is provided. Clients identify the required approval of any type of care as a major problem. A managed care plan may not approve or pay for care that it considers nonessential. If a healthcare provider and a plan consultant disagree about which type of treatment is appropriate, the client often feels caught in the middle. This situation frequently occurs in emergency care. Even when approval is granted, the process may be long and frustrating for both the client and the physician involved.

Some plans require that an individual travels to a designated hospital when an emergency is not life threatening. Thus, a consumer may be denied payment if he or she goes to the closest hospital as may occur when the consumer is away from home.

A managed care company may have a specific formulary or list of drugs that are allowed to be prescribed. The company usually negotiates for drug purchases at lower prices than paid by the general public. For many conditions, there are clear therapeutic equivalents, and medication restrictions are not a concern. For the person with a chronic health condition who has been stabilized on specific medications, however, moving into a managed care plan can pose a real threat to health maintenance if the plan will not approve the client's current drugs.

People on Medicare also have the option of joining managed care plans under an option termed Medicare Advantage. Under such circumstances, the person joins the plan and pays a monthly fee similar to the cost of a supplemental health insurance (**Medigap**) policy (see below). The government makes a single payment for each individual Medicare recipient directly to the plan and the plan provides all care. The amount per individual was calculated as an average of the expenses incurred by Medicare recipients for all costs. Most Medicare Advantage plans have co-payment fees for services and assess charges for prescriptions.

Health Maintenance Organizations

The first managed care organizations were HMOs that originated as an alternative to traditional insurance plans and were nonprofit in nature. Although traditional insurance plans paid for care when subscribers were ill, HMOs were the first to provide payment for care aimed at preventing illness. HMOs provided well-child care, prenatal care, immunizations, gynecologic examinations, and other preventive services when insurance companies did not.

Because the HMO receives the same income (except for modest co-payments) whether a client requires extensive care or very little care, there is a built-in incentive to emphasize preventive care and avoid costly hospitalization. A flat charge per month covers routine preventive healthcare; care for illness; hospitalization and, in some instances, prescription costs; outpatient care; and other services. HMO-enrolled individuals are often responsible for a co-payment. These co-payments support part of the cost of care and give the consumer an incentive to use services wisely. The line between HMOs and traditional insurance plans has blurred as all health plans pay for preventive care services and the term HMO has become synonymous with managed care plan.

State-Administered Health Plans

States may operate a variety of healthcare resources for their residents. All states manage some type of workers' compensation plans for those injured on the job. This plan may be managed as a state monopoly or contracted to private insurance companies. Employers are required to pay premiums based on statistical information about covered injuries and hazards in various job categories. As healthcare reform continues, these state plans may be expanded and modified with federal subsidies for costs.

Most states support state mental hospitals and public health services. Additional public health services may be supplied through county and city governments. Hospitals designed to provide care for those who are indigent may be operated by the city (such as New York City hospitals) or by the county (such as Cook County Hospital in Chicago).

Federal Government Programs

The federal government in the United States is deeply involved in healthcare financing. Federal programs cover older adults, the poor, federal workers, the military, the veterans, and American Indians and Alaska Natives, some through special programs and some through Medicare and Medicaid. Some individuals express concern about government involvement in the United States healthcare system. When all of these programs and agencies are considered together, it is clear that the federal government already controls many aspects of healthcare.

Medicare

In 1965, after years of effort and testimony by many health-related groups (including the American Nurses Association [ANA]), and with widespread public support, an amendment to the Social Security Act was passed. Title XVIII of the Act, which was termed Medicare, provided payment for hospitalization (Part A) and insurance that could be purchased to meet physicians' fees and outpatient costs (Part B) for people over age 65 and certain others who were receiving Social Security payments. In 2004, Medicare Part D, which covers prescription drugs, was approved, and it took effect in 2006.

Participation in Medicare Part A is automatic for those on Social Security, whereas participation in Medicare Part B is optional and a premium is deducted from the Social Security check to pay for Part B. Medicare Part A pays only for acute hospitalization and a limited amount of rehabilitative care that may occur in a nursing home. Medicare does not pay for any long-term or custodial care in a nursing home. Part B reimburses for physician care and outpatient services based on a fixed schedule of payments. Medicare is administered through CMS, which uses contracted insurance companies termed *Medicare carriers* or *Medicare intermediaries* to process claims. Payments from Medicare do not cover the entire cost of the care provided. The amount authorized is determined by CMS. Medicare then pays a fixed percentage of that authorized amount. The individual pays the remaining percentage. If the provider charges more than the authorized amount, that portion of the fee is not recoverable from either Medicare or the client. Many individuals who receive Medicare also pay for supplemental insurance to cover the part of the healthcare bill for which Medicare Parts A and B do not pay. This is commonly referred to as Medigap insurance and is available from many different insurance companies, such as Blue Cross and Blue Shield.

The premium for Part D prescription coverage may be added to the premium for the Medigap policy or Medicare Advantage contract or may be a separate Part D policy. The cost of prescriptions under Part D is subsidized by Medicare. Plans differ in cost and have different benefits and requirements, such as co-pays, deductibles, coverage of different generic and brand name drugs, and additional coverage in the gap or "doughnut hole" (that area of costs currently between $3,310 and $4,850 for which no reimbursement is provided) that is built into the general plan. The ACA has scheduled changes to reduce this gap in coverage. Each plan is free to establish its own formulary of drugs that are covered and may change that formulary once a month. Participants must investigate each plan to determine whether the drugs they currently take are covered. If new drugs are prescribed, the provider will need to check on the plan to learn what therapeutic equivalent drugs may be covered by that particular plan. Participants may change plans once each year. Individuals who belong to Medicare managed care plans have their Part D integrated into that plan. These drug plans have significantly increased the cost of Medicare.

The complexity of filing claims with Medicare and with an insurance company designed to supplement Medicare coverage (the Medigap policy) is problematic for many people because the insurance company will not pay until Medicare has determined coverage and paid its share. If there are many different health claims, the sending and receiving of the various claims requires careful record keeping. Even when claims are filed by the provider, they may be denied payment if they do not conform to specific rules and regulations. Often older people accept an initial denial of payment for the claim as the final decision and do not pursue the matter further. There is a high rate of reconsideration when denials are appealed. Therefore, it is often wise to encourage clients to appeal a denial of payment.

Medicaid

Title IX of the Social Security Act, which was termed Medicaid, provides funds for healthcare for those dependent on public assistance and certain other low-income individuals. Costs for Medicaid are shared between the federal government and each state. Very low-income individuals who are eligible for Medicare may be covered by Medicaid in the same way that those who can pay are covered by Medigap policies. This often is referred to as being dual eligible. Each state is responsible for administering Medicaid: the state determines eligibility and level of coverage. Payments from the federal government to the states are administered by CMS. Benefits vary greatly among states. As healthcare costs rise and state budgets are severely affected by decreased tax revenue, there has been great pressure to cut this program. To avoid federal control, a few states have not participated in the Medicaid program. Some states have requested waivers from the usual regulations of CMS governing Medicaid to allow experimentation with different plans that might help to control costs.

In 1999, the federal government provided a mechanism for states to enlarge their Medicaid programs, so they could enroll children from low-income families who did not qualify for Medicaid and who would otherwise be without healthcare coverage. This State Children's Health Insurance Plan (SCHIP) represented the first time that the United States has supported healthcare as a right for all children. Not all states agreed to participate in the plan because it required their financial contribution and provides for some federal control of the program. All states must provide a method of coverage for children of low-income families.

Problems Facing Medicare and Medicaid

Medicare and Medicaid are important healthcare resources, but they have not been without problems. Costs have been higher and have been rising faster than anticipated at their inception. There has been a great deal of publicity about instances of abuse and even fraud, associated with these two programs.

The Medicare bill contains many provisions that have made a significant impact on nursing. The definition of skilled nursing care in the original bill was narrow and excluded many important aspects of care necessary to maintaining the health of clients. Through later efforts and testimony, nursing organizations were instrumental in convincing legislators to recognize that the definition of skilled nursing care was critical. As a result, a Senate subcommittee asked the ANA to study skilled nursing care, to provide background data for the Senate. Amendments to the Medicare/Medicaid Act of 1972 encouraged the study of alternative ways of providing healthcare to contain costs. These alternatives included the use of nurses in expanded roles and the use of managed care.

In 1982 and again in 1993, Congress revised Medicare to prevent serious financial deficits in the system that escalating costs could create. The ACA contains some modifications of Medicare, but there is still concern that increased demand by an aging population will undermine the financial stability of Medicare and that further cuts in Medicare spending are being proposed.

The growing number of older adults; the rising costs of medications, supplies, and wages; and the widespread use of costly, highly technical diagnostic tools and therapies all have contributed to escalating healthcare costs. With the baby-boomer generation now in retirement years, further strain will be placed on the financial resources of the system. Despite these concerns, Medicare and Medicaid have provided healthcare dollars and services to many people who would otherwise have done without.

Military and Other Federal Healthcare

TRICARE is the healthcare program for uniformed service members. It includes active duty and retired members of the U.S. Army, U.S. Air Force, U.S. Navy, U.S. Marine Corps, U.S. Coast Guard, Commissioned Corps of the U.S. Public Health Service, and the Commissioned Corps of the National Oceanic and Atmospheric Association and their families around the world

(TRICARE, 2017). This program has many different options as well as a pharmacy plan. While care is available in military facilities, most participants receive care in the private sector with TRICARE acting as the health plan.

The U.S. Department of Health and Human Services (DHHS) provides direct healthcare services through the Indian Health Service (IHS), which operates hospitals, health centers, school health centers, health stations, and urban American Indian health centers and provides payments to community providers where no IHS facilities are present (DHHS, 2015). Most other healthcare provided through the DHHS is through payments to community clinics and other support for meeting the needs of low-income and disadvantaged individuals.

The Department of Veterans' Affairs operates many clinics, hospitals, and nursing homes for veterans. These are found across the country. For those who are eligible for care from the VA, benefits are comprehensive. The VA is engaged in a major effort to improve services to veterans. Information on the VA's services is available at www.va.gov.

Patterns of Payment

Understanding the various methods of paying for healthcare services can help you understand what is happening in the organizations and agencies involved in the healthcare system. The following discussion covers those most commonly used methods of paying for healthcare services.

Fee-for-Service Payment

Fee-for-service payment means that each time a service is provided a fee is generated and then billed to the care recipient. The more services provided, the more fees charged. This was the traditional method of charging for healthcare in the United States. Initially, private individuals paid almost all fees. When insurance companies began assisting with payment, the bill was sent to the insurance company and to the client. The insurance company then paid the amount established in the policy (eg, 80%), and the client was required to pay the rest.

As costs rose, insurance companies began setting a standard for reimbursement. Under this system, if a policy stated that a company reimbursed at 80%, this meant 80% of a fee that the insurance company determined was reasonable. If the provider charged more than what was considered reasonable, the client was responsible for the excess, in addition to 20% of the "reasonable" fee. Insurance companies usually set these fees based on statistical analysis of prevailing fees in a geographic area. In a time of rapid inflation, providers complained that there was often a serious discrepancy between the fee used for calculating benefits and the actual fees being charged. This standard fee still provided for paying a fee for each service rendered.

Prospective Payment

A **prospective payment** is a fixed reimbursement amount for all the care required for a particular surgical procedure, an illness, or an acuity category. This reimbursement amount is determined in advance of the provision of service. The predetermined amount is paid without regard to actual services required or the costs of those services in individual situations. Thus, the same payment is made whether the person is healthy and has an uncomplicated hospital stay or whether the person is in poor health and has complications that increase the cost of care or the length of the hospital stay.

Prospective payment is designed to provide an incentive for providers to control costs. Prospective payment has accomplished this as hospitals began to monitor the use of high-cost testing and pharmaceutical products and to limit the length of stay. Another advantage to payers in a prospective payment system (PPS) is that costs are predictable. The system transfers the burden of risk (the probability that an individual may require extraordinary services) from the payer to the provider. Several specific types of prospective payment have particular significance for nurses. These are DRGs and **resource utilization groups** (RUGs).

Diagnosis-Related Groups

The first major change in the method of payment for healthcare services began October 1, 1983, when the federal government stopped using a fee-for-service reimbursement system for Medicare and introduced a PPS using **diagnosis-related groups** (DRGs) to determine the payment for each Medicare client admitted to the hospital. This change was designed to stop the spiraling costs of Medicare and to correct inequities that made the costs of care in one facility very different from those in another facility.

The method of determining the rates to be paid in the Medicare PPS—the creation of DRGs—resulted from a computerized analysis of costs that had been billed for hospitalized individuals in the past and a determination of an average length of stay. This analysis led to the formation of categories of medical diagnoses that require similar treatment and for which costs are similar. Each category (or DRG) has a name and number; for example, DRG 236 is "fracture of the hip and pelvis." In addition, a decision was made to increase the payment for care when another illness or condition is present. This second condition is termed a **comorbidity**. Thus, a person with heart failure whose basic DRG is "fractured hip" is designated "fractured hip with congestive heart failure." A hospital receives greater reimbursement for providing service to this person because care is more complex and costs are higher. Hospitals also receive additional amounts for cases that are determined to be outliers. An outlier is a case in which the client's length of stay significantly exceeds the average. The number of days needed to qualify a case as an outlier is predetermined. For example, the average length of stay for DRG 236, "fractured hip and pelvis," is 6.2 days, but the stay must reach 29 days for the case to be considered an outlier. Pressure is placed on all providers to ensure that the client is discharged within the average length of stay on which payment is based.

Most hospital costs are included in the DRG reimbursement. The actual DRG reimbursement amount is recalculated each year by CMS through a complex formula that considers the area of the country in which care was provided (eg, Northwest, Southeast), the urbanization of the area (eg, rural, suburban), and the type of care required. Some hospital costs still are reimbursed separately.

Most of the controversy surrounding the implementation of DRGs has not been concerned with the incentives for cost control or the prospective reimbursement system itself, but rather how the payment amounts are determined and how the system is being administered. Hospitals with a large population of extra high-risk clients (eg, the very old or the poor) have expressed concern that discharging a client for convalescence in a home with a caring family, good food, and a clean environment is much different from discharging a client to an impoverished environment. Many believe that the individual situation should be considered when determining regulations for length of stay. The proponents of shortened stays point out that shortened stays are effective cost-containment measures. They argue further that a client's lack of a support system is a social problem and that hospitalization cannot be used to solve social problems. Alterations and modifications of the system will continue, but the basic prospective plan is not expected to change.

Resource Utilization Groups

Resource utilization groups (RUGs) are the categories used to determine prospective payment for nursing home clients. Each RUG represents a group of residents who require a similar amount of care and would have a similar cost of daily care. Unlike the hospital prospective payment, which is a flat amount for the entire hospital stay, the prospective payment for nursing home care is a fixed daily rate. This daily rate must include all the services, including medications and treatments, that a resident needs. The actual daily rate of reimbursement to the nursing home is the average of the RUGs for all residents. This is often referred to as the **case mix**.

The basis for determining to which RUG a nursing home resident will be assigned for reimbursement purposes is the comprehensive MDS prepared by the RN. This assessment is transmitted electronically to the appropriate center for review and payment categorization. If the assessment is not completed accurately or in a timely manner, the resident automatically is assigned to the lowest reimbursement RUG category. The facility is then unable to recover the difference between the lowest RUG and the actual RUG to which the resident is eventually assigned. Reassessments are required at specified intervals.

Many nursing homes have reduced staff, changed practice patterns, and made other adjustments to adapt to the effect of RUGs. One unintended result of the move to PPS for the nursing home has been the refusal of nursing homes to admit high-cost residents. For example, an individual with an extensive wound that requires intensive wound care with expensive products might cost more per day for care than that the highest RUG category allows. In the past, it was possible to bill separately for the expensive dressings and topical agents used. When this is not possible, the facility may refuse to admit the client. This actually may increase costs for the payer, because clients remain in the high-cost hospital if no long-term care facility will admit them.

Capitation

Capitation is yet another way of determining payment within the healthcare system. In a capitated system, a fee is paid to a provider organization for each person (each "head," thus the term) signed up for the plan whether that person uses any healthcare services. Global capitation refers to the inclusion of all services, both inpatient and outpatient, including physician costs in the capitated amount. Capitation may also be limited and only include outpatient and physician costs.

Capitation shifts an even greater share of the risk of providing costly healthcare from the third-party payer to the provider organization. Providers in a capitated system have an incentive to guide individuals to low-cost outpatient services or other care environments rather than to the acute care hospital. A goal of this payment system is to encourage preventive services that may make high-cost interventions unnecessary. HMOs were the original capitated systems.

A criticism of a capitated system is that when the provider is at risk for providing care, there may be an unconscious (or even deliberate) attempt to deny medically necessary care to keep costs down. In some capitated systems, consumers have complained that they were unable to obtain services they believed were medically necessary.

Evidence-Based Practice 6.1: Cost of Healthcare

Rosenkoetter, M. M. (2016). Overview and summary: Organizational outcomes for providers and patients. *Online Journal Of Issues In Nursing, 21*(2), 1. doi:10.3912/OJIN. Vol21No02ManOS

Among the 11 industrialized countries of the world, the United States healthcare system was ranked as the most expensive and the least efficient. Healthcare spending was $2.6 trillion in 2010 and is projected to be $4.8 trillion in 2021. The comprehensive reform law, the Affordable Care Act, was intended to reform healthcare coverage, cost, and delivery. There is some controversy about the efficacy of this law.

Several controllable factors contribute to the increasing cost of healthcare. Increasing technology needs to be managed. Some "improvements" are not necessarily better. Decisions to make changes in equipment, practice, or technology need to be driven by valid research. Medical errors are often preventable and measures should be taken to prevent medical errors that often lead to increased hospital length of stay and expense. The focus on collaboration in healthcare is a topic that needs further research and discussion as it has the potential to greatly improve healthcare in decrease overall costs.

COST CONTROL IN HEALTHCARE

Because healthcare costs continue to rise, cost control is a major focus of today's healthcare system. Many factors contribute to the rising costs of health, and many strategies have been used to attempt to limit the rate of increase (Evidence-Based Practice 6.1).

Understanding Increasing Costs

Many factors contribute to the rising costs of healthcare (Box 6.1).

High Technology and New Facilities

One important factor in cost increase is the price of new, more sophisticated technology. The rising cost of technology affects every area of the healthcare field, from the cardiac care unit to the laboratory. Companies that manufacture health-related devices and drugs reportedly have some of the highest profits in any industry. These companies justify their profits as appropriate relative to the risk and cost involved in research and development. However,

---

BOX 6.1 CONTRIBUTING FACTORS IN RISING HEALTHCARE COSTS

- Price of new technology
- Construction of new facilities
- Higher survival rates, leading to greater need for costly intensive or long-term care
- Growing population of older adults requiring healthcare
- Rise in salaries for healthcare providers
- High costs of drugs and health-related equipment

some critics believe that these companies take advantage of the public's dependence on their products. For example, recent evidence indicates that the drug companies spend as much on advertising as they do on research (Swanson, 2015). For those health insurance plans and HMOs providing prescription coverage, the costs of prescription drugs are cited as a key reason for premium increases. The public has expressed concern that drug companies sell identical drugs in other countries for far less money than what they charge consumers in the United States. Drug companies contend that high costs in the United States are essential to support continued drug research, which is very costly. One of the realities contributing to this situation is that other countries place price controls on drugs, and the United States does not.

An increasing population needs a greater number of facilities, and the construction of new care facilities also contributes to rising costs. In addition, existing facilities often require modifications. More space is needed for new technologies both at the bedside and in many hospital departments. Electronic healthcare records require space and infrastructure of wiring and servers as well as the computers and software. The regulations governing hospital construction also have become more stringent, requiring more fire-safety and infection-control measures and protection against environmental hazards. These factors combine to make the per-bed cost of new hospital construction or hospital remodeling increasingly expensive. Additionally, decreases in the length of hospital stay and the move to outpatient services have left many hospital beds unused on a fluctuating basis. Unoccupied hospital beds create a major drain on organizations, because large sums of capital investment are tied up and not returning any income.

Changing Patient Profile

The average length of hospital stay for standard diagnoses has decreased steadily. The typical client in today's hospital is discharged rapidly to convalesce at home or in a long-term care facility, leaving behind only the acutely ill. Many clients who would have died quickly in the earlier years live through a crisis but require long and intensive care. All of these factors make the acuity level of a client today much greater. This in turn requires more intensive observation and care and the use of more specialized equipment.

The population of the United States as a whole is growing older, and, statistically, older adults have an increased incidence of all chronic illnesses. A greater percentage of that population requires healthcare on a regular basis and may depend on medications, treatments, and therapies for continued functioning.

Uninsured Individuals

Health plans in the United States are primarily linked to employment, except for those eligible for Medicare and Medicaid, because the cost of independent plans is prohibitive. Major incentives to pass the ACA were to provide a mechanism for more individuals to be able to purchase insurance, to subsidize those unable to afford insurance, and to reduce the effect of uncompensated care on healthcare providers.

Many healthcare providers have struggled with the financial problem of uncompensated care. Uncompensated care is a particular concern for hospitals. Individuals arrive at emergency rooms, and laws require that they be assessed before they leave. If an acute problem is found, they must be treated. If the client has no insurance and is not able to pay privately (which is the common case for those without insurance), the provider is never compensated for the care given. For hospitals with trauma centers and busy emergency rooms, these cases may be ones that require extensive resources lasting over months. Uncompensated care may threaten the viability of these institutions. The provisions of the ACA have decreased the demand for uncompensated care. However, there will continue to be those not covered by the provisions of healthcare reform, and thus uncompensated care will not disappear altogether.

Other Factors Affecting Costs

Salaries for healthcare workers are part of the cost equation. In the mid-1900s, the salaries of healthcare workers (except for physicians) were far below those of the general society. To remedy this, for a time, salaries of healthcare workers rose more rapidly than the general inflation rate. Physicians also had an increase in income greater than the relative inflation rate, until the mid-1990s, when changes in the system began to affect income levels for physicians.

Lack of competition in the healthcare field is one factor that may contribute to higher costs. Although physicians continue to be primary gatekeepers in the system, the advent of other PCPs, such as NPs, nurse midwives, and PAs, offers alternative and less costly care for many routine problems and normal life processes such as respiratory infections, pregnancy, and well-child care.

Critical Thinking Activity: Cost of Medications
Create a sample client with a chronic illness such as diabetes or congestive heart failure and list of all the medications that this client might receive. Conduct a web search to determine the cost of these medications. Compare the generic and the brand name cost. If a medication is not covered by insurance, or if the patient is uninsured, they may have to pay for the medication out of pocket. How much would the patient have to pay monthly for the most expensive medication on the list you created? What is the total yearly cost of all the medications on the list? What could be done to lower prescription costs?

Strategies for Cost Control

As healthcare costs continue to rise, third-party payers have used several methods to control costs, including changing patterns of payment and controlling the actions of providers. These strategies are often referred to as *cost containment* actions.

Limiting Hospital Costs

With the changes in payment, hospitals have developed many mechanisms to limit costs. Because federal regulations limit the reimbursement to hospitals, physicians are asked to judge carefully the necessity of diagnostic studies and costly procedures for hospitalized clients. Physicians sometimes are asked to consult with a pharmacist before prescribing certain high-cost drugs to determine whether a low-cost therapeutic alternative exists. There is great pressure on physicians to discharge clients by the average length of stay to ensure that costs remain within the established prospective payment amount. Physician practices are monitored, and they have even been threatened with denial of hospital privileges if their clients consistently stay beyond the expected length of stay. These cost-containment measures may interfere with the physician's independent decision-making about what care is needed and when.

To add new high-cost equipment or additional client care facilities, a healthcare institution may be required to apply for a certificate of need from the state. This establishes that there will not be unnecessary duplication of services in an area and that a need for them exists. For example, if every hospital purchased magnetic resonance imaging equipment that was used to only one fourth or one third of its capacity, the cost per use would have to be higher to cover the investment and maintenance costs than if the device were used to capacity.

Preferred Provider Organizations

In an attempt to contain costs, third-party payers such as insurance companies, HMOs, and managed care organizations sometimes negotiate with providers of healthcare to supply certain kinds of care at an agreed-upon, usually lower, price. The third-party payers then provide incentives for clients to use these preferred providers. These incentives may include the waiver of all or part of co-payments by the insured or coverage of additional conditions or situations.

Preferred provider organizations (PPOs) include hospitals, nursing homes, corporations employing care providers, or groups of care providers who have cooperated to negotiate more successfully with third-party payers for these special contracts. The advantage to the provider is the ensured number of clients and the guaranteed income that in a time of competition in healthcare may be significant. Each PPO operates independently. Therefore, the exact structure and contractual arrangements are independently determined.

Case Management

Case management is a technique used to efficiently move an individual requiring major health services through the system resulting in more effective use of services and reduced cost. According to the Case Management Society of America (CMSA), case management is a collaborative process that assesses, plans, implements, coordinates, monitors, and evaluates options and services to meet an individual's health needs through communication and available resources to promote quality cost-effective outcomes (CMSA, 2015).

The case manager is an experienced health professional with knowledge of available resources who oversees or monitors a case to ensure that necessary care is instituted promptly and is provided in the most cost-effective setting. Nurses have often assumed the role of case manager. In this role, the nurse monitors the care as it is provided, ensuring that appropriate referrals are made, changes in the plan of care are instituted appropriately, and the care follows established standards. Because of their understanding of the whole person, both physiologically and psychosocially, and their understanding of how the system works, nurses are particularly well suited to this role. The CMSA provides a system for certifying professional case managers.

Case managers may work as internal case managers where they operate within only one part of the system (eg, managing cases from admission through discharge in a nursing home or hospital) or they may manage cases across all phases of care from outpatient through hospitalization, rehabilitation, and back to outpatient-external case managers. At their best, case management systems ensure that delays in client transfer or breaks in communication do not occur and that costs are minimized through efficiency. Case managers often act as advocates for clients in the system.

Vertically Integrated Healthcare Systems

Organizations contracting to provide managed care are expanding their own control through the development of **vertically integrated systems**, that is, those that provide every level of healthcare service. A vertically integrated system may have contracted physicians, laboratories, a hospital, a subacute facility, a rehabilitation facility, and a home care agency. This allows the contracting organization to offer managed care corporations a package that provides care at all levels for each enrolled member of the managed care plan for a capitated fee. The contracting organization then has an incentive to control costs by decreasing the use of high-cost services and more effectively using low-cost alternatives. It is also in a better position to negotiate with the managed care system about reimbursement.

Using Acuity Measures to Determine Costs

Healthcare providers who negotiate contracts and plan care need accurate data regarding the specific cost of each service. One way of trying to understand and control these costs is through the development of acuity measures. Acuity in this context refers to the severity of illness and the rapidity of change in the client, and thus the intensity of medical and nursing care and other therapies required.

There are various ways of measuring acuity in both acute and long-term care settings. Most systems use categories that reflect the different types of care needed. Each category is assigned a numerical value (eg, a scale of 1 to 4). All applicable category values are summed and compared with a standard. As a person needs more assistance, more points are assigned. Each category is assigned an appropriate number of points, and the total is computed. The points identified for an individual client are then compared with a standard, and the client is assigned an acuity level. Clients with the fewest points are level 1 and require the least care. Those with the most points are level 4 and require the most care. Each system in use has its own scale for determining acuity. Acuity values are sometimes called **intensity measures** because they reflect the intensity of care needed.

In some settings, acuity levels or intensity measures are used as a mechanism for determining the staffing needs of a client care unit. Acuity levels also are used as a means of billing for the level of nursing care needed and are reflected in a variable, rather than flat, charge for the nursing portion of a client's room charge. It also has been suggested that prospective reimbursement might be based on acuity level rather than on medical diagnosis because acuity levels reflect the real impact on resources more accurately than do medical diagnoses. The RUGs developed for prospective reimbursement in long-term care are essentially an acuity measure based on the nursing assessment.

Increasing the Availability of Mid-Level Providers

Because physicians are the most costly healthcare providers, increasing the use of nonphysician PCPs, such as NPs and PAs, is being used to decrease healthcare costs. These are referred to as mid-level providers. The use of mid-level providers relies on the ability to obtain reimbursement for the care these individuals deliver.

Changing Fee Structures

In addition to reducing payments through PPSs, the federal government has sought to control costs for Medicare and Medicaid by establishing higher deductibles (the portions that individual clients must pay) and by limiting the fees that the government will pay. Because older adults and the poor are often unable to pay these deductible amounts, they become liabilities for healthcare providers, who cover these costs by collecting higher fees from those who do pay their bills. Hospitals, physicians, and pharmacies argue that as more limits have been imposed, the limited reimbursement no longer covers the actual costs of care. This jeopardizes the entire system. Medicaid costs also have been contained by tightening eligibility requirements, which shuts more people out of the healthcare system. Healthcare reform relies on expanding eligibility for Medicaid to cover the working poor. Many employer plans are requiring more cost sharing by employees both to reduce the cost to the employer and as an incentive for the employee to use healthcare wisely. Fee structures have historically rewarded procedures and medications with higher reimbursement than teaching or addressing psychosocial needs. Changing fee structures to support actions that promote health and avoid exacerbations of chronic illness has been proposed as one possible source of cost containment.

Controlling Fraud and Abuse

As Medicare and Medicaid have become a larger part of the financing for the healthcare system, fraud has become a larger problem with individual cases responsible for millions in fraudulent payments (Evidence-Based Practice 6.2). HIPAA created a federal Healthcare Fraud and Abuse Control Program that coordinates federal, state, and local law enforcement activities in fighting healthcare fraud and abuse. Information on preventing Medicare fraud is available at the Medicare Web site (www.medicare.gov/) under Forms, Help & Resources.

Other Cost-Containment Measures

In medical facilities, personnel are asked to be more cost conscious. Nursing personnel must be aware of the tremendous cost of any complication or prolonged length of stay. Care pathways specify care and identify outcomes for each day of hospitalization, with the goal of ensuring that resources are used wisely. Cost consciousness involves such ordinary measures as canceling meal trays when clients are discharged, and using expensive supplies with care.

Efforts at reducing costs affect the entire healthcare environment, the decision-making processes, power structures, the kinds of care provided, and the ways that individual healthcare providers practice. Concerns about cost continue to exert pressure for change in the system.

Evidence-Based Practice 6.2: *Medicare Fraud*

Medicare takedown uncovers $712 million in fraud. (2015). *PT in Motion, 7*(9), 53.

Fraudulent Medicare claims are an ongoing problem. In 2015, a large investigation by the United States Department of Justice uncovered $712 million dollars in false billings by 234 individuals. These false claims are a big concern as they result in a waste of resources in an already overburdened system. The Department of Justice described this investigation as the largest coordinated operation in the history of Medicare fraud investigation. In addition to overcharges, there were many charges for services that were not provided or services that were provided by unqualified individuals.

> **Critical Thinking Activity: Cost Control**
> What cost-control measures have you seen in places where you have had clinical practice? Analyze the effects of these cost-control measures on client care.

ACCESS TO HEALTHCARE

Access to healthcare refers to the individual's ability to obtain and use needed services. Access can be an economic, a geographic, or a sociocultural issue. Creating access requires a broad approach that encompasses access to healthcare providers and hospitalization as well as addressing other factors that affect health. In addition to providing a family with a prescription, for example, a provider must determine whether there is a way to fill that prescription. Prescribing a special diet requires learning whether that the individual has the necessary knowledge and resources to follow that diet.

Economic Access

The problem of economic access to healthcare was discussed from a system perspective when the various methods of paying for healthcare were presented. Economic access is often dependent on having a health plan or being eligible for one of the government programs. Some of the decisions made for purposes of cost containment may have unforeseen consequences in terms of economic access. Although giving people an incentive to use services wisely is the stated goal of raising deductibles and co-payments, the result for lower-income families may be the delay or avoidance of timely care. Many of the provisions of the healthcare reform were for the purpose of increasing economic access to healthcare.

Daily Ethical Dilemma 6.1: Use of Resources

Jones, a homeless 58-year-old African-American man, has been in end-stage renal failure for 6 years. He does not have insurance and does not qualify for Medicaid where he lives. He has been receiving hemodialysis, which is paid for by Medicare. He does not have a known drug problem but does have significant mental health issues and prefers to live on the streets rather than shelters or halfway houses that the State has identified as housing for him. During the cold winter months, he makes as many as 10 visits a week to the university hospital emergency department. This is where he receives most of his dialysis treatments as an inpatient. Emergency department physicians have become increasingly frustrated at what they see as abuse of the system. They feel that he is using valuable resources and he should receive palliative care only.

• What is the primary dilemma in this situation?
• How might Jones' care be managed more cost effectively?
• What potential biases if any are evident in this scenario?
• Should physicians be tasked with determining what care each client should receive (gatekeeping) to conserve resources?

Some groups, such as minorities and older adults, that experience disparities in healthcare access are heavily affected by the coexistence of poverty in these groups. Even those eligible for Medicaid-financed care may not be able to find a PCP willing to care for them. The low reimbursement rates and the need to cope with the complex governmental system lead many private providers to opt out of such care.

Geographic Access

Geographic access to healthcare is a special concern for those in rural areas. Changes in the healthcare system have resulted in the closure of some small rural hospitals that cannot compete with large corporate agencies. When a rural hospital closes, area residents lose local access to emergency room care, hospital, and diagnostic services. The need to travel to receive healthcare especially affects older adults and the poor.

Communities without hospitals find it more difficult to recruit physicians and other PCPs. Historically, most healthcare providers have preferred not to work in areas where hospitals are not available to provide diagnostic and treatment services. Many medical schools, with the support of both federal and state funds, developed programs to encourage medical students and residents to consider family practice as a specialty and to practice in a rural location. Although successful in increasing the number of physicians entering rural practice, in some states, the number of physicians leaving rural practice is greater than those entering the profession.

Geographic access may be a concern for those in urban areas as well. Economically depressed areas of large cities have fewer healthcare providers, forcing the residents of those areas to travel long distances, often using inconvenient public transportation, to receive healthcare.

NPs have a long history of moving into underserved areas both rural and urban. Significant support for the education of NPs and for removing barriers to their reimbursement was part of the ACA. As more individuals have economic access, the demand for PCPs is expected to increase. NPs are expected to be major players in providing primary care.

Access to healthcare is affected by whether all services are available in one location. Some organizations now offer all health services in one geographic location. A single healthcare site allows an individual to see a primary provider and a specialist and have diagnostic tests and procedures in one trip to one location. This makes efficient use of the client's time, increases the likelihood that the client will follow through with recommended procedures, and simplifies communication among providers.

Sociocultural Access

Sociocultural differences affect access. When individuals feel uncomfortable in a setting because of their socioeconomic status or because their cultural background and beliefs are not respected, they are reluctant to use the services provided. Making care culturally accessible may mean having available in the care setting translation services, materials in multiple languages, and care providers who understand and are sensitive to cultural differences.

EVALUATION AND ACCREDITATION OF HEALTHCARE AGENCIES

A variety of standards and processes to enforce those standards have been established to evaluate healthcare. Meeting the standards of a state governmental agency is termed approval or *certification*. Meeting the standards of a nongovernment agency is usually designated as

accreditation. Healthcare institutions are often both certified by a government body and accredited by a nongovernment agency. In some instances, government bodies accept accreditation as the equivalent of government standards and do not require an additional approval process. Approval by a specific organization may be required for an agency to receive some types of third-party payment. Therefore, accreditation is important for the agencies involved. Most evaluation processes involve evaluating client outcomes as well as the structure of the organization and the processes used to provide care.

Medicare/Medicaid Certification

Those agencies that seek Medicare or Medicaid funding must meet specific federal standards (termed the *conditions of participation*) and be Medicare certified in addition to meeting the basic state standards for operation. By designating those to whom payment will be given, Medicare effectively exerts control. Because the costs of private care are so high, most people choose to receive care where it can be reimbursed, making other choices when the care is not reimbursed.

Healthcare institutions and agencies may seek accreditation from nongovernment bodies that set standards for high quality and provide guidelines to assist in developing policies and procedures. Medicare and Medicaid have granted several of these nongovernment agencies what is called *deemed status*. This means that the standards of the agency are considered equal to or exceeding the Medicare standard. Therefore, a healthcare agency that has been accredited by the voluntary process from an agency discussed as follows may be deemed as meeting the standards set by Medicare and Medicaid without additional certification.

The Joint Commission

Hospitals, nursing homes, and related organizations may seek accreditation from The Joint Commission. This nonprofit, voluntary organization was established in 1951 by the American College of Surgeons, the American College of Physicians, the American Medical Association, and the Canadian Medical Association (The Joint Commission, n.d.) to set standards for hospital care. Today's organization has a board of directors with members from many healthcare and public occupations. The standards of the organization are comprehensive and involve evaluating the structural aspects of institutions, the processes used within that agency to deliver and monitor care, and the outcomes of care provided. It has deemed status for federal programs. The Joint Commission provides accreditation for a wide variety of healthcare facilities including home care, ambulatory care, and assisted living.

During visits to facilities referred to as *surveys* (done approximately every 3 years), The Joint Commission investigates all aspects of an organization, including the physical plant, the entire delivery of care process, and the evaluation and quality improvement plans being used. It has the power to demand change to maintain accreditation status. In most instances, however, problems that are not of serious danger to clients are noted for remediation and the facility is asked to report on the changes made.

DNV Accreditation

In September 2008, DNV (Det Norske Veritas) Accreditation became the first alternative to Joint Commission accreditation for hospitals. This nonprofit organization has been in existence for many years, working with manufacturing and other industries on developing effective quality improvement processes and managing risk. The expansion into healthcare follows their same model of operation. The surveys are done annually. Those institutions that meet the Medicare/Medicaid COP are accredited but are then guided toward improvement to meet the international standard, which reflects continuous quality improvement and customer satisfaction. DNV does not provide consulting nor does it provide prescriptive processes for institutions. They state that their focus is to help organizations develop their own best practices by focusing on outcomes. While at this writing, only 466 hospitals in the United States are accredited by DNV. This may change as organizations examine their options for accreditation (DNV, 2017).

Community Health Accreditation Program

The Community Health Accreditation Program (CHAP) was established to provide a voluntary accreditation system for community-based health services including home health agencies, hospices, and home medical equipment providers (www.chapinc.org). This is a peer-reviewed process governed entirely by community health agencies with public representation. Medicare and Medicaid do not require a separate Medicare certification for an organization that has CHAP accreditation.

National Committee for Quality Assurance

The National Committee for Quality Assurance (NCQA) reviews and evaluates health plans and provides recognition of plans that meet standards of excellence. NCQA has established a set of statistical measures called the Healthcare Effectiveness Data and Information Set (HEDIS) and is a tool used by more than 90% of America's health plans to measure performance on important dimensions of care and service. This information is available from its Web site, www.ncqa.org. These data provide a standard set of information that both employers and consumers can use to compare and evaluate health plans.

Quality Improvement Organizations

The first systematic evaluation of healthcare services was established through the Professional Standards Review Organization setup by Medicare and Medicaid in the 1980s. These efforts have continued to expand through quality improvement organizations (QIOs). "A Quality Improvement Organization (QIO) is a group of health quality experts, clinicians, and consumers organized to improve the quality of care delivered to people with Medicare" (CMS, 2016).

Areas of concern in terms of quality improvement are patient safety, care coordination or transitions, clinical treatment advancement, and preventive care methods. QIOs also work to promote best practice models and serve as a resource in the areas of health information technology and electronic health records. Consumers may appeal decisions made by healthcare providers to their state QIO (CMS, 2016).

Outcome Measures for Evaluation

Outcome measures refer to actual health results in the clients and communities served. Outcomes now are measured in relationship to hospitals, long-term care facilities, and the population as a whole. Some outcomes have been designated **key indicators**, also termed **quality indicators** (QIs), which are specific, measurable aspects of healthcare that show the effectiveness of the system as a whole. Some of the outcome measures are based on the outcomes identified by *Healthy People 2020* (DHHS, 2017).

Hospital Healthcare Outcomes

The federal government compiles statistics related to hospital healthcare outcomes. These include infection rates and morbidity and mortality rates associated with specific hospitals and procedures. In 1995, the federal government began releasing these figures to the public. These government statistics may be helpful in evaluating some aspects of care. One result of outcome studies has been the recommendation that only hospitals that perform a specified number of highly technical surgeries (eg, cardiac surgeries) each year should offer those procedures. Hospitals that perform fewer procedures per year have higher complication and mortality rates.

The Agency for Health Care Research and Quality (AHRQ) has identified a set of items that could be used as indicators of quality of care and community access to care. It identified three groups of QIs: prevention QIs, inpatient QIs, and patient safety QIs. Since their beginning in the early 1990s, these QIs have been refined through the use of extensive data banks maintained by the HHS (AHRQ, 2016).

Many healthcare agencies are constructing their documentation systems to collect data that demonstrate performance in relationship to these QIs. This is enlarging the purpose of documentation from a focus on the individual client to a focus that includes system concerns.

Institutional Outcomes Measurement

Individual institutions are establishing ways to measure the outcomes of the care they provide. *Outcomes* here refer to data such as the number of clients admitted with a fractured hip who had uncomplicated recoveries leading to effective rehabilitation and the number of clients who had complications or did not recover. Knowledge of outcomes is essential for planning and for effective marketing. Because data only become valuable for planning when they are organized in a useful framework for analysis, healthcare agencies have moved rapidly to the computerization of data and the implementation of standardized protocols for data collection.

One of the standardized tools hospitals use to monitor outcomes is called the **clinical pathway**. This is also referred to as a critical path, a care map, or an anticipated recovery path. The clinical pathway describes the optimum progression through the system of the individual with a particular health problem. By establishing the desired outcome for day 2 of the postoperative client with a fractured hip, it is possible to determine when an individual client is not meeting the desired outcome. The advantage for the client is that care can be modified immediately to address the problem. The advantage for the system is the ability to aggregate data across all clients and examine what is working well and what needs to be changed.

Long-Term Care Quality Measures

Quality measures (QMs) are used in long-term care as part of the regulatory process. QMs differ from QIs "These measures assess the resident's physical and clinical conditions and abilities, as well as preferences and life care wishes" (CMS, 2015). CMS has identified 14 QMs for long-term care residents. These QMs serve as the focus for the state surveyors. Long-term care facilities track these indicators themselves and use them as a focus of improvement.

Home Care Quality Indicators

The home care quality indicators provide tools for measuring quality in home care (AHRQ, 2016). They are based on assessments using the MDS for home care. These indicators can be monitored to evaluate the performance of a home care agency. Examples of indicators are "prevalence of weight loss in individuals who are not palliative care clients" and "prevalence of decrease in ability to dress one's upper body." One area of concern in comparing agencies based on these indicators is that the population served by the agency affects the outcomes of care. Those agencies caring for a greater percentage of the poor and the disadvantaged face challenges in meeting the same outcome standards.

National Health Indicators

In 1992, DHHS and the Public Health Service published *Healthy People (2000), National Health Promotion and Disease Prevention Objectives.* The purpose of this document was to establish national goals to serve as a focus for health promotion and disease prevention activities by individuals, organizations, and the federal government. The *Healthy People* program has continued to guide federal efforts through *Healthy People 2010, 2020* and objectives for *Healthy People 2030* are being discussed (DHHS, 2017).

POWER IN THE HEALTHCARE SYSTEM

Part of trying to understand any system involves examining some of the unique sources of **power** and authority within it. If we define power as the capability of doing or accomplishing something, then understanding how power is distributed and used in the healthcare system can help us function more effectively. Sources of power unique to the healthcare system are the authority to decide who may enter and leave the system, who may practice in it, and how funding is controlled. An understanding of power in the healthcare system provides a foundation for nurses to accomplish their goals for patients and their families. Without this understanding, nurses may find themselves without power and thus unable to accomplish desired goals.

Regulatory Power

The primary regulatory agencies in healthcare are government bodies as discussed earlier. Through regulation, these agencies have a profound effect on how institutions operate. The accrediting bodies (eg, The Joint Commission, CHAP, and NCQA) all have power to stimulate change in the system. If you have the opportunity to be in an institution when accreditation visitors are present, you will note that every aspect of the physical plant, the policies and procedures, and the competence of staff are examined. Preparing for an accreditation visit stimulates the agency to self-evaluate and correct any deficiencies.

Third-Party Payer Power

Because they represent the financial interests of large groups of people and control payments for services, third-party payers have the power to demand changes in the healthcare system. When they were first established, these agencies did not see their role in healthcare as anything beyond a financial relationship. As healthcare costs rose, these agencies began looking for ways of controlling costs to maintain their competitive place in the insurance market and have set increasingly rigid criteria for payment for services. The standard rates set for payment for procedures tend to place some restraints on charges (although actual fees often are slightly ahead of payment schedules). By determining whom they will pay for services, insurance companies reduce the choices available to those who carry insurance, and subscribers usually must select from the choices available if they wish to be reimbursed. Third-party payers therefore exert a more powerful influence over institutions and care providers than do individual subscribers.

Physician Power

Physicians historically had almost unlimited power within the healthcare system. They determined who entered the system and when. They decided whether and when other services and personnel would be used, and they determined when clients would leave the system. As other agencies and professionals in the healthcare system have obtained some power and independence, the overall power of the physician has diminished. Those favoring increased distribution of power have argued that more competition, more choice for consumers, and input from a greater variety of healthcare providers and from consumers will make the system more balanced and more responsive. Despite changes, physicians remain powerful in the healthcare system.

Consumer Power

The sources of power previously discussed present problems because the client is excluded. Clearly, the client is involved in only the most basic aspect of entry into the system: determining that he or she needs care.

Consumers do have rights in the healthcare system. These are stated in different ways by different institutions and groups, but all revolve around the recognition of the healthcare consumer as an individual with the ability and right to be self-determining. Consumers are in a particularly vulnerable position in the healthcare system. Because they put their lives in the hands of those in the system, they are often reluctant to complain or request changes for fear of offending those on whom they depend. In addition, when consumers try to exert power in the system, they may meet with resistance. Consumers are most often effective in exerting power in the system by working in groups and through established committees and agencies.

The American Hospital Association's document "The Patient Care Partnership: Understanding Expectations, Rights, and Responsibilities" (http://www.aha.org/advocacy-issues/communicatingpts/pt-care-partnership.shtml) provides a framework for viewing the rights of individuals within the hospital system. This document, which emphasizes that responsibilities accompany rights, is further discussed in Chapter 8.

Nurse Power

Historically, nurses have had limited power in the healthcare system, a situation that has its roots in many of the traditional aspects of nursing discussed in Chapter 1. Change may not occur as rapidly as desired, and nurses often are frustrated because of their inability to influence the system. Nevertheless, things are changing in nursing. Nursing organizations are working to provide nurses with a voice at higher decision-making levels in healthcare. By understanding the political realities and the ways in which decisions are made, and by working together to speak with a united voice, nurses can increase their power in the system.

There are a variety of implications for nurses in the current cost-control environment. The availability and accuracy of documents that reflect the acuity level and multiple problems of a client when records are audited for compliance is essential (determination of acuity level is discussed earlier in this chapter).

Critical Thinking Activity: Power

Nurses are actively seeking power in the healthcare system. Consider the roles of nurses in the facilities with which you are familiar. How might nurses in these settings increase their power?

IMPLICATIONS FOR NURSES

Nurses have continuing interest and concern in the direction in which healthcare moves. They are most concerned about client well-being in the midst of a powerful system. Who will help consumers cope with their health problems and those of their families? Who will assist them in negotiating the various parts of the healthcare system? Will the individual identities and unique needs of consumers be addressed, or will each person be treated as the "standard client"? A major concern is whether the reimbursement system provides adequate funds for quality nursing care to be delivered.

Another important concern of nurses is whether that aspect of healthcare that we call *nursing*, with its focus on the individual, will be maintained. Will the pressures for demonstrating cost-effectiveness result in a loss of caring because it is not always quantifiable? Will the system recognize the critical thinking skills and abilities of nurses as well as their technical skills? Will many educated and skilled nurses be replaced by unlicensed assistive personnel? The future poses many as yet unanswered questions.

There are ongoing concerns in the healthcare system relating to the actual use of healthcare services by the public and to the structure of the system itself. Several states already have instituted efforts to create a more coordinated healthcare system for their citizens. No one can predict all the details of the future system with certainty, but we have tried to point out the major changes now occurring and the directions in which the healthcare system is moving. Nurses need to remain knowledgeable and involved in the political processes as changes are proposed in the healthcare system.

Critical Thinking Activity: Primary Care Providers

Identify clients you have encountered from a variety of social, cultural, and economic backgrounds. Given these clients' needs and backgrounds, what type of healthcare provider would best meet their needs for primary care? What barriers might they meet in trying to gain access to primary care? What might you do to assist these individuals?

Stegen & Sowerby Stories: Part 2

R emember Molly, the woman whose mental health provider finished his residency and she did not call back to schedule with the new oncoming resident? She came to the clinic to meet the new resident and get refills on her medications. She stated that she was fine but did not keep her next appointment. Read the rest of the story at www.thePoint.com.

Want to Know More?

A variety of resources are available on thePoint® to enhance your learning and understanding of this chapter, such as:

- Full Stegen & Sowerby Stories
- NCLEX-Style Student Review Questions
- Journal Articles
- Case Studies
- Learning Objectives
- Relevant Websites
- And more...

KEY CONCEPTS

- The various types of healthcare services are differentiated by the needs of the client being served and range from specific specialized services to skilled care to custodial care.
- Many different types of agencies provide healthcare services, including long-term care settings, acute care hospitals, ambulatory care centers, home care agencies, and healthcare businesses. There are a wide variety of nursing roles in these different settings. Healthcare agencies are classified according to length of stay, mix of services provided, and ownership of the agency.
- Acute care is centered in the work of the traditional hospital, which has become a hub for healthcare in most communities.
- Long-term care facilities provide many types of care. Nursing homes provide care for those without the ability to manage ADLs and who need ongoing care. Assisted-living centers provide supportive services to those who can manage most of their own ADLs. Rehabilitation centers assist the individual in returning to the maximum level of independence possible.
- Ambulatory care settings provide care on an outpatient basis. This care may range from simple office calls for common illnesses and health promotion activities such as immunizations to the performance of ambulatory surgery.
- Home health agencies offer a wide variety of care services that may include traditional public health services, high-intensity skilled care in the home, and rehabilitation services. Home care agencies offer services within the home that assist individuals in avoiding institutional care settings when they are unable to complete their own ADLs.
- Changes in the healthcare delivery system are creating many problems that affect healthcare workers. Among these are issues related to primary care, accreditation of health professional education programs, and the future of health professional education and licensure.
- The financing of healthcare is complex and involves personal payment, insurance companies, HMOs, preferred providers, and governmental systems, each of which operates differently.
- Through control of financing, third-party payers exert control over all aspects of healthcare.
- Cost increases have created stress in the healthcare system. Understanding the basis of these increases is essential for planning to contain costs.
- Mechanisms for controlling costs and improving patterns of care have been instituted. These have included changing methods of payment, controlling healthcare providers, and manag-

ing care. The federal government has played a major role in the development and implementation of these mechanisms.

- Access to healthcare must be considered in terms of economic, geographic, and sociocultural access. A major concern in the system is those who do not have access.
- Quality of care is maintained by a wide variety of mechanisms. Institutions and agencies providing care receive oversight in the form of governmental approval and accreditation by certifying organizations.
- Quality is evaluated through peer review and the use of outcome measures, including key indicators and individual client outcome standards.
- Power is exerted in the healthcare system by those who control finances, those who control access, and those with special knowledge. Traditionally, nurses and consumers have experienced little power in the system. Both are working to gain recognition and to affect more significantly the way the system functions.
- There are many implications for nurses in the financing and control of healthcare, including cost control, the well-being of the client, the effective use of healthcare resources, and changing the healthcare system.

NCLEX-STYLE PRACTICE QUESTIONS

1. Which of the following is true regarding SCHIP (State Health Insurance Children's Plan)? Select all that apply.

   A. Federally funded
   B. For those not eligible for Medicaid
   C. Mandated by states
   D. For children of single parents

2. What does HIPAA stand for?

   A. Health Information Protection and Accountability Act
   B. Health Insurance, Privacy, and Accuracy Act
   C. Health Insurance Portability and Accountability Act
   D. Health Information Privacy and Accessibility Act

3. The Veterans Administration (VA) system is an example of what?

   A. Private healthcare system open only to veterans
   B. Government owned healthcare system that is federally funded
   C. A health maintenance organization (HMO) owned and operated by the United States government
   D. National healthcare system branch for veterans of the armed services

4. Which of the following statements describes a diagnosis-related group (DRG)?

   A. Categories used to classify patients into groups for the purpose of payment or reimbursement
   B. The testing and medication recommended for group of diagnosis or illnesses that often occur together
   C. An insurance plan that assigns patients to a group based on their health and medical conditions
   D. A support group for patients suffering various conditions to which they are assigned upon diagnosis

REFERENCES

Agency for Healthcare Research and Quality. (2016). *Quality indicators.* Retrieved May 26, 2017, from http://www.qualityindicators.ahrq.gov/

Bostwick, M. (2008). *Florence Nightingale: The making of an icon.* New York: Farrar, Straus and Giroux.

Buerhaus, P. I., Auerbach, D. I., & Staiger, D. O. (2009). The recent surge in nurse employment: Causes and implications. *Health Affairs, 28*(4), w657–w668. (Published online 12 June 2009) doi:10.1377/hlthaff.28.4.w657, Retrieved March 25, 2010.

Bureau of Labor Statistics (BLS), U.S. Department of Labor. (2015). *Occupational outlook handbook, 2016-17 edition, registered nurses.* Retrieved May 25, 2017, from www.bls.gov/ooh/healthcare/registered-nurses.htm

Case Management Society of America. (2015). *Who we are.* Retrieved May 26, 2017, from www.cmsa.org

Centers for Disease Control and Prevention, National Center for Health Statistics. (2014). *Nursing Home Care.* Retrieved May 23, 2017, from http://www.cdc.gov/nchs/fastats/nursing-home-care.htm

Centers for Medicare and Medicaid Services. (2008). *National health expenditure data, Table 13 Nursing home expenditures.* Retrieved October 11, 2009, from http://www.cms.hhs.gov/NationalHealthExpendData/downloads/proj2008.pdf

Centers for Medicare and Medicaid Services. (2016). *Quality Improvement Organizations.* Retrieved May 26, 2017, from http://www.cms.gov/QualityImprovementOrgs

Centers for Medicare and Medicaid Services. (2015). *Nursing Home Quality Initiative.* Retrieved May 26, 2017, from https://www.cms.gov/Medicare/Quality-Initiatives-Patient-Assessment-Instruments/NursingHomeQualityInits/index.html?redirect=/NursingHomeQualityInits/10_NHQIQualityMeasures.asp#TopOfPage

Department of Health and Human Services. (2000). *Healthy people 2010.* Washington, DC: U.S. Government Printing Office. Retrieved June 18, 2010, from www.healthypeople.gov

Department of Health and Human Services. (2015). *Basis for health service.* Retrieved May 25, 2017, from https://www.ihs.gov/newsroom/factsheets/basisforhealthservices/

Department of Health and Human Services. (2017). *Healthy people 2020.* Retrieved May 26, 2017, from http://www.healthypeople.gov

DNV. (2017). *Search Hospitals.* Retrieved May 26, 2017, from http://dnvglhealthcare.com/hospitals

Encyclopedia.com. (2016). *Technology: History of Medical Technology.* Retrieved May 23, 2017 from http://www.encyclopedia.com/science/encyclopedias-almanacs-transcripts-and-maps/technology-i-history-medical-technology

Genworth Financial. (2016). *Genworth 2016 cost of care survey.* Retrieved May 25, 2017, from www.genworth.com/about-us/industry-expertise/cost-of-care.html#

Health Insurance Portability and Accountability Act of 1996. Retrieved June 18, 2010, from http://aspe.hhs.gov/admnsimp/pl104191.htm

Institute of Medicine. (2010). *The future of nursing: Leading change, advancing health.* Retrieved December 3, 2010, from http://www.iom.edu/Reports/2010/The-Future-of-Nursing-Leading-Change-Advancing-Health.aspx

Joint Commission. (n.d.). *The Joint Commission history.* Retrieved December 3, 2010, from http://www.jointcommission.org/assets/1/18/Joint_Commission_History.pdf

Kaiser Family Foundation. (2010). *State health policy.* Retrieved June 16, 2010, from http://www.kff.org/statepolicy/

Merriam-Webster. (2017). *Dictionary.* Retrieved May 25, 2017, from www.merriam-webster.com/dictionary

National Association of Free Clinics. (2016). *What is the NAFC?* Retrieved May 25, 2017, from http://www.nafcclinics.org/

National Institute of Health. (2015). *Early psychiatric hospitals. Diseases of the mind: Highlights of American Psychiatry through 1900.* Retrieved May 23, 2017, from https://www.nlm.nih.gov/hmd/diseases/early.html

Swanson, A. (2015). Big pharmaceutical companies are spending far more on marketing than research. *Washington Post*. Retrieved December 21, 2017, from https://www.washingtonpost.com/news/wonk/wp/2015/02/11/big-pharmaceutical-companies-are-spending-far-more-on-marketing-than-research/?utm_term=.cfd333c4b718

TRICARE. (2017). *About us*. Retrieved May 25, 2017, from www.tricare.mil/About

U.S. Census Bureau. (2011). *The older population 2010*. Retrieved May 25, 2017, from www.census.gov/prod/cen2010/briefs/c2010br-09.pdf

U.S. History.org. (2017). *The Pennsylvania hospital. The Electric Ben Franklin*. Retrieved May 23, 2017, from http://www.ushistory.org/franklin/philadelphia/hospital.htm

Weatherford, D. (n.d.). *The evolution of nursing. National Women's History Museum*. Retrieved May 23, 2017, from www.nwhm.org/blog/the-evolution-of-nursing/

Legal Responsibilities for Practice

After completing this chapter, you should be able to:

1. Differentiate the three general sources of law and explain how they apply to nursing.
2. Explain the role of institutional policies and protocols in legal decision-making.
3. Identify nursing actions that violate criminal law and discuss how such violations may be avoided.
4. Explain liability in relationship to nursing practice, including situations in which liability is shared by employers or supervisors.
5. Analyze the benefits to individual nurses of purchasing professional liability insurance.
6. Explain the nurse's role in supporting client rights through informed consent and advance directives.
7. Identify specific issues that can constitute malpractice and discuss the nurse's responsibility in relationship to them.
8. Identify factors that contribute to a suit being instituted against a healthcare professional, and explain how an individual nurse might prevent legal suits.
9. Explain the various phases of a legal action.
10. Differentiate the possible roles of a nurse when testifying for a legal proceeding.

KEY TERMS

Advance directive
Civil law
Common law
Competence
Constitutional law
Criminal law
Decision maker
Directive to physicians
Durable power of attorney for healthcare
Emancipated minors
Enacted law
Ethics

Expert witness
False imprisonment
Gross negligence
Healthcare proxy
Informed consent
Judicial law (decisional or case law)
Lawsuit
Liability
Living will
Malpractice
Mature minor
Misdemeanor
Negligence

(continued on page 229)

KEY TERMS *(continued)*

Privileged communication
Protected health information (PHI)
Prudent professional
Reckless endangerment

Regulatory law (administrative or
executive law)
Statutory law
Tort

Stegen & Sowerby Stories: Part 1

J oe, a 43-year-old man with a history of hypertension, arrived at the emergency department (ED) with right upper quadrant pain. His blood pressure was 155/85 mm Hg, and his heart rate was 110 beats per minute (bpm). On examination, his right upper quadrant pain was confirmed with difficulty because of his morbid obesity. The ED physician ordered routine laboratory tests and an ultrasound of the right upper quadrant to confirm cholecystitis. The client complained of increasing pain and required several doses of intravenous (IV) morphine to control his pain. This examination, blood work and the ultrasound, took about 7 hours. The ultrasound showed some sludge in the gallbladder but no stones. Over this period, Joe's heart rate and blood pressure both increased to 120 bpm and 175/95 mm Hg, respectively. The blood work results were all in normal range except his creatinine, which was increased from the baseline of 1.1 to 1.8 mg/dL indicating acute kidney injury.

Because of the acute kidney injury, the ED physician ordered a computed tomography (CT) scan of the abdomen without contrast. The CT scan was delayed by about 4 hours for logistical reasons, and it took about an hour for the initial reading to be returned to the ED.

- What was the cause of the abdominal pain?
- Why do you think the blood pressure and heart rate keep increasing?
- What client complaints would you expect with this scenario?
- What are the potential liability issues?

Every newspaper contains reports of sensational cases being considered in our courts and legal arenas. Concerns about lawsuits and liability are voiced in every business. Healthcare remains at the forefront of professions where legal issues constitute a major area of concern. The prudent nurse considers legal issues before a crisis arises and uses sound information to help guide action in situations where questions occur. This chapter provides basic information you will need in that process.

Examples and situations relating to legal issues discussed throughout this chapter are given to help you understand the application of the specific concepts. Many more factors are considered in arriving at an actual legal decision than can be presented in a paragraph or two. It is the interaction of multiple factors that makes it impossible to provide absolute predictions regarding legal outcomes in different situations; that is, data may be interpreted differently by judges and juries, resulting in different outcomes, although cases may appear similar.

UNDERSTANDING THE SCOPE OF THE LAW

Legal issues are those that are decided by law. Law may be defined as "the principles and regulations established in a community by some authority and applicable to its people, whether in the form of legislation or of custom and policies recognized and enforced by judicial decision" (Dictionary.com, 2017). Laws are put in place to preserve public welfare and manage certain relationships (such as contracts) within the society. **Ethics** deals with "values relating to human conduct, with respect to the rightness and wrongness of certain actions and to the goodness and badness of the motives and ends of such actions" (Dictionary.com, 2017). Legal and ethical issues are often discussed together because they go hand in hand, with one supporting the other. In this chapter, we focus on how the law affects nursing practice. Ethics are discussed in more detail in Chapter 8.

SOURCES OF LAW

If nurses know the source of law, then they know how it can be challenged and changed, and how powerful it can be. There are three general sources of law: *statutory law*, *regulatory* (also known as administrative) *law*, and *common law*. All are relevant to nursing practice **(Fig. 7.1)**.

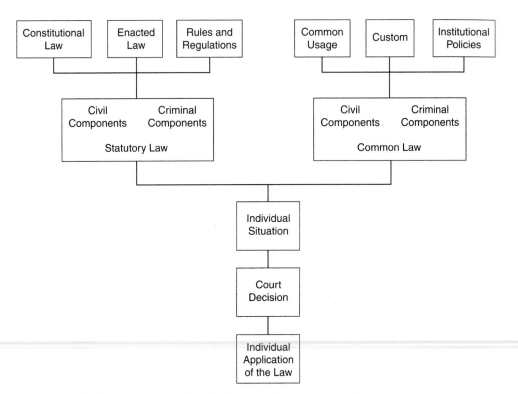

Figure 7.1. Civil law and criminal law both may affect a nursing situation.

Statutory Law

A statute is a written rule or formal regulation established by a government legislative authority, such as the Congress, the state legislature, or the city council. A violation of a statute is legally punishable. **Statutory law** is published in codes that are broken down into specific rules. In the United States, statutory law includes constitutional law and enacted law. All laws fall in a hierarchy of authority, with constitutional law having the greatest authority, and the enacted law the next. Regulatory law, which is discussed later, has less authority than statutory law.

Constitutional Law

Constitutional law is established by the federal government and based on the United States Constitution (**Fig. 7.2**). The Constitution was developed by the Constitutional Convention of 1787, approved by the Continental Congress, and then ratified by all the states. It establishes the general organization of the federal government and specifies the federal power and limitations to that power. The powers that are not specifically given to the federal government in the Constitution are retained by the states. The Constitution can be amended (ie, changed), with the amendments having the same status as the original provisions. Amendments to the Constitution require similar passage and ratification by the states.

In addition, each state has its own constitution that acts as the highest law for that state. Many other nations, such as Great Britain, do not have a constitution or equivalent document. In those countries, the enacted law is the highest level of law.

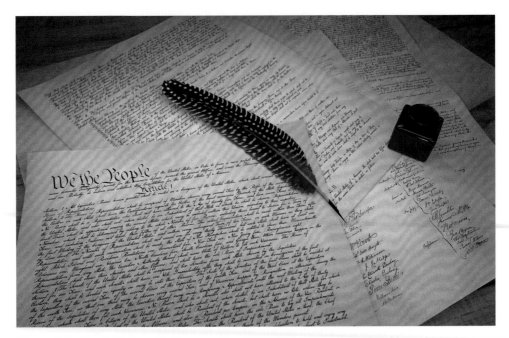

Figure 7.2. The U.S. Constitution provides the basis for all constitutional law.

Enacted Law

Enacted law includes all bills passed by legislative bodies, whether at the local, state or province, or national level. Enacted laws of the United States federal government all carry the designation USC (United States Code) in their official title. The federal Social Security Act (42 USC 401) is an example of federally enacted law. Enacted laws of states or other governing bodies carry a title and number designation specific to each individual state. Nurse practice acts in the various states are examples of enacted laws at the state level.

Regulatory Law

Regulatory law (also referred to as executive or administrative law) includes the rules and regulations established by government agencies to carry out enacted laws. These appear as carefully written rules that apply to everyone. At the federal level, the Center for Medicare & Medicaid Services writes regulations governing the payment of Medicare and Medicaid funds that are authorized through legislation. At the state level, the board of nursing (or its equivalent) is authorized through enacted laws to establish and enforce rules and regulations that govern the practice of nursing in that state. The rules and regulations protect the safety of the public by defining standards for nursing education and practice (see Chapter 3). Rules and regulations of administrative bodies, often referred to as the Administrative Code, can be enforced in court.

Common Law

Common law is derived from common usage, custom, and judicial law (judicial decisions or court rulings). It is based on the English common law. Because it is based on occurrences of events, common law is less clear and exact than statutory law; it is composed of many actions and documents that are not specific written rules that apply to everyone. Common law is fluid and changes over time. In general, statutory law and regulatory law carry more weight in court than does common law.

Judicial Law

Judicial law (also referred to as decisional or case law) is derived from decrees or judgments from the courts. Judicial decisions or rulings in court cases apply statutory, regulatory, and common law to specific situations. These decisions then become precedents for interpretations of all types of law in other cases. A court also has the power to examine the same or a similar issue in a subsequent case and make a different decision, thus creating a new precedent. Court rulings are binding within the jurisdiction of the particular court that determines them but are used in a more general way (as guidelines) in other jurisdictions. In any specific situation, the final determination of the application of all types of law is the decision of the court in that case, although in most instances a decision may be appealed to higher courts.

Common Usage and Custom

As the term seems to imply, courts are empowered through the concept of common law to examine the common usage and custom in a community for patterns that reflect the community's standards for behavior. Common usage and custom are not usually written down and specific. However, written documents can be used to support common usage and custom in specific cases. For example, when examining standards of professional practice in a court case, the court may examine documents that specify standards of professional practice as reflecting common usage. These documents may be changed by the organization writing the standard and thus are not fixed.

The issue of safe medication practice illustrates how common usage applies to nursing. Neither statutes nor regulations are written about how to safely give medications. If a client is harmed by receiving an inappropriate medication, the issue of whether the standard of practice was violated by the individual nurse might be considered in light of the standards of safe medication practice used in the healthcare facility and whether those standards were followed.

OTHER FACTORS AFFECTING LEGAL DECISIONS

In addition to the sources of law discussed above, several other factors can affect how laws are interpreted and enforced. These factors also play an important role in our legal system.

Administrative Rulings

An administrative ruling, also referred to as an advisory opinion, made by a state board or by an attorney general provides a guideline based on an interpretation of the enacted and regulatory law relative to a specific situation. It is not considered a final legal decision and different boards and attorneys general might vary in their opinions. The validity of an opinion stands until the issue is brought before a court and the court rules on the situation and provides a final decision. The court decision may or may not support the advisory ruling.

Rights and Responsibilities in Healthcare

In the United States, client rights within the healthcare system continue to receive considerable attention by both government and consumer bodies. The federal Health Insurance Portability and Accountability Act (HIPAA) of 1996 contains a significant section regarding the privacy of **protected health information (PHI)**. PHI refers to individually identifiable data about a person's health or healthcare. This act made privacy in regard to healthcare a legally supported right at the federal level. Based on this, all healthcare agencies and health plans are required to provide training for all employees in regard to the privacy rules and the procedures that ensure compliance. There are significant monetary penalties for breaches of privacy. Many facilities have adopted employment policies that include dismissal for certain types of breaches of client confidentiality.

Some of the rights of which we commonly speak are not legally supported but are based on ethical values. For example, we often speak of a right to healthcare. There is no legal basis for this right in the United States, but many people believe an ethical basis exists. In some countries, such as Canada and Great Britain, healthcare is a right supported by the law. In these countries, healthcare for all has been established through legislation and administrative rules and regulations.

Responsibilities often accompany rights. If a right is guaranteed, the government and designated others have legally mandated responsibilities to ensure that the right is upheld. In the matter of the right to privacy of medical records, for example, all healthcare workers have legally mandated responsibilities to ensure that privacy is upheld.

Evidence-Based Practice 7.1: Confidentiality and Consent

Newman, A. B. (2016). Critical care nurses' knowledge of confidentiality legislation. *American Journal of Critical Care, 25*(3), 222–227. doi:10.4037/ajcc2016518

The legal regulations can be hard to apply in situations where clients may not be able to give consent for the communication of private health information. This is often the case in critical care environments. Nurses need to understand both state and national regulations that govern the confidentiality of private health information.

In this article, nurses were asked to describe their knowledge of both state and federal regulations regarding confidentiality. It was determined that nurses had a good knowledge of federal regulations regarding confidentiality. They were not as well educated about the state-specific regulations regarding confidentiality and health information. The author recommends that thorough education both before and after licensure be implemented to improve nurses' understanding of both state and federal confidentiality regulations.

Institutional Policies, Protocols, and Procedures

Institutional policies provide guidance in the proper actions to be taken in specific situations, identify the individuals responsible for taking action, and may establish specific timelines for action. Established agency policies may be considered the standard of practice for that agency and, therefore, common usage (common law) by the court and may become important as a basis for legal decisions. Members of the healthcare agency's staff who have expertise in the practice area under consideration usually develop the specific policy. Policies may protect the institution and its employees from legal difficulties if they are based on current practice and sound legal advice.

Protocols, as the term is used in the healthcare environment, provide a list of actions for managing a specific problem that may involve the use of more than one procedure. For example, a protocol on the care of a central venous catheter might include frequency of tubing change, the type of fluid used for flushing, the frequency of dressing change, the type of dressing materials to be used, and other aspects of care. Protocols for nursing often include aspects of care that might be part of the medical orders for client care. Therefore, they are usually developed with consultation between nursing and physician representatives and may be approved by the medical practice committee as well as by a nursing committee before implementation.

Specific institutional procedures outline the steps in a particular task. In the example of the central venous catheter, a procedure would be the list of steps to be taken when flushing the catheter to maintain patency. A procedure for nursing would be developed by the relevant nursing committee or sometimes by a clinical nurse specialist.

The purpose of policies, protocols, and procedures is to ensure that there is consistent, sound practice in an institution. Just as policies must be updated, so should protocols and procedures. Nurses may be in a position to recognize the need for such a change as they use and compare a policy with the latest professional information.

Communication in Action 7.1: *Making Changes in a Procedure*

Stan Wilson, a registered nurse (RN), was reading a nursing journal. He was surprised to learn that, according to an article, the procedure they were using at his hospital for IV site care was specifically not recommended. In fact, that practice was identified as showing an increased incidence of site inflammation. The next day he took the journal with him to work. He said to his coworkers, "Look at this article during your break if you can. It has some information that has made me concerned about our current IV site care procedure. I am going to show this to our manager Nancy and ask if we can start a study process to figure what really is best to do." He contacted the manager and asked for a time to sit down and talk with her about a concern. When they sat down to talk later in the day, he introduced the subject: "Nancy, I just read this article about IV site care. This is a peer-reviewed journal, and the article quotes some impressive research. According to the information here, our IV site care procedure does not meet current standards. Some specific concerns are our cleaning procedure and the ointment we are using at the site. Would you read this article? Then we can talk about the possibility of referring this issue to our evidence-based practice committee." This was a great way for Stan to handle the new information. If Stan had just gone to work and changed the way he did IV site care and told everyone else he worked with to change without going through the established process, he could have been reprimanded. It is always important to involve the appropriate people in discussions about policy and procedure changes.

CLASSIFICATION OF LAWS

Law is divided into civil and criminal components. Both statutory law and common law may be subdivided in this way.

Criminal Law

Criminal law addresses the general welfare of the public. A violation of criminal law is called a crime, and it is prosecuted by the government. On conviction, a crime may be punishable by imprisonment, parole conditions, a loss of privilege (such as a license), a fine, or any combination of these. The punishment is intended to discipline the violator and deter further such actions by this person as well as discourage others from committing the crime. A crime may be classified as either a misdemeanor or a felony. A **misdemeanor** is a lesser infraction of the law and is punishable by a fine or an imprisonment of less than a year. A felony represents a more serious violation of the law and carries heavier fines and longer periods of imprisonment, and, in the most serious of cases, perhaps even execution (Guido, 2013).

Civil Law

Civil law regulates conduct between private individuals or businesses and is enforced through the courts as damages or monetary compensation (Guido, 2013). Private individuals or groups may bring a legal action (a **lawsuit**) to court for breach (or breaking) of civil law. The judgment of the court results in a plan to correct the wrong and may award a monetary payment to the wronged party. Nurses may find themselves involved with both civil and criminal laws, either separately or within the same situation.

CRIMINAL LAW AND NURSING

It is costly to the state to undertake criminal prosecution; therefore, some violations of criminal law are not prosecuted in court. Knowing this, some nurses make the error of believing that "minor" violations are acceptable. Criminal action could result in the loss of a job and a license to practice nursing even when not prosecuted in court.

An example relates to laws regulating the distribution and use of controlled substances such as opioids. Violation of these laws is a crime. Thus, altering or changing controlled drug records is a crime even if no diversion of drugs occurred. Falsification of a controlled drug record may not result in criminal prosecution because of the cost to the state, but it usually would result in loss of a job and reporting to the licensing authority for disciplinary action.

Errors that result in serious injury or death of a client are investigated and may be prosecuted and tried by the criminal courts. These legal actions may be based on such charges as gross negligence, reckless endangerment, or criminal negligence. (See discussion of negligence that follows.) A license to practice nursing may be temporarily withdrawn while such charges are investigated and tried. If the individual is found innocent, the license may be restored. If the individual is convicted of the crime, however, the nursing license may be revoked, in addition to sentencing and other penalties.

Nurses who commit felonies, such as theft, abuse, or deliberate harm, in which a client is a victim, are usually charged under both criminal laws and the laws regulating nursing practice. Nurses who commit felonies outside of the care setting can be prosecuted under criminal law and under the law regulating nursing practice if the felony reflects on their fitness to practice nursing. For example, an individual prosecuted for selling narcotics usually will have action taken under the Nurse Practice Act as well.

CIVIL LAW AND NURSING

Civil law relates to legal disputes between private parties. Malpractice actions brought in healthcare situations involve civil law.

Torts

A **tort** is "a wrongful act, not including a breach of contract or trust, that results in injury to another's person, property, reputation, or the like, and for which the injured party is entitled to compensation, a civil wrong committed against a person or the person's property" (Dictionary. com, 2017; Guido, 2013). The result may be physical harm, psychological harm, harm to livelihood, or some other less tangible value, such as harm to reputation. The action that causes a civil wrong may be either intentional or unintentional.

An intentional tort is one in which the outcome was planned, although the person involved may not have believed that the intended outcome would be harmful to the other person. For example, preventing a client from leaving against medical advice may be based on concern for the client, but it interferes with liberty and causes psychological harm and to do so is an intentional tort.

An unintentional tort is an action causing harm to another person or property that was not intended to happen. The most common cause of an unintentional tort is negligence.

Negligence

Negligence is a general term that refers to "a failure to exercise that degree of care" (Dictionary.com, 2017; Guido, 2013). If harm is caused by negligence, it is termed an unintentional tort and damages may be recovered. Experts differ on what should be termed the *essential characteristics* of negligence. For our purposes, we will identify four main characteristics and indicate common variations.

1. *Harm:* Injury must have occurred to an individual. Injury (which is the basis of harm) and damages (which include the consequences to the person of the injury) are considered separate characteristics by some.
2. *Duty:* The negligent person must have been in a situation where he or she had a responsibility or duty toward the person harmed.
3. *Breach of Duty:* The person must be found to have failed to fulfill his or her responsibility. This might include either doing what should not have been done (commission of an inappropriate action) or failing to do what should have been done (omission of a necessary or an appropriate action). This is also referred to as failing to act as a reasonably prudent person.
4. *Causation:* The harm or injury must be shown to have been caused by the breach of duty.

Gross negligence or **reckless endangerment** includes the same four elements that are present in simple negligence as defined above, but the person's behavior is defined as "failure to use even the slightest amount of care in a way that shows recklessness or willful disregard for the safety of others" (Lectric Law Library, 2017). There have been instances of nurses being charged with gross negligence under criminal law for serious errors resulting in the death of a client. When criminal charges are brought, there is always a charge of negligence and not just a simple error in question. This degree of inappropriate behavior is very difficult for an individual to prove. This distinction becomes important in the discussion of charitable care and responding to community emergencies below.

Malpractice

Malpractice is a term used to identify professional negligence—liability resulting from improper practice based on standards of care required by the profession for which the person has been educated (Guido, 2013). Therefore, malpractice is a term used to describe negligence by nurses in the performance of their duties. The professional person must have had a professional duty toward the person receiving the care. For example, the nurse was performing the professional activities of a nurse for the person needing the care (in either a paid or volunteer capacity). Additionally, the harm that occurred to this person or to the property must be based on a failure to act as a prudent professional and in accordance with professional standards in the situation. This is a higher standard than is required of the general public; it demands appropriate professional judgment and action (Guido, 2013). See Box 7.1.

Just as all parts of the situation are clear in some general negligence situations and not in others, the same can be said of professional duty. The nurse who is assigned to care for a patient in a hospital clearly has a duty to that patient. In some situations, duties overlap and more than one nurse might have a duty toward the same patient, for example, the assigned nurse, another nurse on the unit, and a unit manager. Whether a particular nurse had a professional duty to

---

BOX 7.1 ESSENTIAL ELEMENTS OF MALPRACTICE

- Harm to an individual
- Duty of a professional toward an individual
- Breach of duty by the professional
- Cause of harm is the breach of duty

---

a patient might be in dispute. In general, all nurses within a facility are considered to have a duty toward all patients and even toward visitors, in case of emergency, and are expected to act on behalf of the institution in that regard. For example, if a visitor falls, any nurse present is expected to respond, institute action, and summon help. Again, the court would decide whether a duty was present if any legal action occurred.

Critical Thinking Activity: Family Medical Advice
You have taken a new position as a home health nurse. One of your clients is an older woman who has a leg ulcer and a long history of diabetes. Your role is to assess the client in relationship to her diabetic management and wound care and teach as needed. While you are in the home, her husband tells you that he has been having pain in his knee and asks if you would examine it and tell him whether it is all right to use a heating pad on it, and whether he should take ibuprofen or some Tylenol. Do you have a duty to help him? Why or why not? What will your response be? What legal issues are involved in this situation? If you advise him and your advice turns out to be incorrect, what legal action could he take?

A breach of duty, as mentioned earlier, is a failure to act as a **prudent professional**, that is, according to the standard of care for the profession in a particular situation (Guido, 2013). The various sources of standards of nursing care were discussed above.

The final issue in determining malpractice becomes one of identifying the cause of the harm that occurred. Malpractice is present only if a breach of duty was the cause of the harm. The presence of harm is often clear but the direct cause may not be clear. For example, if the outcome of a situation is a fractured hip, no one will dispute that this is harm. However, the cause of a fractured hip must be determined; it might be the person's own responsibility, the family's failure to call for help, the coffee spilled on the floor by the visitor, or failure of due care by the nurse. Ultimately, a judge and/or jury must often decide whether the breach of duty by the nurse was the cause of the harm.

LIABILITY

A **liability** is an obligation or debt that can be enforced by law. A person found guilty of any tort (whether intentional or unintentional) is considered legally liable, or legally responsible, for the outcome. The person legally liable usually is required to pay for damages to the other person. These may include actual costs of care, legal services, loss of earnings (present and

Figure 7.3. Professional liability insurance is essential for legal protection. A person found guilty of any tort (whether intentional or unintentional) is considered legally liable, or legally responsible, for the outcome.

future), and compensation for emotional and physical stress suffered. Although liability is legally determined by a court, an individual who believes that he or she would be held legally liable if a court were consulted may agree to pay damages (or that individual's insurance company may agree to pay) without actually going to court. Damages may be paid even when the person denies negligence, because a court case would cost more than paying damages **(Fig. 7.3)**.

Personal Liability

As an educated professional, you are always legally responsible or liable for your actions. Thus, if a physician or supervisor asks you to do something that is contrary to your best professional judgment and says, "I'll take responsibility," that person is acting unwisely. The physician or supervisor giving the directions may be liable also if harm results, but that would not remove your personal liability.

Employer Liability

The law holds the employer responsible for hiring qualified persons, establishing an appropriate environment for correct functioning, maintaining correct policies and procedures, and providing supervision or direction as needed to avoid errors or harm. Therefore, if a nurse, as an employee of a hospital, is guilty of malpractice, the hospital also may be named in the suit. The employer's liability may exist even if the employer appears to have taken precautions to prevent error.

It is important to understand that this doctrine does not remove any responsibility from the individual nurse, but it extends responsibility to the employer in addition to the nurse. If, for example, a hospital has a procedure that does not conform to good nursing practice as you know it, and you follow that procedure, you will still be liable for any resulting harm. You are expected to use your education and experience to make sound judgments regarding your work.

Communication in Action 7.2: *Clarifying Your Actions*

The RN who gives medications on a large medical unit at night notes that an order for dopamine is considerably larger than the usual dose. She looks up the medication in a reference book and finds that she is correct about the dosage: The ordered dose is several times the usual dose. The nurse then calls the supervisor and explains the situation and suggests that the physician be called (in this facility, night calls to physicians must be approved by the supervisor).The supervisor double-checks the order with the RN and then states, "Dr. Jones is an outstanding physician. I am sure he has a good reason for ordering this dose. Go ahead and give the medication as ordered. I'll take responsibility. I don't believe it is worth bothering him at night." The RN then gives the medication, and the client suffers a serious reaction. After being reassured that the supervisor would take responsibility for administering what appeared to be an excessive dose of the medication, the prudent nurse might reply, "I know you mean to be reassuring, but if the dosage is wrong I will be liable because I am the nurse administering the drug. I think it is best to call Dr. Jones and clarify the order. He has the same goal that we do: the safety and well-being of the client. I will be glad to make the call now."

Supervisory Liability

In the role of a clinical leader, charge nurse, unit manager, supervisor, or any other role that involves delegation, supervision, or direction of other people, the nurse is potentially liable for the actions of others. The supervising nurse is responsible for exercising good judgment in a supervisory role, including making appropriate decisions about assignments and delegation of tasks. If an error occurs and the supervising nurse is shown to have exercised sound judgment in all decisions made in that capacity, the supervising nurse may not be held liable for the error of a subordinate. If poor judgment was used in assigning an inadequately prepared person to an important task or if oversight was inadequate, the supervisory nurse might be liable for the resulting harm. The extent of the subordinate's responsibility would depend on his or her level of education and training. People with limited education or training might not be liable for some errors; the more education subordinates have, the more likely they will be liable.

Limits on a Client's Claim to Negligence

Several situations may be viewed by the court as a valid defense to a client's claim that negligence has occurred. *Contributory negligence* is based on the concept that the client contributed to the injury by not acting prudently in that circumstance. For example, the client may not have followed instructions, may have provided false information that led to improper treatment, or may not have followed warnings about the side effects of medications. In five states or territories (Alabama, District of Columbia, Maryland, North Carolina, and Virginia), contributory negligence prevents the individual from receiving any compensation for injury. All other states incorporate the use of comparative negligence. This means the court would determine what percentage of the injury resulted from the client's negligence and what part rested with the nurse, and reduce the damage award accordingly (Guido, 2013).

Charitable Immunity

Charitable immunity refers to a situation in which an individual or an organization is held to a lesser standard of care because of the provision of charitable care. This lesser standard is that the person must be guilty of gross negligence (discussed above) in order to be liable. Thus, they are protected from liability for ordinary negligence.

Institutional Charitable Immunity

Historically, charitable immunity covered all the work of some hospitals and churches. Charitable immunity was granted if all the income for the institution was derived from charitable giving. Some laws even provided specific dollar amounts of liability limitation for charitable organizations. This type of immunity for institutions is rapidly disappearing because there are few major hospitals that do not provide both compensated care and uncompensated care. There is also a strong public interest in holding all organizations accountable for the actions of those who work under their auspices.

Charitable Immunity for Volunteers in Health Settings

In 1997, the federal government enacted the Volunteer Protection Act. This law provides for immunity from charges of simple negligence and only allows charges for gross negligence for volunteers in health clinics and other settings. This is an especially important protection for healthcare providers who choose to volunteer. State laws protecting volunteers may provide more protection but cannot limit the protection provided under federal law. This has been done to encourage healthcare providers to volunteer their services where they are greatly needed. If you choose to volunteer your services as a nurse, you should investigate the protections afforded in your state.

Charitable immunity does not mean that a person cannot sue a volunteer care provider; however, it makes it much less likely that they could win and, therefore, less likely that an attorney would help them to pursue such a case. Legislation in some states requires that the clinic inform clients in writing that by accepting free care they are agreeing to the limited liability of the care providers.

Good Samaritan Laws

Another type of charitable immunity is found in laws that relate to people responding to emergencies. These are often referred to as Good Samaritan Laws. These laws are meant to encourage anyone to render assistance in an emergency situation without fear of liability for simple negligence. Liability is only for gross negligence. The nurse rendering aid in an emergency must behave as a reasonably prudent nurse in that situation. Thus, the standard is higher than for the nonprofessional person. For example, a person on the street might bend an injured person's neck in an effort to help the person, but a nurse might be found to be reckless for doing that because the nurse has more formal education regarding proper actions in accidents. An additional aspect of the professional responsibility is to not abandon the person until care can be turned over to another competent person. So the professional may relinquish responsibility to emergency services personnel who arrive on the scene, but not to a simple bystander. In reality, healthcare providers have not been sued for rendering aid in emergency situations.

Each nurse must make an individual decision about rendering emergency aid in a specific situation unless the local law mandates that people respond to emergencies. Vermont (Title 12,

Chapter 23; SS 519, 1968) and Minnesota (Minn. Stat. Sec. 604A.0 1, 2003) both require that a person encountering an emergency render assistance unless it would put themselves in danger.

The decision to render aid involves ethical as well as legal considerations. If the profession of nursing is a public trust and nurses are truly involved in the business of caring, then failure to aid an individual who is in serious danger is an ethical violation of that trust. Professional liability insurance does provide coverage when assisting in this way, which may make a nurse feel more comfortable about rendering emergency aid.

LIABILITY INSURANCE

Liability insurance transfers the legal and any settlement costs related to a suit from the individual to an insurance company, which spreads the risks to a large group of policy holders. The expectation is that most individuals will not be sued and that the pool of premiums collected from policy holders, therefore, will adequately cover the costs of those who are sued, the administrative costs of managing the policies, and the profit for the insurance company. Individuals benefit by transferring risk from themselves to the insurance company for the cost of the insurance policy.

A liability insurance crisis exists in the United States. The cost of liability insurance for primary healthcare providers (such as physicians and nurse practitioners) has escalated at an extraordinary rate. Some of the factors that have caused this are the large judgments that have been made, the number of suits that have been brought, the large fees that attorneys receive, and the high profits of insurance companies. Advanced practice nurses have been especially affected by the increase in premiums, because their incomes have traditionally been moderate and they cannot charge fees sufficient to cover insurance costs that may equal those of physicians. Nurses who are not employed in advanced roles are able to obtain malpractice insurance for a modest cost.

Some states have initiated legislation that allows for awards to cover actual losses and costs of care, while limiting awards for pain and suffering and other nontangible factors. Sometimes this legislation has been accompanied by restrictions on insurance company rates. Laws in some states are being amended to restrict the monetary liability of any party according to the percentage of responsibility. Liability laws continue to be a major concern for nurses, because nurses are being named in an increasing number of suits, although the total number is still low.

Institutional and Individual Insurance

Many hospitals and other institutional employers carry liability insurance that covers both the institution and its employees. Some hospitals may limit the coverage that their policies provide for individual employees in an effort to hold down costs. Even if an employer carries liability insurance, it is usually advisable for the individual professional to carry an independent policy. If a legal action is instituted against you, your individual liability insurance policy provides an independent attorney who is focused on your welfare.

An independent policy provides coverage in voluntary activities as well as on the job. It moves with you as you transfer from one employer to another. If the institution has charitable immunity and nurses are paid employees, the policy supports the individual nurse who may be sued when the institution is protected from a lawsuit. Many nursing liability policies also provide coverage for legal expenses incurred in defending your license in a disciplinary proceeding. Some policies may provide for personal liability in your home (for such things as a person tripping on a rug and being injured) as well as professional liability.

Keep in mind that insurance is not the only source of payment for a judgment in a legal action. Judgments may be levied against most tangible assets, including houses, cars, and savings; judgments also may be levied against future earnings. Married nurses who reside in community property states should realize that one half of the assets of a couple may be vulnerable to a judgment. Community property states at this time include Arizona, California, Idaho, Louisiana, Nevada, New Mexico, Texas, Washington, and Wisconsin. These factors combine to support the need for the individual professional to carry liability insurance that will provide an attorney and protection in the case of any judgment.

Analyzing Liability Insurance Coverage

Individual liability insurance for RNs is available from a variety of insurance companies (directly through their agents) and through professional organizations that offer coverage as a service to members. When investigating individual liability insurance, ask the agent or company the questions in Box 7.2. Of particular importance is the difference between a *claims occurred* and a *claims made* policy. A *claims occurred* policy is safer because if you subsequently drop the policy, it will still be in effect for any incident that occurred while you were covered. If a *claims made* policy was chosen, then the coverage for any claim ends when the policy premium is no longer being paid. Because the time limit on liability claims

---

BOX 7.2 QUESTIONS TO ASK REGARDING LIABILITY INSURANCE

1. In what situations would I, as an individual, be covered?
2. In what situations would I not be covered?
3. How is my coverage affected by my actions? For example, if I failed to follow hospital policy, would I still be covered?
4. What are the monetary limits of the policy?
5. Does the policy provide me with an attorney?
6. Does the insurance cover incidents that occurred while the policy was in force, regardless of when the claim is brought (claims occurred insurance coverage), or does it cover incidents only if I am currently insured (claims brought insurance coverage)?

Additional Questions Regarding an Individual Liability Policy
1. Is it renewable at my option? What factors affect renewability?
2. What is the cost compared with other policies?

Additional Questions Regarding an Institutional Liability Policy
1. Does the policy provide me with a personal attorney, or will the same attorney be working for the hospital?
2. At what point would the hospital no longer be responsible and would I become personally responsible?
3. How would my job be affected if a lawsuit was filed or payment awarded based on an action against me? (Check institutional policy as well as the insurance company policy.)
4. Does the insurance company have the right to seek restitution from me if it pays a claim based on my actions?

is substantial, you would have to continue to hold the policy and pay the premiums even if you were no longer employed in healthcare. Because the cost of nursing professional liability insurance is so low, any difference in cost between the two types of policies would be slight.

The nurse should carefully investigate liability insurance coverage carried individually or by the hospital. The questions in Box 7.2 can help you to compare policies from different insurance carriers. When coverage appears equal, you might ask how long a company has been in business and how long it has been providing nursing liability insurance. You want to be insured with a reliable, stable company. Questions 1 through 8 in Box 7.2 apply to individual insurance policies. For an institutional policy, ask the questions 1 to 6 and 9 to 12.

Critical Thinking Activity: Liability Insurance
You are accepting a position in a clinic. When might you ask about professional liability insurance coverage? Formulate specific questions. Identify the person who would be the best source of this information. How will you proceed if this person does not have the information you seek? If the interviewer tells you that the clinic is well covered by liability insurance, will you purchase personal malpractice insurance? Why or why not?

LEGAL ISSUES COMMON IN NURSING

Some legal issues recur frequently in nursing practice. It is wise for the nurse to understand these particular issues as they relate to individual practice.

Duty to Report or Seek Medical Care for a Client

A nurse who cares for a client has a legal duty to ensure that the client receives safe and competent care. This duty requires that the nurse maintain an appropriate standard of care and take action to obtain an appropriate standard of care from other professionals when necessary. For example, if a nurse assesses a client and determines that the attention of a physician is essential but fails to make every effort to obtain that attention, the nurse has breached a duty to the client. *Failure to rescue* is shorthand for failure to prevent a clinically important deterioration, such as death or permanent disability, from a complication of an underlying illness or medical care (Agency for Health Research and Quality AHRQ, 2017) and is considered a nursing-sensitive outcome. Reductions in *failure to rescue* rates are associated with low client-to-nurse ratios. Monitoring clients to identify deterioration and intervening to assure care are critical RN functions.

Nursing Responsibility for Medical Orders

The nurse has a responsibility to critically examine medical orders that are written for a client. Although the nurse is not responsible for the medical order itself, the nurse's education provides a background to identify obvious discrepancies or problems. In one reported case (Anonymous, 1997), two doctors left conflicting orders, which the charge nurse then transcribed. The court

Communication in Action 7.3: *Obtaining a Telephone Order*

Evan Wilson was an RN on a medical unit. He called Dr. Marie Steven regarding the needs of a patient Esther Moran. The nurse in Dr. Steven's office answered the phone. Evan stated, "Hello, this is Evan Wilson, an RN on 4W at Mercy Hospital. I am caring for Dr. Steven's client Esther Moran, who was admitted this morning for management of her heart failure. She is complaining of indigestion and has asked for an antacid, which Dr. Steven has directed her to use while at home. I would like to speak with Dr. Steven about this." The nurse replied, "Dr. Steven is with a client now, but I am familiar with Mrs. Moran and I am sure that Dr. Steven would order the antacid. Go ahead and give it to her. I will talk with Dr. Steven and get her O.K. as soon as she is available." Evan replied, "I appreciate your interest in facilitating care for Mrs. Moran, but I can only accept an order that the physician has initiated after assessing the situation. It will be fine if you call me back after talking with Dr. Steven. If needed, Dr. Steven can call me on my cell phone for additional information. Thanks for your help."

ruled that the nurse had a duty to understand the client's plan of care and to communicate with the doctors who had written the conflicting orders. While this case happened some time ago, courts of today are likely to expect this level of critical thinking by the nurse.

Another area of important nursing responsibility is in relationship to telephone orders. The Joint Commission discourages these whenever possible, encouraging instead written orders that are faxed or communicated in writing in some other way (such as a secure online connection). However, there are emergencies when telephone orders are essential to timely care. In these instances, there should be clear guidelines as to how orders are documented and verified. The preferred method is for the nurse to speak directly to the prescriber, write down the order as received, and then read it back to the prescriber for verification. The prescriber must then review and sign the order as soon as practical. When it is entered into a computer system by the nurse, there is some method for the physician to verify the order at the next visit (National Coordinating Council on Medication Error Reporting and Prevention, 2017).

Confidentiality and Right to Privacy

Confidentiality and the right to privacy with respect to one's personal life are basic concerns in our society. All information regarding a client belongs to that client. This right has been inferred from interpretation of the federal constitution but is explicitly stated in some state laws. HIPAA demands major efforts of all healthcare providers in regard to protecting client privacy. In theory, the rights identified in HIPAA should protect a client's privacy. Healthcare agencies are required to provide clients with a document on the agency's privacy policies. These policies are often multipage documents that may include a variety of ways in which an individual's health information is used and many clients do not read them carefully. Policies usually indicate that information will be used for business operations. Because third-party payers (such as insurance companies and health maintenance organizations) will not reimburse for care if they do not receive records documenting diagnoses and care provided, clients often must sign statements giving approval for all needed information to be sent to their insurance company. They may be unaware of exactly what information is sent or who may see it.

When computerized records are transmitted to insurance companies, they no longer contain only a brief statement of diagnosis and treatment; they may also contain detailed accounts of interactions between a client and a mental healthcare provider, health information of a sensitive nature, and genetic information that could be used inappropriately. Because increased use of computerized records can result in easier retrieval and cross-referencing of records from many sources, the general public, healthcare providers, and government officials are becoming more concerned about potential invasions of privacy. Safeguards must be built into all computerized medical record systems that prevent unauthorized access and the tracking of those who do access the system.

Only those professional persons involved in the client's care who have a need to know about the client are allowed routine access to the record. A physician, nurse, or any other employee who is not involved in the client's care or who does not have an administrative responsibility relative to that care is not allowed routine access. Persons not involved in care may be allowed access to the record only by specific written authorization of the patient or by court order. Be cautious about what information you share verbally and with whom.

Medical records professionals state that it is not uncommon for attorneys, family members, media representatives, or law enforcement officials to request access to client records or specific client information without having express consent from the client or a legal court order to view the records or be given information. Those unfamiliar with laws regarding privacy sometimes reveal information inappropriately. If you are ever approached for client information by someone who purports to have authority, your best course of action is to refer that individual to appropriate administrative personnel, who can determine the validity of the request.

Other areas of concern are the Internet, e-mail, and fax machine transmissions. Through these avenues, a healthcare provider may consult with other professionals to provide the best diagnostic and treatment services to the client. However, online computer communications are not private. Those with the necessary skill may intercept and read any e-mail or Internet message. Facilities receiving faxes may not adequately safeguard faxed information. Therefore, the identity of clients must be protected in any such communication. Some online documents are shared through encryption and password protection within a protected computer system that may be accessed from remote locations. A level I trauma center computer system was hacked in the summer of 2017, leaving the facility without computer access for six weeks. A cyber security firm was hired to get the systems back online. A representative from that firm said attacks like these are just the beginning (https://www.cbsnews.com/news/cbsn-on-assignment-hackers-targeting-medical-industry-hospitals/).

In a world where electronic communication such as Facebook, Snapchat, Tumblr, Twitter, and text messaging have become common, healthcare providers may inadvertently breach privacy by comments made in an electronic posting or message. The safest approach is that no references of any kind regarding any client should be made on an online site or in a message. Additionally, care should be taken to not disclose information regarding the healthcare facility itself. Once sent, messages and postings cannot be withdrawn and may be widely distributed without your consent or knowledge. When you are seeking employment, having made comments about clients even in general terms or about potential employers may be considered as showing poor professional judgment.

Defamation of Character

Any time that shared information is detrimental to a person's reputation, the person sharing the information may be liable for defamation of character. Written defamation is called libel. Oral defamation is called slander. Defamation of character involves communication that is malicious and false. Sometimes such comments are made in the heat of anger. Occasionally, statements written in a client's chart are libelous. Severely critical opinions may be stated as fact. An example of such a statement might be, "The client is lying," or "The client is rude and domineering." Clients may charge that comments in the chart adversely affected their care by prejudicing other staff against them. The astute nurse will chart only objective information regarding clients and give opinion in professional terms, well documented with fact.

Libel and slander may also be charged when written comments or verbal statements are made regarding another healthcare provider. Thoughtless or angry comments that impugn the abilities of a physician or that might cause a client to lose trust in a physician can be slander. In conversations, the prudent nurse carefully considers any comments about other healthcare providers before making them. There are accepted mechanisms for confidentially reporting inappropriate care or errors; be sure to use them and do not make critical statements to uninvolved third parties. In many states, licensed professionals are required to report poor practice or illegal acts on the part of other professionals. Criticism reported without malice and in good faith, through the appropriate channels, is usually protected from legal action for defamation. If you have such a concern, you should investigate the appropriate channels to be used in your setting.

Privileged Communication

Privileged communication refers to information that is shared by an individual client with certain professionals but that does not need to be revealed, even in a court of law. This professional is said to possess "privilege"—that is, has the privilege of not revealing information. All states consider certain types of communication (between client and attorney, between client and doctor, or between an individual and a member of the clergy) privileged. Not all states recognize the nurse–client relationship as one in which privileged communication takes place; even those states that recognize nurse–client communication as potentially privileged do not consider *all* communication between clients and nurses to be privileged. Privilege is a limited concept reserved for information given in confidence to the nurse within the nurse–client

---

Communication in Action 7.4: Accurate and Responsible Documentation

William Whittier was caring for a client who was brought in by an ambulance after being found unconscious on the sidewalk. There was considerable side discussion among the staff about whether the client was intoxicated. In his documentation, William notes, "Skin red, flushed, and warm. Strong breath odor that resembles alcohol. Client responds only to shaking and loud verbal stimulation." Later, when the client has become more responsive and awake, he documents, "Client states, 'Boy, am I hung-over! What happened?'" This provided factual information for the reader without making potentially libelous accusations.

professional relationship. Only a court can determine whether privilege exists in any specific case. If a court does not determine information is privileged, then you are legally obligated to testify about the communication.

Informed Consent

Every person has the right to either consent (agree) to or refuse healthcare treatment. The law requires that a person give voluntary and **informed consent**. Voluntary means that no coercion exists. Informed means that a person clearly understands the choices being offered.

Consent for Medical Treatment

Consent for medical treatment is the responsibility of the medical provider (eg, physician, dentist, and nurse practitioner). Informed consent contains information on:

- The nature of the decision/procedure
- Reasonable alternatives to the proposed intervention
- The relevant risks, benefits, and uncertainties related to each alternative
- Assessment of client understanding (University of Washington School of Medicine, 2014)

Consent (the acceptance of the intervention by the client) may be either verbal or written and indicates a client has decided to go ahead with the procedure based on a clear understanding of the options. Written consent usually is preferred in healthcare to ensure that a record of consent exists, although a signature alone does not prove that the consent was informed. A blanket consent for "any procedures deemed necessary" usually is not considered adequate consent for specific procedures. The form should state the specific proposed medical procedure or test.

The law places the responsibility for obtaining consent for medical treatment on the provider who will perform the procedure. It is the responsibility of the provider to provide appropriate, accurate, complete, and correct information, and the provider is liable if the client charges that appropriate information was not given. A nurse may present a form for a client to sign, and the nurse may sign the form as a witness to the signature. This does not transfer the legal responsibility for informed consent for medical care to the nurse. If the client does not seem well informed, the nurse should notify the provider so that further information can be given to the client. Although the nurse would not be liable legally for the lack of informed consent, the nurse has ethical obligations to assist the client in exercising his or her rights and to assist the provider in providing appropriate care.

Consent for Nursing Measures

Nurses must obtain a client's consent for nursing measures undertaken. This does not mean that exhaustive explanations need to be given in each situation, because courts have held that clients can be expected to have some understanding of usual care. Consent for nursing measures may be verbal or implied. The nurse may ask, "Are you ready to ambulate now?" The client answers, "Certainly," providing verbal consent. Alternatively, the nurse may state, "I have the injection the doctor ordered for you. Will you please turn over?" If the client turns over, this is implied consent.

Similarly, consent for care should be requested in emergency situations, such as those mentioned earlier in the discussion of Good Samaritan policies, if the injured is able to give that consent. A simple statement such as, "I am a registered nurse. Do you want my help?" is sufficient.

The nurse should remember that the client is free to refuse any aspect of care offered. Like the physician, the nurse is responsible for making sure that the client is informed before making a decision. Good nursing care requires that you use all means at your disposal to help the client comprehend the value of proposed care. For example, the postoperative client needs to understand that getting into a chair is part of the plan of care, not a convenience for the nurse or simply a change to prevent boredom. Thus, a client's refusal of care is accepted only after the client has been given complete information. The nurse would then carefully document this situation.

Competence to Give Consent

A person's ability to make judgments based on rational understanding is termed **competence**. Dementia, developmental disabilities, head injuries, strokes, medications, and illnesses creating loss of consciousness are common causes of an inability to make judgments. Determining competence is a complex issue. The client's illness, age, or condition alone does not determine competence. Legal competence is ultimately determined by the court. The general tendency of the courts has been to encourage whatever decision-making ability an individual has and to restrict personal decision making as little as possible.

When a person is determined legally to be incompetent, a legal guardian is appointed and consent is obtained from the legal guardian. A legal guardian is constrained from making some types of decisions. An example would be the decision about discontinuation of dialysis for an incompetent individual. If a person left a living will or a detailed document naming a durable power of attorney for healthcare that included wishes regarding end-of-life issues, the guardian might be allowed to decide to end dialysis. When such an individual leaves no clear indication regarding personal wishes or never had the capacity to make such decisions, the healthcare providers might insist on getting a court decision before accepting the consent of the guardian to terminate the dialysis.

Healthcare providers often encounter clients for whom no legal determination of competence has been made but who do not seem able to make an informed decision; examples include the very confused older person, the inebriated person, and the unconscious person. There are usually institutional guidelines to follow in determining that a person cannot give his or her own consent. The guidelines may require examination by a physician and documentation of the client's condition. More than one physician may be required to examine the client.

Competence may change from day to day, as a person's physical illness changes. The person who has had major surgery and is receiving large doses of narcotics for pain may not be able to reason clearly. Forty-eight hours later, this same individual may be perfectly alert and capable of considering complex issues. An individual may be competent to make some decisions, such as "I don't like rice and I won't eat it!" but incompetent to make others, for example, decisions regarding financial matters. These differences in competence require care providers to adjust their own planning to incorporate patient self-determination whenever possible, even when the person is legally incompetent. If a person truly is not capable of making decisions, the nurse should attempt to present necessary nursing actions in a way that elicits cooperation and avoids confrontation over decisions. For example, rather than asking the cognitively impaired person if she wants to take her medications, the prudent nurse simply states, "Here are your medications. It is time to take them."

Withdrawing Consent

Consent may be withdrawn after it is given. People have the right to change their minds. Therefore, if after one IV infusion a client decides not to have a second one started, that is the client's right. As a nurse, you have an obligation to notify the physician if the client refuses a medical procedure or treatment.

When individuals are participating in any type of research protocol for care, they are free to withdraw from the research study at any time. When caring for individuals who are part of a research process, you have obligations to protect the client's right to make decisions, even if they are contrary to the interests of the researcher. You would have an obligation to inform the researcher of the client's decision.

Consent and Minors

The parent or legal guardian usually provides consent for care of a minor. You also should obtain the minor's consent when he or she is able to give it. Increasingly, courts are emphasizing that minors be allowed a voice when it concerns matters that they are capable of understanding. This is especially true for the adolescent, but this consideration should be given to any child who is 7 years of age or older. Often courts do not seek consent from minors, but rather an indication that they understand the purpose of the care. For adolescents, the court may ask that negotiation with minors occur. When minors refuse care and legal guardians have authorized that care, do not proceed until legal clarification is given. Consult your nursing supervisor. This may be an issue for an ethics committee as well as for legal representation.

Minors who live apart from their parents and are financially independent, or who are married, are termed **emancipated minors**. In most (but not all) states, emancipated minors can give consent to their own treatment. Some states have specific laws relating to the **mature minor**, allowing sexually active minors to give personal consent (without also obtaining parental consent) for treatment of sexually transmitted infection or for obtaining birth control information and supplies. Be sure of the law in your state if you practice in an area where this is a concern. Most institutions have developed policies to guide employees in making correct decisions in this and other areas dealing with consent.

Advance Directives

Advance directives are legal documents stating the wishes of individuals regarding healthcare in situations in which they are no longer capable of giving personal informed consent. These documents are completed in advance of the situation in which they might be needed, and they direct the actions of others. There are several types of advance directives, such as a living will and a durable power of attorney for healthcare. For more information, see Evidence-Based Practice 7.2.

The Living Will

A **living will** or **directive to physicians** provides information on preferences regarding end-of-life issues such as types of care to provide and whether to use various resuscitation measures. The basis of a living will is an if-then plan. Most commonly, it declares that if "I am terminally ill and not expected to recover," then "I want this care given and do not want that care given." The *if* condition may also include the fact that the person is in a persistent vegetative state and not expected to recover function and capacity. Many states require that two physicians must agree that the person is terminally ill or in a persistent vegetative state. Although living wills

Evidence-Based Practice 7.2: Advance Directives

The powers that be: Understanding powers of attorney, conservators, guardianships and more: A primer. (2017). *ISNA Bulletin, 43*(3), 10–15.

There are many different legal documents designed to make clients' wishes known in the event they are unable to speak for themselves. There are also documents that designate someone else to make decisions in the event of a medical emergency. Most nurses do not routinely deal with legal documents but it is important to understand how each type of document might be used.

The Indiana State Nurses Association published this study guide to help nurses understand what each type of document is for and how it can be applied. By careful study of this guide, you can familiarize yourself with the various legal documents regarding advance directives and what you need to know about the various applications of these documents.

or directives were originally advisory for families and physicians as they made decisions, some states have now passed laws requiring that these documents be honored. If the physician does not agree with the decision of the client, then the physician in that state is obligated to withdraw from care and refer the case to another physician.

Living wills or directives to the physician may address other aspects of care in addition to resuscitation efforts. For example, they may indicate whether the individual wants to be tube fed if he or she is in a persistent vegetative state, whether surgery should be used in certain instances, or whether IV fluids or ventilator support should be used. Some advance directives are several pages long, as the person addresses many different possible concerns. Aging with Dignity, an organization in Florida, has developed and disseminated, in conjunction with the Robert Woods Johnson Foundation, an advance directive document called the Five Wishes. This document addresses not only life-sustaining therapies that are desired or not desired but also other aspects of end-of-life care, such as the desire for people, for touch, for music, and so forth. The five wishes that form the structure of the document are listed in Box 7.3. The Five Wishes document is an accepted legal advance directive in the majority of states. The Five Wishes Web site lists states that accept this as a legal document. In other states, the Five Wishes document may be used as an addendum to the legally accepted advance directive document to inform healthcare providers of personal wishes for end-of-life care.

BOX 7.3 FIVE WISHES FOR END-OF-LIFE CARE

- Which person do you want to make healthcare decisions for you when you can't make them?
- What kind of medical care you want or don't want?
- How comfortable you want to be?
- How you want people to treat you?
- What you want your loved ones to know?

Aging with Dignity: www.agingwithdignity.org/5wishes.html

Durable Power of Attorney for Healthcare

A **durable power of attorney for healthcare** (DPOA-Healthcare) is a document that legally designates a **decision maker**, should the person be incapacitated. This document may also be referred to as designating a **healthcare proxy**. This document provides individuals with the opportunity to identify a preferred legal decision maker if they are incapacitated. The DPOA for healthcare is activated only when the person becomes incapacitated. It may be combined with a living will that contains specific advance directives, such as those discussed above, thus providing directions for that designated decision maker regarding preferences.

If an individual has designated a decision maker for healthcare, this supersedes all general legal designations for decision makers. In a society where there are many different family relationships, durable power of attorney for healthcare is an important personal decision. For example, individuals who live in life partnerships other than marriage must have a durable power of attorney for healthcare to provide that life partner with decision-making ability for emergencies or critical situations. For the adult with no living parents or spouse and multiple siblings, the designation of one person as a decision maker may diminish family conflict and facilitate the provision of the care the individual wishes.

Physician Orders for Life-Sustaining Treatments

Limitations on resuscitation in the event of a cardiac or respiratory arrest may take many forms. These orders are generally referred to as Physician Orders for Life-Sustaining Treatments (POLST). The most comprehensive is the order that reads "Do Not Resuscitate (DNR) or No Code, meaning that no resuscitation efforts of any kind are to be made and the client be allowed to die naturally. There would be no cardiopulmonary resuscitation (CPR), no resuscitative drugs, and no mechanical ventilation. This is often the choice of the person who has a life-threatening disease such as terminal cancer and for whom resuscitation would only serve to prolong illness and discomfort. In some instances, the person may request a limited resuscitation effort, such as CPR and medications but no mechanical ventilation. Facilities may have a variety of ways to designate these limitations on resuscitative efforts and to communicate these directions to those providing care. An important understanding for nurses is that in the absence of a written order from a physician, other care providers are obligated to initiate resuscitation if an arrest occurs.

In an attempt to "effectively communicate the wishes of seriously ill patients to have or to limit medical treatment as they move from one care setting to another," the POLST organization at the Oregon Health Sciences University developed a set of standardized orders regarding CPR, medical interventions, antibiotics, artificially administered nutrition, and a summary (POLST, 2017).

An advance directive (or living will) provides information that the physician can use as a basis for deciding when an order limiting life-sustaining treatment is appropriate. In many states, there are laws that designate under what circumstances a physician may write an order limiting treatment in the absence of an advance directive. If the client has not completed an advance directive and is not expected to recover, the physician may determine that resuscitation would be futile. Futile means that it would not add appreciably to life or have the potential for success. Laws or policies usually require the agreement of two physicians that resuscitation would be futile. After this medical determination, then the person who legally is the designated decision maker is consulted, provided information regarding the client's condition, and asked to consent to the physician's DNR order. This entire process must be documented in the client's record.

All care providers must understand that a DNR order does not limit other types of care that will be provided. Treatment of wounds to promote healing, pain management, resolution of other physical problems (such as nausea or constipation), antibiotic administration to control treatable infections, and oxygen to ease breathing are all examples of care that will still be appropriate. Even radiation therapy might be determined appropriate to reduce tumor growth and increase comfort. This type of care is referred to as palliative treatment: therapy designed to relieve or reduce the intensity of painful symptoms but which is not designed to cure a condition.

In some instances, an order may be written that specifies "comfort care only." This order again occurs after consultation with the client as able and family as appropriate. When this order is written, treatment of infections and other problems may not be initiated unless it would increase comfort. The focus becomes maximum comfort in the face of impending death. The client for whom comfort care only is ordered should receive the same concerted focus on end-of-life care that would occur in a hospice setting.

Nurses sometimes find themselves in situations in which they believe that the client's condition is futile and that a DNR or comfort care only order would be appropriate, but the physician has not made this determination or, having made this determination, has not consulted with the family and written a DNR order. In other instances, family insists on continuing all care options including resuscitation and ventilator support. Such situations can be difficult for nurses because they have no decision-making authority, and yet they are the ones who legally must carry out the resuscitation. Much depends on the nurse–physician working relationships, care provider–family relationships, and the ability to discuss difficult issues together. Some care facilities encourage care conferences where these matters can be raised for discussion. Nurses can be effective advocates for increased communication and discussion of these difficult issues.

Patient Self-Determination Act

In 1990, the United States Congress passed the Patient Self-Determination Act (PSDA). This Act took effect in 1992 and required that on admission to any healthcare service (hospital, long-term care center, or home care agency), clients be given an opportunity to determine what lifesaving or life-prolonging actions they want carried out. Much of the impetus for this legislation was the belief that many individuals were having their lives prolonged in situations in which they would have preferred this not be done. As indicated by the nursing theorist Dorothea Orem (2017), all clients want to be able to care for themselves (see the following Nursing Theory Alert).

Theory Alert   *Dorothea Orem*

Dorothea Orem was born in Baltimore, MD, in 1914. She completed her nursing diploma studies at Providence Hospital School of Nursing in the 1930s. She later completed both a Bachelor's and Master's of science in nursing at the Catholic University of America in Washington, DC. She made many contributions to the science of nursing before her death in 2007. Orem's theory, called the Self-Care Deficit of Nursing Theory, proposed that all clients want to care for themselves. Her theory includes the concept that clients recover more quickly and holistically if they are able to perform their own care as much as possible. If a client is unable to perform self-care, a self-care deficit is identified. A nursing care plan is then devised to complete the needed care and help the client to recover the ability to care for self. Nurses and clients work together to ensure that clients receive quality care and regain the ability to care for themselves.

The PSDA requires the agency to provide adequate information for the individual to make an informed decision regarding these important matters. As a result of this legislation, agencies reviewed and revised policies and protocols regarding consent. In many agencies, a nurse has the responsibility to provide the education and obtain a signature on a document indicating preferences. Some difficulties arise in this process when the person giving the information does not clearly understand that the decision about resuscitation is not based on the *current* situation but upon a client's choice of what should happen in a *possible* situation where the client becomes terminally ill and is not being expected to survive. Clients may become concerned that they will be abandoned if an untoward event happens. Clear communications can alleviate these concerns and assist the client to make important decisions regarding end-of-life care while he or she is healthier and still able to make the decision for himself or herself.

Emergency Care

Care in emergencies has many legal repercussions; therefore, the judgment that an emergency exists is important. Certain actions may be legal in emergencies and not legal in nonemergency situations. In emergencies, the standard procedures for obtaining consent may be impossible to follow. Further, in emergencies, personnel must sometimes take on responsibilities that they would not undertake in a nonemergency situation. Critical thinking on the part of all healthcare providers is essential when differentiating an emergency from a nonemergency.

Most facilities that provide emergency care have policies and procedures designed to ensure adequate support for claiming that an emergency exists. Thus, the policy will often state that at least two physicians in the emergency department must examine the client and concur that the emergency requires immediate action, without waiting for consent. This ensures maximum legal protection for the physician and the institution.

Consent in Emergencies

If a true emergency exists, consent for care is considered to be implied. The law holds that if a reasonable person were aware that the situation was life threatening, he or she would give consent for care. An exception to this is made if the person has explicitly rejected such care in advance; an example is a Jehovah's Witness carrying a card stating his personal religion and that he does not wish to receive blood or blood products. This is one reason why emergency department nurses should check a client's wallet for identification and information related to care. Checking a client's wallet should be done with another person, and a careful inventory of contents documented and signed by both. There should be little concern about liability in taking emergency action if this is completed.

Standards of Practice and Emergencies

Standards of practice in emergencies differ from those in nonemergency situations. In hospital emergencies, the nurse sometimes may be in the position of identifying an emergency and whether a needed action is one that only a physician usually performs. The hospital is expected to have a policy and protocol, which the nurse would follow, to verify and document the situation fully. This usually involves consultation with a supervisory nurse and verification of the emergency situation, as well as attempts to obtain medical assistance. Again, critical thinking by the nurse is essential to determine whether a true emergency exists. Review the information on scope of practice in Chapter 3 to help you with decision making in regard to emergency actions.

When life or limb is truly in danger, the courts have held that a nurse can do those things immediately necessary, even if they usually are considered medical functions, provided the nurse has the essential expertise to perform the actions safely and correctly. The matter of having essential expertise is crucial; this is why all members of an emergency response team must learn all aspects of the code procedure. If, for any reason, the physician were unable to respond to the code, a nurse who was prepared with this essential expertise would assume the role of the leader of the code team.

Protocols and Emergencies

Most healthcare agencies have established protocols for nursing action in a variety of emergency or even urgent situations. These provide directions for nursing action that would usually be a physician's order. For example, if the client's blood pressure drops precipitously, the protocol might indicate that the nurse would start an IV infusion with a specified fluid to maintain circulating volume and to provide IV access for emergency drugs. The administration of oxygen to a person suffering acute respiratory distress is another situation frequently covered by a protocol. When emergencies occur, nurses are protected from a charge of practicing outside the scope of the RN by following the protocol that was approved by the medical staff.

Noninstitutional Emergency Care

In many states, official emergency personnel must render all possible aid, including all resuscitative measures, when they are called to an emergency situation. This has sometimes resulted in the resuscitation of a terminally ill person who had previously stated that resuscitation was not desired. As more individuals receive terminal care in their homes, this has become an increasing concern.

Legislation allowing for client self-determination regarding emergency responders has now been passed in most states. The law usually stipulates the precise circumstances under which an individual may provide an advance directive regarding emergency procedures, and how that directive must be documented so that emergency personnel can honor it. For example, the individual may be required to wear a specific armband and the DNR order may be posted on the door of the refrigerator or other prominent position in the home. All emergency responders must be aware of their responsibilities regarding advance directives.

Fraud

Fraud is deliberate deception for the purpose of personal gain and is usually prosecuted as a crime. However, it may also serve as the basis of a civil suit. Situations of fraud in nursing are not common. One example would be trying to obtain a better position by giving incorrect information to a prospective employer. By deliberately stating (falsely) that they have completed a nurse practitioner program to obtain a position for which they would otherwise be ineligible, individuals are defrauding the employer. This may be prosecuted as a crime, because they are placing members of the community in danger of receiving substandard care. Individuals also may commit fraud by trying to cover up a nursing error to avoid legal action.

Courts tend to be harsher in decisions regarding fraud than in cases involving simple malpractice, because fraud represents a deliberate attempt to mislead others for one's own gain and could result in harm to those assigned to that individual's care.

Assault and Battery

Assault is saying or doing something to make a person genuinely afraid that he or she will be touched without consent. Battery involves touching a person when that individual has not consented to the action. Neither of these terms implies that harm was done; harm may or may not occur. For an assault to occur, the person must be afraid of what might happen because the individual appears to have the power to carry out the threat. "If you don't take this medication, I will have to put you in restraints" is an example of an assault. For battery to occur, the touching must occur without consent. Remember that consent may be implied rather than specifically stated. Therefore, if the client extends an arm for an injection, he cannot later charge battery, saying that he was not asked. But if the client agreed because of a threat (assault), the touching still would be considered battery because the consent was not freely given.

Assault and battery are crimes under the law. However, most of these cases in healthcare are instituted as civil suits by the injured party, rather than as criminal cases by government authorities. Assault and battery are most commonly treated as criminal cases when they involve suspected abuse of a client. Most of us in healthcare are shocked and dismayed to learn of instances in which care providers were abusive. Individuals who have difficulty with impulse control and anger may become frustrated with a client and threaten, push, shove, or otherwise harm the individual. Most jurisdictions have laws requiring that anyone who knows of abuse to an individual, whether a child, a developmentally delayed adult, or an older person, report that abuse to the proper authorities. Within an institution, there should be policies and procedures for this type of reporting. Appropriate authorities must conduct a careful investigation to ensure protection of the rights of the person accused and the person harmed.

False Imprisonment

Making a person stay in a place against his wishes is **false imprisonment**. The person may be forced to stay either by physical or by verbal means. It is easy to understand why restraining a client or confining a client to a locked room could constitute false imprisonment if proper procedures were not first carried out. Again, false imprisonment is a crime, but when it occurs in healthcare, it is most often the basis of a civil suit rather than a criminal case.

The law is less clear about keeping a client confined by nonphysical means. Removing clients' clothing for the express purpose of preventing them from leaving could make a nurse liable for false imprisonment. Threatening to keep people confined with statements such as, "If you don't stay in your bed, I'll sedate you" can also constitute false imprisonment. If people need to be confined for their own safety or well-being, it is best to help them understand and agree to that course of action.

In a conventional care setting, you cannot restrain or confine responsible adults against their wishes. All persons have the right to make decisions for themselves, regardless of the consequences. The client with a severe heart condition who defies orders and walks to the bathroom has that right. You protect yourself by recording your efforts to teach the client the need for restrictions and by reporting the client's behavior to your supervisor and the physician.

In the same context, the client cannot be forced to remain in a hospital. The client has the right to leave a healthcare institution regardless of medical advice to the contrary. While this might not be in the best interests of the person's health, the client has the right to decide to leave against medical advice. Again, document your efforts in the record and follow applicable policies to protect the facility, the physician, and yourself from liability.

False imprisonment suits are a special concern in the care of the psychiatric client. Particular laws relate to this situation. In the psychiatric setting, you may have clients who have voluntarily sought admission. The same restrictions on restraint or confinement in the general care setting apply to these clients. Other clients in the psychiatric setting may have been committed involuntarily according to the laws of the state. Specific measures may be used to confine the involuntarily committed client. Laws in terms of situation, type of restraint allowed, and the length of time restraining may be used often define these measures. If you work in a psychiatric setting, review specific policies regarding restraint to protect clients and to assist staff in functioning within the legal limits.

FACTORS THAT CONTRIBUTE TO MALPRACTICE CLAIMS

A suit usually does not always follow the poor results or harm that may on occasion occur in the course of nursing practice. An understanding of the factors that enter into whether a suit is instituted may be helpful to you.

Consequences of the Error

When an error results in serious consequences, such as prolonged hospitalization, disability, or even death, individuals are likely to institute legal action. The aim may be to cover costs such as needed care, lost wages, and other costs associated with the error. There also may be a wish to have the individual or organization pay for the pain and suffering experienced. For example, the person who was severely burned by a cautery used incorrectly in surgery would experience lost productivity and wages due to time off for care and healing. Additionally, the person would experience severe pain and suffering and might have permanent scarring. That person might seek compensation for these nonmonetary losses. In other situations, when no one seems to take responsibility for the error or people do not seem to care or feel regret for what happened, there may be a wish to punish those involved. Punitive damages may be awarded when the court determines that the injury reflects not just a single incident but a pattern of unsafe care.

Social Factors

Much is being written about changes in the public's attitudes toward healthcare providers. Healthcare is big business, and clients complain increasingly of not being accepted and respected as individuals. In general, clients are more willing to bring suit against someone who is part of a large, impersonal system.

Health costs are high, and some people think hospitals and physicians have the ability to pay large settlements, whether directly or through insurance. If a client's own income is lessened or disrupted by an illness, he or she might bring suit as a solution to economic difficulties. Increased public awareness of the size of monetary judgments that have been awarded also may be an economic incentive to initiating a suit.

Suit-Prone Clients

Some people are more likely to bring suit, for real or imagined errors. By recognizing these people as suit-prone clients, it is possible for you to protect yourself through increased vigilance regarding care and thorough record keeping. Although it is important to guard against stereotyping, the following general descriptions may help you to avoid problems. Suit-prone clients usually are identified by overt behavior in which they are persistent faultfinders and critics of healthcare providers and of all aspects of care. They may be uncooperative in following a plan of care and sensitive to any perceived slight.

Persons who exhibit hostile attitudes may extend their hostile feelings to the nurses and other healthcare providers with whom they have contact. The nurse who becomes defensive when faced with hostility only widens the breach in the nurse–client relationship. It is necessary to pay careful attention to those principles of care learned in psychosocial nursing that deal with how to help the hostile client. Assisting clients in solving their own problems and offering support are the best forms of protection for the nurse.

Another type of client who appears more suit prone is the very dependent person who uses projection to deal with anxiety and fear. These individuals tend to ascribe fault or blame for all events to others and are unable to accept personal responsibility for their own welfare. Again, meeting these clients' needs with a carefully considered plan of care is the answer.

A common error is to withdraw and become defensive or the other extreme of becoming more authoritarian and directive when confronting a suit-prone client. This reaction occurs partly because a situation is unpleasant and partly because a staff member feels personally threatened by the client's behavior. This reaction tends to increase the client's feeling of separation and distance from the staff and increases the likelihood of a suit if a poor outcome occurs.

When staff members are helped to view the client as a troubled person who manifests his or her problems in this manner, sometimes they find it easier to be objective. The client is in need of all the skill that the thoughtful nurse can bring to the emotional problems. The entire health team needs to develop a careful and consistent approach, which provides security and stability to the client and family. The suit-prone client does not always end up suing; much depends on the response of healthcare providers.

Suit-Prone Nurses

Nurses may also be suit prone. Nurses who are insensitive to the client's complaints, who do not identify and meet the client's emotional needs, or who fail to recognize and accept the limits of their own practice may contribute to suits instituted not only against the nurse but also against the employer and the physician. The nurse's self-awareness is critical in preventing suits (Fig. 7.4).

Staff members may contribute to a client's distrust of care through complaining about working conditions, telling clients about problems occurring on the unit, and disparaging other healthcare providers. There is a distinction between informing a client that you must meet someone else's needs, and therefore will not return for a specified period of time, and giving the client the impression that you do not have time to attend to his or her needs.

Figure 7.4. Certain things can be done to prevent malpractice suits.

PREVENTING MALPRACTICE CLAIMS

A variety of things can be done to prevent malpractice claims from ever happening. Many of these actions are ones that you can take as an individual, while others require the involvement of the entire healthcare team.

Maintaining Excellent Standards of Care

The most significant thing you can do to prevent malpractice claims is to maintain a high standard of care. To do this, work at improving your own nursing practice and also the general climate for nursing practice where you work. You can do this in many ways. An important aspect of high-standard care is excellence in communication with patients and families. Therapeutic communication skills including listening, clarifying, and problem solving are especially critical.

Communication in Action 7.5: Talking With an Upset Family

Mr. Jenkins had been at the desk every hour demanding something for his very ill wife. Sometimes it was pain medication and at other times it was something such as a glass of water. He has said, "You people need to take better care of Mildred! If I weren't here, who knows what would happen to her?" Jennifer Tompkins approached Mr. Jenkins in his wife's room. "You seem really concerned about your wife's care," she said. "I would like to talk with both of you about it and see if together we can make some plans that help you both in this very difficult situation you are facing here."

Self-Awareness

Identify your own strengths and weaknesses in practice. When you identify a weakness, seek a means of growth. This may include education, directed experience, or discussion with colleagues. Be ready to acknowledge your limitations to supervisors, and do not accept responsibilities for which you are not prepared. For example, the nurse who has not worked in pediatrics for 10 years and accepts an assignment to a pediatric unit without orientation and education is setting the stage for an error to occur. The standard of care does not change for an inexperienced nurse. As a professional, do not accept a position if you cannot meet the criterion of being a reasonably prudent nurse in that setting. In instances of true emergency (eg, disaster or flood), courts may be more lenient, but "we need you here today" does not constitute an emergency.

Adapting Proposed Assignments

As discussed previously, nurses may find themselves assigned to units where they have little or no experience with the types of client problems they will encounter. It is reasonable to be assigned to assist an overworked nurse in a special area if you can assume duties that are within your own competence and allow the specialized nurse to assume the specialized duties. It is not reasonable or safe for you to be expected to assume the specialized duties. Thus, if you were not prepared for coronary care, you might go to that unit, monitor the IV lines, take vital signs, and make observations to report to the experienced coronary care nurse; the experienced nurse then would be able to check the monitors, administer the specialized medications, and make decisions. Note that this does fragment the client's care, and it would not be appropriate as a permanent solution but could alleviate a temporary problem in a safe manner.

Following Policies, Procedures, and Protocols

It is your responsibility to be aware of the policies, procedures, and protocols of the institution that employs you. If they are sound, they can be an adequate defense against a claim, providing they were carefully followed. In all circumstances, avoid shortcuts and "work-arounds."

For example, the medication procedure may involve checking all medications against a medication administration record (MAR). If you do this and there is an error in the MAR, you might not be liable for the resulting medication error because you followed all appropriate procedures and acted responsibly. The liability would rest with the person who made the error in transcribing the medication from the physician's orders to the MAR. If, however, you had not followed the procedure in checking, you might also be liable because you did not do your part in preventing error. As discussed previously, policies are often designed to provide legal direction.

Changing Policies, Procedures, and Protocols

As nursing evolves, changes are needed in policies, procedures, and protocols. Part of your responsibility as a professional is to work toward keeping these up to date. Are there written policies to deal with emergency situations? Statements such as, "Oh, we've always done it this way" are not adequate substitutes for clearly written, officially accepted policies. Often, facilities that are reluctant to make changes based on the suggestions of individual nurses are much more receptive to new ideas when the legal implications of outmoded practice are noted. References such as the guidelines produced by the Agency for Healthcare Research and Quality and articles with research results may provide strong support for needed changes in practice.

Effective Documentation

Nurses' records are unique in the healthcare setting. They cover the entire period of hospitalization or long-term care, 24 hours a day, in a sequential pattern. Your record can be the crucial factor in avoiding litigation. Documentation in the record of observations made, decisions reached, and actions taken and the evaluation of the client's response are considered much more solid evidence than verbal testimony, which depends on one's memory.

Because each case is determined by the facts as well as by the applicable law, clear documentation of all relevant data is important. For legal purposes, observations and actions that are not recorded may be assumed not to have occurred. Documentation needs to be factual, legible, and clearly understandable. Only use approved abbreviations. Make sure narrative notes have clear statements and correct errors according to the policy of the facility. In paper records, liquid erasing fluid, erasures, and heavy crossing out may be interpreted as attempted fraud in record keeping. In computerized charting, there are usually approved methods of making corrections after an entry has been made. Be sure to follow those processes carefully. Avoid any statement that implies negligence on the part of any healthcare provider. Nurses should be aware that their notes protect not only themselves but often other members of the healthcare team and the facility.

Properly kept records also may protect you from becoming liable for the error of another, by demonstrating that you did everything in your power to prevent harm, including consulting with others. These records might include a complete log of telephone calls to a physician and consultation with any relevant supervisor. Documentation should support that you followed all relevant policies and procedures when an emergency occurred. Although it is easy to become impatient with the time required by paper work and record keeping, complete and clear documentation is often the basis of a successful defense against a claim of malpractice.

One concern about problem-oriented records and charting by exception (ie, only noting when there is a change from the expected outcome or when an intervention is omitted) is that these formats may provide less-detailed information and may be less helpful in defense against litigation. This does not have to be the case. You can use any system of charting and record keeping to create appropriate and adequate documentation of care. If you identify something that needs to be recorded and cannot find a provision within your system to make that recording, you can be sure that others have experienced the same difficulty. You might begin making inquiries toward establishing a clear mechanism for the record keeping that concerns you. When nurses serve on committees to review and plan charting procedures, it is wise for them to seek consultation with the attorney for the facility. This helps to ensure that the plan for record keeping is legally sound as well as professionally useful.

ELEMENTS OF A LEGAL ACTION

An individual begins legal action by consulting an attorney and bringing suit against all of those who might have been responsible for the problem. Once the suit has been filed, the next step in legal action is the process of discovery. From there, it may be dropped, settled out of court, or settled by trial.

Discovery

In a civil lawsuit (one between parties for the recovery of damages), a lengthy discovery process commences. Discovery involves gathering information through documents (such as previous medical records and results of mental and physical examinations), interrogatories (written

---

BOX 7.4 GUIDELINES FOR TESTIFYING

- Listen carefully to the entire question before answering and pause to let your attorney object if appropriate.
- Answer only the questions asked and frame your answer in your mind before beginning to speak.
- Do not volunteer additional information.
- Admit if you do not remember.
- Refer to your written documentation to support your answers.
- Be brief and direct.
- Do not use medical or technical terminology unless essential—then explain your terms.
- Explain when a simple yes or no would be misleading.
- Note differences between hypothetical cases presented and the one under consideration.

---

questions answered under oath), and depositions (verbal questions answered under oath and recorded by a court reporter). Testimony refers to an individual's verbal or written account of a situation.

A deposition is a formal proceeding in which each attorney has an opportunity to question a witness outside of court, and a sworn verbatim record is made by a court reporter. On occasion, the deposition may be videotaped. Depositions in healthcare cases often are held in attorneys' offices or in the healthcare facility for the convenience of the witnesses. Sometimes depositions are taken to preserve the testimony of a witness for trial and are used in place of live testimony at trial. Most depositions in which you would participate, however, would be depositions for discovery purposes. The same guidelines that apply to testifying in court apply to giving a deposition (Box 7.4).

Settlement Out of Court

Often, cases are settled before trial because of information obtained during the discovery process. The person bringing suit may be persuaded that no malpractice occurred or that it cannot be proved and may drop the suit. On the other hand, the persons or institutions being sued (or their insurance companies) may determine that it is in their best interests to avoid a trial and agree to pay damages; often, this is done without admitting that malpractice occurred. A settlement may require that no party to the settlement reveals its terms to others. Often, the cost in time and money to defend a malpractice case exceeds the cost of a settlement. However, any settlement must be reported to the National Practitioner Data Bank. This has made many healthcare professionals reluctant to settle a legal action for reasons of finances and convenience; however, the insurance company may have the authority to settle the case. Consult the policy at your facility to determine whether you would have a voice in determining any settlement.

Trials

A trial is a legal proceeding that takes place in a courtroom and is presided over by a judge. Some trials are settled before the judge (or panel of judges) alone, and others also have a jury present. In most instances, a trial is a public hearing, and anyone can attend and listen to the proceedings. The various witnesses may appear in person or, when agreed to by both sides, a deposition may be accepted in place of in-person testimony. The judge has full authority over all that takes place in the courtroom.

The plaintiff is the individual bringing suit. The defendants are all those being named in the suit. Each side presents its witnesses, who are examined (questioned) by the attorney. The attorney for the other side then is able to cross-examine (question) that witness about any of the information presented. The final decision is made by a vote of the jury meeting privately or by the judge, who considers all the information and makes a ruling. Monetary awards may be made at the time of the decision or may be established by further deliberation.

THE NURSE AS WITNESS

In the course of your practice as an RN, a time may come when you are asked to serve as a witness in a legal proceeding. Several kinds of cases may involve the nurse as a witness to fact or as an expert witness. When you become involved in any legal action, be sure that you understand both your rights and your obligations in regard to legal action. Always consult an attorney before talking to anyone about a matter in which you have been asked to testify, especially a malpractice action.

The Nurse as Witness to Fact

A witness to fact is an individual who has firsthand knowledge of the specific situation that forms the basis of the legal action. A witness to fact (also referred to as a lay witness) testifies to the exact situation and circumstances of the event or events in question. For example, as a nurse, you might be asked to testify as a witness to fact when a person was injured in an automobile accident and you or your organization were involved in the care of that person. Your testimony in such a case might be on behalf of the injured person, to help describe the injuries and the care received for those injuries.

Daily Ethical Dilemma 7.1: Confidentiality

Hilary works at a behavioral health facility that is currently involved in a lawsuit. On one occasion, she observed a physician and a client arguing. Later the client sued the physician for injuries that were allegedly sustained during the argument. Hilary is not named in the lawsuit and is not sure what she can do but she wants to be helpful. When the risk management department of her facility suggests she speak with defense counsel about her observations she readily agrees.

- What information does Hilary possess that might be helpful?
- What information does she possess that might not be helpful?
- Do you think she should speak with the defense counsel?

The attorney for the client learns that Hilary made a statement and he is very angry that he was not present for Hilary's questioning and files a HIPAA complaint against Hilary for violating client confidentiality.

- What should Hilary do now?
- What do you think her employer will do?
- What could she have done differently to avoid this situation?

New Mexico Nurse. (2017). Nursing liability and HIPAA ex-parte patient discussions. *New Mexico Nurse, 62*(1), 8.

Another situation involving the nurse as a witness to fact is one in which a client brings a lawsuit against persons or organizations who have provided healthcare that the client believes was below the standard of the community. Medical malpractice is alleged in such a situation. For example, the nurse may have to give evidence regarding medical record notes or care given to the client in the days before the alleged malpractice occurred. Sometimes a nurse is asked to provide information regarding the usual practices of the unit staff.

In both of these situations, the nurse's concern is with the specific factual details of a particular case. Nurses will testify only to what they have observed or done, not to hearsay or opinion. When nurses are asked to testify as to the facts of a situation, they sometimes believe that because they have done nothing wrong they do not need legal counsel. The law is complex, and you could jeopardize the position of an institution for which you work, or even jeopardize yourself and your professional future, with unwise statements. The person who is bringing suit may alter or amend the original complaint to involve new defendants, including you. If you have liability insurance, advise your insurance company of your role as a witness and an attorney will be assigned to talk with you. If you are covered by an employer's policy, consult with the appropriate administrative representative immediately to obtain legal counsel. This attorney should assist you in understanding the questions in the case, your role, and how you can protect yourself in the situation. However, they cannot tell you what to say, that would be illegal (Fig. 7.5).

Every witness is required to swear (take an oath) or affirm to tell the entire truth. Failure to tell the entire truth is perjury, which is a crime. As a witness, you are expected to answer the questions asked of you to the best of your ability; however, you do not have to provide an answer that would incriminate yourself, nor do you have to answer a question for which you

Figure 7.5. When testifying in court, you should answer only the questions asked. Do not introduce other information.

do not remember or know the answer. It is perfectly permissible to state, "I do not remember" or "I do not know" if you do not.

It is helpful to use words and terms that can be understood by those who are not familiar with medical terminology, or to explain medical terminology when its use is essential. Be brief and direct when answering questions. Answer the question asked of you. In clinical practice, nurses often use rephrasing techniques to gain information from clients. This is not appropriate when giving testimony. Do not volunteer additional information that has not been asked for by the attorney. You may open up entire areas of inquiry that would not be considered without your comments. However, be cautious about simply answering "yes" or "no." In some instances, an explanation is essential; a simple answer may sound as if you did not perform appropriately. It is the attorney's job to ask the questions to bring out the facts to which he or she wants you to testify. The opposing attorney will have an opportunity during cross-examination to ask you additional questions that the attorney believes are necessary for the facts of the case.

The Nurse as Expert Witness

A nurse also may be involved in a lawsuit as an expert witness. An **expert witness**, under Rule 702 of the Federal Rules of Evidence (accepted in the federal courts and many state courts), is defined as "a witness qualified as an expert by knowledge, skill, experience, training, or education who may testify in the form of an opinion or otherwise." An expert nurse witness may have long experience in a particular area of practice, be certified in the area, possess higher education in the area being considered, or have other evidence of special expertise. For example, in a case involving a client's care in a critical care unit, the expert nurse witness may be certified in critical care, have a master's degree with a focus in critical care, and have worked in high-intensity critical care for 20 years.

The purpose of testimony as an expert witness is to provide information and opinion that can be used by the judge or jury to understand complex areas of care and make a decision. A nurse may provide a professional opinion, related to his or her area of expertise, on the appropriate care for a given situation. The expert witness may review the record and give an opinion as to what that record states and the meaning of the data found there.

Stegen & Sowerby Stories: Part 2

Remember Joe, the man in the ED with suspected cholecystitis? After waiting 7 hours for initial screening and another 5 hours to get the CT scan and have the results read, a diagnosis of possible aortic dissection was returned but the results were unclear. After a consult with several other physicians, a CT of the lower abdomen and pelvis was ordered and a dissection of the descending aorta was diagnosed. Read the rest of the story at www.thePoint.com.

Want to Know More?

A variety of resources are available on the Point® to enhance your learning and understanding of this chapter, such as:

- Full Stegen & Sowerby Stories
- NCLEX-Style Student Review Questions
- Journal Articles
- Case Studies
- Learning Objectives
- Relevant Websites
- And more...

KEY CONCEPTS

- Law includes those rules of conduct or action recognized as binding or enforced by government.
- Statutory law includes all written laws and government codes.
- Constitutional law, which has the greatest authority in any jurisdiction, is found in the United States Constitution and in state constitutions.
- Enacted law includes those laws passed by legislative bodies.
- Regulatory law, also referred to as administrative or executive law, includes those rules and regulations established by administrative bodies within the government.
- Common law includes judicial law, also referred to as case law, and common usage or custom.
- Civil law encompasses those laws regulating private conduct between individuals.
- Criminal law regulates actions having to do with the safety of the community as a whole.
- Violations of criminal law are considered crimes, whereas violations of civil law are considered torts.
- Legal rights are derived from constitutional guarantees and carry with them responsibilities. Other rights are ethically determined and, while not supportable by law, do govern the behavior of healthcare professionals.
- Malpractice actions brought against healthcare workers involve civil law. Nurses may be involved in cases related to intentional torts, negligence, or malpractice.
- Individuals who are negligent or have committed malpractice are legally liable for the effects of that action. This means there is an obligation to the individual wronged.
- Liability may be focused on the individual, supervisor, or employer.
- Liability insurance may be purchased that transfers the cost of being sued and the cost of any settlement from the individual to a large group.
- A number of legal issues recur in nursing. Among these are the duty to report or seek medical care for a client, protection of the client's confidentiality and right to privacy, defamation of character, privileged information, issues related to informed consent, medication administration, and issues related to different types of emergency care.
- Many legal issues surround consent for care by the client or by a decision maker. These include the provision of advance directives (orders to the physician), such as living wills, durable power of attorney for healthcare, and physician orders for life-sustaining treatments.

- Nurses can be involved in criminal cases related to fraud, assault and battery, and false imprisonment. In some cases, however, a civil suit may be brought against a nurse for these issues and they may not be prosecuted as crimes.
- Many factors contribute to malpractice claims. These include seriousness of the error, social factors, characteristics of suit-prone clients, and characteristics of suit-prone nurses.
- A nurse can do many things to prevent malpractice claims. Being aware of your own practice; accepting only those assignments for which you are prepared; following policies, protocols, and procedures; and properly documenting care are among the most important.
- A legal action may include a process of discovery, dropping the action, settlement out of court, or a trial.
- Nurses may be called as witnesses in trials because of personal knowledge of the case (witness to fact) or because of their expertise in a particular area (expert witness). You must understand both your rights and your obligations regarding legal action before giving a deposition or testimony.

NCLEX-STYLE PRACTICE QUESTIONS

1. To be an effective advocate for a client, the nurse must give safe and effective care in accordance with what?
   A. The State Board of Licensure
   B. The office of the Chief Nursing Officer (CNO) of the employing facility
   C. The National Council of State Boards of Nursing (NCSBN)
   D. The Nurse Practice Act

2. As a new nurse, you help a coworker put a combative client who is a danger to himself and others in restraints before getting an order. What may you be guilty of doing?
   A. Assault
   B. Illegal detainment
   C. Battery
   D. Unsupervised detention

3. You discover that a primary care provider has ordered a very large dose of a pain management medication for one of your clients. What should you do?
   A. Call the primary care provider.
   B. Notify the pharmacy.
   C. Hold the medication and chart not given.
   D. Give the medication and chart your concerns.

4. You stop at the scene of a motor vehicle accident. After identifying yourself, what actions are appropriate? (Select all that apply.)
   A. You must know the Good Samaritan Laws in your state.
   B. You can offer to help but you cannot insist.
   C. After assisting, you can leave the scene to get help.
   D. You cannot be held liable unless there is gross negligence.

REFERENCES

Agency for Health Research and Quality. (2017). *Glossary, "F."* Retrieved May 16, 2017, from https://psnet.ahrq.gov/glossary/f

Anonymous. (1997). Court case: A failure to communicate. *Nursing, 97,* 27(2), 32.

Dictionary.com. (2017). *"Law" and "Ethics."* Retrieved May, 16, 2017, from http://dictionary.com

Guido, G. W. (2013). *Legal and ethical issues in nursing* (6th ed.). Upper Saddle River, NJ: Prentice Hall.

Lectric Law Library. (2017). *Gross negligence.* Retrieved May 16 2017, from www.lectlaw.com/def/g020.htm

Minnesota Statutes. (2003). Section 604A.0 1. retrieved May 31, 2018, from https://www.revisor.mn.gov/statutes/?id=604a.01.

National Coordinating Council on Medication Error Reporting and Prevention. (2017). *Recommendations to reduce medication errors associated with verbal medication orders and prescriptions.* Retrieved May 16, 2017, from http://www.nccmerp.org/recommendations-reduce-medication-errors-associated-verbal-medication-orders-and-prescriptions

Newman, A. B. (2016). Critical care nurses' knowledge of confidentiality legislation. *American Journal of Critical Care, 25*(3), 222–227. doi:10.4037/ajcc2016518

Physician Orders for Life-Sustaining Treatments. (2017). *POLST.* Retrieved May 18, 2017, from http://polst.org/wp-content/uploads/2017/05/2017.03.27-POLST-Paradigm-Handout.pdf

The powers that be: Understanding powers of attorney, conservators, guardianship and more: a primer. (2017). *ISNA Bulletin, 43*(3), 10–15.

University of Washington School of Medicine. (2014). Informed consent. In *Ethics in Medicine.* Retrieved May 18, 2017, from http://depts.washington.edu/bioethx/topics/consent.html

Vermont Statutes. (1969). *Title 12, Chapter 23; SS 519* (1968).

Ethical Concerns in Nursing Practice

After completing this chapter, you should be able to:

1. Discuss the concepts of ethics and morality and how they are applied in the healthcare field.
2. Explain how nurses and their clients benefit from an understanding of bioethical issues.
3. Describe four ethical theories that may be used to guide ethical decision making and give an example of each applied to a nursing situation.
4. Explain the ways in which personal religious and philosophic viewpoints, the Codes for Nurses, and documents addressing clients' rights are used as a basis for ethical decision making.
5. Analyze ways sociocultural and occupational factors affect ethical decision making for nurses.
6. Outline a framework for ethical decision making.
7. Discuss how ethical standards are associated with commitment to the client, personal excellence, and the nursing as a profession.
8. Analyze how ethics affect specific work situations, particularly your obligations related to a chemically impaired nursing colleague.
9. Analyze the multiple factors in right-to-die issues, including physician-assisted suicide and the difference between active and passive euthanasia.
10. Analyze the various points of view related to withholding and withdrawing treatment.
11. Discuss the ethics that establish the foundation for providing clients with informed consent and involving them in decisions regarding treatment.
12. Discuss the importance of recognizing and adhering to boundaries with clients.

Advance directive
Autonomy
Beneficence
Bioethics
Boundary violations
Chemically impaired professional
Code of ethics
Cultural relativism

Deontology
Distributive justice
Ethical dilemma
Ethics
Euthanasia—negative and positive
Fidelity
Futile
Justice

(continued on page 270)

KEY TERMS   *(continued)*

Living will	Standard of best interest
Moral distress	Theory of social justice
Morals	Utilitarianism
Nonmaleficence	Values
Paternalism	Values clarification
Rationing of healthcare	Values conflict
Right	Veracity
Right to die	Whistle-blowing
Right to refuse treatment	Withdrawing/withholding treatment

Stegen & Sowerby Stories: Part 1

Kristen, 25 years old, started her first job out of training in the operating room (OR) at a local hospital. During the routine screenings for hire, it was discovered that Kristen was hepatitis C positive, meaning that she was carrying the disease. This did not preclude her employment, and she started working. Unfortunately, shortly after hire, Kristen had become addicted to drugs. She saw an opportunity to have easy access to medications by injecting the drugs labeled for client use and refilling the syringes with sterile water prior to the patient receiving the medications (Brown, 2010).

What are the legal and ethical violations in this scenario? What are the legal ramifications for Kristen? What are the legal ramifications for the hospital? Do you think anyone in the OR noticed unusual behavior in Kristen?

Have you ever overheard a physician discussing with a client's family whether to start an older comatose client on a series of antibiotics to treat pneumonia? Or have you been present at a nurses' conference at which attendees discussed an order to stop enteral therapy on a client who has shown no response to stimuli? Or perhaps you have observed a staff nurse leaving the unit after completing the shift with a pocket full of pens, Band-Aids, or tape. These are examples of situations that involve moral and ethical judgments—judgments as to what is right, what is wrong, and what one ought to do in a given situation.

Ethics in organizations can be viewed from two different perspectives, individualistic or communal (Brown, 2015). While each individual is responsible for his/her decisions and actions, as part of an institution, the organization is "partially responsible for the behavior of their members" (Brown, 2015, para 4). This is especially true for nursing and healthcare organizations where situations that call for judgments requiring serious consideration of what is right or best for our clients, their families, and the community are impossible to escape. Although some of these decisions can be based on clinical knowledge, many will require additional expertise in the realm of ethical and moral decision making.

Fortunately, there are guiding principles to assist us in the process. As you work at the process of applying critical thinking to your ethical nursing decisions, look seriously at the assumptions that have been made. Assumptions often are based on ethical and moral values.

All of these are good reasons why we need knowledge of ethics, morality, and the process of ethical decision making.

Bioethics is defined in the Merriam-Webster Online Dictionary (2017a) as a "discipline dealing with the ethical implications of biologic research and applications, especially in medicine." This area of study is also called biomedical ethics because of its association with medical practice. It is a subdiscipline within the larger discipline of ethics, which is the philosophic study of morality, or what is right and what is wrong. The word bioethics was coined by the biochemist Van Rensselaer Potter (1911–2001), a researcher at the University of Wisconsin in Madison, in 1970.

Today more than ever, nurses and their clients need to keep pace with the technologic changes occurring in healthcare. It should be read, studied, and discussed within the framework of the information concerning ethical decision making. It is not possible in this text to explore the topic of ethics and bioethics in depth; however, we provide an overview of the topic in this chapter. To assist you in understanding some of the terminology used in the discussion of ethics (and as a point of reference), we have provided a list of definitions in Table 8.1. We also discuss some of the approaches to ethical decision making and give examples of its

Table 8.1   Terminology Related to Ethics

Term	Definition
Absolutism	View that there is only one correct moral principle or code for which there are no exceptions
Altruism	Behavior motivated by concern for the well-being of others and that is intended to benefit others
Amoral	State or quality of being indifferent to morality
Categorical imperative	From Immanuel Kant's ethics, the view that for an act to be moral, it must be able to be applied to everyone
Cultural relativism	View that there is enormous variety in the mores and morals of people in different cultures and times, and no single cultural position is correct
Descriptive ethics	Focuses on what people actually do in given situations
Ethics	Specific area of study of morality that concentrates on human conduct and human values (from the Greek ethos, meaning character, habitual uses, and customs)
Ethical/moral egoism	When one considers only his or her own good or self-interest
Ethical/moral nihilism	View that no universally valid or true moral principles exist
Ethical/moral objectivism	View that universally valid and true moral principles exist
Ethical/moral relativism	View that no universally valid or true moral principles exist but, rather, that all moral principles are valid relative to culture or individual choice
Ethical/moral skepticism	View that we cannot know whether there are universally valid moral principles
Ethics of care	Focuses on those traits valued in intimate personal relationships, such as compassion, love, sympathy, and trust
Hedonism	View that good can be defined as that which is pleasurable
Metaethics	Deals with the extent to which moral judgments are reasonable or justifiable

(Continued)

Table 8.1   Terminology Related to Ethics (continued)

Term	Definition
Moral	Generally accepted as dealing with what is good and what is bad, what is right and what is wrong
Moral agent	Person capable of making distinctions between what is right and what is wrong
Moral philosophy	Branch of philosophy that examines beliefs and assumptions about the nature of certain human values
Moral thought	Individual cognitive evaluation of right and wrong, good and bad
Naturalism	View of moral judgment that regards ethics as dependent on human nature and psychology
Normative ethics	Examines individual rights and obligations as well as common good
Philosophy	Intense and critical examination of beliefs and assumptions (from the Greek words *philia*, meaning love or friendship, and *sophia*, meaning wisdom)
Practical ethics	Use of ethical theory and analysis to examine commonly occurring moral problems
Situational ethics	View that one's actions are governed entirely by the situation rather than by principles or rules
Subjectivism	View that moral principles are applicable to the agent alone, that what is right for one might not be right for another
Virtue ethics	Places emphasis on the agents or people who make choices and take actions

application in healthcare. Some direct application to your performance as a nurse and to personal decision making is provided. As you read about ethical/bioethical issues and conflicts, and discuss them in your classroom or with a classmate, respect others by listening carefully to what they have to say and honestly attempting to understand their positions and their accompanying values and beliefs. Only by considering all aspects of an issue can we seek and find understanding for ourselves.

UNDERSTANDING THE CONCEPT OF ETHICS AND BIOETHICS

Since the time of Socrates and the Golden Age of Greece, philosophers have attempted to provide a logical approach to the questions of human conduct that arise in our lives. Why do we act the way we do? What constitutes good and evil, ethical and unethical behavior? What are the factors that result in various cultures embracing different values? How are we to be guided in our decision making? How will the ethics of care affect our professional performance?

When we talk about **morals**, we are referring to the basic standards for what we consider right and wrong that typically are based on religious beliefs, social influences (including education), group norms, culture, and life experiences. If we are of good moral character, we would not steal from a neighbor or cheat on an examination. This word, derived from the Latin *mores*, means custom or habit.

In the formal sense, ethics is a branch of philosophy (the study of beliefs and assumptions) referred to as moral philosophy. The word *ethics* is derived from the Greek term *ethos*, which means customs, habitual usage, conduct, and character. Ethics offers a formal process for answering the question about what one ought to do in a given situation. Understanding some of the basic ethical principles and guidelines assists us in making logical and appropriate decisions. It helps us identify the motives for action and define relationships between human beings.

As we work at sorting out those behaviors that we typically describe as good, **right**, desirable, honorable, fitting, or proper (or the direct opposite), we also are dealing with values. Perceptions are based on values, and each of us (and each society) has a differing set of values. Generally speaking, **values** are important and enduring beliefs or ideals shared by the members of a culture about what is good or desirable and what is not that exert major influence on the behavior of an individual and serve as broad guidelines in all situations (Business Dictionary, 2017). Values are most commonly derived from societal norms, religion, and family orientation, and they provide the framework for making decisions about the actions we take every day. For example, if you were born in the United States, you may have been raised to believe it is unethical to restrict women's right to vote. Those in another society may have been raised to believe that this is the ethical (and logical) way to structure public life.

We all have been in a situation in which we experienced a **values conflict**. This occurs when we must choose between two things, both of which are important to us. For example, if you are a new mother, you probably value caring for your child on a full-time basis; however, if you also must help provide support for the family and your values support the concept that this is your responsibility, leaving your child to go to work results in a values conflict.

Most of the time we do not think about our values—we just accept them. We are most likely to think about them when we have a difficult decision to make, when something goes wrong, or when we find ourselves in a conflict because of differing values. In nursing, we work with a diverse client population and therefore are exposed to a variety of values and ethical standards. The need to give conscientious care to all clients often forces us to examine the principles in which we believe.

The process of becoming more conscious of and naming what one values or considers worthy is known as **values clarification**. We examine what we believe is good, bad, beautiful, worthy, meaningful, and so forth and explore the process of determining our personal values. This increases our self-awareness or understanding of ourselves and assists us in making choices. It facilitates decision making, because we have a better grasp of our own value systems.

Having a good understanding of yourself will be helpful when you are faced with an ethical dilemma. If you spend a few minutes checking definitions of an ethical dilemma on your computer, you will find a variety of definitions. Some would suggest that it involves choosing between two unfavorable alternatives; others would say it requires choosing from among two or more morally accepted courses of action when one choice prevents selecting the other. We define **ethical dilemma** broadly: any situation in which guiding moral principles cannot determine which course of action is right or wrong. Examples abound: who should receive a needed heart transplant—a young 34-year-old male with a wife and two children or a 78-year-old gentleman who also has diabetes? Should assisted suicide be an alternative for an individual experiencing great pain and suffering from terminal stages of cancer when the focus of healthcare is to save lives? Should abortion be an alternative for a 14-year-old impregnated as the result of rape?

Ethical dilemmas usually have no perfect solution, and those making decisions may find themselves in direct conflict with another. Should you experience such a situation, be constructive (rather than destructive) in the methods you choose to work toward resolving the differences. Listen carefully without interrupting, and be willing to hear what others have to say. Seek clarification using gentle questioning. Respect cultural differences, and be attentive to body language. Explain the context of your point of view, and try to picture the other person's perspective of what you are saying.

The History of the Evolution of Bioethics

A number of factors contributed to the interest in and the development of bioethics. Evolving in the last decades of the 20th century, awareness of bioethical issues was heightened by abuse of human subjects who were unknowingly coerced into participating in research and by the rights movement for self-determination that occurred in the 1950s and 1960s. Media addressing the topic drew attention to practices that many believed were wrong.

Some would suggest that the birth of bioethics occurred with the publication of a magazine article in *Life* titled "They Decide Who Lives, Who Dies" (Alexander, November 9, 1962). This article told the story of a group of individuals in Seattle whose duty it was to select clients for the first hemodialysis program to treat chronic renal failure. Many more clients needed treatment than could be accommodated; those not selected would likely die. This event was followed several years later by an article about the ethics of medical research that provided the impetus for examining these issues.

Soon after, centers for research in bioethics emerged, most notably the Institute of Society, Ethics, and the Life Sciences, located in Hastings-on-Hudson, New York (often called The Hastings Center), which was founded in 1969, and the Kennedy Institute of Ethics, located at Georgetown University in Washington, DC. The Kennedy Institute of Ethics, founded in 1971 by Joseph and Rose Kennedy, is a teaching and research center that provides ethical perspectives on major policy issues. It boasts the largest university-based faculty in the world devoted to research and teaching biomedical ethics. Journals such as the *Hastings Center Report* and the *Journal of Medicine and Philosophy* have come into being, and an encyclopedia, *The Encyclopedia of Bioethics*, has been published. Web sites devoted to the topic of bioethics are so numerous that they cannot be listed in the confines of this textbook. Today, bioethicists are included in many important task forces and special committees.

Entire textbooks have been devoted to bioethical considerations. Initially, most of these were written for medical students, but now just as many are written for nursing students. Some nursing programs include a course in ethics and bioethics in the curriculum. This chapter can only introduce the topic and, we hope, broaden your perspective and deepen your interest. You are encouraged to read about and study these issues further as they affect your nursing practice.

Most of the bioethical issues have evolved as a product of the technologic advances occurring in medical practice and research and were not a concern 50 years ago. Table 8.2 lists some of the significant medical milestones that have occurred since 1920, some of which we have come to take for granted (eg, antibiotics and deoxyribonucleic acid, that is, DNA). You readily can see that in 1960 there was no quest for human organs or critical decisions regarding the life status of a possible donor. We were not able to fertilize ova outside the human body and transfer the fertilized eggs into a woman's uterus until 1978. Certain

Table 8.2   Some Medical Milestones of the 1900s

When	Who	What
1928	Alexander Fleming	This British bacteriologist noticed that one of his culture plates had grown a fungus and the colonies of staphylococci around the edge of the mold had been destroyed. Because this fungus was a member of the *Penicillium* group, he named it penicillin.
1938	Howard Florey and Ernst Chain	These two pathologists took up the work of Fleming and demonstrated the efficacy of penicillin in treating infection. In 1945, the three were jointly awarded the Nobel Prize for Physiology of Medicine.
1951	Forrest Bird	The first Bird breathing device was developed (Bird Mark 7), and breathing treatment machines were introduced. Inhalation (respiratory) therapy rapidly developed as a health profession (Pilbeam, 1998).
1953	James Watson and Francis Crick	These two geneticists deciphered DNA's double-helix structure. Researchers began to focus on the internal functioning of the cell, and molecular biology developed as a specialty.
1954	Physicians in Boston	Transplanted the kidney from one twin to the other, thus moving kidney transplantation from the experimental stage it had occupied since 1902. Kidney transplantations have been the most successful of transplantations (Kidney Transplantation: Past, Present & Future, n.d.)
1955	Jonas Salk	Public health officials began immunizing children against polio with Dr. Salk's vaccine, which contained dead virus.
1957	Albert Sabin	A polio vaccine was developed, which was based on weakened live virus that could be administered orally.
1967	Christiaan Barnard	This South African surgeon performed the first human heart transplant.
1972	British engineers	The computed tomography (CT) scanner, which assembles thousands of x-ray images into a highly detailed picture of the brain, was developed in England. It was later expanded to provide scans of the entire body.
1978	English physicians	The process of in vitro fertilization (IVF) was developed. Louise Brown became the first person to be conceived in a test tube, and then implanted into her mother's uterus.
1979	World Health Organization	This group declared that smallpox had been eradicated 2 years after the last known case was identified. This occurred because of worldwide immunization against the disease.
1981	Physicians in San Francisco and New York	Doctors from these two cities reported the first cases of what would later become known as acquired immunodeficiency syndrome (AIDS). To date, no cure exists.
1982	The U.S. Food and Drug Administration	The first drug developed with recombinant DNA was approved by this group. It was a form of human insulin; its availability saves thousands of lives.
1995	Duke University surgeons	Hearts from genetically altered pigs were transplanted into baboons, proving that cross-species transplantations can be done. Transmission of animal viruses to humans emerges as a serious concern.
1998	James Thomas and scientists from University of Wisconsin—Madison	Culture embryonic stem cells (cells that are the parent cells of all body tissues) from donated human blastocysts, opening the door to potential repair or replacement of diseased tissues or organs (All About Popular Issues, 2002–2010).

Source: Material for this table was gathered from an article by Sherwin B. Nuland, Time Special Issue, Fall 1996 except as otherwise noted.

lifesaving machines (eg, ventilators) and miracle drugs (eg, some of the chemotherapeutic agents used today) were not available to offer extension of life. Technologies such as magnetic resonance imaging, which gives us information about the structure of tissues and allows for early diagnosis and treatment, were not available. Positron emission tomography was to follow. As advances occur in medical practice and technology, we must challenge ourselves to think through our own beliefs and feelings about these practices, especially as they relate to quality of life and patients' choices.

Major Areas Where Bioethics Is Applied

The bioethical issues surrounding the delivery of healthcare grow in number each year, constantly changing and taking on new scope and proportions. For years, we have debated issues related to birth and death; today, those topics represent just the tip of the iceberg. Of equal or greater concern are such matters as universal access to healthcare and insurance for all, **rationing of healthcare**, cost containment and quality of care, where and how federal dollars should be spent with regard to the nation's health, and the obligation of others to assist the homeless. Our media thrive on issues created by recent biomedical research, such as concerns regarding stem cell research. Biotechnology opens many doors, and as more possibilities become realities, new issues must be addressed. How far should a society go in memory boosting or its suppression? Is it appropriate to carry out sex selection? What about cloning? Should assisted reproduction be regulated? To what extent should drugs be used on children to control their behavior? Should we extend life through age retardation? These are but a few of the questions for which our society must find answers.

Each year, the percentage of America's gross domestic product (GDP) spent on healthcare increases. The Centers for Medicare and Medicaid Services (CMS) estimate that the national health spending grew 5.8% to reach $3.2 trillion or $9,990 per person in 2015, raising the health share of GDP to 17.8%. Healthcare expenditure continues to rise faster than the GDP, in part, because of government healthcare subsidies and the aging of the baby boomer population (CMS, n.d.).

Because of lifestyle changes and medical breakthroughs, more people today live to reach old age, thus placing a greater burden on an already stressed system. Life expectancy has increased 1 to 2 years in each recent decade. In the United States, the life expectancy for females born in 2013 is 81.2 years and for males it is 76.4, compared with 47 years at the beginning of the 20th century (Centers for Disease Control [CDC], 2015). Diseases such as Alzheimer's and multiple sclerosis, for which cures are still being sought, have increased in prevalence. With globalization have come new threats to our well-being, such as that created by the H1N1 influenza pandemic and the Ebola virus.

New technologies have led to treatments that were not available even 5 years ago. Rather than decreasing healthcare needs, the new technologies have resulted in increased needs because these specialized services are in high demand. Many treatments require use of technologies so expensive that they are priced beyond what an individual or family can afford without help from third-party payers. Finding new and better ways to treat life-threatening conditions challenges medical researchers, and the treatments that become available often invite debate among bioethicists. For example, stem cell research is forcing our society to make distinctions about life's beginnings that have enormous scientific and religious implications.

> **Critical Thinking Activity: Values in Conflict**
> Identify situations you might confront in nursing in which your personal religious or philosophic values would be involved. What would be the consequences of following the dictates of your value system? Do conflicts exist between your value system and actions required by the situation? If so, how will you recognize the differences and how will you deal with them? Are there any other alternatives? What might they be?

BASIC ETHICAL CONCEPTS

The most frequently addressed ethical concepts include autonomy, beneficence and nonmaleficence, justice, fidelity, and veracity. Let's examine each one.

Autonomy

Autonomy involves the right of self-determination or choice, independence, and freedom. It comes from the Latin *auto*, meaning self, and *nomy*, which means control. Many consider autonomy to include respect for the individual with the expectation that each person will be treated as unique and equal to other people. Other words often associated with autonomy include dignity, inherent worth, self-reliance, individualism, and power.

In today's healthcare delivery system, it is important to respect clients' rights to make decisions about and for themselves, even when we do not agree with those decisions (rights are discussed later in this chapter). This is closely tied to informed consent because it requires that clients be provided clear and sufficient information to make good decisions for themselves. Even when the information is provided, you may have difficulty accepting the client's decision, for example, the decision of a new mother, who is a Jehovah's Witness and whose life is in danger because of blood loss, to refuse to have a blood transfusion.

As with most other rights, there may be restrictions on the right to choose—autonomy does not mean that individuals can do anything they want. When one person's autonomy interferes with another individual's rights, health, or well-being, limitations may be imposed. For example, should an individual have the right to choose a certain expensive treatment if that choice would unjustly deny money to another person for another treatment; should an expensive bone marrow transplant be administered when the physician does not believe a positive outcome is realistic? Does the autonomy of a client with a highly communicable disease take precedence over the right of the community not to be exposed to the disease? And if rights are to be limited, who defines and enforces those limitations?

For some individuals, autonomy may be less important than values related to the family and community. Is this acceptable? Who decides how much autonomy is enough? Once again, we must consider the idea that autonomy is predominantly a Western value. Many cultures have deeply held values about the family, rather than the individual, as decision maker. So what happens when the family decision is not what health providers think is best for the client?

Communication in Action 8.1: Exercising Autonomy

Joan Wagner often studied with a group of classmates as they prepared for examinations. An examination on medications and dosages was scheduled, and Joan believed she would profit most from studying independently because study sessions often strayed from the content being studied. Additionally, her time was very limited on the evening study was planned. As the group discussed study plans, Joan said, "I really appreciate the opportunity to study with you, but I believe I need to approach this material individually. I need to be sure I can independently master some of the areas related to dosage. Perhaps we can study together later for the content of our next unit." In addressing her own needs, Joan expressed autonomy.

Beneficence and Nonmaleficence

Beneficence comes from the word beneficent, meaning doing or producing good, especially performing acts of kindness and charity (Merriam-Webster Online Dictionary, 2017b). The concept of beneficence extends from promoting good to **nonmaleficence** (the prevention of intentional harm). As far back as Hippocrates, physicians were entreated to do no harm. Florence Nightingale stated that the client should be no worse for having been nursed. The *Code of Ethics for Nurses with Interpretive Statements* (ANA, 2015) addresses this issue when it clearly delineates the steps to be taken to remove harm or evil. Some examples include reporting unethical practices of a colleague to appropriate authorities or expressing concern to the individual who is engaged in practices that result in substandard practice.

In healthcare, we recognize that sometimes we unintentionally do harm to individuals. For example, the discomfort associated with debridement of wounds, adverse drug reactions, and the side effects of such treatments as irradiation and chemotherapy for cancer are certainly harmful to the individuals who experience them. In many cases, given the alternatives, a client will opt to have the treatment (eg, chemotherapy) in spite of the adverse effects. The ethical mandate is that we refrain from intentionally inflicting harm. Sometimes, it is difficult to accept that a side effect of a particular treatment might result in harm to a client. Concern for the possible, although rare, reaction to vaccination for pertussis (whooping cough) is but one example.

Even more problematic is the continued use of medical therapies when they are **futile**, that is, do not have the potential for creating a positive outcome but clearly have the potential for adverse outcomes. Additional chemotherapy in the client with terminal cancer may fall into this category. Deciding when a treatment is medically futile is a physician's decision, but there are many areas of gray in which one physician might identify a treatment as futile and another suggest that there is at least some possibility of effectiveness. Futility is discussed in greater detail later in this chapter. *Good* is a general term of approval or commendation, and may be defined as that which is "of a favorable character or tendency" (Merriam-Webster Online Dictionary, 2017d). Thus, we tend to think of it as something that promotes life, development, and fulfillment. We view it as good when a friend makes a quick recovery from surgery, when a child graduates from high school or college, or when aging parents are able to take that long-awaited trip they have been planning for years.

It is sometimes difficult to decide who will determine what is good for a specific person in a specific situation. In most instances, we expect that people will make their own decisions about what is good for them (autonomy). But who decides for the infant regarding procedures such as immunizations that inflict some degree of pain and a low risk of side effects, but have long-lasting benefits? Who decides for the individual who is unconscious or mentally incompetent?

Another problem centers on how we identify what is good. There are often competing values that challenge our concept of good. Is the ongoing support of life good if that life is filled with pain? If giving good care to one client means that lesser care will be given to another (a situation encountered more frequently in today's healthcare environment), how can we defend such an action? What if giving good care means violating good nursing economics (ie, cost containment)? There are no simple answers, and the answers are not the same for everyone.

The issue of sanctity of life is of major concern in the healthcare arena. Some would argue that all life is good. Others would adamantly assert that life is not good when the quality of life is greatly diminished; this latter belief has led to serious discussions regarding euthanasia and assisted suicide, has supported the establishment of such groups as the Hemlock Society, and has resulted in a few states legally permitting assisted suicide.

According to the NHS (2014) Web site, there are four primary arguments against assisted suicide: (1) on religious grounds, (2) it violates medical ethics, (3) we are on slippery slope that could create unintended consequences, and (4) we should be doing better palliative care and are therefore failing the client if he or she chooses suicide (NHS, 2014).

The argument in favor of assisted suicide is twofold: (1) an ethics-based assertion that autonomy and freedom of choice are fundamental rights and (2) passive euthanasia is already widespread so we should attempt to regulate it (NHS, 2014). Each person must evaluate his or her own values and beliefs in order to decide being for or against assisted suicide.

Another example of a situation in which quality-of-life issues emerge can be seen in an instance in which parents are advised at a prenatal check-up that the fetus has a life-compromising condition such as meningomyelocele. The parents must weigh the quality of the life and the complications inherent in the meningomyelocele in relationship to beliefs in the sanctity of all life when making decisions about terminating the pregnancy. Surrounding all issues regarding the sanctity of life are religious views and values that look upon all life as sacred. Certainly arguments regarding the sanctity of life play a major role in discussions regarding abortion, whether supported by religious beliefs or personal value systems. The sanctity of life also affects our personal beliefs about capital punishment.

Closely aligned to the issue of sanctity of life is the concept of medical futility mentioned briefly earlier in the chapter. Medical futility is a term applied to situations in which interventions are judged to have no medical benefit or in which the chance for success is low (Segen's Medical Dictionary, 2011). This concept is often applied to cardiopulmonary resuscitation and to do not resuscitate (DNR) orders but also relates to situations in which a client exists in a persistent vegetative state. The issue is further complicated by the fact that no set definition of the concept exists and that personal values affect the determination of futility. Should the decision regarding futility of treatment be different based on age, cost, or the ability to pay? Thus, it can be said that although the topics of the sanctity of life and medical futility are widely discussed, there exists little consensus about them. As a nurse, you will often encounter difficult situations in the care of your clients in which opposing values play against one another. Understanding your own values, which may change over time, is important in these situations.

> ### *Communication in Action 8.2:* *A Case of Unwashed Hands*
>
> You enter the women's lounge and notice a fellow healthcare provider is there. After using the toilet, that individual walks to the door to leave the area without first washing her hands. You said, "Hey, Judy! You were heading out without washing your hands before returning to work. You must have a lot on your mind this morning!" Preventing harm through speaking up reflects an ethical value.

Justice

Justice, sometimes referred to as fairness, refers to the quality of being just or fair; conformity to truth, fact, or sound reason; or treating like cases similarly (equity) and looks at the concepts of moral rightness in action or attitude (The Free Dictionary, 2017). We must ask, "How is fairness defined?" Does fairness mean that people should always be treated the same? In terms of access to healthcare, is it just for one person to receive more resources than another receives? If so, what makes it just, and how does that relate to the distribution of scarce medical resources? Does age make a difference in what we consider just? Should it? Does justice imply that the government should provide the resources or services individuals are unable to provide for themselves? Can we measure fairness in any objective sense? What should occur when one person's rights interfere with the rights of another? The object of **distributive justice** is to distribute rewards and punishments to everyone according to his/her merits or demerits (The Free Dictionary, 2017). The expectation is that all individuals have an equal opportunity to access scarce resources and healthcare organizations and health plans will provide to individual recipients the care and service each is due. This has been a major issue in the United States as Congress struggles to establish healthcare for all (see Chapter 6). Several criteria have been used to define the just distribution of limited medical resources: need, equity, societal contribution, ability to pay, effort, and merit. The use of these criteria is controversial. Need involves known medical need, not elective procedures. Equity addresses trying to distribute equally to all in need. Contribution considers what an individual might be expected to give to society at a future date. (This approach has met with concern over labeling those who are disabled or unable to contribute as less worthy and thus can be discriminated against.) Ability to pay is self-explanatory, but to deny needed health services because an individual cannot pay contradicts the concepts of charitableness that exist in our society. Client effort deals with a client's adherence or nonadherence to medical advice. For example, should a client who refuses to quit smoking be eligible for a heart transplant? Merit (the good to be received) addresses the potential that exists for benefit from the additional investment of limited health resources, for example, the investment of federal dollars in cancer treatment. Who will decide about the future potential for a current investment? These six criteria have not always provided a strong basis for decision making, and the ethical issues related to allocation of scarce resources promise to become more complex in the coming years as people live longer and technology provides more alternatives.

Fidelity

Fidelity refers to the obligation to be faithful to the agreements, commitments, and responsibilities that one has made to oneself and others, both implicitly and explicitly. Fidelity is the foundation of the concept of accountability that we hear about so often in nursing today. What are the responsibilities of healthcare personnel to individuals, employers, the government, society, and each other? When these responsibilities conflict, which should take priority? In reality, which do take priority? Are nurses obligated to provide care to all clients? Under what circumstances, if any, might this be challenged? What are the nurse's promises to society? Would it also cover areas such as competence? Abiding by institutional policies? Operating within the profession's code of ethics?

Disasters are examples of when nurses experience a conflict between obligations to work and obligations to family. What should the nurse do during a disaster? The nurse has a professional responsibility to report for duty and provide care for the community in their time of need but the nurse also has a responsibility to his or her family. The *ANA Code of Ethics* (2015) is conflicting since provision two states that the nurse's primary responsibility is the client (community) but provision five states that the nurse owes the same duty to self as to others. During a disaster, the nurse will need to assess and prioritize needs of the community against his or her own family to determine the correct course of action. Another situation that often challenges us in healthcare is that of confidentiality. Is maintaining confidentiality a moral/ethical issue as well as a legal issue related to fidelity? Are there any instances when it is acceptable to violate the principle of confidentiality? If you are working with an impaired colleague, is it appropriate and ethical to violate a confidential situation in the interest of client well-being? We discuss this issue in detail later in the chapter.

Veracity

Veracity refers to telling the truth or not intentionally deceiving or misleading clients. From childhood, we are all admonished to tell the truth and to avoid lying. When we are children, this seems straightforward. As we become adults, we see more instances in which the choices are less clear. For example, do you tell the truth (veracity) when you know the truth will cause harm to an individual (beneficence vs. nonmaleficence)? Do you tell a lie when it would make someone less anxious and afraid? You might see this as beneficence (doing good), but then you have abandoned the principle of veracity. Failing to be honest is considered by some as leading to a slippery slope, because when we conceal the truth from a client, it suggests to all others involved (eg, family members, friends, nursing assistants, housekeeping staff) that health practitioners lie. This deception is later remembered, and the concept that one cannot rely on health professionals pervades. In other words, it diminishes one's esteem and reliability and erodes trust, which is an essential element of the nurse–client relationship. Lying also diminishes oneself. Lying can change your concept of yourself as an honest person and may adversely affect future behavior if practice in lying makes it easier to lie in the future. Not all societies value telling the truth to the ill person. In some societies, such as Japan, the client is to be protected from bad news or information that would provoke anxiety. Therefore, to lie and provide false reassurance may be considered doing good (beneficence) and avoiding harm (nonmaleficence). When health professionals relate to families with a different view of truth telling to the ill person, their values may come in conflict.

Truth Telling and Healthcare Providers

The issue of whether to share specific information with a client may not carry the emotional and bioethical impact that one experiences with concerns such as euthanasia, but it is often encountered in the healthcare environment. Although informed consent has forced a more straightforward approach between the physician and client, the problem of having the client fully understand the outcome of care still exists. Sometimes, the question about telling the client the expected outcome of care results from a request made by a close relative, but most of the time, it results from the persistence of past medical practices.

In such instances, the physician operates in a paternalistic role in relation to the client. Under this model of care, the locus of decision making is moved away from the client and resides with the physician. "Benefit and do no harm to the patient" is the dictum often cited as the ethical basis for this approach. It rationalizes that complete knowledge of his or her condition would place greater stress on the client. More recent discussions of medical ethics explore the rights of clients, particularly their right to make their own medical decisions. These discussions emphasize that in our pluralistic society, which also has fostered medical specialization to keep up with advances in knowledge and technology, physicians may be unable to perceive the best interests of their clients and to act accordingly.

Physicians do not agree on how much information should be provided to clients regarding their conditions. We usually experience a major controversy relating to this issue when a client has a terminal diagnosis such as cancer. Physicians may feel concerned that sharing bad news will result in unhappiness, anxiety, depression, and fear, and that the client suffering from a terminal illness will give up. In some cultures, such as Japan, this approach is widely considered appropriate, and both physicians and families strongly believe that those who are ill should be protected from bad news.

Physicians who argue the other side of the issue state that there exists a common moral obligation to tell the truth. They believe that the anxiety of not knowing the accurate diagnosis is at least as great as knowing the truth, especially if the truth is shared in a humane manner. These physicians also argue that one needs to have control over one's life and, if the news is bad, to have time to get personal affairs in order.

Regulations regarding informed consent and more aggressive treatment for all life-threatening conditions have minimized situations in which clients are not provided full knowledge of their condition. However, these situations still arise. Sometimes, healthcare providers are challenged as to the best ethical and legal approach when a family is from a different cultural background and strongly disagrees with giving full information to a client.

Another instance of veracity and beneficence coming into conflict is in the obstetric area of the hospital and deals with sharing information with the parents of a newborn who is critically ill or who has a malformation. Sometimes, physicians want to spare the mother unpleasant news until the mother is stronger. This occurs frequently enough for obstetric nurses to have labeled it "spare-the-mother syndrome." In some instances, the physician may want to delay giving information until suspicions can be validated. If the doctor is waiting for the return of laboratory tests to confirm suspicions of genetic abnormalities, several days may be required. If good communication exists between the nurse and physician, so that the nurse is well informed, the nurse can provide emotional support and meet the client's need for information.

Another situation in which sharing the truth may be a concern occurs when a parent is diagnosed with a degenerative disease (such as Huntington disease) for which there is no cure and that is an autosomal dominant trait (ie, there is a 50% chance that an offspring also will develop the disease). Should this information be shared with the offspring? Because there is

Communication in Action 8.3: To Tell or Not to Tell

You assessed your client every hour because of elevated blood pressure. The fourth time you checked it during your shift, you noted that the reading was 195/105, more elevated than previously. The client asked you, "How was the reading this time?" You replied, "This time I got a reading higher than before. I am going to check it again in 15 minutes and, in the meantime, notify your physician of my findings. I will return in just a few minutes." The choice of the nurse was to tell the truth to the client even if it caused anxiety. The nurse also knew that the client's anxiety may have been increased by feeling that information was being denied to him or by the uncertainty of not knowing. He may be reassured that action was being taken.

also a 50% chance they will not develop the condition, is it wrong to compromise the individual's good life with bad news? What if the parent does not want the information shared and the physician believes it should be? Is ignorance bliss? What about the right to make informed choices and decisions?

Although to tell or not to tell (or to delay telling) is a problem that exists between client and physician, nurses often become involved. Because the nurse is in contact with the client for a more extended time, he or she may be put on the spot by the client's questions. The nurse may feel that hedging on a response compromises the ethics of nursing practice. In such instances, a conference, whether formal or impromptu, that would involve the physician, nurses, and other appropriate members of the healthcare team, may help everyone deal with the situation. The nurse who is a novice in the healthcare system should realize that anyone may initiate a client care conference, although appropriate channels of communication should be followed in organizing it.

The question of whether to tell has been applied to another issue in the healthcare delivery system in recent years. That controversy pits the rights to privacy of the individual who is human immunodeficiency virus (HIV)-positive against society's right to be protected. Many express concerns about privacy and confidentiality. If universal testing for HIV/AIDS were to be mandated, what would be next? Others argue that if healthcare providers exercise proper precautions, little danger exists. Still others would find the cost of universal testing too great to make it realistic. There is no agreement among healthcare providers, activists, civil libertarians, and all concerned citizens regarding this issue, and the controversy is certain to continue.

ETHICAL THEORIES

It is not our intent to delve with any depth into the writings of early philosophers. However, because ethical theories are mentioned frequently in the literature that deals with bioethical issues, some background information follows.

An ethical theory is a moral principle or a set of ethical concepts and moral principles that can be used to assess what is morally right or morally wrong in a given situation. Over the years, many people have called on the theories of philosophers to guide in decision making. The most widely used theories are presented in Table 8.3. You are encouraged to consider various ethical approaches and discuss with your classmates when each might be used appropriately.

Table 8.3 Major Ethical Theories and Theorists

Title of Theory (Other Names)	Theorist Associated With Work	Basic Principles of Theory
Natural Law (objectivism)	St. Thomas Aquinas (1225–1274)	Actions are morally right when they are in accord with our nature and end as human beings. Good should be promoted, evil avoided, and ethics grounded in our concern for human good.
Deontology (formalistic system, the principal system of ethics, or duty-based ethics)	Immanuel Kant (1724–1804)	Ethical decision making is based on moral rules and unchanging principles (or motivations that are derived from universal values), considered separately from the consequences. The fundamental principle is called the categorical imperative, unconditional commands that must be applied similarly in all situations without exception.
Utilitarianism (often referred to as teleology, consequentialism or situation ethics, although there are some differences)	Jeremy Bentham (1748–1832) and John Stuart Mill (1806–1873)	An act is right when it is useful in bringing about a desirable or good end. A second principle allows the end to justify the means. Fits well into Western society's values regarding work ethic and the behavioristic approach to education, philosophy, and life. Applicable to research.
Social Equity and Justice	John Rawls (1921–2002)	Sets forth principles of justice developed in 1971. Allows social and economic positions to be to everyone's advantage and open to all. Introduces a "veil of ignorance" whereby persons making choices would not have any specific information regarding those involved, thus choosing the alternative that supported the most disadvantaged person. Supports justice and equal rights for everyone.
Ideal Observer	Raymond W. Firth (1901–2002)	Requires that decisions be made from a dispassionate, disinterested, and consistent viewpoint with full information about the situation and the consequences available.

An application of utilitarianism (or consequentialism) as seen in the healthcare industry would be the justification of capitation in the managed care organization (MCO). Because the MCO pays a certain amount of money per member per month to a contracted provider, the MCO would argue that it has provided the greatest good for the greatest number of members. In public life, it would be illustrated by the public health department fully funding immunizations and providing only limited funding for episodic care of illness. Preventing communicable disease will benefit many more people in the community than will caring for individual illnesses.

An example of deontology might be applied to a situation in which all persons involved in a research study have a complete understanding (informed consent) of the study and its purposes. The participant is treated as a moral being with freedom of decision making and not simply a means to an end. The participant who has a bad result might be immediately dropped from the study because the well-being of the individual participant is considered more important than the study itself.

In applying Rawls' (1971) **theory of social justice**, one could not ethically justify using income inequalities or the ability to pay to determine a client's eligibility for access to health-care. According to social justice, the most disadvantaged person should receive the preferential benefit.

Critical Thinking Activity: Which Ethical Theory Do You Like?
Of the ethical theories provided in this chapter, select the one that is of greatest inter-est to you and describe the aspects of the theory that make it most attractive. Examine factors that bring you to this point of view. What are your biases? What are the conse-quences of supporting this ethical theory on your professional practice? Which of the theories do you believe is most critical in the healthcare arena?

APPLYING BASIC CONCEPTS

The basic ethical concepts discussed so far have many applications to the way we live our daily lives and how we interact with others, as well as how we perform as professional nurses. A major application of these concepts is how we view the rights of an individual, a concept tied to the concept of autonomy.

Rights

The discussion of ethical concepts is founded on the belief that people are entitled to certain rights or privileges. Typically, we think of a right as a just claim or entitlement, or as something that is owed to an individual on a legal, moral, or ethical basis. Most rights are based on the concept of autonomy of the individual. In common usage, this is often extended to include privileges, concessions, and freedoms. Rights are associated with many different areas of our lives. We tend to think of ourselves as having civil and political rights such as the right to assembly, to vote, to own property, and to speak freely. We have economic, social, and cultural rights, such as the right to healthcare, the right to education, and the right to work. Rights form the basis of most professional codes and legal judgments (see Chapter 7 for more discussion of rights as used in the legal sense). Legal rights include the right to due process and trial, and we have personal rights, such as the right of an individual to self-determination and privacy. Problems occur when one individual's rights come in conflict with the values of others. For example, if a client is admitted to a hospital and refuses treatment, and there is a strong indica-tion that with treatment the client could recover, should the physicians and nurses respect the client's right to self-determination? The conflict of rights provides us with many challenges and dilemmas. Although it is not within the confines of this text to discuss all of the circumstances, consider some of the major areas in which you may deal with rights in your role as a nurse.

Right to Self-Determination

Federal legislation has been passed to ensure that individual rights are respected. The Patient Self-Determination Act, also known as the Danforth amendment, is discussed in Chapters 7. This act was created because of our society's fundamental belief in the individual's right to decide. However, this act does little to recognize cultural diversity and sensibility to groups that have a unique set of values and well-defined role relationships, in which the role of family in making healthcare decisions is strongly valued.

Rights and Cultural Relativism

Cultural relativism is the principle that what an individual believes and does makes sense in terms of his or her own culture. Cultural relativism embraces the notion that groups and individuals hold different sets of values that must be respected. The principle was made popular by anthropologists who wanted to compare and contrast a wide range of cultures in a systematic and even-handed manner. It gained greater popularity when the Commission of Human Rights of the United Nations began preparing the Universal Declaration of Human Rights. The Commission struggled to formulate a statement of human rights that would take into account the individual as a member of a social group of which he or she was a part.

Individuals raised in the Western culture have difficulty imagining the prospect of performing as a suicide bomber, as witnessed in news broadcasts from the Middle East where such behaviors are viewed as heroic by some groups. Consider also female circumcision, also referred to as female genital mutilation. In some cultures, concerns about virginity, ability to attract a husband, the husband's sexual pleasure, and religious beliefs dictate that female children be circumcised. Western countries have acted to make this practice illegal, indicating that it is outside the bounds of what can be accepted as simply a cultural difference.

An example of a legal practice is *coining*, a traditional practice in China and other South East Asian countries that uses a hard object with a smooth edge to create bruising in a linear pattern in order to rid the body of negative energies. Without knowledge of this practice, it could appear to be caused by abuse.

Rights of the Unborn and the Pregnant Woman

There are many times when we grapple with whose rights should be respected. The most obvious example of this situation occurs when we consider the rights of the unborn to life versus the right of the mother to make choices regarding her own body. This issue is one that has continued to divide members of our society and is often an issue brought forth when candidates run for election or when appointments are made to the Supreme Court. The concern becomes even more contradictory, paradoxical, and convoluted when we consider that some states will permit a late-term abortion; however, in that same state, if an automobile accident occurs in which a pregnant woman is killed (thus also killing the fetus she is carrying), the offending driver can be charged with two cases of manslaughter—both the mother and the unborn child.

Right to Privacy and Right of Confidentiality

An area receiving much attention today is that of the rights of the client to privacy and the confidentiality of medical information. Privacy may be thought of as the right to be left alone or free from intrusion. It also includes the right to select desired care based on personal values and beliefs and to have control over how sensitive information is shared.

Confidentiality deals with not sharing information. This has surfaced as a major concern, because sensitive health records are now computerized and can be e-mailed, telecommunicated, faxed, or copied to various individuals or groups who may have an interest in the information. This information, which could include individually identifiable health data, might be readily available to anyone who logs on to a computer. People are concerned that exposure of personal health information, especially that related to genetic tests or communicable illnesses such as sexually transmitted infections or HIV, could result in loss of or denial of health insurance, or could result in embarrassment or discrimination in the work environment.

In 1996, Congress passed legislation in the Health Insurance Portability and Accountability Act (HIPAA). It required that steps be taken or legislation passed to ensure the privacy of individually identifiable health information.

The ANA has been concerned about this issue for some time and continues to work with other national groups on the issue of privacy and confidentiality. Table 8.4 identifies some of the activities in which the ANA has been involved related to this issue.

The ANA Code of Ethics for Nurses with Interpretive Statements (2015) and the International Council of Nurses Code of Ethics for Nurses (2012) both address the issue of client confidentiality. As a student and future nurse, remain ever mindful of your responsibility to maintain client privacy and confidentiality in all matters.

The Standard of Best Interest

When a decision must be made about a client's healthcare and the client is unable to make an informed decision, the decision may be made based on the **standard of best interest**. As the name implies, it is based on what the healthcare providers or family believes is best for that individual, taking into account tangible factors such as how the client may be harmed, how the client may benefit, and any physical and fiscal risks. This is an application of the concepts of beneficence and nonmaleficence. Such decisions may be based on the individual's expressed wishes and preferences as noted in verbal statements or by written documents such as living wills if they are available. Healthcare professionals strive to avoid unilateral decisions and work hard to educate clients and families to include them in making the best possible decisions. Unilateral decisions often imply that the decision maker knows what is best for the client. This is referred to as **paternalism**, or the deliberate treatment of people in a fatherly manner, especially by caring for them but not allowing them to have rights or responsibilities. In instances where parents have denied their children lifesaving care, the courts have occasionally overturned the parent's decision on the best-interest standard.

Ethics and Financial Compensation

Another issue receiving attention, discussion, and review is the practice of rewarding physicians (monetarily or not) for limiting care as was first seen in the advent of diagnosis-related groups under Medicare that established limits for payment for services. Recently, health maintenance organizations have come under fire for rewarding physicians who maintain lower

Table 8.4 ANA Activities Regarding Patient Privacy

Date	Ana Group	Activity
1994	House of Delegates	Approved a policy called Privacy & Confidentiality related to electronic data
1998	Board of Directors	Endorsed the Core Principles of Telehealth intended to regulate technology used to provide long-distance care and client data
1999	ANA membership	Developed position statement on privacy and confidentiality
2006	Board of Directors	Revised and accepted updated position statement on client privacy

costs of care or for penalizing those who do not. The impact this might have on nurses who are involved in the care of clients perceived to be receiving less than adequate treatment and the nurse's obligation to serve as an advocate for the client is yet to be determined. It certainly emphasizes the importance of all nurses understanding ethics and ethical principles.

FACTORS THAT INFLUENCE ETHICAL DECISION MAKING

Ethical decisions are not made in a vacuum. Many factors influence us as we seek appropriate answers to the dilemmas that we face with new problems and new realities of today challenging yesterday's answers.

In determining their own bases for making ethical decisions, some individuals rely on formal philosophic or religious beliefs that define matters in relation to what is believed to be the truth or good or evil. Others make decisions based on personal life experiences or on the experiences of those close to them. Still others rely on professional codes of ethics to give guidance on ethical issues. In reality, ethical decision making often involves a combination of all of these factors.

In studying ethical issues, it is important for you to understand the many forces that are operating simultaneously in our society. These forces are not independent or mutually exclusive, but act and react with one another in a constantly changing milieu, causing evolutionary changes in all segments of society **(Fig. 8.1)**. The following is a discussion of some of the factors that affect ethical decision making in the healthcare environment.

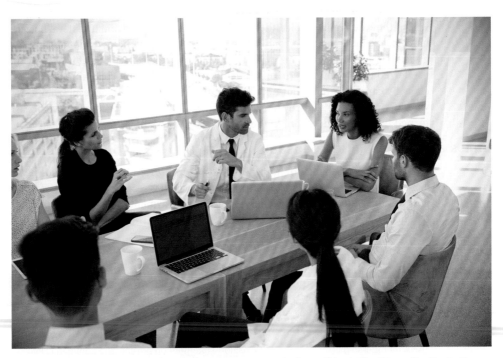

Figure 8.1. Decisions made in relation to one aspect of an ethical situation will affect all other aspects of the problem.

Codes for Nurses

Through their professional organizations, nurses have developed some common guidelines to use in making ethical decisions. They are contained in the ANA's code for nurses, the International Council of Nurses (ICN) code for nurses, and the National Association for Practical Nurse Education and Service's (NAPNES) Standards of Practice for licensed practical/vocational nurses (LPNs/LVNs). Each attempts to outline the nurse's responsibilities to the client and to the profession of nursing.

The ANA code is unique among professional codes because it addresses specific issues and does not confine itself to matters of etiquette or broad general statements. Although identifying the need for a code of ethics as early as 1896, it was not until 1950 that a code of ethics was adopted after accepting tentative codes in the 1920s, 1930s, and 1940s. This code has been revised several times since then. Early versions stated that a nurse had an obligation to carry out a physician's orders; later versions, however, stress the nurse's obligation to the client. This includes protecting the client from incompetent, unethical, or illegal practice. The nine primary provisions of the code for nurses without explanatory provisions are presented in Box 8.1. You can view the entire code, including the preface, by visiting the ANA Web site, http://nursingworld.org, and searching for "Code of Ethics for Nurses."

BOX 8.1 PRIMARY PROVISIONS OF THE ANA CODE FOR NURSES

1. The nurse practices with compassion and respect for the inherent dignity, worth, and unique attributes of every person.
2. The nurse's primary commitment is to the patient, whether an individual, family, group, or community, or population.
3. The nurse promotes, advocates for, and protects the rights, health, and safety of the patient.
4. The nurse has authority, accountability, and responsibility for nursing practice; makes decisions; and takes action consistent with the obligation to promote health and to provide optimal care.
5. The nurse owes the same duties to self as to others, including the responsibility to promote health and safety, preserve wholeness of character and integrity, maintain competence, and continue personal and professional growth.
6. The nurse, through individual and collective effort, establishes, maintains, and improves the ethical environment of the work setting and conditions of employment that are conducive to safe, quality health care.
7. The nurse, in all roles and settings, advances the profession through research and scholarly inquiry, professional standards development, and the generation of both nursing and health policy.
8. The nurse collaborates with other health professionals and the public to protect human rights, promote health diplomacy, and reduce health disparities.
9. The profession of nursing, collectively through its professional organizations, must articulate nursing values, maintain the integrity of the profession, and integrate principles of social justice into nursing and health policy.

Reprinted from American Nurses Association. (2015). *Code of ethics for nurses with interpretive statements*. Washington, DC: American Nurses Publishing, American Nurses Association, with permission.

The ICN first adopted a code in 1953, and the code has been revised and reaffirmed several times since then. The most recent revisions occurred in 2012. The preamble of this code addresses the general responsibilities of the nursing profession. Four sections follow, dealing with the more specific concerns of people, practice, the profession, and coworkers. In addition, the ICN provides suggestions for use of its code and a chart to assist nurses in translating the standards into action. The four elements of the ICN code are presented in Box 8.2. The full document is available at the ICN Web site, http://www.icn.ch/who-we-are/code-of-ethics-for-nurses/

Critical Thinking Activity: Compare Two Nursing Ethical Codes
Compare and contrast the value statements found in the ANA Code of Ethics for Nurses with Interpretive Statements and the ICN Code of Ethics for Nurses. What topics are included in each? Which are not? What does the inclusion of similar topics signify to the profession of nursing? How do you account for topics that are not included in both?

Since 1941, NAPNES has set standards for nursing practice of LPNs; they were last published in 2007. These standards also incorporate moral, ethical, and legal components to guide the practice of the practical nurse. The standards can be viewed online by visiting https://napnes.org/drupal-7.4/sites/default/files/pdf/standards/standards_read_only.pdf

The Client's Rights

The client's rights, as discussed earlier, are another consideration in decision making. Ideally, we have always recognized them in some way. As early as 1959, the National League for Nursing formulated a statement regarding patient rights. For many years, however, healthcare professionals assumed that they knew what was best for clients and made many decisions without consulting or considering the rights of the client. For example, a client with a specific disease was not offered information about possible treatment alternatives, even when valid alternatives did exist. The client's physician decided which treatment method was preferable, and that was the only one presented to the client. This is another example of paternalism, discussed earlier in this chapter.

As the health consumer movement became more active, greater attention was paid to the rights of the client. Today, clients may expect to be informed of all alternatives for treatment and often want to participate in choosing a type of treatment, weighing the possible benefits and risks of the treatment methods presented. For example, a client with a diagnosis of ovarian cancer may want to be involved in the decision whether to first start treatment with chemotherapy or surgery. Many research their health problems on the Internet and come to the physician with questions about specific therapies and approaches to treatment. The law also has supported the right to informed decision making.

In 1973, the American Hospital Association (AHA) published *A Patient's Bill of Rights* (AHA, 1992), which outlined the rights of the hospital client and served as a basis for making decisions about hospitalized clients. Some criticized this document, saying it is rather innocuous because it simply reminded clients of their rights (such as privacy, confidentiality, and informed

BOX 8.2 ICN CODE FOR NURSES—ELEMENTS OF THE CODE

Nurses and People

- The nurse's primary responsibility is to people requiring nursing care.
- In providing care, the nurse promotes an environment in which the human rights, values, customs, and spiritual beliefs of the individual, family, and community are respected.
- The nurse ensures that the individual receives accurate, sufficient and timely information in a culturally appropriate manner on which to base consent for care and related treatment.
- The nurse holds in confidence personal information and uses judgment in sharing this information.
- The nurse shares with society the responsibility for initiating and supporting action to meet the health and social needs of the public, in particular those of vulnerable populations.
- The nurse advocates for equity and social justice in resource allocation, access to healthcare, and other social and economic services.
- The nurse demonstrates professional values such as respectfulness, responsiveness, compassion, trustworthiness, and integrity.

Nurses and Practice

- The nurse carries personal responsibility and accountability for nursing practice and for maintaining competence by continual learning.
- The nurse maintains a standard of personal health such that the ability to provide care is not compromised.
- The nurse uses judgment regarding individual competence when accepting and delegating responsibility.
- The nurse at all times maintains standards of personal conduct that reflect well on the profession and enhance public confidence.
- The nurse, in providing care, ensures that the use of technology and scientific advances are compatible with the safety, dignity, and rights of people.
- The nurse strives to foster and maintain a practice culture promoting ethical behavior and open dialogue.

Nurses and the Profession

- The nurse assumes the major role in determining and implementing acceptable standards of clinical nursing practice, management, research, and education.
- The nurse is active in developing a core of research-based professional knowledge that supports evidence-based practice.
- The nurse is active in developing and sustaining a core of professional values.
- The nurse, acting through the professional organization, participates in creating a positive practice environment and maintaining safe, equitable social and economic working conditions in nursing.

Nurses and Coworkers

- The nurse sustains a collaborative and respectful relationship with coworkers in nursing and other fields.
- The nurse takes appropriate action to safeguard individuals, families, and communities when their health is endangered by a coworker or any other person.
- The nurse takes appropriate action to support and guide coworkers to advance ethical conduct.

consent) but said nothing of hospitals that fail to act in accordance with these rights. The AHA revised this document in 1992 to speak more forcefully to the hospital's responsibility for providing medically indicated care and services and to emphasize the collaborative nature of health maintenance. In April 2003, the AHA Bill of Rights was updated with a version titled *The Patient Care Partnership*. This document outlines what clients may expect during a hospital stay and encourages clients to ask questions if they have concerns. *The Patient Care Partnership* can be reviewed at http://www.aha.org/advocacy-issues/communicatingpts/pt-care-partnership.shtml

Social and Cultural Factors

Changes in the attitudes of society as a whole profoundly influence each of its segments. For example, the changing roles of women, the shifting attitudes toward marriage and the family, and the increasing emphasis on culturally competent care and evidence-based practice have all required nurses to reexamine their personal feelings and alter their approach to providing nursing care.

Ethical concerns are the by-products of many factors at work in our society today, including the role of the individual and the family. In the healthcare field, this is illustrated by the use of the terminology *healthcare* as opposed to *medical care*. Healthcare suggests much greater involvement of others in care delivery, whereas medical care places the physician in the key role. We see similar language being applied to *telehealth* as opposed to *telemedicine*. The meaning of *consumer unit* is shifting from an individual to a whole family or even a whole community. The focus of care also has shifted from disease to prevention and wellness, even when encountering chronicity.

The size of the group being affected by ethical decisions has a bearing on the decision-making process. The smaller the group, organization, or society involved in or affected by the decision making, the easier the process of arriving at an acceptable alternative. When a larger group is affected by a decision, it becomes more complex because more divergent views are encountered. Many of our ethical considerations now involve our society as a whole or, in some cases, the world; therefore, solutions are difficult. An excellent example is the difficulty the United States has encountered in trying to develop and implement a national health plan. The value a society places on the individual or the family directly influences the standard of care **(Fig. 8.2)**. In Western

Figure 8.2. In providing care, the nurse respects the beliefs, values, and customs of the individual.

society, we believe in each person's right to exercise choice based on individual beliefs and conscience. We also place high value on preserving individual life; therefore, we often use tremendous resources to try to achieve additional years, months, or even days of life, for example, in the case of heart transplantation. A society that placed greater emphasis on the community good than on the individual may not choose to use resources in that way. The standard of care might aim for comfort without the use of expensive treatment modalities.

A culture's religious values and belief in an afterlife directly affect ethical issues. A person who believes that an outcome is predetermined by fate will probably not choose to commit major resources and efforts toward altering that outcome.

The population, or, more accurately, the overpopulation, of a country relative to its resources also may have a direct bearing on how resources are allocated. The material resources to provide many health services may not be available. Decisions may be made to eliminate certain costly healthcare procedures even though they are known to be effective and desired by individuals. Limited resources are frequently an issue around the globe and decisions must be made on how to best utilize what is available in a way that helps the most people.

Critical Thinking Activity: Consider Your Personal Experience
Identify two sociocultural factors with which you have had personal experience that could affect ethical decision making. How is your view of this different than it might have been 5 years ago? In what ways have your views remained the same? Why do you think your views have changed or remained the same? What implications does this have for the way you will view things in the future? If you are comfortable doing so, discuss these with a classmate.

Science and Technology

Scientific advancement and technology have left us wrestling with concerns that would have been considered science fiction 50 years ago. Before the development of kidney dialysis, we accepted the fact that people with nonfunctioning kidneys would soon die. After machines that could filter body wastes were invented, a genuine dilemma arose over who would have dialysis and who would not; the number of people needing treatment far exceeded the personnel, time, and equipment available to treat them. As the technology increased the availability of equipment to treat those needing it, the ethical questions refocused on decisions to end treatment rather than on issues related to initiating treatment.

Other technologies have had similar effects. The advent of machines that could artificially breathe for someone challenged the medical and legal professions to examine their definitions of life, and brought into focus problems of whether and when to turn off a ventilator. Heart and lung machines that could adequately perfuse the body while the heart was stopped for surgical procedures enabled operations to be performed that could not be considered in times past. Fetal monitors provide a continuous readout of the status of the fetus during the labor process. Such monitoring has resulted in a greater number of infants delivered by cesarean section. The transplantation of organs from one individual to another has created untold ethical dilemmas. Stem cell research using embryos challenges us at a national level. Individuals with AIDS have a shortened life expectancy even with the best of healthcare. Should they be encouraged to participate in research that is sometimes risky in an effort to advance scientific knowledge and the possibility of future benefit to others? How far should experimentation go? Advances in science and technology continue to offer us some of the greatest ethical challenges.

Legislation

Social change and legislation interact constantly. Legislation may follow changes in society's attitudes, converting new ideas into law. For example, a greater acceptance of infants born to single mothers has resulted in legislation that changed the wording of birth certificates and dropped the word *illegitimate*. Similarly, attitudes are being challenged regarding parenting by members of the lesbian/gay/bisexual/transgender/queer (LGBTQ) population, through either artificial insemination or adoption. Some individuals who disagree with these actions seek legislation to ban them. When social change is desired, legislation may be actively sought to require people to talk and behave in new ways. This was true for civil rights legislation. A change in society was desired, and supporters of civil rights sought legislation as one step toward change. Laws were created to make discrimination illegal and represented the first step in the change process. Attitudes and behaviors do not necessarily change with legislation but do provide legal recourse for those being discriminated against with the hope that more changes will come. Another example is the legislative action that addressed the needs and opportunities available to the disabled that brought about changes in public policies, procedures, and even architecture.

Judicial Decisions

The judicial system provides a major avenue for debating and trying to solve ethical problems. More issues are being taken to court, and judicial decisions are used more often as the basis for determining appropriate action. As you continue to study this topic, note that we have cited landmark decisions regarding ethical issues. The process does not stop there, however. Some people may disagree with a judicial decision and continue to oppose it, appealing the decision to a higher court. Higher courts may overturn judicial decisions. Meanwhile, the questions regarding the individual's role in carrying out a judicial decision remain. For example, although the law in the past forbade abortions (prior to the Roe *v* Wade Supreme Court decision in 1973), some physicians believed strongly in the right of the individual to have the procedure done. These physicians were upset by the results of abortions performed by individuals who lacked the necessary education and skill to do it safely, and therefore were willing to perform abortions despite the law prohibiting the procedure. These physicians were, of course, liable to prosecution if it were discovered they were performing illegal abortions, and some were prosecuted. The issues of abortion and government funding of the procedure are still controversial, and it is unlikely that these issues will be resolved in a way that is satisfactory to everyone.

Funding

The financing of healthcare represents a major area of conflict that has ethical dimensions. The government has become increasingly involved in providing funds for healthcare. Some people are asking how much time, money, and energy we should allocate to healthcare, and how those resources should be divided. How obligated are we as a society to make some form of healthcare available to all? Should that care be provided to illegal immigrants who live in this country as well as to legal residents? What is it that healthcare can and cannot provide? Which is more important, prevention or cure? Healthcare includes controversial procedures (abortion, sterilization, gene therapy) as well as high-cost options (transplantation). This challenges the basic values of some taxpayers who do not ethically sanction these procedures and do not want their tax dollars used to fund them.

Personal Religious and Philosophic Viewpoints

Religious beliefs form the basis for ethical decision making for most people; however, a person who is a member of a particular religious group may not ascribe to all of the beliefs of that group. Some individuals make their own decisions regarding each situation, which, in some cases, may not parallel the doctrines of their religious group. For example, some religions or cultures require same sex healthcare workers. They would find any healthcare setting that did not respect this belief to be in conflict with their basic values.

Your personal viewpoint and possible bias certainly will be factors that influence your ethical decision making. As stated earlier, values are the product of our life experiences and are influenced by family, friends, religion, culture, environment, education, and many other factors. It is important to be aware of your own beliefs and biases in order to provide culturally competent care to clients where you accept and respect cultural differences.

PERSONAL VALUES AND THE WORK ENVIRONMENT

Nursing offers a variety of job opportunities to the new graduate, and you will want to consider your personal values when choosing a position after graduation. You certainly cannot expect to avoid all conflict or problem situations, but you will want to avoid working in an area in which conflict is constant.

Seeking Employment

Before you accept a position, consider whether it has the potential to conflict with your basic beliefs. For example, if you believe that no individual should be denied lifesaving techniques, you might be unhappy working in a research institution where the effects of treatment or no treatment are studied. In this situation, making your views known and refusing certain assignments after you begin employment might result in termination, because the employer may justifiably assert that you agreed to fulfill all the responsibilities of the position when you accepted employment.

Similarly, you might choose to work in an area that supports your personal value system or strong ethical commitment. For example, religious groups that saw value in the life of the dying person began the hospices for the dying in England. Their religious beliefs were and have continued to be part of their approach to care. It is important to find a work environment that is congruent with your values and beliefs regardless of the type of organization. This will reduce conflict and moral distress for you.

Workplace Influences

By virtue of the positions they hold in the healthcare system, nurses experience special pressures as they try to make decisions. An awareness of these factors may help you as you grapple with personal problems in decision making and will be significant in your choice of jobs.

Status as an Employee

Most nurses are not in independent practice but are employed by hospitals, nursing homes, community agencies, or outpatient facilities. Codes do not speak of responsibilities to the employer, yet, from an ethical standpoint, you have certain loyalties and obligations to the employer who pays your salary and makes decisions regarding your work. You may feel pressures of loyalties divided among your client, your employer, and yourself.

When discussing ethical decisions in the abstract, most people say that, of course, the client's best interest should be the only priority. In real situations, however, the issues often are not so clearly defined. If a nurse's decision affects the employer adversely, the result may be job loss, poor references, and a severely curtailed economic and career future.

When nurses are consistently faced with situations such as the one described above, it is referred to as the human condition of **moral distress**. Jameton (1984) first described moral distress as occurring when one knows the ethically correct action to take but feels powerless to take that action. The sources of moral distress are many and varied, but Saver (2009) has listed three common areas: end-of-life situations (particularly where there is disagreement about treatment), fair distribution of resources, and protecting clients' rights. Situations in which the client or family makes decisions that the nurse does not agree with and yet require the nurse's participation fall into this category.

Collective Bargaining Contracts

Collective bargaining contracts can protect nurses in making ethical decisions. By formalizing reasons and procedures for termination of employment, and outlining grievance measures to provide a mechanism by which the individual nurse can be protected, a contract may provide greater freedom. Others believe that contracts hamper individual freedom because of the lengthy processes that are required. See Chapter 5 for more discussion of collective bargaining and grievance measures.

Daily Ethical Dilemma 8.1: Blank Surgical Permits

Carrie Lipton works on a surgical unit in a community hospital. At the request of one of the chief surgeons, it is the practice on that unit for the nurses to sign blank surgical permits on admission to the unit. Carrie does not believe that it is ethical to require clients to sign blank documents because they are not informed of alternative methods of treatment or possible complications in writing. She discusses her concerns with the surgeon. He becomes angry and complains to the hospital administration, stating if something isn't done he'll take his surgeries elsewhere. Carrie is called to the office of the Chief Nurse Executive to discuss the issue.

If the surgeon goes elsewhere, this might create a considerable economic loss for the hospital, and, depending on the action of the hospital administrator, Carrie might be labeled a troublemaker and discharged to placate the physician. If you were in Carrie's position, what would be your next step? What are your alternatives? Who might serve as your advocate in this situation? Is there any other way the situation might have been handled for a more positive outcome? What would that have been?

Collegial Relationships

An excellent climate for ethical decision making can be provided when nurses who work together support one another, share in decision making, and present a unified approach to others. All too often, such relationships are lacking in healthcare institutions, especially as we move into a time when several generations of nurses are working in the same unit. Nurses feel alone and are not experienced in seeking and providing support to one another. Greater collaboration and support on the part of all nurses in this area might be rewarding and is certainly long overdue. This is discussed in greater detail in Chapter 11.

Authoritarian and Paternalistic Backgrounds

The historically authoritarian and paternalistic attitudes of physicians and hospitals often have relegated nurses, most of whom are women, to dependent and subservient roles. These role differentiations have discouraged nurses from taking independent stands on issues and continue to affect relationships in the healthcare field. In some settings, ethical decisions are made without the participation of nurses, yet nurses are expected to implement the decisions.

More nurses are speaking out against an approach that leaves them out of the decision-making process. Nurses today might expect a physician to discuss the possibly futile treatment of a critically ill client with the client, family, and nursing staff. The client would be encouraged to express personal needs, the family's views would be included, and the nurses' input would be part of the decision-making process regarding the medical plan of care. The advent of ethics committees, in which nurses have a voice, has created a positive environment for discussions in many institutions.

Institutional Supports for Ethical Behavior

An institution or organization that recognizes the individuality of all employees and treats them with respect in regard to decisions may provide a working climate that supports ethical behavior. When nurses are respected and there is no fear of reprisal or adverse response, ethical concerns can be voiced and issues raised.

For years, many hospitals have had ethics committees composed of physicians. With a major goal of monitoring physician behavior, they acted when a physician's inappropriate behavior, such as arriving at the hospital intoxicated, was reported to them. Today, the structure and mission of ethics committees have enlarged considerably. Composition of the committee often includes physicians, nurses, social workers, hospital administrators, a community representative, an ethicist, a chaplain or minister, and perhaps an attorney.

Three major roles of the ethics committee include education, policy review and development, and case review. Through case review, the group provides guidance to the hospital community, clients, and their families on matters that may involve ethical concerns such as end-of-life care, consent for medical interventions when the client is unable to participate in the discussion or decisions regarding the termination of treatment. Using their expertise and experience, the members of ethics committees help individuals who must make ethical decisions to identify whether they have all the relevant information, to determine other options they have not considered, and to compare the situation with basic ethical principles and theories. Often, the committee acts in an advisory capacity to medical staff members and families struggling with difficult decisions.

Consumer Involvement in Healthcare

With consumer involvement in healthcare, nurses again may face situations in which they are expected to take action based on the conclusions of others. Many nurses may find this problematic. For example, an older adult diabetic who has gangrene of the foot may refuse amputation, saying, "If I'm going to die, I'm going to die whole." The nurse, recognizing the lifesaving benefit of the amputation, may have difficulty maintaining effective communication and rapport with the client and family because of his or her own conviction that an amputation is the best treatment. Mental health is another area in healthcare in which nurses may struggle. Clients may refuse to adhere to the recommended treatment and, as a result, live in a homeless, psychiatrically unhealthy situation. This also is very difficult for family members.

A FRAMEWORK FOR ETHICAL DECISION MAKING

When faced with ethical decisions, most of us hope to find the right answers. Unfortunately, a right answer may not exist for everyone or every situation; such is the nature of dilemmas. However, you can proceed from a basic framework that encourages you to look beyond your first thoughts or feelings to basic issues. A great deal has been written about the decision-making process. Along with this, several models have been developed to assist us when ethics are involved (Curtin, 1978; Jameton, 1984; Milner, 1993; Thompson & Thompson, 1981; Velasquez, Moberg, Meyer, et al., 2009). Over time, the steps have remained somewhat alike, and you will see a similarity to the steps of the nursing process with which you are already familiar. When clients and families must make ethical decisions, you may assist them in working through this process within the framework of their own values.

Identify and Clarify the Ethical Problem

To define the ethical concern, the situation needs to be reviewed so as to gain as clear a perception of the problem as possible. What is the decision to be made? Does the decision involve a choice between good and bad? Two "goods"? Two "bads"? Could this be damaging to someone or some group? Who are the relevant parties to this decision? What are their values? Are there legal or institutional concerns? Consider what ethical principles might be involved. Are those principles in conflict? Who should assume responsibility for this decision? Is this an individual's decision or is it one in which a collaborative decision must be made? What is your role and relationship to the problem? Are there time constraints on making this decision? What other factors influence the decision? Once a clear picture of the problem has been achieved, more information can be gathered about the situation.

Gather Factual Data

It is important to have as much information about the unique situation as possible. The facts of the situation make a difference in what options are possible. Remember that there is no magic pattern or formula to facts in most situations; they are screened through each person's background and experience. What clearly appears to be a true fact to one person may seem to be opinion to another or perhaps even a falsehood. Therefore, seeking other viewpoints may help everyone involved to see the situation more clearly. Who are the relevant people in the situation and what are their concerns and perspectives? Have they all been consulted? Consider whether legal cases might affect decision making in this case.

Identify and Evaluate Options

Most ethical problems have more than one possible solution. If only one solution existed, there would be no ethical dilemma because there would be no choice. In some cases, more than one solution may be satisfactory; in others, none of the options will seem satisfactory. The more options identified, the more likely those involved will find one they can support. What is the range of actions that could be taken? What would be the anticipated outcome of those actions?

For each option, consider its impact on each person involved. Also think about the impact on society as a whole if this option were chosen. Consider the ethical theories presented and explore how each option compares with the basic principles of each theory. In this way, it might be determined that one option is basically a utilitarian approach (seeking the greatest good for the greatest number), whereas another clearly supports a deontologic position of doing one's duty. Which option does the greatest good while at the same time doing the least harm? Which option respects the rights and dignity of all persons involved? Is one approach more appropriate than another in this situation? Is this approach in keeping with your own moral and ethical position? Helping others to explore these questions (without necessarily using the terminology of formal ethical theories) requires personal involvement and interpersonal skill.

Make a Decision

At some point, a decision must be made. Clients and families, as well as healthcare providers, may find this difficult and, in some instances, painful. However, to not make a decision is, in fact, making a decision. There will never be enough time, data, or alternatives in some situations. No matter how thorough the analysis or how carefully people weigh all competing claims, there may still be uncomfortable feelings. When dealing with these feelings, it is helpful to plan ahead to the action that will be taken. What would a respected and admired individual say? This strategy may be helpful to you as well as to clients and families.

Act and Assess

Once a course of action is chosen, it must be carried out. This may involve working with others or personally carrying out plans. Clients and families need ongoing support as they carry out their decisions. Assess the outcomes as the processes go forward. Unforeseen outcomes are common in ethical situations. Share your thoughts and concerns with others as you proceed, and continue to seek new insights into the situation.

As you assess the outcome in any particular situation, consider its relevance for a wider range of situations and concerns. Use this situation as a foundation from which to grow and develop. Ask yourself, "What have I learned from this experience that will be useful in the future?" "What would I do in another situation?" "What would I change?"

SPECIFIC ETHICAL ISSUES RELATED TO THE PROFESSION OF NURSING

Some ethical issues of concern to nurses relate specifically to the nursing profession; others relate to bioethical issues confronting all of society. In this section, we discuss the issues facing nurses through commitment to the client, commitment to personal excellence, and commitment to the nursing profession as a whole. We present a definite viewpoint regarding ethics in the nursing profession. We feel strongly about the individual nurse's responsibility for nursing practice and place high value on personal integrity in professional relationships.

Commitment to the Client

Nursing has a strong history of being committed to the well-being of clients who need care. Both codes of ethics—from the ANA and ICN—clearly point out the nurse's obligation to fulfill this commitment. In the past, this obligation has been used to try to persuade nurses that they must not be concerned for themselves, their working conditions, their salaries, or other aspects of their employment. However, rejection of the handmaiden philosophy and the adoption of more nurse autonomy do not require rejection of a basic philosophy that nursing is focused on providing clients and their families with support for growth toward maximum health and well-being. Clients can never become the objects of nursing care but must be approached as unique individuals who deserve concern, respect, and culturally competent care that evolves from evidence-based practice.

Commitment to Your Employer

Once you have accepted a position in a healthcare organization, you also have accepted the responsibilities that the position encompasses. Some of these responsibilities may be spelled out in the contract, if a formal contract exists between the employer and the employee. Others are more or less taken for granted. It is these latter responsibilities that can present problems.

Responsible Work Ethic

First, it is understood that you will arrive at work on time. When you arrive late, you obligate others to remain overtime to ensure continuous client care. If you find yourself in an emergency situation that is going to cause you to be delayed, it is important that you notify your supervisor that you are going to be late.

Second, it is also expected that you will not abuse breaks or sick leave. When one extends a break beyond the usual time allowed, it jeopardizes the opportunity for others to have a full break. Your clients also receive less than optimum care if you are unavailable. Likewise, the fact that you have a given number of paid sick days each year does not mean that you are entitled to that many more days off. They are intended for use if you are ill. Often, it is difficult to find replacements when staff members do not report for work. This means that others must pick up additional work assignments and that the quality of care provided that day may be less than desired.

Many healthcare facilities operate 24 hours a day, 7 days a week. This means that there are at least two or three shifts to be covered, as well as weekends and holidays. Be prepared to take your share of weekend and holiday shifts, as well as evening and night rotations, without grumbling if this is part of the staffing pattern. Most employers have developed some system of rotation, with employees able to make requests for the time that works best for them. Some employees for whom the holiday carries less significance may prefer to work, especially if there is additional pay for those days.

If you work in an area where you have a fair amount of privacy, remember that you should not conduct personal business during your work shift. Scheduling appointments, telephoning friends or business associates, writing notes, and similar activities should occur during your break or after you have finished your shift.

When you decide to terminate your employment, it is expected, as part of professional behavior, that you will give appropriate notice. Please refer to Chapter 4 for further discussion regarding resignation.

Responsible Use of Supplies

Pilfering includes stealing in small amounts or stealing objects of little value. Many people who are scrupulously honest in other aspects of their lives do not recognize that taking small items from a place of employment is indeed theft. Employees often take home adhesive bandage strips, pens, and other such objects so routinely that they do not even consider whether this is right or wrong. This constant petty theft may total thousands of dollars, the cost of which must be passed on to those who pay the bills—the patients. As a leader in the care setting, the registered nurse (RN) is often in a position to communicate clearly to all employees that pilfering is unacceptable. The nurse can set an example of careful stewardship of the hospital supplies.

Sometimes removing supplies is an oversight rather than a planned action (Fig. 8.3). To make efficient use of time, nurses commonly place many small items such as alcohol wipes, extra Band-Aids, and pens in their pockets. One hospital unit found that its yearly supply budget for black pens was almost exhausted in the first 6 months of the year. The simple action of placing a basket in the lounge into which nurses dropped everything from their pockets before leaving cut the pen costs dramatically. Perhaps you can be equally creative in helping to solve such problems in your work setting.

As the costs of healthcare soar, it is important that everyone associated with healthcare be mindful of the use of resources. You can help reduce costs by being judicious in your use of resources. For example, supplies that will not be used should not be taken into client rooms,

Figure 8.3. Many people who are otherwise scrupulously honest do not recognize that taking small items from a place of employment is theft.

only to be discarded later. Using extra linens such as bath towels to clean up spills adds to costs. Determining that a clean glove is acceptable rather than reaching for sterile gloves reduces costs. Ensuring that all charges are processed for supplies that are used is also important. Operating equipment in a knowledgeable manner to reduce breakage or repairs is the responsibility of all workers. When all people do their part, the cumulative effect can be significant.

Commitment to Your Colleagues

It has been suggested that a strategy to improve the nurse shortage is to improve the quality of the work environment. Many factors influence the climate of the work environment. One of the most noteworthy is our relationship with colleagues. As a new graduate, what effect do you have on this?

One approach is to model those behaviors that you wish to see in others. Develop a collaborative approach. Maintain a positive attitude; respond to others in a pleasant, courteous manner; be sensitive to others; and be a positive ambassador for nursing. Be supportive of others and avoid opportunities to gossip about your colleagues and their activities. Compliment others on things they do well and provide assistance with things they are still learning. This is especially important as you become a more seasoned employee and have responsibility for helping to orient others. Give new employees time to learn skills that are new to them and to become efficient in their execution. Show care and compassion to fellow workers as well as to your clients.

Today, the workforce in nursing consists of individuals from four different generations, resulting in differences in attitudes, beliefs, work habits, and expectations (see Chapter 11). This can result in greater conflict in the workplace. All nurses must assume shared accountability for establishing and maintaining intergenerational relationships that foster a positive work environment. Nurses must seek to understand each generational cohort, communicating in a manner that will accommodate and capitalize on generational differences.

Commitment to Personal Excellence

Nurses must be committed to personal excellence and assume responsibility for maintaining competence. You are the one who is best able to identify your weaknesses and practice deficits as well as your strengths. Your careful and genuine self-evaluation is the client's best protection against poor or inadequate care.

When we are truly honest with ourselves in the self-evaluation process, we often uncover areas we wish were not there. These weaknesses, once identified, provide the greatest opportunity for growth and improvement. Fortunately, when it is done informally, these weaknesses do not have to be shared with anyone. On the other hand, do not hesitate to ask for assistance if you think you need it.

Many institutions now include self-evaluation and the establishment of personal goals in the formal evaluation of employees. In this process, you might be asked to prepare a written self-evaluation that will be shared with your immediate supervisor and may be incorporated into your records.

So how do you proceed? One approach to self-evaluation is the use of the nursing process format. Begin with a thorough personal assessment, objectively gathering data about your own performance and keeping notes on yourself. For example, if you want to increase your efficiency in carrying out treatments, you may want to time yourself on several occasions to determine how long you are taking and whether you improved with performance.

After data have been collected, give yourself time to analyze it thoroughly. The self-assessment outline includes questions you should ask yourself (Box 8.3); however, the criteria

BOX 8.3 SELF-EVALUATION PLAN

Assessment of Client
- Do I gather enough data about clients and families, including both strengths and deficits?
- Is there sufficient depth and breadth in the data I gather?
- Do I listen closely to the client and attend to what is being said?
- Do I regularly use all available sources for information about my clients (eg, client, family, other staff, chart, Kardex)?
- Have I recognized problems quickly so that they did not become worse through inattention?
- Do I recognize physiologic, social, and psychological problems?
- Is my assessment free of personal biases and viewpoints?
- Do I separate relevant from irrelevant data?

Planning for Client Care
- Do I routinely seek more information on which to base decisions about client care?
- Are my assumptions correct?
- Do I include the client in decision making whenever possible?
- Do I consult with others on the healthcare team when planning?
- Are my written plans clear, concise, and reasonable to carry out?
- Do I take into account the realities of the situation when planning care?
- Are my plans for care sound and appropriate to the individual client?
- Do I employ principles from the biologic and social sciences in planning?
- Have I considered all alternatives?

Intervention
- Is my work organized and finished on time?
- Do I maintain optimum safe working habits?
- Do I perform technical skills in an efficient and safe manner?
- Do I communicate clearly and effectively with clients, family, and staff?
- Do I use therapeutic communication techniques appropriately and effectively?
- Do I use teaching approaches appropriate to the individual client and family?
- Do I keep accurate and complete written records?
- Do I understand and perform any administrative tasks that are my responsibility (eg, ordering supplies, planning for laboratory tests)?
- Do I make the effort to learn about new techniques and procedures?
- Do I function as a team player?
- Do I incorporate critical thinking into all of my activities?

Evaluation
- Do I routinely evaluate the effectiveness of the nursing care I give?
- Do I effectively assist in evaluation of the patient's response to medical care and to ordered therapies?
- Do I encourage the client to participate in evaluating both the process and the outcome of care?
- Have I evaluated all aspects of care fair-mindedly?

(Continued)

BOX 8.3 SELF-EVALUATION PLAN (continued)

Personal Growth and Relationships
- Have I established a sound trust and working relationship with coworkers?
- Do I support and assist my coworkers when possible?
- Do I communicate effectively with others on the healthcare team?
- Do I seek answers to questions for which I have no answer?
- Have I sought opportunities for learning and personal growth?
- Is my attitude helpful and productive?
- Do I have sound working habits (eg, appearing on time, limiting coffee and lunch breaks to the correct time)?
- Is my appearance appropriate to the working environment?
- Do I use appropriate channels of communication within the institution?
- Do I handle criticism constructively?
- Do personal biases interfere with the care that I provide or my relationship with colleagues?
- Am I doing my share in overall professional activities (eg, serving on committees, assisting with development projects)?
- Am I honest with myself, being neither too harsh nor too easy on myself?
- Do I have personal values and beliefs that interfere with providing quality nursing care?

that you use to determine whether your answers reflect the quality of performance you want to attain are not included. Those specific criteria must be individualized to the setting in which you work and the nature of your role in that setting. For example, the breadth of data that represent excellent practice for the nurse in the emergency department differs from what would represent excellence for the nurse working in a rehabilitation setting. Thus, criteria specific to your work situation are needed.

Your analysis can reveal strengths, weaknesses, and areas for growth or improvement. Congratulate yourself on the strengths identified and then clearly delineate those areas in which you want to change or to improve. Identifying and stating the problems or growth needed helps you to plan more effectively, just as it has in nursing care planning.

Next, establish a plan of action. The plan will be more helpful to you if it contains clearly defined goals. Once the goals are set, you will be better able to plan the appropriate action and timeline to meet them. You might consider such things as requesting in-service education, taking continuing education courses, consulting with colleagues, and doing independent reading and study. Some plans need to include specific things related to your daily nursing care. To do this, you may want to request assignments that provide opportunities for practice of the desired skills. Perhaps you are interested in transferring to a specialty area of care. This will involve communication with your immediate supervisor and may involve enrolling in special classes.

Implementing this plan will require you to remain focused on what you are trying to accomplish. Keeping records on your progress is often helpful and provides positive reinforcement when you realize that some of your goals have been met.

Periodic evaluation of your progress is necessary so that you do not become discouraged. Sometimes it is hard to identify gradual change. Any records you have kept are valuable for this purpose. Plan rewards for yourself for improvement that occurs. Try not to become discouraged if you do not see the improvement you desire. Remember that just as a reassessment and a new plan are often necessary in patient care planning, a revised plan also may be needed in the self-evaluation process. Keep in mind that your overall goal is personal excellence in nursing practice.

Commitment to the Nursing Profession

Commitment to the nursing profession requires that each nurse be concerned not only about personal performance but also about how nursing is practiced. This involves participation in formal and informal evaluation of nursing care, dealing with poor care, and identifying the impaired nurse. Nurses always have evaluated one another in both formal and informal ways. The main purpose of peer evaluation is to maintain consistent high-quality nursing care and not simply noting error or deficiency. This is an ethical, professional obligation.

Formal Evaluation

Formal evaluation of nursing care occurs in most settings under the title of quality assurance and quality improvement. *Quality assurance* is a planned program of evaluation that includes ongoing monitoring of the care given and outcomes of care. It includes a mechanism for instituting change when problems or opportunities for improvement are identified. Quality assurance programs are required by The Joint Commission (see Chapter 6). Special nursing projects such as the work done on nursing outcomes (see Chapter 1) have a focus on the quality of care provided.

All types of evaluation first call for establishing specific criteria to be used in the evaluation. These criteria may refer to process, outcome, or both. The creation of the criteria is a professional nursing responsibility. The process begins by determining whether the nursing actions taken are complete and appropriate. Criteria developed to evaluate this aspect are called process criteria. One basis for developing process criteria is *Nursing: Scope and Standards of Practice*, published by the ANA (2015), which is a revised version of *Standards of Clinical Nursing Practice*, published in 1991 and again in 1998, 2004, and 2010. General standards refer to all settings; more specific ones exist for more than 20 specialty areas of nursing. Some specialty organizations, such as the Intravenous Nurses Society, also have published standards that refer to their specialty.

Another basis for formal evaluation is the use of outcome criteria for client care. Outcome criteria are specific, observable client behaviors or clinical manifestations that are the desired results of care. Typically, nurses working in groups consult nursing literature so that they develop and establish the appropriate criteria. Several methods have been used to evaluate both the process and the outcomes of nursing care. These may include conferences designed to discuss the matter to be evaluated, interviews with clients or staff, direct observation of clients, and review of the record. This record review, which is gaining wider acceptance in nursing, involves comparing the client record with the criteria and is often completed by medical records personnel. The accuracy of the review depends on the adequacy (ie, the completeness) of the documentation. If information does not appear in the record (other than situations in which charting by exception are employed), then, for the purposes of the audit, the appropriate observations were not made or the actions were not taken.

This is just one of the reasons why you must recognize the importance of your documentation and make sure that you maintain a high standard in records. The record review has raised serious concerns, which have resulted in greater attention to documentation and even revision of record systems. Nurses then have taken the initiative to determine the meaning of the data in relationship to enhanced client well-being. Changes in policies and procedures and in-service education classes often occur. Once remedial action has been taken, reevaluation is done to determine its effectiveness.

Informal Evaluation

An important day-to-day evaluation of client care occurs informally as peers observe the performance of others. Watching other nurses also helps you to grow in your own practice. When you observe coworkers, strive for objectivity. A common mistake is to let personal feelings influence what we see, such as viewing a close friend in a positive light or seeing only the negative aspects of a nurse with whom we have a poor relationship. Remember to examine the results or outcomes of care. Two nurses may use different approaches or techniques in similar situations, but both may achieve positive results. In most instances, you will see good care. Do not hesitate to commend others and share your positive feelings. Everyone benefits from positive reinforcement of skill; it helps nurses to create a good climate for personal growth and sharing.

Addressing Substandard Care

Concern for the welfare of clients requires that nurses acknowledge the existence of substandard care and work toward improving that situation. It is not a matter of whether the nurse should become involved, but rather how to most effectively accomplish the goals of better care.

If faced with a situation where client care is less than desired, consider whose care you are criticizing. If it is the care of another nurse, or a care provider with less educational preparation than you possess, the situation is more straightforward. If you have questions about medical care delivered or the action of a physician, it becomes more difficult, because medical actions are outside the scope of practice of nursing. Be careful about how you proceed, referring to hospital policy manuals, trusted colleagues, your supervisor, or possibly the chief of the medical staff for advice before taking action.

When you observe a colleague practicing what you think is poor client care, such as poor sterile technique, it is not as difficult. The action you choose to take will depend on the seriousness of the situation you have observed. Usually, the simplest and most effective solution is to go directly to the person involved and discuss what you have observed. As mentioned in other sections of this textbook, this should occur in a private setting, away from others, and as soon after the occurrence as possible. This approach allows the nurse to give a rationale for the action taken. When you understand the situation more fully, you may have a different point of view. If you disagree with your colleague and the situation is not critical, you might want to state simply that you disagree. If the situation is critical, the two of you will want to seek resources that will outline the best approach. If you observe poor care a second time, and it has been determined that your colleague's care is substandard, you should again approach the person. State what you have seen and note that it is the second time. If the person still disagrees that a problem exists, state that you feel obligated to discuss this with your immediate superior because it is not in the best interest of the client. You should then follow through on this.

If you have a reputation on the unit for maintaining a focus that enhances the welfare of clients, and you have been quick to praise the good care provided by others, your action in response to poor care will be more readily accepted. Remember that your attitude when approaching another nurse is crucial. Facial expressions and tone of voice, as well as words, need to be considered. If you are perceived as friendly and caring, your comments probably will be accepted in a far different manner than if you are seen as being negative and critical. However, you cannot always count on this reaction. Many nurses feel threatened by the idea of evaluation or have had bad experiences in which evaluation only involved pointing out deficiencies. These nurses may be angry and upset with any colleague who considers evaluation part of the colleague role. Therefore, it is wise to have thought out how you will proceed.

A Basic Pattern for Action

The first step to be taken in any situation in which you believe substandard care exists is to collect adequate, valid information on behavior that you have personally observed. Do not make decisions based on gossip, hearsay, or an isolated instance, unless the single incident was very serious. If this is the case, be certain of your facts before taking action.

Also be certain you understand both the formal and the informal systems of authority and responsibility within your facility and the laws of the state in which you practice. In some states, laws exist requiring that poor practice be reported directly to the relevant licensing board. In others, reporting to your supervisor is considered adequate reporting. You need to know which people have the authority to make decisions and changes, what the official prescribed route of change is, and what the hidden priorities of the institution might be. It is most commonly recommended that once you are certain of your data and know how the system works in your organization, you should take concerns to your immediate supervisor, who would forward the concern until it reached the individual or body with the authority and duty to act. Many people believe that reporting to a supervisor fulfills your ethical responsibility as well as your legal responsibility.

When you approach a supervisor, give specific information that includes the dates, the situations, and the action you took. Do not indulge in generalities or sweeping statements; stick to specific observed instances by simply describing what you saw. Let the supervisor know that you have talked with the person under discussion and have informed the person that you would speak with the supervisor. It is important to specify the action you would like to see occur. You might ask the supervisor to discuss the matter with both of you, or you might ask the supervisor to discuss the matter with the other nurse or observe the nurse. It is also important to remember that once you have initiated this action, you may or may not be involved in some follow-up. You may never learn what was done, even when positive action was taken, because of the constraints of confidentiality for the affected employee. If the manager decides to observe and take corrective action, that will be confidential for the employee involved. Occasionally, results emerge only much later, when a change in procedure and policy occurs.

If you observe an incident that has the potential to cause a client danger (eg, an unreported medication error) or one that has legal ramifications (eg, the falsifying of narcotic records), you have a legal as well as an ethical responsibility to go immediately to a supervisor with your information. In a situation that has the potential for legal involvement, keep an exact personal record of your observations and actions. Include in the record the times and dates of incidents and of your reporting efforts (see Chapter 7).

Alternative Approaches for Action

At times, the system does not always work as expected. Your concern regarding what you perceive as poor practice may be dropped or ignored at any one of many points. Often, there are good reasons for this. Perhaps, the persons in authority want to collect more specific data about a situation, with as little general discussion as possible. Sometimes, there are aspects of a legal contract or a collective bargaining contract of which you are unaware that must be considered in the actions that are taken. Other times, professional confidentiality may make it seem that nothing is being done, when, in fact, steps have been taken to correct a situation. It is easy as a newcomer to the healthcare scene to see only part of a picture. Simply checking back with a manager, acknowledging that information may be confidential, and asking for reassurance that the matter is being addressed may be an appropriate action.

If your initial approach is not effective, a formal route for seeking further change would lead you through the official lines of authority within your facility. After discussing your concern with your immediate supervisor and receiving no satisfactory response, tell the supervisor formally that you intend to carry your concern to the next higher authority. Informing your supervisor of your plans should help to avoid problems, but be prepared to listen to some words of warning from the supervisor or efforts to discourage you from taking action. There are reasons this individual has chosen not to pursue the issue; some of these may be valid.

However, there are times when an alternative approach is more appropriate than formal action. Another route for seeking further change is through designated committees or procedures within your facility. As hospitals move into models of shared governance, this may be your best alternative. Discussing or sharing a problem (without naming names) with a particular committee might require a carefully written and documented report explaining your concern. You then might be called to answer questions that the committee believes are important.

You may volunteer to serve on committees that deal with peer review. If there are no such committees, you may work to have them established, perhaps through a bargaining unit. This route of action will require a considerable investment of your own time and effort, a factor you need to consider.

Another alternative approach is to use the informal system within the facility. You may discuss your concern with a trusted person (or mentor) who has influence within the system. You may learn that you are not alone in your concerns, that efforts toward change are being made, and that your input of data is welcomed. Another approach would be to seek the assistance of another individual with power within the organization. However, we must caution you about using informal systems, as they can backfire. Therefore, we suggest that you use these alternative approaches only when the ones suggested earlier have failed to bring about the desired results.

A final alternative to a problem in your work setting is to offer your resignation if a change is not made. Continuing to work in an environment in which poor practice exists may place you in conflict with your ethical standards and values. If you find it necessary to do this, be careful that you do not jeopardize your own future with angry letters or intemperate remarks. Render your resignation in a polite and professional manner, even when expressing dissatisfaction with the system.

Reporting directly to a state licensing board or professional organization's disciplinary committee is an avenue of action outside of the employment setting. The licensing board exists to assure the public of safe practice; therefore, these organizations and agencies usually deal with serious problems that represent a breach of the public trust or serious harm. They may not have the capacity or desire to pursue minor (though still important) problems. The same constraints apply when reporting to these organizations. Remember that their investigation and decisions may be done in a judicial or legal manner. This may involve the requirement that you provide legal testimony regarding your complaints.

Personal Risks in Reporting

If you decide to pursue any of these routes, be fully aware of the possible consequences. You may be labeled a troublemaker, or worse. You may lose the opportunity to be promoted because you are seen as being antagonistic to the system. Although officially it should not happen, it is possible that you could lose your job for raising too many issues. We do not mean to be unduly discouraging, but we want to warn you that the role of change agent is not easy, and you should be aware of the consequences and weigh them before you decide to act. Above all, be certain that your perceptions are correct and that your concerns are well grounded.

Whistle-Blowing

The ultimate step one might take in a situation in which negligence or maltreatment is allowed to persist would be whistle-blowing. **Whistle-blowing** is when an employee or past employee reports a violation of the law that is considered fraud or abuse so that it may be investigated by the state or federal government (Little & Brownstein, 2014). In healthcare, Ray (2006) has identified whistle-blowing as the revelation of an ethical failure in which the organization has lost its moral compass. Lachman (2008) emphasizes the importance of establishing an ethical organizational culture. In the business world, whistle-blowing that resulted in high-profile cases involving manipulation of gas prices, breast implants, accounting fraud, and insider trading alerted the public to ethical wrongdoing.

If you encounter a situation that you consider so serious that whistle-blowing actions need to be taken, do so only after thoughtful consideration, because exposing unethical and incompetent healthcare providers is not without risk. The worst-case scenario might be legal retaliation; an individual identified as giving substandard care might sue you for slander, which could be expensive to defend. There may be unpleasant reactions from coworkers or you may place your job in jeopardy. Some states have enacted legislation that protects nurses and other healthcare staff members from retaliation when they report a case, but others have not. Section 11(c) of the OSH Act is a federal mandate supporting other whistle-blower statutes that prohibit employers from discriminating against employees who raise safety or health concerns (Occupational Safety and Health Administration, n.d.). Because there can be serious ramifications to whistle-blowing, do not go public until all the avenues to address concerns through the system have been exhausted, with no response. The following should guide your activities:

- Consider contacting an attorney before taking any steps.
- Learn as much as you can about your state's policies by contacting your state nurses association, the ANA, or your state board of nursing.
- Be certain of your facts and have them well documented. Be confident that a wrongdoing has occurred.
- As you pursue your concern within the system, follow the healthcare organization's chain of command.
- Be professional when dealing with others.

Recommending a Care Provider

Clients and acquaintances may ask you to recommend a physician or other care provider because they believe that, as a nurse, you have special knowledge and insight in such matters. If you have no personal knowledge about the requested information, then honestly tell the individual requesting information that you have no personal or professional knowledge regarding a particular care provider. However, if you do have knowledge, you could recommend several competent persons, pointing out characteristics of each that might be factors in personal choice.

For example, your next-door neighbor exuberantly greets you when you return from work one afternoon with the news that she believes she is pregnant. Because you work in the birthing rooms at the local hospital, she asks you if you can recommend an obstetrician. After letting her know you, too, are excited about the news, you state, "There are three who are very popular at our facility. One is an older physician who has a fairly traditional approach to childbirth, another is a young and innovative physician who strongly advocates partner participation and natural childbirth, and the third is new in the community but appears to allow clients a great deal of choice in their approach to childbirth." After this, you explore with her some of her expectations regarding care and allow her to make a personal choice.

If you are asked specifically about a physician whose care you believe to be less than satisfactory, you are faced with a different dilemma. Making severely critical statements might leave you open to a legal charge of slander by the physician (see Chapter 7). However, saying nothing is ethically a problem because you are not acting to protect the client. A safe approach is to state, "I personally would prefer to see Dr. N or Dr. O rather than Dr. X." If pressed to give reasons, you are legally more secure if you say that you would prefer not to discuss specifics or to focus the conversation on the strengths of the doctors you have recommended.

Be careful that any recommendations are not based on hearsay or gossip. If you do not have solid information on which to base a referral, do not be drawn into making one. Being a nurse does not obligate you to be an expert on all healthcare questions.

THE CHEMICALLY IMPAIRED PROFESSIONAL

Chemically impaired professional is a term used to describe that person whose practice has deteriorated because of chemical abuse, specifically, the use of alcohol and drugs. The terms addiction, drug addiction, alcoholism, chemical dependency, and chemical impairment are all names that we associate with the dependence on alcohol, drugs, or other substances. Addiction has been defined as compulsive need for and use of a habit-forming substance (such as heroin, nicotine, or alcohol) characterized by tolerance and by well-defined physiologic symptoms upon withdrawal (Merriam-Webster Online Dictionary, 2017c). Dependency refers to the "state of relying on or being controlled" by a substance such as drugs or alcohol. There is a strong possibility that if you remain active in the profession, at some time, you will find yourself working with a chemically impaired colleague; perhaps you already have.

Chemical Impairment in Healthcare Professionals

One would like to believe that nurses, who have studied the physiologic effects of alcohol and drugs on the system, would avoid such abuse. However, this is not the case. As a result of increasing concern about the problem, in the 1980s, nurses began to collect data on the topic (Bissell & Haberman, 1984; Bissell & Skorina, 1987; Sullivan, Bissell, & Williams, 1988). Later studies explored the probable use of alcohol among nursing students (Campbell & Polk, 1992; Marion, Fuller, Johnson, et al., 1996; Sullivan, Bissell, & Leffler, 1990; McCulloh Nair, Nemeth, Williams, et al., 2015). Some studies would suggest that the prevalence of substance abuse is no higher in healthcare professionals than in the general population, but certain professions such as the emergency room workers, anesthesiologists, and psychiatrists experience higher rates of drug abuse (Physician Health Program, 2015).

Why are nurses affected by this problem? Factors that lead to chemical dependency include the stress of the nursing profession, particularly in intensive care units and emergency departments. Frequent shift changes and staffing shortages resulting in excessive overtime add to the situation. Musculoskeletal injuries and pain and knowledge of medications also contribute to the abuse as do unrealistic personal expectations, frustration, powerlessness, anxiety, and depression. Once the problem exists, denial is a big part of the disease.

All areas of the profession are affected by the problem of chemical dependency in nursing. A significant financial impact, in the forms of sickness, absenteeism, tardiness, accidents, errors, decreased productivity, and staff turnover, is realized by institutions that employ nurses with dependency problems. Problems related to drug abuse are complicated by the fact that the nurse often obtains drugs from the supply available on the hospital unit and is therefore in violation of the Controlled Substances Act. As with other healthcare conditions, early recognition and treatment have been recommended to help offset this problem.

Since 1981, the ANA has worked with the problems of chemical abuse, first establishing a task force to review the concern and then, in 1990, developing suggested state legislation focusing on voluntary treatment rather than disciplinary action (ANA, 1990). Many states have alternatives to discipline programs for nurses with substance use disorder. The programs vary by state, range from three to five years, and may include peer assistance and recovery monitoring. Information on each state with links to program information can be located on the National Council of State Boards of Nursing Web site; https://www.ncsbn.org/alternative-to-discipline.htm.

Recognizing the Chemically Impaired Nurse

The concerns about the chemically impaired nurse are twofold. The first is a personal concern for the nurse who is afflicted: The illness may go undetected and untreated for years. The second concern is for the client, whose care is jeopardized by the nurse whose judgment and skills are weakened, thus increasing the possibility of errors.

The major avenue for identifying impaired nurses is through nonimpaired coworkers. However, nurses, by virtue of their education, are socialized into caring roles and have not always dealt with the problem in a straightforward fashion. The impaired nurse was often protected, transferred, ignored, and, in some instances, promoted. None of these actions helped solve the problem. As you enter the nursing field, be aware of the following characteristics, which are commonly seen in impaired nurses or healthcare practitioners (O'Neil, 2012):

- Mood swings
- Slurred speech
- Tardiness and frequently leaving work environment
- Frequent days off for implausible reasons
- Noncompliance with acceptable policies and procedures
- Deteriorating appearance

- Inconsistent job performance
- Inadequate documentation
- Involvement in discrepancies of controlled substances in the workplace
- Alcohol or marijuana on breath
- Poor judgment, concentration
- Dishonesty
- Belligerence to supportive inquiries

Reporting the Chemically Impaired Colleague

As an RN, what should you do if you suspect that a colleague has a chemical dependency problem? First of all, you need to know what the law in your state requires of you. In many states, every professional is legally obligated to report a chemically dependent healthcare professional. This reporting most commonly is done through channels at the place of employment but also may be done directly to the state board of nursing. If you do not know the requirements, you should immediately learn what they are. In some states, failure to report can result in disciplinary action toward you.

When planning to report, you do not have to be sure beyond any doubt that a problem exists. You need to have enough data to present a reasonable concern. The investigation to clearly establish the problem is the responsibility of the employing agency or the state board. To establish reasonable concern, collect and document data, including objective facts, dates, and times when the situation occurred. For several good reasons, you should not confront the person whom you suspect at this time.

First, the person may become more secretive about the behavior because of the danger of being caught. This will make collection of data difficult, if not impossible. Personal defenses and denial may become stronger. The suspected person may ask for a transfer to another shift or to a different part of the facility, or, if truly feeling threatened, may seek employment in another facility.

Second, the person may feel attacked and rejected. To ensure that it will not end in a disaster, a confrontation needs the support of an appropriate and knowledgeable healthcare professional to ensure that the individual is guided to appropriate choices for treatment and rehabilitation. If the person is someone you know well, who confides in you regarding personal problems and is likely to follow your suggestions, you might use those occasions to refer the individual to appropriate resources for personal assistance and counseling.

Another reason why you should not confront the suspected person at this time is that you are still collecting data and documenting them. You cannot be sure from a single observation that a problem exists. There are often reasons why things are not what we initially perceived them to be.

Once you feel you have data to support a realistic concern, report them to a supervisor to validate your observations. Usually, once you have notified your supervisor, he or she will assume responsibility for the problem, but may ask for your continued assistance with data collection or with confrontation (see earlier discussion on reporting to your supervisor).

Once adequate information has been gathered, agency administrative personnel will notify the state board of nursing. In addition, they usually must notify the state board of pharmacy if drugs are involved. More investigation will be carried out; records will be examined. If a problem exists, actions appropriate to the situation will be taken. These usually include a carefully planned confrontation by an intervention team, a requirement that treatment be sought, and a presentation of the consequences of not seeking treatment.

The worst thing you can do if you suspect a problem is to ignore it or help a colleague cover for inadequacies. The colleague will not get better if the problem is not recognized and treated. The longer the delay, the greater the chance that an innocent patient will be placed in jeopardy.

Fortunately, help and rehabilitation are being made available to those who need it through state nurses associations and state licensing authorities. These programs usually provide a specific contractual agreement regarding professional practice during the treatment and monitoring period. This is often done without formal disciplinary proceedings. The goal of this process is restoration of the individual to effective functioning.

In some states, the licensing boards may institute formal disciplinary proceedings to suspend a license or issue a license with limitations on practice, and to provide monitoring and supervision while the individual seeks treatment. When treatment is completed, the board may reinstate the license with temporary limitations and continued monitoring and support. The goal is the eventual full rehabilitation of the healthcare professional to the service of the community. Reporting a chemically dependent colleague may be the most caring action you can take.

If, as a nursing student, you suspect that a fellow classmate (or worse yet, an instructor) has a problem with chemical abuse, you would be wise to discuss your concerns with your instructor (or with the director of the program if you suspect an instructor). Because such problems typically worsen with time, the earlier they are addressed and corrected, the better it is for everyone. Again, it is important that you have accurate information to report, along with times, dates, and examples of the behavior that caused your concern.

Critical Thinking Activity: Chemical Dependency
Assume that you have serious concerns that a colleague is delivering poor client care because of problems with chemical dependency. Where would you begin? What is your personal responsibility? What is your responsibility to your colleague? What is your responsibility to the clients? What steps should you take? Do you have a personal liability in the situation?

Theory Alert   *Hildegard E. Peplau*

Hildegard E. Peplau developed a theory that helped explain the phases of interpersonal processes with four sequential phases: orientation, identification, exploitation, and resolution. Dr. Peplau was born in 1909, attended a diploma program in 1931, received a BA in interpersonal psychology in 1943, an MA in psychiatric nursing from Colombia University New York in 1947, and an EdD in curriculum development in 1953. She taught at Rutgers University and developed the first postbaccalaureate program in nursing.

Dr. Peplau published Interpersonal Relations in Nursing in 1952, which is a middle range descriptive classification theory also called psychodynamic nursing. The works of Harry Stack Sullivan's theory of interpersonal relations (1953), Percival Symonds, Abraham Maslow, and Neal Elgar Miller influenced her theory. When dealing with ethical dilemmas, the nurse must have excellent interpersonal communication skills, a part of which relates back to the nurse taking time to examine his or her own values and beliefs in order to understand one's self (Current Nursing, 2012).

BOUNDARY VIOLATIONS

The term **boundary violations** is used to refer to situations in which nurses move beyond a professional relationship and become personally involved with a client and the client's life. It is of particular concern because it represents a violation of the trust relationship that exists between the client and the nurse. In nurse–client relationships, the nurse necessarily holds power, creating a vulnerable situation for the client. The nurse also has access to confidential and privileged information about clients and their families. It is the nurse's responsibility to define the boundaries of the relationships and ensure that they are maintained. The nurse must be warm and empathetic but should not try to be friends with the client **(Fig. 8.4)**.

Perhaps the most extreme boundary violation is professional sexual misconduct. Professional sexual misconduct has been defined as "any behavior that is seductive, sexually demeaning, harassing or reasonably interpreted as sexual by the patient" (National Council of State Boards of Nursing, 2014, p. 5). This overinvolvement is unethical, can cause loss of employment, and can cause possible criminal charges depending on the severity of the misconduct.

Although sexual misconduct is the major focus of this concern, boundary violations expand into other areas of conduct, such as overidentifying with a particular family member or moving into pseudofamily relationships with the client's family. If this happens, the family may question the nurse's motives, wondering whether the nurse is looking for a bequest in a will or other tangible benefit. Such overinvolvement will interfere with the nurse's personal life and even could result in legal actions on the part of the family.

Figure 8.4. Maintaining appropriate professional boundaries prevents confusion and unwanted consequences.

Some early indications that boundaries are beginning to break down include situations in which the nurse spends extended time with a client beyond assigned duties or visits the client when not on duty. Showing favoritism or possessiveness of a client, meeting clients in isolated areas in a manner that has nothing to do with direct client care, or personal disclosure by the care provider are other indicators that boundaries are being violated (National Council of State Boards of Nursing, 2014).

It is important that you are able to recognize situations in which a colleague may cross sexual boundaries. If you believe sexual misconduct is occurring on the unit where you are employed, the steps you would follow are similar to those you learned to use in dealing with chemical abuse. It is extremely important that you document the behavior carefully, noting dates, times, and the names of the individuals involved. Keep your documentation focused on factual information and objective data. You would then share this information with your immediate supervisor.

BIOETHICAL ISSUES CONCERNING DEATH

One of the most important and most common areas of ethical debate in which nurses experience ethical dilemma involves the topic of death and dying. As mentioned earlier, the advent of lifesaving procedures and mechanical devices has required redefinition of the term *death*, caused us to examine the meaning of quality of life, and created debates about death with dignity.

Also associated with the issue of death are several companion concerns that did not exist before the technologic advances that occurred over the past 30 years. Some of these concerns relate to euthanasia, the right to refuse treatment, and the right to die. Other concerns relate to organs retrieved from the dying, because of the scarcity of these medical resources. Generally, the demand for donated organs far exceeds the number of organs available to meet the needs. Superimposed on all these issues is that of informed consent.

Death Defined

Until recently, the most widely accepted definition of death was from *Black's Law Dictionary*, which defines death as the irreversible cessation of the vital functions of respiration, circulation, and pulsation. This traditional view of death served us well until the development of ventilators and other advances in medical science that made it possible to sustain life functions. We also have learned that various parts of the body die at different times. The central nervous system is one of the most vulnerable areas, and brain cells can be irreversibly damaged if deprived of oxygen, while other parts of the body will continue to function.

Newer definitions of death have been built around the concept of human potential—meaning the potential of the human body to interact with the environment and with other people, to respond to stimuli, and to communicate. When these abilities are lacking, there is said to be no potential. Because this potential is directly related to brain function, the method most often used to assess capability is electroencephalography. Brain activity, with few exceptions, is said to be nonexistent when flat electroencephalographic tracings are obtained over a given period, often 48 hours. After this point, the person may be considered dead, although machines may be supporting the vital functions of respiration and circulation. Many institutions now accept this definition of cerebral death and use it as a basis for turning off respirators and stopping other treatments. It is also used as a basis for determining death when there is a desire to recover organs from the client.

Planning for End-of-Life Issues

Increasing emphasis is being placed on prior planning for end-of-life issues. Identifying futile treatments is one aspect of this process. Another important consideration relates to client self-determination regarding these issues. Many hope that the use of such planning will decrease the ethical dilemmas in end-of-life situations.

Futile Treatments

Futile treatments (medications, devices, or therapy) are those that are evaluated by the health-care team, the family, or both as being nonbeneficial or harmful to the client inasmuch as they bring no benefit to the client (Jecker, 2014). For example, when an individual is dying from terminal cancer, treatment for a respiratory infection may be deemed futile because it will not alter the fact that the person is dying and will not restore a satisfactory quality of life. Identifying whether further treatment is futile may be extremely difficult. It is related to many assumptions about quality and quantity of life and, based on the best interest principle, places high demands on the individual responsible for decision making. However, Schneiderman, Jecker, and Jonsen (1996) suggest that if, in the past 100 cases of the same nature, there was no change in the outcome based on the treatment, it can be considered futile. Others take a position that treatment never can be declared futile. In their thinking, the future cannot be predicted accurately, and if there cannot be absolute certainty about the outcome, then futility cannot be clearly identified.

Other problems may arise when futility is declared. To what extent should the client be involved in the decision making? Does a client have a right to treatment even if it has been identified as futile? What about cost considerations? Should insurance companies be required to pay for treatment that has been classified as futile? What about Medicare or Medicaid? Should there be differences in decisions based on age or quality of life?

Critical Thinking Activity: Futility of Treatment
Do you think that factors such as ability to pay, treatment of children or younger adults versus older adults, the cost of the treatment, and the percentage of time the treatment is effective should be issues considered when deciding whether treatment is futile? Provide a rationale for each answer. What are your biases?

Client Self-Determination: Ethical Issues Surrounding Advance Directives and Living Wills

In December 1991, the federal Patient Self-Determination Act (PSDA) went into effect. Passed by Congress in 1990, this legislation requires that all Medicare and Medicaid providers inform clients on admission of their right to refuse treatment. The intent of this legislation was to enhance an individual's control over medical treatment decisions by promoting the use of advance directives (see Chapter 7). The entire process has not been without its problems.

The time of admission to a healthcare facility is often filled with anxiety, making it almost impossible to consider such matters.

The American Nurses Association emphasized that nurses should facilitate informed decision making and should occupy a critical role in education, research, client care, and advocacy. The organization's 1991 position statement of nursing and client self-determination remains in effect but was updated in 2010 with *The Nurses Role in Ethic and Human Rights: Protecting and Promoting Individual Worth, Dignity, and Human Rights* position statement.

In an attempt to gain greater control over the area of dying, several documents have been developed to assist with this process. **Advance directives** are legal documents that indicate the wishes of an individual with regard to end-of-life issues and were described and discussed in Chapter 7. A **living will**, a form of advance directive, allows individuals to identify what measures to include in care if they become terminally ill. The living will is often used to request that no extraordinary measures be implemented, although it can be used to indicate a preference that all possible actions should be taken.

Some have voiced concern that advance directives have failed to achieve their goals. Often, this is because they are not available or are misunderstood, are not clear, or are not as specific as needed. There is also a tendency for family members, when faced with the real situation, to say, "Well, he didn't really mean that." It is essential to prevent confusion, distress, and ethical dilemmas at the end of life that clients and families understand advance planning in order to have their wishes met. Nurses, with the care team, should provide education and resources to support clients and families to understand and complete advance directives.

Another approach being used with increasing frequency is the signing of a *durable power of attorney for healthcare*. In this type of an agreement, an individual (referred to as the principal) may designate another person to have the power and authority to make healthcare decisions for the principal should the principal be unable to make those decisions. Durable power of attorney documents were discussed in detail in Chapter 7.

 ### Evidence-Based Practice 8.1: *Palliative Care*

Temel, J. S., Greer, J. A., Muzikansky, A., et al. (2010). Early palliative care for patients with metastatic non-small-cell lung cancer. *New England Journal of Medicine, 363*, 733–742.

Researchers conducted a study of 151 subjects divided into randomized groups that received either palliative care with the standard oncology care or standard oncology care alone. The group receiving palliative care reported less depression, improved quality of life, and lived an average of three months longer than the control group. Interestingly, the palliative care group was also less likely to have received aggressive interventions, which represents a potential cost savings for clients and insurers.

Euthanasia

Euthanasia, meaning good death, may be classified as either negative or positive. The word, as it is generally applied, refers to the act or method of causing death painlessly so as to end suffering.

Negative Euthanasia

Negative, or passive, euthanasia refers to a situation in which no extraordinary or heroic measures are undertaken to sustain life. The concept of negative euthanasia has resulted in what are called _no codes_ or DNR orders in hospital environments. In these situations, hospital personnel do not attempt to revive or bring back to life persons whose vital processes have ceased to function on their own.

It is difficult to describe what constitutes extraordinary measures and to determine on whom they should or should not be used. Is it one thing to defibrillate a 39-year-old man who is admitted to an emergency department suffering from an acute heart attack, and quite another to defibrillate a 95-year-old man whose body is riddled with terminal cancer and whose heart has stopped? Often, people who are involved in giving medical and emergency care develop an almost automatic response to lifesaving procedures and may have difficulty accepting dying as an inevitable part of the life process. This is particularly true when emergency personnel receive a 911 call and rush to the home of an individual who has requested that no extraordinary measures be taken to sustain life. Often, cardiopulmonary resuscitation or other such efforts are started before the rescuers know of the request.

It is difficult to know when it is permissible to omit certain life-supporting efforts, or which efforts should be skipped. If the 95-year-old man who is dying of terminal cancer were also to develop pneumonia, should his physician prescribe antibiotics? This brings us to the distinction between stopping a particular life-supporting treatment or machine, and withdrawing treatment or not starting a procedure in the first place—that is, withholding treatment.

Some ethicists do not differentiate between **withholding treatment** in the first place and **withdrawing treatment** once it has been determined to be inappropriate or futile. They would see both as having the same position in terms of right and wrong. Those who support negative euthanasia support both withholding and stopping treatment. The general public often sees these as separate issues and may support withholding treatment, while not supporting the termination of treatment once it has begun. Increasingly, the legal system has supported withdrawing treatment that is determined to be futile. A landmark case in 2005 was that of Terri Schiavo, who was in a persistent vegetative state following a heart stoppage due to a chemical imbalance that occurred 5 years earlier. Her husband wanted her feeding tube removed, which would ultimately result in her death; her parents wanted the treatment continued. Finally, the courts decided that the husband was the legal decision maker. He then had the feeding tube removed.

Positive Euthanasia

Positive, or active, euthanasia occurs in a situation in which the physician prescribes, supplies, or administers an agent that results in death. On some occasions, a physician prescribes strong narcotics for a terminally ill client and requests that the medication be given frequently enough to keep the client comfortable. Although this is not legally considered positive euthanasia, nurses may be reluctant to administer a medication that they realize has a potentially fatal effect when given in that dosage. Medications given for the comfort of the dying client may be ethically justifiable even if they hasten death to some extent. This is based on the ethical concept of double effect, in which the acceptable effect (such as pain relief) is the purpose of the medication and the secondary effect (such as depressing respiration) is not the intended effect. When nurses have difficulty with this issue, a client conference with an oncology specialist or with a nurse skilled in the area of death and dying can help the staff to clarify values and deal with individual feelings.

Rights Issues Surrounding Death

Rights issues surrounding death are gaining much more attention than in previous years. These include the right to refuse treatment, a right to death with dignity, the right to choose the time and manner of one's death, and even a right to assisted suicide. These may be grouped together under the terminology **right to die**.

A great deal of controversy surrounds the issue of maintaining the lives of persons considered to be in a persistent vegetative state. Some of the issues that arise are the client's rights stated above (if their wishes are known), the family's wishes, and the cost to society. In most cases, the problems emerge when the life of a person is being maintained through support measures that might be considered extraordinary. Healthcare providers and families may fail to communicate effectively when physicians continue to emphasize that the client may be helped to *survive* while not clearly explaining that this does not indicate that there will be *recovery* to any prior level of function.

Withdrawing and Withholding Treatment

Withdrawing treatment is defined as stopping treatment that is considered medically futile, that is, will not provide a cure or control the disease. Withholding treatment occurs when this type of treatment is not provided at all. Although withholding and withdrawal of therapies have been described mainly in situations related to technical interventions (ventilator, hemodialysis), they can also be applied by extension to chemotherapy, artificial hydration, and nutrition as long as the aim of these therapies is to prolong life beyond expectation, to delay death. Landmark cases are numerous with some of the most notable ones being the case of Karen Quinlan, a young comatose woman on a ventilator whose parents sought to have the treatment stopped, and the Terri Schiavo case mentioned earlier.

Of particular concern to nurses are their own feelings when a decision is reached to remove life-supporting measures, whether the measures are tube feedings or ventilators. Strong emotional attachments often form between the nurse and client, even when the client is in a vegetative state. Nurses who have worked to preserve the client's dignity have great difficulty letting go. It is important to support colleagues during these times. Support groups or counseling may be necessary to help staff cope with grief.

Positions on Withholding and Withdrawing Treatment

Several organizations and groups have issued guidelines for their members and others who would find them useful, with regard to the issue of withholding or withdrawing treatment. Key to all of these guidelines is whether the patient is legally competent (able to make decisions for himself or herself) or incompetent (in need of someone else to make those decisions). Table 8.5 outlines the date, organization, and major tenets of some of those positions.

Assisted Suicide

Assisted suicide involves helping another end his or her life. In June 1997, the United States Supreme Court rendered a decision on physician-assisted suicide (PAS). This decision took

Table 8.5 Positions on Withholding and Withdrawing Treatment

	Organization	Position
1983	President's Commission Report—*Deciding to Forego Life-Sustaining Treatment*	Focused on the ethical, medical, and legal issues in treatment decisions. Distinguished between withholding (not starting) and withdrawing (stopping after it started) treatment without making a moral distinction between the two. Suggested that withholding may require more justification because the positive effects would not be known.
1986	American Medical Association—*Statement on Withholding or Withdrawing Life-Prolonging Medical Treatment*	Stated that life-prolonging medical treatment and artificially or technologically maintained respiration, nutrition, and hydration could be withheld from a client in an irreversible coma even if death was not imminent (Fry, 1990).
1986	Office of Technology Assessment of the US Congress—*Life-Sustaining Technologies and the Elderly*	Issued the results of its study on the use of life-sustaining technologies on the elderly. Report noted that the most controversial of the technologies was that of nutritional support. Identified that the most troublesome aspect of nutritional support is whether it is intravenous feeding and hydration or a tube feeding (Fry, 1990).
1987	Hastings Center—*Guidelines on the Termination of Life-Sustaining Treatment*	Provided clear definitions of key terms and a general guideline for making decisions regarding treatment. Viewed nutrition and hydration as medical interventions, much as other life-sustaining measures. Placed emphasis on the client's ability to make decisions and required case-by-case assessment (Fry, 1990).
1988	American Nurses Association—*Guidelines on Withdrawing or Withholding Food and Fluid*	Indicated that there were few instances under which it would be permissible for nurses to withdraw food or fluid from their clients. No distinction was made between withdrawing and withholding (ANA, 1988).
1992	American Nurses Association—*Position Statement on Foregoing Medically Provided Nutrition and Hydration*	Stated that the decision to withhold medically provided nutrition and hydration should be made by the client or surrogate with the healthcare team. The nurse continues to provide expert and compassionate care to clients who are no longer receiving medically provided nutrition and hydration. Distinguished between medically provided nutrition and hydration and the provision of food and water (ANA, 1992).
1994	Alzheimer Association	Stated that if such a client is unable to receive food and water by mouth, it is ethically permissible to choose to withhold nutrition and hydration artificially administered by vein or gastric tube. Spoon-feeding should be continued if needed for comfort (Alzheimer's Association, n.d.).
2009	American Pediatric Association	Supported the position that withdrawal or withholding medical interventions is morally permissible when requested by competent clients, or, in the case of clients without decision-making capacity, when the interventions no longer confer a benefit to the client or when the burdens associated with the interventions outweigh the benefits received (Diekema & Botkin, 2009).
2010	National Hospice and Palliative Care Organization (NHPCO)	Indicated that is always acceptable to withhold or withdraw artificial nutrition and hydration when a competent client refuses or when adequate evidence exists that an incompetent client would have found the balance of risks and potential benefits to be unacceptable or when it is in the client's best interest (NHPCO, 2010).

the position that there was no constitutionally protected right to PAS on behalf of terminally ill clients.

The activities of a retired Michigan pathologist, Jack Kevorkian, who is alleged to have assisted clients in their suicides, received much media attention in the 1990s. Although eluding criminal charges for a number of years, in March 1999, Dr. Kevorkian was convicted of second-degree murder and the delivery of a controlled substance after CBS televised a video showing him administering lethal drugs. Dr. Kevorkian's release from prison in 2007 brought renewed attention to the issue of assisted suicide.

In April 2001, the Netherlands became the first nation to fully legalize euthanasia, a process that was 3 years in the making, but has specific rules and requires that the client give informed consent. In 2003, Belgium legalized voluntary euthanasia, while Germany and Switzerland allow assisted suicide but prohibit the physician from assisting other than prescribing the medication.

As of 2016, five states, California, Colorado, District of Columbia, Vermont, Washington, and Oregon, have set aside the Supreme Court ruling to the extent that residents have supported Death with Dignity Acts allowing PAS, and California has proposed such legislation at least once. On December 31, 2009, the Montana Supreme Court determined that nothing in state law prevents clients from seeking PAS, making Montana the third state that will allow the procedure. The Montana law falls far short of the reform standard established by the other states where the legislature has protected doctors from having to stand trial if challenged so long as they comply in good faith with a set of rigorous procedures (Bowden, 2010). Oregon first passed such legislation in 1997 and reconfirmed it in 1994; Washington's legislation became effective on March 5, 2009. The ANA has developed a position statement in which it states that the nurse should not participate in assisted suicide. Such an act is viewed as a violation of the Code for Nurses. It is the position of the ANA that the challenge for nurses should not be in legalizing assisted suicide. Rather, the role of the nurse should be directed toward reversing the despair and pain experienced in the last stages of life, and in fulfilling the obligation to provide competent, comprehensive, and compassionate end-of-life care (ANA, 2013). The ANA published a *Call for Action: Nurses Lead and Transform Palliative Care* in the spring of 2017 in an effort to improve palliative care, which is comprehensive, compassionate, and client-centered care. Many argue that good palliative care would reduce the desire for assisted suicide by improving quality of life and providing support to the client and family.

The Right to Refuse Treatment

The **right to refuse treatment** is an issue closely aligned with the right to die. However, it carries special implications that require separate consideration. Although we discussed some of the parameters of this issue in the previous section on the right to die, other aspects can create even bigger problems for the nurse. Support of the right to refuse treatment is based on a basic belief in and respect for the autonomy of the client. Cases such as one in which a client refuses to have a leg amputated, despite the fact that not having the surgery undoubtedly will result in death, often will make the news. When the client refuses treatment but does not withdraw from the role of being the client, the matter becomes more complex. By refusing one type of treatment, the client is essentially demanding alternative medical management. An example would be the client who refuses to have a gangrenous toe surgically removed and demands to

Figure 8.5. People working in the healthcare field are frequently confronted with the dilemma of clients who may wish to refuse treatment.

have it treated otherwise. One form of treatment may be more accepted than another, but both may be successful.

When children are involved, it is even more newsworthy and again points out that there is as yet no consensus about when minors should be allowed to refuse treatment. Often, cases involving children are related to cases in which the parents refuse to have the treatment started, many times because of religious beliefs. The courts usually become involved in reaching a decision. When time is not a factor, the court may recommend that treatment be delayed until the child is 15 or 16 years old and can make a decision as an older minor. Other judges will rule just the opposite, deciding that it is cruel to place the burden of the decision on this older minor.

Because nurses have the most contact with clients, they must examine their own feelings and attitudes when clients refuse treatment. Nurses must recognize that clients also have the right to attitudes and beliefs. If a nurse decides that his or her feelings are so strong that they might interfere with the ability to give compassionate care, it would be wise to ask to be assigned to other clients (Fig. 8.5).

Stegen & Sowerby Stories: Part 2

Kristen was eventually caught and fired after infecting at least 18 patients with hepatitis C. Charges were pressed and Kristen had to testify in a court of law. Read the rest of the story at www.thePoint.com.

Want to Know More?

A variety of resources are available on thePoint° to enhance your learning and understanding of this chapter, such as:

- Full Stegen & Sowerby Stories
- NCLEX-Style Student Review Questions
- Journal Articles
- Case Studies
- Learning Objectives
- Relevant Web sites
- And more...

KEY CONCEPTS

- Ethics is a branch of philosophy referred to as moral philosophy. It seeks to provide answers to some of the questions of human conduct that arise in our life and attempts to determine what is right or good.
- Inherent in the study of ethics is an appreciation of individual values that are derived from societal norms, religion, and family orientation. We can better understand our own value system through the process of values clarification.
- The basic ethical concepts of beneficence, nonmaleficence, autonomy, justice, fidelity, veracity, and the standard of best interest underlie ethical decision making and may be in conflict in an individual situation.
- The ethical theories of utilitarianism, deontology, natural law, and social equity and justice may be used to examine the implications of ethical decisions.
- The concept of justice has been expanded to include distributive justice that is applied in situations requiring the allocation of scarce resources. The problems associated with the allocation of scarce resources are expected to increase in the near future.
- Ethical decision making may be based on personal religious and philosophic viewpoints, but must always be grounded in professional standards seen in the Codes for Nurses and the statements of client rights.
- A variety of social and cultural factors including attitudes, science and technology, legislation, judicial decisions, and funding all influence ethical decision making.
- The nurse's status as an employee, collective bargaining contracts, collegial relationships, the authoritarian and paternalistic backgrounds of healthcare, deliberations of ethics committees, and consumer involvement create pressures regarding ethical decision making.
- A basic framework for ethical decision making emphasizes identifying and clarifying the problem, gathering data, identifying options, making a decision, acting, and assessing.
- Nurses have ethical obligations to the client and to the employer and must maintain an objective stance regarding other healthcare providers, and when confronting substandard care. Commitment to personal excellence and to the profession of nursing are also desired characteristics of the professional nurse.

- In serious situations, when using the chain of command does not invoke response to voiced concerns, one might use whistle-blowing to bring attention to the circumstances. This should be used as a last resort because of the possible ramifications to the individual blowing the whistle.
- The chemically impaired nurse is a concern to the profession and a danger to clients. All nurses have an obligation to report those who demonstrate chemical impairment and to assist impaired colleagues in finding treatment and rehabilitation.
- Boundary violations, a situation in which the nurse moves beyond a professional relationship and becomes involved with clients and their families, have become a concern in nursing. Educational programs to increase understanding of this problem and to help avoid its occurrence are being conducted.
- End-of-life issues are some of the most common ethical and bioethical dilemmas routinely faced by nurses. While state laws may support assisted suicide, the ANA code of ethics guides nurses to relieve suffering and despair to support quality end-of-life care instead.
- Surrounding the discussion of right to die are many issues, including those related to client self-determination, futile treatment, withholding or withdrawing treatment, assisted death, and the right to refuse treatment

NCLEX-STYLE PRACTICE QUESTIONS

1. The nurse reviews the medications for possible interactions before administering them. This is an example of which ethical concept?

    A. Autonomy
    B. Veracity
    C. Nonmaleficence
    D. Beneficence

2. You are scheduled to work tomorrow, but your friends want you to call in sick. You go to work as scheduled. Which ethical concept does this demonstrate?

    A. Veracity
    B. Fidelity
    C. Justice
    D. Nonmaleficence

3. If you suspect a colleague is chemically impaired, what is the first thing you want to do?

    A. Immediately report to your supervisor
    B. Collect data, document, and report
    C. Talk to your colleague about concerns
    D. Speak to other coworkers for validation

4. Prioritize the steps of the ethical decision-making process.

    A. Gather factual data
    B. Identify and clarify problem
    C. Make a decision
    D. Act and assess
    E. Identify and evaluate options

5. Which of the following symptoms could indicate that a colleague is chemically impaired?
   A. Occasional fatigue
   B. Boundary violations
   C. Occasional missed work
   D. Inconsistent job performance

REFERENCES

Alexander, S. (1962). They decide who lives, who dies. *Life, 53*, 102–125.

Alzheimer's Association. (n.d.). *Ethical issues in Alzheimer's disease: Assisted oral feeding and tube feedings*. Retrieved June 6, 2018, from https://www.alz.org/alzwa/documents/alzwa_Resource_EOL_FS_Oral_Feeding.pdf

American Nurses Association. (1988). *Guidelines on withdrawing or withholding food and fluid*. Washington, DC: Author.

American Nurses Association. (1990). *Suggested state legislation: Nursing Practice Act, Nursing Disciplinary Diversion Act, Prescriptive Authority Act* (Pub. No. NP-78). Washington, DC: Author.

American Nurses Association. (1992). *Position statement on foregoing medically provided nutrition and hydration*. Washington, DC: Author.

American Hospital Association. (1992). *A patient's bill of rights*. Chicago, IL: Author.

American Nurses Association. (2013). *Position statement: Euthanasia, assisted suicide, and aid in dying*. Retrieved May 26, 2016 from http://www.nursingworld.org/euthanasiaanddying

American Nurses Association. (2015). *Code of ethics for nurses with interpretive statements*. Silver Spring, MD: Nursingworlds.org.

Bowden, T. (2010). *Montana addresses physician-assisted suicide*. Retrieved August 11, 2010, from http://blog.aynrandcenter.org/montana-addresses-physician-assisted-suicide/

Brown, J. (2010, February 24). *Hospital tech who spread Hep C via drug thefts get 30 years. Denver Post*. http://denverpost.com/2010/02/24/hospital-tech-who-spread-hep-c-via-drug-thefts-gets-30-years/

Brown, M. (2015). *Ethics in organizations. Markkula Center for Applied Ethics: Better Choices*. Retrieved from https://www.scu.edu/ethics/ethics-resources/ethical-decision-making/ethics-in-organizations/

Bissell, L., & Haberman, P. W. (1984). *Alcoholism in the professions*. New York, NY: Oxford University Press.

Bissell, L., & Skorina, J. (1987). 100 alcoholic women in medicine. *Journal of the American Medical Association, 257*(2), 939–944.

Campbell, A. R., & Polk, E. (1992). *Legal and ethical issues of alcohol and other substance abuse in nursing education*. Atlanta, GA: Southern Council on Collegiate Education for Nursing.

Centers for Disease Control and Prevention (CDC). (2015). *Heath, United States, 2015: With special feature on racial and ethnic health disparities*. Retrieved from https://www.cdc.gov/nchs/data/hus/hus15.pdf#014

Centers for Medicare and Medicaid Services (CMS). (n.d.). *National health expenditure projections 2016–2025: Forecast summary*. Retrieved June 4, 2017, from https://www.cms.gov/Research-Statistics-Data-and-Systems/Statistics-Trends-and-Reports/NationalHealthExpendData/Downloads/proj2016.pdf

Current Nursing. (2012). *Theory of interpersonal relations. Nursing Theories: A companion to nursing theories and models*. Retrieved June 4, 2017, from http://currentnursing.com/nursing_theory/interpersonal_theory.html

Curtin, L. (1978). A proposed model for critical ethical analysis. *Nursing Forum, 17*(1), 12–17.

Diekema, D. S., & Botkin, J. R. (2009). *Forgoing medically provided nutrition and hydration in children. American Pediatric Association*. Retrieved from http://pediatrics.aappublications.org/content/124/2/813

Distributive Justice. (2017). Retrieved June 4, 2017, from http://legal-dictionary.thefreedictionary.com/Distributive+justice

Fry, S. T. (1990). New ANA guidelines on withdrawing or withholding food and fluid from patients. In C. A. Lindeman & M. McAthie (Eds.), *Readings: Nursing trends and issues* (pp. 499–507). Springhouse, PA: Springhouse.

International Council of Nurses. (2012). *The ICN code of ethics for nurses.* Geneva, Switzerland: Author.

Jameton, A. (1984). *Nursing practice: The ethical issues.* Englewood Cliffs, NJ: Prentice-Hall.

Jecker, N.S. (2014). *Medical futility. Ethics in Medicine: University of Washington School of Medicine.* Retrieved from https://depts.washington.edu/bioethx/topics/futil.html

Kidney Transplantation: Past, Present, and Future. (n.d.). *History.* Retrieved June 6, 2018, from https://web.stanford.edu/dept/HPS/transplant/html/history.html

Lachman, V. D. (2008). Whistleblowing: Role of organizational culture in prevention and management. *Demotological Nursing, 20*(5), 394–396. Retrieved August 10, 2010, from http://www.medscape.com/viewarticle/582796_5

Little, K., & Brownstein, J. (2014). Primer on whistleblowing in healthcare. *The Ambulatory M&A Advisor.* Retrieved from http://www.ambulatoryadvisor.com/primer-on-healthcare-whistleblowing/

Marion, L. N., Fuller, S. G., Johnson, N. P., Michels, P. J., & Diniz, C. (1996). Drinking problems of nursing students. *Journal of Nursing Education, 35*(5), 196–203.

McCulloh Nair, J., Nemeth, L. S., Williams, P. H., Newman, S. D., & Sommers, M. S. (2015). Alcohol misuse among nursing students. *Journal of Addictions Nursing, 26*(2), 71–80.

Milner, S. (1993). An ethical nursing practice model. *Journal of Nursing Administration, 23*(3), 22–25.

Merriam-Webster Online Dictionary. (2017a). *Addiction.* Retrieved June 4, 2017, from http://www.merriam-webster.com/dictionary/addiction

Merriam-Webster Online Dictionary. (2017b). *Beneficence.* Retrieved June 4, 2017, from http://www.merriam-webster.com/dictionary/beneficence

Merriam-Webster Online Dictionary. (2017c). *Bioethics.* Retrieved June 4, 2017, from http://www.merriam-webster.com/dictionary/bioethics

Merriam-Webster Online Dictionary. (2017d). *Futility.* Retrieved June 4, 2017, from http://www.merriam-webster.com/dictionary/futility

National Association of Practical Nurse Education and Service. (2007). *NAPNES standards of practice for licensed practical/vocational nurses.* Falls Church, VA: Author.

National Council of State Boards of Nursing. (2014). *A nurse's guide to professional boundaries.* Retrieved from https://www.ncsbn.org/ProfessionalBoundaries_Complete.pdf

National Hospice and Palliative Care Organization. (2010). *Commentary and position statement on artificial nutrition and hydration.* Retrieved from https://www.nhpco.org/sites/default/files/public/ANH_Statement_Commentary.pdf

NHS. (2014). *Euthanasia and assisted suicide-Arguments.* Retrieved June 4, 2017, from http://www.nhs.uk/Conditions/Euthanasiaandassistedsuicide/Pages/Arguments.aspx

Occupational Safety and Health Administration. (n.d.). *The whistleblower protection programs. United States Department of Labor.* Retrieved June 9, 2017, from https://www.whistleblowers.gov/

O'Neil, M. G. (2012). *You suspect that your coworker is impaired—What should you do? Medscape.* Retrieved from http://www.medscape.com/viewarticle/769388

Physician Health Program. (2015). *Drug-addicted doctors & health care professionals.* Retrieved June 9, 2017, from http://www.physicianhealthprogram.com/addiction-news/drug-addicted-doctors-health-care-professionals/

Rawls, J. A. (1971). *Theory of justice.* Cambridge, MA: Harvard University Press.

Ray, S. L. (2006). Whistleblowing and organizational ethics. *Nursing Ethics, 13*(4), 438–445.

Saver, C. (2009). *Life-and-death scenarios lead to moral distress in nurses.* Retrieved August 18, 2009, from http://news.nurse.com/apps/pbcs.dll/article?AID=/20090601/NATIONAL01/90529002/-1/

Schneiderman, L. F., Jecker, N., & Jonsen, A. (1996). Medical futility: Response to critiques. *Annals of Internal Medicine, 125*(8), 669–674. doi:10.7326/0003-4819-125-8-199610150-00007

Segen's Medical Dictionary. (2011). *Medical futility*. Retrieved June 5, 2018, from https://medical-dictionary.thefreedictionary.com/medical+futility

Sullivan, E., Bissell, L., & Leffler, D. (1990). Drug use and disciplinary actions among 300 nurses. *International Journal of the Addictions, 25*(4), 375–391.

Sullivan, E., Bissell, L., & Williams, E. (1988). *Chemical dependency in nursing: The deadly diversion*. Menlo Park, CA: Addison-Wesley.

Thompson, J., & Thompson, H. (1981). *Ethics in nursing*. New York, NY: Macmillan.

Values. (2017). Retrieved June 4, 2017, from www.businessdictionary.com/definition/values.html

Velasquez, M., Moberg, D., Meyer, M. J., Shanks, T., McLean, M. R., DeCosse, D., et al. (2009). *A framework for thinking ethically*. Retrieved June 4, 2017, from http://www.scu.edu/ethics/practicing/decision/framework.html

Safety Concerns in Healthcare

After completing this chapter, you should be able to:

1. Identify at least three national organizations that have studied the issue of adverse events and medical errors in healthcare and describe the findings of each study.
2. Discuss the safe practices as outlined by the National Quality Forum and indicate how each would play a part in decreasing errors.
3. Describe actions taken by The Joint Commission to encourage healthcare organizations to reduce the incidence of errors.
4. Explain what is meant by the term *sentinel event*.
5. List at least five occurrences that could be labeled adverse events.
6. Describe what a *time-out* involves.
7. Analyze the relationship between *failure to rescue* and nurse staffing.
8. Describe the sources and types of medication errors and explain how medication errors can be interdisciplinary.
9. Discuss the role of the nurse in preventing errors and providing a safe healthcare environment.
10. Describe the role of the Quality and Safety Education for Nurses (QSEN) project in nursing education.

KEY TERMS

Culture of safety
Failure to rescue
Handoff
National Patient Safety Goals (NPSG)
Root cause analysis (RCA)

Safe practices
Sentinel events
Serious reportable events (SRE)
Time-out
Universal Protocol

Stegen & Sowerby Stories: Part 1

J oan, a 34-year-old pregnant woman, began feeling very ill. She was concerned for the safety of her unborn baby and went to her local hospital emergency department. She was experiencing abdominal cramping, fever, and shortness of breath. Because she was near term and the fetus was in distress, she was given intravenous (IV) antibiotics and rushed to surgery for a cesarean delivery. Upon delivery, the amniotic fluid was foul smelling and chorioamnionitis, an infection of the amniotic sac, was diagnosed.

After delivery, she was transferred to the postpartum floor as a standard postcesarean client. Several hours later, she was found to be lethargic with a low blood pressure. Blood cultures were drawn and IV fluids were administered. Several hours later, the blood worked revealed that the client had gram-negative bacteria and the team realized that she was in septic shock.

- What was the cause of the septic shock?
- Why do you think septic shock developed?
- What client safety concerns do you have with this scenario?
- What potential medical errors could have occurred?
- What communication errors might have occurred?

No one—client, family, or healthcare provider—enters a healthcare setting anticipating that an error will alter that experience and have potentially life-threatening effects. Despite the best intentions, however, a high rate of largely preventable adverse events and medical errors occurs that cause harm to clients. There is no immunity from these mistakes: adverse events and medical errors may occur in any healthcare setting and in any community in this country. In this chapter, we discuss some of the more common errors and the nurse's role in prevention of those errors. Nurses, as managers of client care, must be actively involved in preventing medical errors.

NATIONAL ORGANIZATIONS AND ACTIONS

As providers, as well as the general public, became increasingly concerned about the errors occurring in the healthcare environment, organizations whose focus was data collection and advising initiated studies to gain information about the problem. Some of the major organizations involved in this process are described in Table 9.1.

Institute of Medicine Study

In response to the growing concern about medical errors, in November 1999, the Institute of Medicine (IOM) released a groundbreaking report estimating that between 44,000 and 98,000 clients die as the result of preventable medical errors in hospitals each year (IOM, 2000). The data presented in the 1999 IOM study caught the attention of the general public as well as that of healthcare providers. Neither clients, providers, nor payers (insurance companies, Medicare, Medicaid, and health maintenance organizations) were totally aware of the safety concerns or, if aware, had not recognized their responsibility to create change. The study also reported that hospital-acquired infections (HAIs), many of which can be prevented, take another 100,000

Table 9.1 Major Organizations Studying Healthcare Errors

Organization	Description	Goal
Health and Medicine Division	Called the Institute of Medicine until 2016. The Health and Medicine Division (HMD) is a division of the National Academies of Sciences, Engineering, and Medicine (the National Academies). The National Academies are private, nonprofit institutions that provide independent, objective analysis and advice to the nation and conduct other activities to solve complex problems and inform public policy decisions related to science, technology, and medicine. The National Academies operate under a 1863 congressional charter to the National Academy of Sciences, signed by President Lincoln (www.nationalacademies.org).	To help the government and the private sector make informed health decision by conducting research to provide reliable evidence.
National Quality Forum	Private, nonprofit, open membership public benefit corporation established in 1999 that brings together leaders from every sector of the industry in national dialogue.	To set national priorities, endorse national consensus standards for measuring and publicly reporting on performance, and promoting attainment of national goals through education and outreach.
The Joint Commission	Independent, nonprofit organization that accredits and certifies more than 17,000 healthcare organizations in the United States.	To improve healthcare.
Center for Medicare and Medicaid Services	Established in 2001 and previously known as the Health Care Financing Administration, a federal agency within the U.S. Department of Health and Human Services.	To administer the Medicare program and work in partnership with state governments to administer Medicaid, the State Children's Health Insurance Program, and health insurance portability standards.

lives (IOM, 2000). In 2016, preventable medical errors resulted in over 400,000 deaths in the United States alone. At a cost of $1 trillion, these preventable deaths are the third largest killer of Americans after heart disease and cancer (Zikhani, 2016).

National Quality Forum

In 2002, the National Quality Forum (NQF) created and endorsed a list of **serious reportable events (SRE)**—also referred to as adverse or *never events*—to increase public accountability and consumer access to critical information about healthcare performance. Initially, 27 events were identified; in 2006, one additional occurrence was added. The 28 were each classified under one of six categories of events: surgical, product of device, client protection, care management, environment, or criminal. The most recent SRE report in 2011 lists 29 events that are clearly defined and preventable. A listing of the SREs can be found at http://www.qualityforum.org.

In 2003, the NQF, with support from the Agency for Healthcare Research and Quality (AHRQ), identified 30 **safe practices** that evidence shows can work to reduce or prevent adverse events and medical errors. The original safe practices were updated in 2006, 2009, and 2014. The latest audit of the 2010 report, published in 2014, lists 34 practices that are organized into seven functional categories for improving client safety (Box 9.1). An executive summary detailing the 34 safe practices can be found at http://www.qualityforum.org/Publications/2014/05/2010_Safe_Practices_Audit.aspx.

BOX 9.1 CATEGORIES FOR IMPROVING CLIENT SAFETY

- Creating and sustaining a culture of safety
- Informed consent, life-sustaining treatment, disclosure, and care of the caregiver
- Matching healthcare needs with service delivery capability
- Facilitating information transfer and clear communication
- Medication management
- Prevention of healthcare-associated infections
- Condition- and site-specific practices

The Joint Commission

To address concerns about errors in healthcare, The Joint Commission established patient safety goals for each year beginning in 2002 through the present time (The Joint Commission, 2017a, 2017b). Agencies that were accredited by The Joint Commission were required to begin targeting high-incidence preventable safety problems, such as falls, misread physician orders, and communication errors. The Joint Commission requires that accredited institutions investigate all sentinel events. A **sentinel event** is an unexpected occurrence involving death or serious physical or psychological injury or the risk thereof. Serious injury specifically includes loss of limb or function. The phrase "or the risk thereof" includes any process variation for which a recurrence would carry a significant chance of a serious adverse outcome. Serious adverse outcome is defined as instances of error that have the potential for serious harm or death to the client (The Joint Commission, 2017c). Some examples of sentinel events, both errors and near misses, are presented in Box 9.2. As you can see, not all sentinel events are errors; rather, some can be considered a near miss. More information can be obtained on sentinel events by visiting www.jointcommission.org and clicking on Sentinel Events. At this site, the number of specific events can be found along with recommendations for prevention.

As a critical method by which to promote and enforce major changes in client safety in thousands of participating healthcare organizations, The Joint Commission has established **National Patient Safety Goals** (NPSG). There is a separate set of safety goals for each type

---

BOX 9.2 EXAMPLES OF POTENTIAL SENTINEL EVENTS

- Surgery on the wrong body part
- Tubing and catheter misconnections
- Overdosing with commonly used anticoagulants
- Death resulting from a treatment-related or medication error
- Client suicide occurring in a setting in which around-the-clock care is provided
- Assault, rape, or homicide of clients or visitors perpetrated by staff, other clients, visitors, or intruders
- A maternal death
- Discharge of an infant to the wrong family
- Unprofessional provider behavior

---

of agency providing care; the goals are structured in the same way for each type of agency and have used a consistent numbering system. Each year, The Joint Commission re-examines the sentinel event data and the safety goals and revises them by deleting those that have been largely achieved and adding new safety goals. When a goal appears to be no longer an area of concern or is not appropriate to that type of agency, the goal and the number are omitted and moved to standards. These patient safety goals are available online at www.jointcommission.org.

In efforts to reduce sentinel events and adverse outcomes, in 2002, accredited hospitals began collecting data on standardized—or *core*—performance measures. In 2004, The Joint Commission and the Centers for Medicare and Medicaid Services (CMS) began working together to align measures common to both organizations. These standardized common measures, called Hospital Quality Measures, are integral to improving the quality of care provided to hospital clients and bringing value to stakeholders by focusing on the actual results of care. With these oversight organizations working together, institutions benefit because the same data set can be used to satisfy both CMS and The Joint Commission requirements, thus decreasing the cost of collecting and reporting.

Centers for Medicare and Medicaid Services

In October 2008, CMS demonstrated their commitment to safety by announcing that they would not reimburse hospitals for the costs associated with six serious hospital-acquired complications. The initial six conditions include pressure ulcers, two HAIs (catheter-associated urinary tract infections [CAUTIs] and *Staphylococcus aureus* septicemia—methicillin-resistant *Staphylococcus aureus* [MRSA]), and three *never events* (air embolism, blood incompatibility, and foreign object left behind in a surgical client).

The underlying rationale was a belief that these are preventable complications and denying reimbursement provides a strong incentive for quality improvement actions to avert them. Some have argued that conditions such as pressure ulcers may have begun before admission and that for some debilitated clients, those conditions may not be avoidable. However, the plan went into effect, and health insurance plans in several states adopted similar policies.

Federal Safety Legislation

Almost immediately after the 1999 IOM report was released, federal legislation was introduced in relation to client safety. Although bills were submitted in the House of Representatives and Senate each year, it was not until 2005 that the Patient Safety and Quality Improvement Act was finally passed by both legislative bodies and signed into law by President George W. Bush (Patient Safety and Quality Improvement Act, 2005). The goal of the act was to improve client safety by encouraging voluntary and confidential reporting of events that adversely affect clients. This law provided protection for individually identifiable healthcare data that might be used to assess safety concerns and created and provided for the certification of client safety organizations to collect, aggregate, and analyze confidential information reported by healthcare providers. It also set up a plan for a network of client safety databases that could be used for research and development without fear of disclosure of data about individual organizations and established mechanisms to provide technical assistance to facilitate work on client safety data **(Fig. 9.1)**.

Quality and Safety Education for Nurses

In 2005, the Quality and Safety Education for Nurses (QSEN) project began. There were three phases from 2005 to 2012, during which time investigators identified the knowledge, skills,

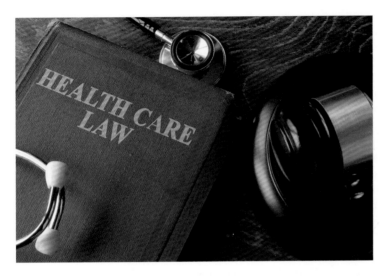

Figure 9.1. The goal of the Patient Safety and Quality Improvement Act of 2005 was to improve client safety by encouraging voluntary and confidential reporting of events that adversely affect clients.

and attitudes (KSAs) needed by future nurses. This information, called the QSEN competencies, is now widely used in nursing education to better prepare nursing students for their role in improving quality and safety in the healthcare system.

ADDRESSING SAFETY CONCERNS

Although it is not possible within the scope of this chapter to discuss each of the categories and guidelines that have been set forth for safe practice, we want to expand on those that most seriously affect nursing practice.

Organizational Culture

One of the areas identified among the 34 safe practices listed by the NQF that affects healthcare organizations is the need to create a culture of safety. The culture of an organization is a product of its history, its mission and values, its beliefs and customs, the structure of the organization, and the manner in which providers of healthcare carry out their roles (see Chapter 1). A **culture of safety** is one in which trust and mutual respect encourage healthcare providers to report errors, near misses, and other adverse events without fear of retribution (Evidence-Based Practice 9.1).

In response to the recommendation regarding a culture of safety, The Joint Commission requires a **root cause analysis**, a comprehensive, in-depth process that seeks to identify all the underlying factors that contribute to an error and to identify their role in causing the error. For example, if a nurse were to give the wrong medication to a client, what were all the aspects surrounding the error? Did the nurse fail to follow the six rights? Was he or she interrupted while preparing the medication? How was the medication stored? How was it labeled? How was it obtained from the pharmacy? How was the order received and transcribed? These are a few of the factors that might affect the outcome. There are many factors that contribute to error. Identifying those factors is the first step to error prevention (Martin, 2016). In order for error reporting and follow-up to be truly effective, it is critical that nonpunitive actions be taken. Individuals who are worried about job security, embarrassment, and legal ramifications are less likely to report an error.

Evidence-Based Practice 9.1: Client Safety

Arnetz, J. E., Zhdanova, L. S., Elsouhag, D., Lichtenberg, P., Luborsky, M. R., & Arnetz, B. B. (2011). Organizational climate determinants of resident safety culture in nursing homes. *The Gerontologist, 51*(6), 739–749. doi:10.1093/geront/gnr053Summary

Creating a culture of safety where workers feel safe to report errors and near misses is an important factor in many aspects of safety. Employees feel safe in that they are not risking their employment by reporting errors or near misses. Clients have increased safety because any errors can be addressed and processes can be examined to improve client safety.

The authors of this article analyzed data from four different nursing homes to determine what aspects of an organization were predictors of safety culture. They determined that goal clarity was a predictor of communication about incidents and that work stress was linked to a lack of compliance with procedures.

Most facilities encourage individuals to report near misses where error could have occurred. An example could be two medications stored side by side in a crash cart that have similar-looking labels but very different actions. A nurse may mistakenly pick up the wrong one and prepare to give it but on the third check note the discrepancy and give the correct medication. Noting this as a near miss might result in changes to the crash cart to decrease the likelihood that this error could occur in a stressful situation.

As a new graduate, you may feel that there is little you can do as a newcomer to the scene to influence a culture of safety. That is not the case. You will soon have the responsibility for directing, overseeing, and evaluating the care provided by those with lesser preparation than you have. There will be occasions when you will need to advise or correct members of your team. How you go about that is critical. When you make suggestions and corrections, keep them system oriented rather than person focused. As mentioned above, use this as an opportunity to improve the quality of care the client receives rather than a time to let a team member know what he or she is doing wrong. Working with team members is discussed in detail in Chapter 12.

Matching Needs With Delivery Capability

Another practice identified by the NQF was to match healthcare needs with service delivery capability. Research has consistently demonstrated that clients undergoing certain high-risk procedures have lower-than-expected mortality rates in hospitals that perform large numbers of those procedures and, conversely, higher-than-expected mortality in institutions that perform low volumes of those procedures. Some examples of high-risk procedures include coronary artery bypass graft, coronary artery angioplasty, abdominal aortic aneurysm repair, pancreatectomy, and esophageal cancer surgery. Safe practice guidelines require that clients be fully informed of the reduced risk at high-volume institutions and encourage their referral to such facilities.

Communications

The area of communication is discussed in many areas of this text and in detail in Chapter 11. This said, it so significantly affects client safety that we will discuss some specific areas where communicating effectively is critical to safe practice.

Figure 9.2. Communication failures can result from hierarchy differences, conflicting roles, ambiguity in responsibilities, and power struggles.

Breakdowns in communication have been cited as a root cause in the majority of cases reported to and studied by The Joint Commission's Sentinel Event Database since 1996. Within the healthcare environment, communication failures can result from a variety of issues including hierarchy differences, conflicting roles, ambiguity in responsibilities, and power struggles (Ammouri, Tailakh, Geethakrishnan, et al., 2015, Fig. 9.2). It has been estimated that communication errors, especially at handoffs, are factors in more than 80% of sentinel events (Joint Commission, 2012). This has resulted in the inclusion of the need to improve the effectiveness of communication among caregivers in The Joint Commission's NPSG every year since their inception in 2005. Links to the safety goals can be found at www.jointcommisson.org/PatientSafety/NationalPatientSafetyGoals/.

Client Safety During Handoffs

In our fast-paced and technologically enhanced healthcare systems, clients are frequently transferred from one area of the hospital to another. An individual admitted through the emergency department could easily have received care in at least five different areas of a hospital. Each time that client is moved, clear and detailed information sharing is required. This is referred to as a **handoff**—a process in which information about the client or resident is communicated from one healthcare provider to another. Handoffs typically occur at change of shifts, which occur two or three times a day, 7 days a week. If team communication skills have been developed, practiced, and maintained, it can mean the difference between an optimal outcome and an adverse event (Birmingham et al., 2015).

In 2012, The Joint Commission released the Targeted Solutions Tool for handoff communications. They defined handoff as "a process in which information about client/resident care is communicated in a consistent manner" from one healthcare provider, called the "sender," to the next care provider, the "receiver" (Joint Commission, 2012). This tool will help healthcare institutions to develop shift-to-shift reports that efficiently and effectively communicate the client's condition, needs, and plan of care. In an effort to attain better communications, the healthcare industry has taken a lesson from the military. The technique known as situation–background–assessment–recommendation (SBAR) was used as a method for communicating information concisely between all ranks in the U.S. Navy. This strategy is very effective for communicating client status information during handoff reports. The first two components address objective facts and relate succinct briefings regarding the client situation. The last two are subjective information that can include opinion and a specific intervention. This system builds in a pattern to the relaying of information that allows the receiver to quickly notice the omission and ask for correction.

Critical Thinking Activity: SBAR Report

Using the information you receive during morning handoff report, create an SBAR briefing.

Mr. Jones was in an auto accident 3 days ago. He has significant pain and has a lower leg fracture of both bones. He had to have surgery to repair the bones after he was seen in the emergency department. His vital signs need to be assessed every hour because he is on morphine 2 mg IV for pain. He is in room 25. His circulation, motion, and sensation (CMS) checks have been good. His leg is elevated. His pain is now a 2 of 10 after receiving morphine 30 minutes ago. He can start on oral pain meds when he is no longer having nausea and is taking fluids well.

Systems such as SBAR are effective because they are easy to understand and follow. Using a structured and repetitive system such as this, the person receiving the information can respond indicating acknowledgment of the data. These forms of sharing information during handoff can be practiced or rehearsed so that all members of the nursing team become familiar with the process.

Tools to Improve Communication

Nurses and physicians work closely to foster positive outcomes with those for whom they care. Yet, they sometimes have difficulty communicating. Nurses have been educated to be narrative and descriptive in their messages. Physicians, on the other hand, may be action oriented and want the main subject matter of the problem so prompt action can be taken. In facilities that lack a structure or procedure for verbal reports, individuals differ in what they see as critical to report. Communications frequently are interrupted or pressured by time. In 2016, a study by Galleta, Carta, D'Aloja, et al. (2016) found that ineffective communication between physicians and nurses resulted in job dissatisfaction and voluntary turnover on the part of nurses. In efforts to better this situation, many healthcare institutions have initiated specific programs to improve communication.

A whole-system approach to communication that is adapted to the unique characteristics of an organization provides the best results because the culture of the organization is a critical component of safe care. Team training must be provided, elements contributing to organizational hierarchy eliminated, roles and responsibilities delineated, and a zero-tolerance policy enforced with regard to disruptive behavior. All healthcare team members are educated about professional behavior and are held accountable to modeling desirable behaviors.

One such program that helps an organization make changes resulting in efficient and respectful exchanges of information that improve client safety and nurses' job satisfaction is the TeamSTEPPS (Team Strategies and Tools to Enhance Performance and Patient Safety). It was developed in 2006 by the U.S. Department of Defense Patient Safety Programs and AHRQ. It is based on the concept of a "just culture" (mentioned earlier) in which all persons—including the client—regardless of their place in the hierarchy are expected to monitor and speak out about the care provided. TeamSTEPPS targets four competencies: team leadership focusing on a positive environment, situation monitoring in which the entire team must be aware of the environment and team performance at all times, mutual support, and communication.

Adopting Safe Practices in Specific Clinical Care Settings

Certain areas of healthcare facilities experience unique problems by virtue of the service provided in that area. Surgery departments are prime examples. To reduce the incidence of wrong site, wrong procedure, or wrong person surgeries, a **Universal Protocol** (which is part of the NPSG) has been developed by The Joint Commission that must be followed by accredited hospitals and surgery centers. The protocol involves three steps to be taken prior to the surgery and includes conducting a preprocedure verification process, marking the procedure site, and performing a *time-out* as described later. When possible, the client is involved in the process. Each facility must develop an individualized plan for the steps as they will be used for their facility.

A standardized list is used for the preprocedure verification process, which includes checking for coexisting health problems that might be of consequence and assuring that medications, supplies, blood, and fluids needed before, during, and after the surgery have been obtained. All test results should be on the record and available.

Sites on which the surgery is to be performed are marked (unless it is on bilateral structures), ideally by the licensed independent practitioner who is ultimately accountable for the procedure and will be present when the procedure is performed although the responsibility for doing the marking may be delegated to a medical resident, physician assistant, or advanced practice nurse.

The standardized *time-out* is conducted immediately before starting any invasive procedure or making the incision. The **time-out** involves the immediate members of the procedure team: the individual performing the procedure, anesthesia providers, circulating nurse, operating room technician, and other active participants who will be involved in the procedure. All relevant members of the team actively communicate during the time-out and agree, at a minimum, that the client identity is correct as is the site and the procedure to be done. The surgical procedure is not started until all questions or concerns are resolved. If more than one procedure is to be done or the person performing the procedure changes, another time-out needs to be done. Completion of the time-out must be documented.

Infection Control

It has been estimated that about 1 of every 25 clients admitted to acute care hospitals and long-term care facilities in the United States develop a healthcare-associated infection (HAI). This type of infection was also called a hospital-acquired (formerly nosocomial) infection. One of the reasons these infections are such a concern is that they frequently occur in people whose health is already compromised by disease, age, or injury. More than 1 million people are affected by HAIs annually. The Centers for Disease Control of the U.S. Department of Health and Human Services has shown that about 36% of these infections are preventable through the adherence to strict guidelines when caring for clients. A study conducted by the U.S. AHRQ showed that incidence of HAIs decreased by 17% between 2010 and 2013 (https://psnet.ahrq.gov/primers/primer/7/health-care-associated-infections).

Many hospitals have adopted a series of practices called a *bundle* to address each type of HAI. The use of all the practices in the bundle has been shown to decrease the incidence of the target infection even though the evidence for each part of the bundle may be limited. For example, many hospitals are adopting a bundle approach to preventing central line-associated bloodstream infections (CLBSI). This bundle includes the entire procedure for insertion, the daily cleaning protocols, and the protocols for use of the central line catheter. Failure to use all the measures prescribed in the bundle may adversely affect client outcomes. Although the cost of implementing a bundle can be significant, its effectiveness in improving quality of care may offset the cost.

Although issues such as staffing are problems to which the hospital administration must respond, as a new graduate, there are steps you can take to reduce the incidence of infection. You will want to practice all the precautions you have been taught during your years as a nursing student. New graduates have the advantage of having the most recent exposure to nursing literature. Perhaps, there are nurses working on your unit who are unfamiliar with evidence-based practice or are uncomfortable seeking information even if the tools for doing so are on the unit. It is no longer acceptable for nurses to carry out a procedure using techniques that reflect a "that's the way we have always done it" philosophy **(Fig. 9.3)**.

Failure to Rescue and Nurses' Time at the Bedside

Considered a client safety indicator by AHRQ, **failure to rescue** has been defined as "the inability to prevent death after the development of a complication" (AHRQ, 2017). Failure to rescue has been tied to the amount of time that the nurse spends at the bedside with incidence of failure to rescue decreasing when nurses spend more time at the bedside and less on other activities. After an IOM report in 2004 estimated that registered nurses (RNs) working a 12-hour shift are only in client rooms for 1.5 hours, facilities endeavored to increase the amount of time nurses spend at the bedside. Table 9.2 identifies successful strategies discussed by Hendren (2010) and outlines how they can be helpful. If life-threatening conditions are to be prevented or immediately treated before irreversible damage is done, they need to be recognized. If early recognition is to happen, the nurse must be with the client. Studies show a direct correlation between increasing the number of nursing hours spent with clients and the reduction of complications such as urinary tract infections and pneumonia experienced by the client.

Figure 9.3. Some nurses are uncomfortable using new methods or equipment.

Table 9.2   Strategies to Increase Nurses' Time at the Bedside and Benefits

Strategy	Benefit
Rounding hourly	Clients understand their nurse will be around regularly and therefore do not use the call bell as often.
Conducting bedside change-of-shift report	Saves time over taping report and allows the nurse coming on duty to ask questions. Improves client safety by involving the client and ensures the client and nurse are working together.
Streamlining documentation	With the help of technology, this improves client safety and saves time.
Addressing medication administration inefficiencies	Electronic medication administration records and bedside medication administration improve safety and remove inefficiencies if developed with input from users.
Using standardized tools for client handoffs	Tools, such as SBAR, provide communication checklists and ensure complete information transferred efficiently.
Keeping supplies in close reach	Reduces the time nurses spend hunting and gathering supplies. Locating supply closets in central locations decreases the miles nurses walk each day.
Outsourcing discharge follow-up calls	Assigning to others the task of follow-up calls to discharged clients frees the nurses on the unit.
Seeking physician input	Having physician involvement at the development of system improvements helps assure success of the project.
Asking nurses	The easiest way to learn what will help nurses save time is to ask them. It also decreases frustration.

Adapted from Hendren, R. (2010). Ten ways to increase nurses' time at the bedside. *Health Leaders Media*. Retrieved July 5, 2010, from http://www.healthleadersmedia.com/content/NRS-248033/Ten-Ways-to-Increase-Nurses-Time-at-the-Bedside.

Nurse Staffing

The quality of care provided to clients is dependent on the healthcare workforce. RNs comprise the largest single component of hospital staff and are the primary providers of hospital client care—61% of RNs in the United States work in state, local, or private hospitals (BLS.gov, 2017). Because of the key role nurses play in client safety and quality of care, the U.S. DHHS and the AHRQ conducted several studies to examine the association between nurse staffing and client outcomes. The result of the investigation indicated that higher RN staffing was associated with less hospital-related mortality, failure to rescue, cardiac arrest, hospital-acquired pneumonia, and other adverse events.

Keeping clients safe and caring for the whole person are the focus of Jean Watson's nursing theory. Read more about this theorist in the following Theory Alert.

Theory Alert *Jean Watson*

Jean Watson explored the science of caring. Born in the 1940s in West Virginia, she earned her nursing degree in 1961. She continued her education, completing a bachelor's degree, master's degree in psychiatric and mental health nursing, and ultimately earning a PhD in educational psychology and counseling in 1973.

Watson's theory, called the Philosophy and Science of Caring, focuses on the ways nurses care for their patients. She believed that caring could be demonstrated and practiced by nurses. Key to her theory was the belief that a holistic approach was vital to the practice of caring in nursing. She was proponent of using the nursing process to create a framework for nursing care. By first assessing the patient, then identifying the problem, a plan of care could be developed. After developing a plan of care, implementation of that plan and evaluation of effectiveness provide the nurse with information that then leads to the next assessment and a repetition of the process.

Watson was a great proponent of the value of caring in healing. She felt that caring in nursing practice produced better health results than a simple medical cure. In 2008, she created the Watson Caring Science Institute to promote her theory and ideas.
(Source: www.nursing-theory.org)

Also tied to nurse–client ratios and staffing, safety is a matter of client satisfaction. Berkowitz (2016) found that the nurse–client ratio was significantly associated with clients' satisfaction ratings. One attempt to improve client experience has been to link reimbursement to client satisfaction scores. Berkowitz reviewed a literature suggesting that improving nurses' work environments, including nurse staffing, may improve the client experience and quality of care (Berkowitz, 2016).

The American Nurses Association (American Nurses Association [ANA], 2017) has campaigned strongly for safer staffing patterns supporting nurses who rank staffing as their biggest problem. Linking insufficient nurse staffing with poorer client outcomes, lengthened hospital stays, and increased chance of client death, the ANA advocates solving the problem by requiring hospitals to set nurse staffing plans for each hospital unit based on changing conditions:

- Client acuity (severity of illness)
- Client numbers

- Nurse skills and experience
- Support staff
- Technology

Using this as a foundation, the organization is working with legislators to pass a legislation that empowers direct care nurses to contribute to staffing plan development through hospital staffing committees. As of May 2017, 14 states had passed nurse safe staffing laws that mirror ANA's approach.

Preventing Falls

Falls occur in all types of healthcare institutions and to all client populations, making them a common cause of morbidity and the leading cause of nonfatal injuries and trauma-related hospitalizations in the United States. Client falls are among the most common occurrences reported in hospitals and are a leading cause of death in people aged 65 or older. Nearly half of all residents in nursing homes fall each year, with many sustaining fractures. Fall-related injuries account for an estimated $31 billion in Medicare costs each year (CDC, 2016).

Clients fall for several reasons. They may trip, slip, or fall because of a failure of equipment or by environmental factors such as moisture on the floor. Falls may also occur due to physiologic conditions, such as fainting, a seizure, or a pathologic fracture of the hip. These types of falls usually cannot be anticipated. Clients can also fall from causes that can be anticipated such as a weak or impaired gait, use of a walking aid, presence of IV lines, impaired mental status, or a history of previous falls.

Facilities often have a very specific fall assessment tool. This includes a thorough and sound assessment of clients, their abilities and limitations, and knowledge of side effects of the medication(s) they are taking. Based on the data obtained through this tool, a graduated series of fall prevention measures are instituted. These are termed the *fall prevention protocol*. This might include environmental changes such as using bed or chair alarms, placing the bed in a low position and putting foam pads on the floor, or locating the client next to the nurses' station. Nursing care modifications might be instituted such as toileting every 2 hours, visual checks at least hourly, or the provision of assistance any time the client gets out of bed.

No single prevention plan is effective for all clients. Although some prevention strategies are obvious and may be used with most clients, other clients present a greater challenge and demand more creative and innovative solutions to ensure client safety, particularly in long-term care settings. Fall prevention remains a nursing challenge and a nursing responsibility.

Increasing Safe Medication Administration

Da Silva and Krishnamurthy (2016) reported that adverse drug events were among the most common medical errors, affecting approximately 7 million people every year across all medical settings. The extra medical costs of treating these adverse drug events are estimated at $21 billion a year, and this estimate did not take into account lost wages and productivity or additional healthcare costs (Da Silva & Krishnamurthy, 2016).

In 1995, U.S. Pharmacopeia spearheaded the formation of the National Coordinating Council for Medication Error Reporting and Prevention (NCCMERP). The NCCMERP defined a medication error as any preventable event that may cause or lead to inappropriate medication use or client harm while the medication is in the control of the healthcare professionals, clients, or consumers. In seeking solutions for medication errors, experts in the healthcare field have recommended key areas on which healthcare professionals focus their efforts. These include elimination of ambiguous abbreviations, computerized physician order entry (CPOE), computerized decision support systems (CDSS), computerized adverse drug event monitoring (CADM), barcode point-of-care (BPOC) medication safety systems, and IV administration smart pumps.

Eliminating Ambiguous Abbreviations

The FDA and the ISMP have launched a national education campaign to eliminate the use of ambiguous medical abbreviations that are frequently misinterpreted and lead to mistakes that result in harm to the client. The goal of the campaign is to promote safe practices among those who communicate medical information (USFDA, 2009).

The Joint Commission has established a NPSG that specifies that certain abbreviations must appear on an accredited organization's "do-not-use" list; ISMP has highlighted those items on their list with a double asterisks (**). You may be aware of some of the abbreviations that are easily confused such as IV and IU. Other issues in writing out dosage abbreviations are included in this list such as errors in dosage from a misreading of decimal points. Thus, there is the requirement that leading zeros before the decimal point always be included and trailing zeros after a decimal point never be used. A listing of the abbreviations identified as problematic by ISMP can be found at http://www.ismp.org/tools/errorproneabbreviations.pdf.

Computerized Physician/Provider Order Entry

Computerized physician/provider order entry is defined as the computer system that allows direct entry of medical orders by the person with the licensure and privileges to do so. The computer system accepts the prescriber's order electronically rather than in writing and checks that order against standards for dosing, interactions, and allergies with other medications the client may be taking and warns the prescriber about potential problems. Directly entering orders into a computer has the benefit of reducing errors by minimizing the ambiguity of handwritten orders (CPOE, 2017). Use of CPOE is being increasingly encouraged as an important solution to the challenge of reducing medical errors and improving healthcare quality and efficiency. Usage has been increasing since the 2009 federal Health Information Technology for Economic and Clinical Health (HITECH) Act was passed to encourage meaningful use of health information technology.

Some of the additional benefits of CPOE include current information that helps physicians keep up with new drugs as they are introduced into the market, drug-specific information that eliminates confusion among drug names that sound alike, improved communication between physicians and pharmacists, and reduced healthcare costs due to improved efficiencies.

Computerized Decision Support Systems

CDSSs provide a review of orders as they are written and compare new and existing orders while scanning for possible drug interactions and appropriate dose schedules and alert the provider to pertinent lab results. This information will have an impact on the physician's decisions and the plan of care for the client. A CDSS can enhance clinical performance related to prescribing practices and provide important reminders and alerts. This system can also recommend less expensive alternative medications to decrease client care costs and has the means to identify and prevent duplications related to medications, testing, and imaging.

Computerized Adverse Drug Monitoring

Adverse drug events continue to be the single most frequent source of healthcare errors that place clients at risk of injury. This can be anticipated because drug treatment is the most common medical intervention, and medication use is a highly complex process. It is also multidisciplinary involving the skills of the provider, the pharmacist, and the nurse and is largely a manual process. Historically, the process for assessing the actual safety of drug use has been difficult, mainly because traditional methods such as chart audits and voluntary reporting of data have been shown to be expensive, insensitive, and largely ineffective for detecting mistakes in drug administration and drug-related adverse clinical events (ADEs). The process has been simplified by using computerized methods for detecting ADEs when computerized client records are in use. The computerized systems employ sentinel words or triggers in a client's medical record. Although these CADMs are effective, they are expensive and require customized software linkage to pharmacy databases. CADM has been a feature in most hospital pharmacy information systems for years although in a limited form. It is now moving beyond pharmacy as a standard offering in CPOE and electronic health record systems.

Barcode Point of Care

BPOC systems use a bedside computer, a server with interfaces to the admission–discharge–transfer and pharmacy systems, and medication administration software to cross-check barcodes printed on client wristbands, nurse identification badges, and medication labels. The

---

Daily Ethical Dilemma 9.1: Medication Administration

Jasmine, a pregnant 16-year-old, arrived in labor at St. Mary's Hospital. Admitted to the hospital, she was in her room when the nurse came in to care for her. She selected a bag of medication from two that were already in the room, and she hooked a bag of what she assumed was penicillin, ordered for the client, to Jasmine's IV line. Jasmine's heart failed and her baby was delivered by emergency cesarean. The baby survived but Jasmine did not recover.

- What do you suspect has happened?
- Identify the potential problems in this scenario.

A review of the case found that the nurse had not put an identification bracelet on the client for use with the hospital's barcode system. Two medications, similar in appearance, and both ordered for the client had been brought to the client's room, penicillin for IV administration and bupivacaine meant to be given as an epidural. The epidural medication was accidentally hooked to the client's IV access resulting in her death. The nurse was also tired from working 16 hours the previous day, then sleeping at the hospital for 7 hours, and returning to the floor for work.

- What action do you think the employer will take?
- How could this mistake have been avoided?

Landro, L. (2010, March 16). New focus on averting errors: Hospital culture. *Wall Street Journal (Online)*.

system matches the provider's orders with the client identification and verifies the *six rights of medication safety* by comparing the barcode on medications with the prescribed medications. BPOC software systems have varying levels of sophistication; some systems offer additional clinical alerts regarding sound-alike/look-alike medications or other clinical advisories particular to a specific medication. Following proper dosage administration, some BPOC systems produce an electronic medication administration record, providing legal documentation of the facts of the administration. BPOC is expensive and carries the additional cost of educating employees in its proper use and monitoring that use.

Smart Pumps

Smart pumps are becoming more prevalent as older IV pump systems are replaced. For several years, infusion pumps have been manufactured with software that can alert users to potential errors. The pumps with this additional software are often referred to as *smart pumps* or intelligent infusion devices. The software associated with the pumps allows an organization to create a library of medications that provides medication dosing guidelines, by establishing concentrations, dose limits, and clinical advisories. Because it can be programmed, it can be tailored for the specific needs of an organization and for different client groups within the facility, based on client location, acuity, or weight. The smart pumps provide clinical advisories, soft alerts, and hard stops. Clinical advisories contain relevant information about a specific medication that is displayed on the smart pump screen when the drug is selected from the library. Soft stops notify the user that the dose selected is out of the anticipated range for this medication. However, soft stops can be overridden by the user, and the medication can still be infused without changing the smart pump settings. Hard stops notify the user that the dose is out of the institution-determined safe range and will not allow the infusion to be administered unless the pump is reprogrammed within the acceptable range. These alerts are especially critical when medications classified as *high-alert medications* are being given because the smart pump can reduce administration errors associated with miscalculated doses.

Smart pump technology is not without limitations. If the smart pump drug library is bypassed, and the infusion rate and volume are manually entered, the dose error reduction software will not be in place to prevent a potential error. There is also a risk of choosing the wrong medication from the stock or selecting the wrong medication from the smart pump's drug library. Alerts can be overridden. Hard stops that are not set appropriately can create a barrier to care delivery and may result in nurses using work-arounds (to be discussed later) such as programming the infusion device using the rate/volume mode rather than using the drug library. Failure of users to understand or critically evaluate the information provided by the alert can also result in an error. Organizational resources must also be considered when selecting smart pumps due to the time that must be set aside to develop, maintain, and update drug libraries and to review other data (ISMP, 2017).

Nurses' Role in Medication Safety

Safe medication administration is not a new topic to you. From your first practice laboratory sessions to where you are today, your instructors have emphasized the importance of the six rights (right client, right drug, right dose, right route, right time, and right documentation) and other techniques that will prevent medication errors from occurring. However, there are many factors that play a part in that error other than mistakes made by the nurse. Table 9.3 identifies some of the other areas that contribute to medication error.

Table 9.3 Common Areas That Contribute to Medication Errors

Area of Concern	Reason for Concern
Calculation errors	Studies have indicated that one in six medication errors involves a calculation error.
Look-alike–sound-alike medications—similar packaging	Many medications sound alike when spoken and/or look alike when dispensed.
Catheter and tubing misconnections	Improper connections and control of intravenous medications result in serious problems.
Interruptions and distractions during time of administration	Medication errors decrease significantly when nurses can administer medications with minimum interruption.
Illegible written medication orders	Handwritten orders are often difficult to read and decipher.
Unclear verbal orders	The pressure of busy units in which verbal orders are frequently given results in increased errors.
Failure to check the client's name with MAR	Studies have identified this as a frequent cause of medication error despite the six rights.
Overly tired nurses	Errors increase when the individual giving the medications is overly tired.
Inadequate staffing and high nurse–client ratios	When nurses are rushed or have responsibility for too many clients, errors increase.
Dispensing of medication	In the United States, medications are generally dispensed on client-specific basis. Internationally, only 18% of the countries require unit dose dispensing.
Verifying the absence of drug allergy	National Patient Safety Agency reported that 5.4% of errors leading to harm or death were associated with allergy.
Absence of pharmacists in client care area	Administration error rates decrease when pharmacists make daily visits to the units.
Confusing or misleading drug labeling	Drugs must be properly labeled to ensure safe administration.

IV, intravenous.

Because the administration of medications is one of the major responsibilities of the nurse, many of the medication errors are made by nurses. As the healthcare environment has become more complex and demanding, the error rate has increased. In response, various steps have been taken to reduce the opportunity for errors to occur. There are many places in the process of providing a medication to a client for mistakes to take place. For example, the provider can err in the drug or dosage ordered, the handwritten order may be difficult to read, it may be inaccurately transcribed, or it could be improperly dispensed or labeled by the pharmacist. However, the final step in most healthcare settings is the administration of the medication by the nurse.

The incidence of medication error can be reduced. When administering medications, always be certain you are giving the right medication to the right client. Rely on at least two pieces of information, such as name and date of birth, which can be verified both on a medication administration document and on the client's wristband or from the client's verbal statement, to ascertain accurate client identification.

If you offer a client a medication and that person questions it or says, "I've never taken a pill that looks like this before," stop and listen to what is being said. When a client objects to or questions whether a particular drug should be administered, the nurse should listen. Answer any questions the client may have and (if appropriate) double-check the medication order and product dispensed before administering it to ensure that no preventable error is made. If a client refuses to take a prescribed medication, that decision must be documented in the appropriate client records. All medications must be labeled, including those in syringes, cups, and basins.

Assuming that you conscientiously and consistently follow all the information you have acquired while being a nursing student regarding safe medication administration, what other factors in the healthcare environment may make you subject to error? One of the occurrences most frequently reported by nurses is that of interruptions while administering medications. One study found that when there were 2 or 3 interruptions, procedural errors happened in 100% of cases, and when there were 4 or 5 interruptions, clinical errors were observed 70% of the time (Evidence-Based Practice 9.2; Hayes, Jackson, Davidson, et al., 2015). Interruptions require an individual to switch attention from one task to another.

Evidence-Based Practice 9.2: Medication Safety

Hayes, C., Jackson, D., Davidson, P. M., & Power, T. (2015). Medication errors in hospitals: a literature review of disruptions to nursing practice during medication administration. *Journal of Clinical Nursing, 24*(21/22), 3063–3076. doi:10.1111/jocn.12944

Medication errors are the most common type of error reported in direct client care settings. Interruptions during medication administration have been identified as a major factor in medication administration errors. It is important to identify how nurses manage interruptions in an effort to improve practice.

The authors of this article reviewed the literature to determine the relationship between interruptions and errors in medication administration. Also reviewed were the methods that were effective in reducing those interruptions. Borrowing from the airline industry practice of eliminating distractions in the cockpit during takeoffs and landings, a "no inter-ruption zone" (NIZ) was shown to reduce overall interruptions by over 40%.

In some facilities, nurses are addressing this concern by alerting others that they are not to be interrupted during the time they are administering medications. Creating a NIZ is another idea borrowed from the aviation industry. Some hospitals have set aside areas for medication preparation that are not to be entered by those not preparing a medication. Posting Please Do Not Disturb signs on the automated medication dispensing machines and medication carts has proved helpful (Fig. 9.4). In still other settings, the nurse wears a vest, a hat, an apron, or some other visual indica-tors that they are in the midst of medication administration and are not to be disturbed.

Additional Responsibilities of the Nurse for Safety

As an individual working in healthcare, you are greatly affected by the attitudes toward cli-ent safety that exist in the workplace. Part of your role as an RN includes your recognition of responsibility for the safety of all clients. It is not enough to make sure that you are per-sonally careful. You need to look at systems and processes to identify areas that need to be studied and changed to be safer. An example is the storage locations for look-alike or sound-alike drugs, especially in emergency areas. Look-alike drugs may be mistakenly confused and

Figure 9.4. No interruption zones reduce medication administration errors.

administered. While as an individual nurse you might focus on more careful reading of the label, addressing the system concern toward moving the storage areas would protect all clients.

In light of these concerns, another pitfall for the nurse is the attempt to become faster and more efficient by omitting some of the safeguards that the institution has put in place because they are time consuming. These shortcuts are sometimes referred to as *work-arounds* because the person is working around rather than within the system. Work-arounds also are used when something else in the system is not functioning well, such as pharmacy deliveries being routinely slow so that needed therapy is delayed. If safety precautions are too burdensome, the issue needs to be addressed through processes established by the agency to determine quality of care. Omitting safety features or bypassing system safeguards puts the client in jeopardy.

Communication in Action 9.1: *Refusing to Adopt a Work-Around*

Joyce Means had recently begun working as a new RN on 7-Center. Her regular preceptor was out sick, and she was working with Melody, another nurse on the unit. As she was beginning to prepare her 9:00 AM medications from the automated machine, Melody said, "Oh, you know you will never get everything done if you go in and out of that machine every time you turn around. When the drawer opens for 9:00 AM, I just take out stuff for other times during the day, put them in a little container, and put them in the cupboard right here with the client's name. It saves tons of time." Joyce replied, "I guess I'll just have to learn to be faster at the machine, because I wouldn't be comfortable doing that. The safeguards in the machine help me to not make mistakes, and I really appreciate that. I think it is safer for my clients, too."

Stegen & Sowerby Stories: Part 2

R emember Joan, the pregnant woman who had an emergency cesarean delivery and then went into septic shock? It was discovered that the emergency department physician had prescribed a one-time dose of antibiotics almost 24 hours earlier, and no further treatment had been ordered. Read the rest of the story at www.thePoint.com.

Want to Know More?

A variety of resources are available on thePoint® to enhance your learning and understanding of this chapter, such as:

- Full Stegen & Sowerby Stories
- NCLEX-Style Student Review Questions
- Journal Articles
- Case Studies
- Learning Objectives
- Relevant Websites
- And more...

KEY CONCEPTS

- The Joint Commission has taken steps to encourage hospitals to reduce the incidence of errors and has established NPSG as well as a list of sentinel events that must be reported by hospitals wanting to maintain accreditation.
- A sentinel event is an unexpected occurrence involving death or serious physical or psychological injury or the risk thereof. Serious injury specifically includes loss of limb or function. The phrase "or the risk thereof" includes any process variation for which a recurrence would carry a significant chance of a serious adverse outcome.
- Serious adverse events or outcomes are defined as instances of error that have the potential for serious harm or death to the client. This could include occurrences of things such as surgery on the wrong body part, a maternal death, tubing and catheter misconnection, overdose with commonly used anticoagulants, or discharge of an infant to the wrong family. They are what The Joint Commission refers to as sentinel events.
- The Universal Protocol includes preprocedure verification process, marking the surgical site and performing a time-out before each surgery when all members of the team review a checklist developed to prevent surgical errors from happening.
- Nursing practice must support safe practices. This could include modifying the organizational culture, participating in effective communications, carrying out infection control, preventing failure to rescue, identifying staffing issues, and assuring safe medication administration.

- Failure to rescue is decreased when there is more nursing time spent at the client's bedside.
- Nurse–client ratios play a significant role in client safety with lower nurse–client ratios contributing to positive outcomes. ANA strongly campaigns for safer ratios and nurse input into staffing patterns.
- Many healthcare workers are involved in the process of providing medications to clients including those who order the medications, those who dispense the medication, and those who administer the medication. Nurses are largely responsible for the administration of medications in healthcare facilities.
- The types and sources of medication errors are many and varied. Technologic approaches have been used to decrease the number of errors that occur. These include eliminating ambiguous abbreviations, CPOE, CDSS, CADM, BPOE, and use of smart pumps.
- Additionally, nurses have devised methods to reduce errors.
- Work-arounds jeopardize client safety by eliminating steps in a process or creating ways to manage outside of the system.
- Because nurses constitute the largest proportion of healthcare workers, their role in the prevention of errors is critical. In one way or another, they touch all aspects of client care from fall prevention to infection control or safe medication administration.

NCLEX-STYLE QUESTIONS

1. Which statement is true about medication errors?

   A. Medication errors only happen to new, inexperienced nurses.
   B. Medication errors are the reason malpractice insurance is needed.
   C. Medication errors are the number one cause of medical errors in the inpatient setting.
   D. Medication errors are primarily the result of data entry errors.

2. Which of the items listed is not a procedure-related accident?

   A. Ground level fall
   B. Intravenous therapy error
   C. Improper use of surgical equipment
   D. Infection of the catheter insertion site

3. What can you do to avoid accidents with equipment in the hospital (select all that apply)?

   A. Never use equipment without a person to help you.
   B. Always lock wheels after using rolling equipment.
   C. Never operate equipment without prior instruction.
   D. Never work around safety measures.

REFERENCES

Agency for Health Care Research and Quality. (2003). *Safe practices for better healthcare: Summary.* Retrieved April 13, 2011, from http://www.ahrq.gov/qual/nqfpract.htm

Agency for Healthcare Research and Quality. (2017). *Guide to patient safety indicators.* Retrieved June 4, 2018, from http://www.qualityindicators.ahrq.gov/

American Nurses Association. (2017). *Nurse staffing measures*. Retrieved June 4, 2017, from https://www. nursingworld.org/practice-policy/health-policy/regulatory/nurse-staffing-measures/

Ammouri, A., Tailakh, A., Geethakrishnan, R., & Al Kindi, S. (2015). Patient safety culture among nurses. *International Nursing Review, 62*(1), 102–110. doi:10.1111/inr.12159

Berkowitz, B. (2016). The patient experience and patient satisfaction: Measurement of a complex dynamic. *OJIN: The Online Journal of Issues in Nursing, 21*(1), 1.

Birmingham, P., Buffum, M. D., Blegen, M. A., & Lyndon, A. (2015). Handoffs and patient safety. *Western Journal of Nursing Research, 37*(11), 1458–1478. doi:10.1177/093945914539052

Bureau of Labor Statistics. (2017). *Occupational outlook registered nurse*. Retrieved May, 11, 2017 from https://www.bls.gov/ooh/healthcare/registered-nurses.htm#tab-3

Centers for Disease Control and Prevention. (2016). *Falls are the leading cause of injury and death in older Americans*. Retrieved May 11, 2017, from https://www.cdc.gov/media/releases/2016/p0922-older-adult-falls.html

CPOE.org. (2017). *Welcome to CPOE*. Oregon Health & Science & University. Retrieved May 11, 2017, from http://www.cpoe.org/

Da Silva, B. A., & Krishnamurthy, M. (2016). The alarming reality of medication error: A patient case and review of Pennsylvania and National data. *Journal of Community Hospital Internal Medicine Perspectives, 6*(4). doi.org/10.3402/jchimp.v6.31758

Galleta, M., Portoghese, I., Carta, M. G., D'Aloja, E., & Campagna, M. (2016). The effect of nurse-physician collaboration on job satisfaction, team commitment, and turnover intention in nurses. *Research in Nursing & Health, 39*(5), 375–385. doi: 10.1002/nur.21733

Hayes, C., Jackson, D., Davidson, P. M., & Power, T. (2015). Medication errors in hospitals: A literature review of disruptions to nursing practice during medication administration. *Journal of Clinical Nursing, 24*(21/22), 3063–3076. doi:10.1111/jocn.12944

Hendren, R. (2010). Ten ways to increase nurses' time at the bedside. *Health Leaders Media*. Retrieved July 5, 2010, from http://www.healthleadersmedia.com/content/NRS-248033/Ten-Ways-to-Increase-Nurses-Time-at-the-Bedside

Institute of Medicine. (2000). *To err is human: Building a safer health system*. Washington, DC: National Academies Press.

Institute of Safe Medication Practices. (2017). *Proceedings from the ISMP summit on the use of smart infusion pumps: Guidelines for safe use*. Retrieved May 11, 2017 from https://ismp.org/Tools/guidelines/smartpumps/default.asp

Martin, E. (2016). Preventing patient harm: Achieving a culture of safety in 2016. *Texas Nursing, 90*(1), 13–16.

Patient Safety and Improvement Act of 2005. (2005). Retrieved April 13, 2011, from www.ahrq.gov/qual/psoact.htm

The Joint Commission. (2012). Joint commission center for transforming healthcare releases targeted solutions tool for hand-off communications. *Joint Commission Perspectives, 32*(8). Retrieved May 9, 2017 from https://www.jointcommission.org/assets/1/6/tst_hoc_persp_08_12.pdf

The Joint Commission. (2017a). *National patient safety goals: 2017 critical access hospital and hospital national patient safety goals*. Oak Brook Terrace, IL: Author.

The Joint Commission. (2017b). *2017 National patient safety goals*. Retrieved May 3, 2017, from http://www.jointcommission.org/PatientSafety/NationalPatientSafetyGoals/

The Joint Commission. (2017c). *Sentinel events*. Retrieved May 11, 2017, from http://www.jointcommission.org/. Type sentinel events in search box.

U.S. Food and Drug Administration. (2009). *Drugs: Medication errors*. Retrieved July 1, 2010, from http://www.fda.gov Type medication errors in search box

Zikhani, R. (2016). Seven-step pathway for preventing errors in healthcare. *Journal of Healthcare Management, 61*(4), 271–281.

CHAPTER 10

The Nursing Profession and the Community

After completing this chapter, you should be able to:

1. Outline how moving care into the community will affect nursing practice.
2. Analyze the philosophy behind community-based care to determine how that relates to your own philosophy of nursing.
3. Explain approaches to client empowerment.
4. Differentiate primary, secondary, and tertiary prevention and how these concepts can be applied in different nursing settings.
5. Outline the various components of disease management and how those provide for health promotion.
6. Discuss how *Healthy People 2020* priority areas and leading health indicators relate to the goals of *Healthy People 2020*.
7. Explain the nurse's role in disaster response in the community.
8. Differentiate the major categories of complementary/alternative medicine.
9. Discuss major issues that surround the use of complementary/alternative medicine.
10. Describe ways in which you could use your knowledge of complementary/alternative therapies when working with clients.

KEY TERMS

Alternative healthcare
Biologically based practices
Community-based nursing
Complementary healthcare
Continuity of care
Disaster management
Disease management
Energy medicine
Health disparities
Healthy People 2020
Herbal medicine
Homeopathy

Integrative medicine
Manipulative and body-based
    practices
Medication reconciliation
Mind–body medicine
Naturopathy
Primary prevention
Secondary prevention
Tertiary prevention
Transition planning
Triage

Stegen & Sowerby Stories: Part 1

Jared is a registered nurse (RN) caring for Ms. Jeffrey who has heart failure and is scheduled to be discharged in the next couple of days from the hospital. Ms. Jeffrey has had three admissions over the last 6 months. The hospital has instituted a new program to assist with the transition to home to provide continuity of care and decrease hospital readmission rates. Prior to discharge, Jared must educate Ms. Jeffrey on self-care, plan for postdischarge medications, reconcile medications, and check on follow-up appointments. Ms. Jeffrey is anxious to go home to her cat and worried about being able to care for herself.

What types of self-care do you think Jared will be teaching? What would be important things to learn about Ms. Jeffrey in order to provide comprehensive teaching and planning for holistic care?

The emphasis in healthcare has increasingly moved out of the institutional setting and into the community. Individuals are treated in ambulatory centers or even in workplaces and return to their homes or perhaps to work. This has both financial and health advantages. Care in a hospital inpatient setting is the most expensive type of care. While the high-technology care and constant surveillance are essential for the seriously ill, for the less seriously ill, that environment poses a myriad of hazards such as infection, medication errors, and lack of rest. In the home, family members must become caregivers, and healthcare workers have a new relationship with clients and families. In all settings, healthcare has moved to a promotion and prevention model, and goals are broader than simply curing illness. This whole movement has had an impact on nursing in many ways.

UNDERSTANDING COMMUNITY-BASED NURSING

The nursing profession has unique privileges that include a trusted relationship with clients and families, access to individuals when they are most vulnerable, and legal status as a profession. In response, as the community's needs change, the nursing profession has an obligation to expand its knowledge base for practice, enlarge its repertoire of skills and abilities, and commit to meeting newly identified needs in innovative and creative ways.

Community-based nursing refers to the wide variety of settings other than inpatient institutions in which nursing is practiced. Public health, home health, ambulatory care, occupational health, and school nursing all reflect community-based practice. From the inception of modern nursing, community-based care has been part of the nursing profession. Graduate nurses of the first hospital training schools worked in homes nursing the sick. In the early part of the 20th century, the public health nurses working in settlement houses in the immigrant neighborhoods of New York and other large cities brought health education, direct care, and advocacy skills to bear on the many health problems confronting the community. As more aspects of healthcare moved into hospitals and other institutional settings, more nursing took place in those environments. However, public health and home care continued the long tradition of nursing in the community.

Care in the community is cost-effective and often more acceptable to the client because it causes less disruption in life. New opportunities arise as the understanding of care in the community enlarges. The principles of community-based care include an emphasis on advocating for clients, promoting client education and self-care, focusing on health promotion and disease prevention, and recognizing the importance of the family, culture, and community.

Community-based care requires effective communication and collaboration. The key in all of these community settings is that the client is in charge. The client decides to work with the nurse, to accept or reject advice and suggestions, and to enter and leave care. The nurse serves as an educator, a guide, a resource person, and an advocate, but health action is taken by the client and family. In addition to those who see themselves as working in a community-based setting, all nurses need to be aware of the community in which the client resides and be able to provide care that fits within the scope of the person's life rather than simply an episode of illness. Care must be family-centered and culturally competent. Nurses working in all environments must be aware of community health organizations, knowledgeable about availability and accessibility of services and supplies, and familiar with the location and specialty of healthcare providers. An interdisciplinary team approach in which the nurse may serve as a collaborator and coordinator takes on new meaning. As all nurses become more community-focused, the boundaries between the institutional nurse and the community-based nurse blur. All need an understanding of how the client functions in each setting, and each setting must adapt to facilitate transitions from one care environment to another.

CLIENT EMPOWERMENT

A community-based philosophy rests on a fundamental belief in the right of the client to control his or her life, including situations related to healthcare. Giving over control to clients removes healthcare professionals from a position of power over others and requires instead that they participate by empowering clients and families. It requires a partnership or alliance between the nurse and the individual and family that is much different from the traditional hierarchical nurse/client relationship.

Empowering others requires possessing knowledge of the alternatives available, the ability to teach based on that knowledge, and the skills to help others make decisions and take appropriate action based on their decisions. Nurses can empower others when they assure that those people have the information necessary to make choices within their lives and when they enable clients and families to make their own choices and manage their own health.

Clients are often fearful of making healthcare decisions because so much is unknown. In addition, not everyone has the same interest in decision-making. While some clients want to make decisions and need the information to do that, others do not want the burden of decision-making. Nurses must navigate these difficult situations and recognize that the client's decision to *not* have information or to not be burdened with certain types of decisions also represents the client's autonomy. In such situations, determining what type of information and the depth of information a client wishes to receive is an important aspect of providing care. The nurse then has the additional responsibility of determining to whom the client has delegated decision-making.

Empowerment supports clients in remaining who they are, not in remaking them into some ideal of a person. The older adult woman who asks that her son make decisions for her is empowered when caregivers respect her enough to allow her to live her life as she chooses. Trying to persuade this woman to change who she is and become the model of an independent person does a disservice to her and increases the distance between her and her caregivers when she most needs to be able to trust in them **(Fig. 10.1)**.

Figure 10.1. Teaching people to manage their own health, giving them the information to make choices within their lives, and helping them to carry out those choices empower them.

HEALTH PROMOTION AND DISEASE PREVENTION SERVICES

Health promotion and disease prevention have long been the major focus of public health nurses, who concentrate on entire populations. This same focus on health promotion and disease prevention is now expanding to nursing in every setting. By recognizing that the determinants of health lie outside of the institution and are found in the community, nurses in the acute care setting enlarge their practice to make it more community-based in philosophy. The various levels of prevention can be addressed wherever the nurse practices.

Primary Prevention

Primary prevention involves the efforts to prevent disease from ever occurring. Primary prevention can be aimed at stopping the cause of disease. On a community-wide level, water treatment and sanitation prevent the spread of communicable diseases by eliminating their sources for the entire population. Helping individuals to be more successful in resisting disease and maintaining health represents another aim of primary prevention. Generalized efforts to educate people regarding healthy diets are aimed at this type of primary prevention. Some efforts involve the individual client and family as the primary focus, although they may benefit the entire community. Immunizations prevent disease not only in the people immunized but also in others by lowering the overall existence of communicable disease throughout the community. Smoking cessation campaigns are aimed at primary prevention and help the individual who quits smoking but also benefit those who might otherwise be subject to second-hand smoke.

Primary prevention can be a focus of nurses in acute and long-term care settings as well as those who work in the community. Nurses need to think in terms of life span development and identify the common preventable diseases and disorders that occur at any point in life. For example, when the client must stop smoking to have surgery and remain in the hospital, the impetus may exist to stop smoking for good. Nurses may help clients to examine their options, consult with physicians for medications to manage withdrawal, point out available smoking cessation programs, and in other ways help clients to quit smoking. Some facilities focus on each contact with a client as an opportunity to review immunization history and encourage updating of immunizations before leaving the hospital. This is particularly important in ensuring that older adults have pneumococcal pneumonia immunization or flu vaccine. When planning for discharge, nurses can build in teaching regarding better dietary practices and help clients understand how those will help in long-term health as well as recovery from the current episode of illness.

Long-term care environments have steadily increased their emphasis on health promotion for even the most disabled individuals. Immunizations, fall prevention through strengthening and balance exercises, and activity programs to prevent social isolation and the accompanying depression serve as primary prevention interventions. Nurses are typically the professionals championing these programs, teaching clients and their families, and increasing public awareness of the concerns.

Secondary Prevention

Secondary prevention involves early identification of health problems through screening and the prevention of complications and adverse consequences of illness. Nurses in ambulatory settings help clients to identify screening tests that are important for them and facilitate scheduling those tests. When admission histories are obtained, the nurse in the acute care setting can attend to information about screenings that are needed and encourage the client to value that activity. To do this effectively, the nurse must understand the current recommendation for screening in specific groups within the population. Asking about screening emphasizes its importance to clients and reinforces other information they may have. It may also create an opportunity for clients to gather additional information. Similarly, in the long-term setting, it is important that nurses continue their focus on prevention activities among the residents. Screening of the older adult population includes different priorities based on the incidence of problems in that age group and the potential years left.

Complications of illness greatly increase morbidity and mortality. Nurses in both acute and long-term care focus on preventing complications as a consistent part of their practice. Careful assessment and timely nursing intervention can prevent the formation of pressure ulcers, development of hypostatic pneumonia, and occurrence of falls. These are only a sample of the many secondary prevention actions taken in the institutional care environment.

Tertiary Prevention

Tertiary prevention focuses on preventing long-term disability and restoring functional capacity. Rehabilitation efforts often have been singled out as the major place where tertiary prevention occurs. However, long-term care has a regulatory mandate to prevent deterioration of older individuals. Although some argue that decreased functional status is a realistic process that happens at the end of life, the increased emphasis on maintenance of function has revealed that even the extremely debilitated older adults may be helped to avoid the complications of dependency and to maintain functional independence in the face of disability longer than was previously thought.

Disease Management

One approach to increasingly sophisticated and targeted prevention services is found in disease management programs. **Disease management** focuses on providing the best evidence-based care for an individual with a specific chronic illness, such as diabetes. These programs are often instituted by health plans or clinics that recognize that failure to manage chronic illnesses knowledgeably results in increased rates of hospitalization, increased demand on the system for high-cost care, and increased incidence of potentially life-altering complications.

By targeting high-impact diseases such as diabetes for special attention, the aim is for both secondary and tertiary prevention. The person with diabetes who is enrolled in such a program receives comprehensive nutrition education, teaching regarding the management of blood glucose through medication and activity, and regular diagnostic evaluations that include hemoglobin A1c and blood glucose measurements to monitor blood sugar control over time, urine analysis to identify renal function, regular eye examinations to identify and treat retinal complications, and regular foot exams to prevent and treat lesions that might progress to gangrene and amputation. While the intensive involvement in prevention services is costly, the process saves overall through the lowered incidence of hospitalization, blindness, renal failure, and amputations, not to mention the cost of human suffering, all of which have monetary costs as well.

Computerized documentation systems facilitate the activities of nurses who are charged with tracking individuals enrolled in a disease management program. They alert the nurse to contact the person through telephone calls, e-mails, or letters when screening services are needed. This same nurse meets with the person to discuss test results. By providing a consistent contact person, the client can develop a trusting relationship and feel more comfortable asking questions and will be more motivated to maintain needed health practices and lifestyle changes.

Theory Alert   Betty Neuman

Dr. Betty Neuman developed a nursing theory that was centered around holistic care with a focus on the person and not the disease and is excellent for community nursing. Dr. Neuman was born in 1924 and earned her diploma as an RN in 1947 in Akron, Ohio, from the Peoples Hospital School of Nursing. She went to the University of California, Los Angeles, where she completed a Bachelor of Science in Nursing and a Master of Science in Mental Health. In 1985, she completed her PhD in clinical psychology from Pacific Western University.

Dr. Neuman started developing her systems model in 1970 to teach nursing students how to view clients holistically, and in 1974, the model was published in *Conceptual Models for Nursing Practice* and titled "The Betty Neuman Health-Care Systems Model: A Total Person Approach to Patient Problems." The model directs nurses to maintain a client's system by using three levels of prevention: primary, secondary, and tertiary. Primary prevention strengthens the flexible line of defense; secondary prevention strengthens the internal lines of resistance, while tertiary prevention helps to stabilize and return the client to wellness. The model uses physiologic, sociocultural, and developmental aspects to provide a holistic overview.
(Source: www.nurses.info/nursing_theory_person_neuman_betty.htm)

HEALTHY PEOPLE 2020

The nation has been addressing health objectives for the whole population through a series of efforts that began with its first set of goals published in 1980 as *Healthy People 1990*. These have been updated at 10-year intervals, and **Healthy People 2020** was released in January of 2010 (US-DHHS, 2010). While the goals of each campaign have not been reached, attention has been focused on them and strategies to work toward them are being refined. A progress update in 2014 showed that four indicators had been met, ten indicators were improving, eight indicators showed no change, and three indicators were getting worse (DPHP, 2014).

Vision, Mission, and Goals of *Healthy People 2020*

Box 10.1 presents the statements of vision, mission, and goals of the *Healthy People 2020* campaign. The vision provides a single comprehensive statement that defines the entire *Healthy People* effort. The mission points to actions that will be needed to achieve the goals. The overarching goals provide a framework in which outcomes can be developed.

Achieving these goals will require a policy focus at all levels of government. Healthcare providers, both individual and institutional, will need to examine their processes and policies. In addition to the roles they have in client teaching, health professionals must recognize the importance of motivation in taking action to improve health. Exploring motivation and the structures that support positive health behaviors will facilitate the engagement of individuals in health promotion activities. To achieve the goals of *Healthy People 2020*, individuals must become aware of their own responsibility for their health. They need to be knowledgeable about what promotes health and what interferes with health. They must make informed choices that lead toward greater health.

BOX 10.1 *HEALTHY PEOPLE 2010–2020* VISION, MISSION, AND GOALS

Vision: A society in which all people live long, healthy lives.

Mission: To improve health through strengthening policy and practice, Healthy People will:
- Identify nationwide health improvement priorities.
- Increase public awareness and understanding of the determinants of health, disease, and disability and the opportunities for progress.
- Provide measurable objectives and goals that can be used at the national, state, and local levels.
- Engage multiple sectors to take actions that are driven by the best available evidence and knowledge.
- Identify critical research and data collection needs.

Goals:
- Eliminate preventable disease, disability, injury, and premature death.
- Achieve health equity, eliminate disparities, and improve the health of all groups.
- Create social and physical environments that promote good health for all.
- Promote healthy development and healthy behaviors across every stage of life.

USDHHS, *Healthy People 2010*, www.healthypeople.gov/hp2020/advisory/PhaseI/summary.htm

Priority Areas of *Healthy People 2020*

The priority areas for action under the *Healthy People 2020* plan include promotion of healthy behaviors, promotion of a healthy and safe community, improvement in the systems for personal and public health that will provide access and eliminate **health disparities** (preventable differences in access for and care of disadvantaged populations), and the prevention or reduction of major diseases and disorders that account for a large proportion of the healthcare problems in society. All of these areas for action will help to achieve the four overall goals.

Healthy behaviors are easy to identify and hard to put into practice. These include adding physical activity to life, managing nutrition well, avoiding being overweight and obese, ceasing tobacco use, practicing safe sexual behaviors, being judicious in the use of alcohol, reducing injury and violence, and maintaining a healthy environment. These are primary prevention behaviors that nurses in all settings can address. The challenges of behavioral change on a large scale have led to increased use of media, such as television advertisements, to impart to individuals information regarding healthy behavior. However, behavioral change is a complex phenomenon and whether these broad strategies are effective is not clear.

Promoting healthy and safe communities has long been considered the province of public health departments. As our understanding of safe communities broadens, the role of domestic violence as a health problem has become more prominent. Many agencies promote awareness of what constitutes domestic violence through posters in public rest rooms, through television spots that highlight resources for help for those facing this problem, and by adding routine assessment for abuse to health histories.

Addressing individual behavior is only successful when the systems of the community support it. Access to health services is essential for people to obtain the screenings and preventive care they need. For example, family planning services contribute to the health of both mothers and infants. Medical products must be safe, and a public health infrastructure must be in place to support a healthy community. Nurses recognize that many individuals never visit a dentist and that assessment of oral health can be part of physical assessment done in other settings, with referral to dental professionals when obvious problems are identified.

While the number of different diseases and conditions fills volumes of books, there are a limited number of conditions that account for the majority of illness and disability. The successful identification and treatment of these diseases create a substantial move toward greater health and quality of life for millions.

Leading Health Indicators for *Healthy People* Initiatives

Leading health indicators are classifications for measurement to determine the success of the *Healthy People* initiatives (Box 10.2). Measures for each category have been devised and are being tracked to determine trends and to evaluate specific strategies for targeted groups. Some are indicators for which a decrease indicates progress, such as tobacco use. For others, an increase indicates success, such as access to healthcare. Specific measurements that will reveal prevalence in the population must be devised for each indicator.

Nurses' Roles in Supporting Healthy Communities

While many nurses work professionally in the community, all nurses can personally support the health of their communities. One personal role is as a supporter and advocate for political measures that would improve the health of the community. This might include contacting

BOX 10.2 THE LEADING HEALTH INDICATORS

- Physical activity
- Overweight and obesity
- Tobacco use
- Substance abuse
- Responsible sexual behavior
- Mental health
- Injury and violence
- Environmental quality
- Immunization
- Access to healthcare

USDHHS, *Healthy People 2020.*

representatives at local, state, or national levels and advocating for passage of important health-related laws or projects. Strategies for this are discussed in Chapter 14.

Another personal role includes being active as a community service volunteer in a homeless shelter, school, or other community agencies. Blood drives, blood pressure screening events, and educational programs may all seek the services of nurses as community volunteers. Within a neighborhood, church, or other settings, nurses are often asked to be resource persons for health-related questions. While nurses need to be careful not to give medical advice

---

Communication in Action 10.1: *Talking With a Neighbor About Health Concerns*

Joe Reynolds is a nurse who works on the surgical unit of a local community hospital. While he works in his yard, a neighbor approaches him and begins to chat. After a few minutes of talking about yard maintenance, the neighbor says, "Uh—Joe, do you know much about these PSA tests?" Joe replies, "A bit. Do you have a question about them?" "Well, I went in to see my doctor. He did some tests and said my PSA is too high and I should go see a urologist. What the heck is it anyway and why should I see another doctor?" Joe asks, "What explanation did the doctor give you?" The neighbor replies, "Well, he talked about numbers and said something about cancer and then I don't remember what else he said." Knowing that even hearing the word cancer can cause enough stress that a person might not hear the remainder of the doctor's explanation, Joe decides to do some simple teaching. He explains, "Well, the test means that something is going on in your prostate. It is an important test, but the results can be positive even when you don't have cancer; other things can cause the readings to be high. However, it really should be checked out so that you get the proper treatment. A urologist specializes in this kind of problem and will do more tests to find out exactly what is going on and then talk to you about whether you need treatment." The neighbor says, "Thanks, Joe. Guess I should make that appointment." Joe replies, "Yes, I think you should. Let me know if there is anything I can help with."

or make recommendations without adequate information, they can advise healthy behaviors, suggest health-related screening, help identify that a problem exists, suggest seeing a healthcare provider for a problem presented, help individuals understand the directions given to them by their physician, and teach people about their medications. Some have suggested that nurses can also be role models of healthy lifestyles for those around them. Although many nurses reject the idea that their lives should be lived with this in mind, others recognize that actions often speak to others much louder than words. The nurse who persists in smoking has less credibility when suggesting healthy lifestyle behaviors to others. Some nurses have used this situation to illustrate their understanding of the difficulty of undertaking lifestyle changes and have entered into groups that work together on healthier living.

MAINTAINING CONTINUITY OF CARE

Continuity of care for the individual means that there is an uninterrupted process across settings in which a person seeks care. In an ideal world, there would never be a duplicated test, a failure to account for medications currently prescribed, or a lack of information upon which the care provider could make decisions. However, the current system is far from ideal. When a mother with young children goes to the emergency room and does not have immunization information, this may affect the care provided. When a person leaves the hospital and does not understand the discharge instructions, that person's health is compromised. When an older adult resident moves from the nursing home to the hospital and information on medications for chronic illnesses does not accompany that person, serious complications may result. The Joint Commission requires that the institutions it accredits study this problem and establish effective policies and procedures to ensure continuity of care. The electronic health record (EHR) is helping to decrease problems but has not eliminated this problem of lack of continuity of care.

Transition Planning

Transitions are the movement of the client from one care environment to another, such as from home care to hospital, from hospital to nursing home, or from one unit in a hospital (such as the intensive care unit [ICU]) to another (such as the general medical unit) as needs for care change. **Transition planning** refers to the planning process that takes place to assure that the client's well-being is maintained throughout the time of transition. As noted in Chapter 9, the actual actions of healthcare providers during the transition are often termed the *handoff*. Many facilities are establishing policies and protocols on exactly what actions must be taken during a handoff. Medication reconciliation, discussed below, is a critical part of the handoff.

The transition to a new care environment has been identified as a time in which the potential for error rises. Whether moving from home to an outpatient setting or between units in the same facility, transition planning is critical to effective care. While physicians usually have the authority to prescribe the move, the nurses are the ones who usually serve as the coordinators of transitions.

Discharge Planning

Planning for a transition often begins when a decision is made for the client's care to be moved to another setting. Some transitions can be predicted before the decision about timing is made. For most clients, discharge from a hospital is an expected event; therefore, planning for discharge begins immediately upon admission, if possible. Upon admission to a hospital, a projected timeline for care may contain specific outcomes to be met along a care pathway. A discharge coordinator may be charged with following the client to assure that planning is accomplished in a timely manner. The discharge coordinator may be a nurse or a social worker. This person works with the family to arrange the appropriate setting for postdischarge care.

All nurses assume responsibility for ensuring that medical orders and nursing plans move with the client to the next location. Written materials that document these orders and plans are essential for accuracy. Teaching is incorporated throughout the process. When discharge is to a nursing home or rehabilitation setting, the goal is that the receiving setting is prepared to provide the care needed. When the person is going home, the nurse is often responsible for ensuring that needed referrals have been arranged and for providing discharge teaching. Clients going home also need written materials to refer to in relationship to self-care. Family members, when available, are integrated into the planning for discharge. The nurse in the institutional setting may follow up with the client after discharge to ensure that the client's healthcare needs are being met in the new environment and that communication has been clear. Appropriate documentation of this process is essential.

Transfers

Whether an individual moves from one unit within an institution to another or from the hospital to a nursing home, a careful plan is still needed. While some transfers occur because of sudden changes in a client's condition or because the demand for beds has accelerated transfers out of a particular unit, most are part of the ongoing therapeutic plan. For a client admitted for surgery, this might include an admitting unit, the surgical suite, the postanesthesia care unit, and the surgical unit, before discharge to home or a rehabilitation setting.

Many facilities now have a separate transfer form that is initiated by the nurse in the unit where the client's care begins. This form identifies all the key transition information. During the handoff, the transferring professional and the receiving professional can quickly review the key information, assess the client, and enter the receiving assessment and acknowledgment of the information on the form. This same process also might be used for the ambulance personnel handing off to the nurse in the emergency department or the nurse handing off to a nurse in a nursing home (although this latter process might occur over the telephone, with written documentation, or e-mail). The advantage of this process is that the receiving nurse does not need to spend a lengthy time trying to find the most important information in a voluminous medical record. Both people are accountable for ensuring that the key information is identified and acted upon.

Medication Reconciliation

One of the major areas of concern for client safety at the time of any transition is the continuity of medications that the client has been taking for the successful management of health problems. The recognition of the importance of this with regard to client safety has resulted in the process called **medication reconciliation**, which occurs after a person is admitted to a care facility. This process is the result of recommendations by The Joint Commission Patient Safety Goals and the Institute for Safe Medication Practices (The Joint Commission, 2017).

Medication reconciliation at admission involves carefully documenting all the medications, and their dosages, including prescribed medications, over-the-counter medications, vitamin/mineral supplements, and herbal products, the person was taking before admission to the care setting. These are then compared with what has been ordered for current care. Any differences are brought to the attention of the medical care provider in order for the best care decision to be made.

This same process is used at all times of transition. Medications change when a person leaves an ICU. Nurses on a surgical unit must be aware of the medications a client received while in the operating room. When a client is admitted through an emergency room, the medication given there will affect ongoing care. If additional medications are ordered in that setting, the nurses must know whether they were given or must still be given after the client comes to the care unit.

Facilities develop a standardized form on which medication reconciliation is documented. These records become part of the client record and are also used to document quality improvement in maintaining safe medication administration by ensuring appropriate continuity of medication orders across transitions.

Critical Thinking Activity: Maintaining Continuity of Care
A charge nurse in a nursing home is planning for the transfer to the hospital of an 87-year-old resident who fell and fractured her hip. This resident has a history of congestive heart failure, osteoarthritis, and osteoporosis but had been ambulatory using a cane and cognitively intact before the fall. What concerns should be addressed before the transfer occurs? What are the issues that will be of concern during the transfer? What information will the receiving nursing unit need in order to provide effective care?

Continuity of Care Documentation

Historically, medical records for any individual may be scattered among the various offices of a primary care physician, a number of specialty physicians, one or more pharmacies, a physical therapist's office, and a hospital. If an individual has geographically moved more than once, these healthcare record sites are multiplied by the number of cities or areas in which the person lived. This may result in discontinuity in care. Clients may not remember exactly what tests were done or their exact results. They may find it difficult to pinpoint whether a particular episode of symptoms occurred 3 or 5 years ago. Although everyone is encouraged to keep a current list of prescription medications and their dosages with them, how many actually carry through with this? When seeking past records is too cumbersome, tests may be redone; there may be no baseline against which to compare results, or significant problems may be overlooked.

The hurricanes of 2005 that saw tens of thousands of individuals displaced from the Gulf Coast region of the United States brought these concerns to the forefront. Cancer clients were evacuated but needed to continue treatment; however, their records remained in flooded hospitals. Individuals with chronic illnesses ran out of prescriptions and were unable to get needed medications. These and many other problems occurred because health records were no longer accessible. This issue remained a problem with Hurricane Harvey in 2017 as electronic medical records struggled to maintain security and ease of access. Healthcare providers use many different systems creating islands of information for clients that cannot be easily accessed by new providers. Combined with physical displacement, the lack of power and/or Internet access also disrupts the ability to access electronic medical records. New systems are being investigated and tested to try to solve this continuing problem.

While EHRs that encompass the documentation of a particular health system, including both inpatient and outpatient settings, are becoming more common, many people still receive care where these are not available. Even an excellent EHR will not be available outside of the system.

The purpose of these computer programs is the creation of an electronic document that "provides a core data set of the most relevant administrative, demographic, and clinical information facts about a client's healthcare, covering one or more healthcare encounters. (It) includes a summary of the client's health status (eg, problems, medications, allergies) and basic information about insurance, advance directives, care documentation, and the client's care plan" (ASTM International, 2005). While the EHR has improved communication and care, a lack of compatibility and interoperability between different systems remains a barrier to "achieving higher quality, increased safety, and lower cost" (Pennic, 2016; **Fig. 10.2**).

As individuals and healthcare agencies become more reliant on EHRs, the expectation is that there will be increased use of them and nurses will be required to access and use the information contained in this record.

Figure 10.2. In an ideal healthcare system, every person would have a "Continuity of Care Record."

DISASTER RESPONSE IN THE COMMUNITY

Potential disasters have always been a concern in communities, but they have become a greater focus of attention since the 9/11 collapse of the World Trade Center Twin Towers in New York City, Hurricane Katrina in New Orleans, the 2010 earthquake in Haiti, and hurricanes in the Atlantic such as Harvey, Irma, and Maria. Box 10.3 lists the 11 major causes of community disasters. Some disasters, such as a fire, may occur in any community; others, such as an earthquake or a hurricane, occur more frequently in one part of the country than in another. **Disaster management** refers to the plans that are in place designating the community's response to a disaster.

Volunteers in Disaster Response

Many communities have plans in place to mobilize volunteers for some roles in a disaster. For example, in areas with earthquake potential, community planning focuses at the neighborhood level, with volunteers responding to neighbors. Provision of basic first aid and management of food, water, and shelter cannot wait for professional rescuers to arrive in the event of widespread damage to roads, power, and other infrastructures. Nurses might take a leadership role in their own neighborhoods because they understand issues of both public health and disease management. Their ability to respond to people's emotional needs as well as physical concerns provides a foundation for effective leadership. There are federal government resources available to help individuals and families to make personal disaster plans. In most disasters, personal advanced planning can make an enormous difference. See the Disaster Planning and Federal Emergency Management Administration (FEMA) websites listed for help in individual planning (www.ready.gov/; www.fema.gov/).

Disaster response volunteers may include Red Cross workers. The Red Cross is designated by the federal government as the key disaster response voluntary agency. Although there is a central paid staff, the majority of Red Cross workers are volunteers. The Red Cross provides training and organization for both healthcare professionals and others who are willing to respond to disasters. It manages shelters and serves as a conduit for donated funds, services,

---

BOX 10.3 TYPES OF COMMUNITY DISASTERS

- Acts of terror
- Disease—especially epidemic disease
- Drought
- Earthquake
- Fire
- Flood
- Food contamination
- Hazmat (hazardous material spill)
- Hurricane
- Power outages
- Tornado

---

and government assistance to help those who are victims of disaster. They have also produced, in conjunction with FEMA, publications with information regarding disaster preparedness for many types of disasters (American Red Cross, 2017).

Other voluntary and nonprofit organizations also respond to disasters. One of the largest and most widely known is The Salvation Army, a Christian group that provides a wide array of social services at all times. During disasters, The Salvation Army workers are active in setting up shelters, providing meals, and helping affected individuals to rebuild their lives. Other religious and disaster response organizations may also be mobilized depending on the size of the disaster. Médecins Sans Frontieres (MSF or Doctors Without Borders) is an international organization devoted to providing emergency aid and medical care globally for people affected by natural disasters, armed conflicts, or other healthcare crises that is independent of religion and politics (http://www.msf.org/en/about-msf).

Institution and Agency Disaster Response

Firefighters, police officers, ambulance drivers, the National Guard, and health professionals are all part of response plans. Most of these individuals are trained for disaster response by their employers.

Firefighters are often the frontline responders to those injured in a disaster. They provide the rescue and emergency medical response skills to save lives. As first responders, firefighters risk the potential for serious injury, smoke or dust inhalation, carbon monoxide poisoning, and heat-related illness from the wearing of protective gear in hot environments. Nurses working in triage must be cognizant of this risk to emergency workers.

Hospitals often serve a pivotal role in managing injuries or illness related to a disaster. Each hospital has plans in place for both internal disasters (such as a fire in one wing of the hospital) and external disasters (such as a tornado in the community). In communities with multiple hospitals, coordination in disaster planning and preparation is essential. Based on their locations and services, each might be designated for a different role.

Learning about their agency's disaster plans should be part of the orientation of all employees. Nurses in hospitals have major roles in responding to disasters. Current clients will be discharged as quickly as possible to open up beds for disaster victims or may have to be moved if the institution is located in an affected area. Units will be reorganized to enable the acceptance and treatment of multiple victims. Nurses may be asked to move to emergency departments to be part of teams that will provide triage. **Triage** involves the initial screening of victims for the purpose of prioritizing treatment and making the most effective and efficient use of both human and material resources. When major triage is no longer needed, nurses may then return to units for client care.

Part of a disaster plan for any agency is a call-in system. This system is a planned process for notifying staff not on duty that there is a disaster and they should report to work. Building such a call-in list is usually the responsibility of the manager of each unit. There may be a telephone tree with people designated to call others within their neighborhood or geographic area, in order for everyone to be notified more quickly. Healthcare professionals sometimes face an ethical dilemma regarding being called in for a disaster. Their own families and neighborhoods may need them, but the hospital is treating the most seriously injured or ill and needs everyone.

Specific Disaster Concerns

In 2017, Hurricane Harvey showed improvements in coordination for the United States compared with Hurricane Katrina on the Gulf Coast in 2005. However, Puerto Rico struggled after Hurricane Maria. These disasters continue to point out the tremendous challenges of managing a widespread disaster when the local resources for response are destroyed. Without hospitals, fire departments, and other agencies, all help has to come from outside the community. Transportation and communication are major problems. Moving large numbers of people, arranging for shelters, and communicating among those trying to provide emergency help can overwhelm communication systems. As a consequence of Hurricane Katrina, communities looked more closely at their disaster planning and requested that both the federal and state governments develop better contingency plans, which was evident with Hurricane Harvey. However, work on disaster planning must continue, and much work is needed for Puerto Rico and outlying areas. The federal government operates a website that is an entry point for learning about the federal government's disaster planning and services (www.ready.gov/.).

Communicable diseases that strike large numbers of individuals in a community are considered *epidemics*, while those that strike large numbers around the world are termed *pandemics*. Influenza is considered a pandemic when a new strain arises to which most people are susceptible and cases arise in large numbers in multiple countries such as that occurred with the H1N1 strain in 2009. Nurses need to become knowledgeable about transmission methods for communicable diseases and the role of immunizations. They must be prepared to give accurate information to those who express concerns. They also need to understand their personal role in any institutional plan for response to an epidemic. The World Health Organization has a Global Outbreak and Response Network (GOARN) that works to identify, alert, and respond to outbreaks, such as Ebola in 2014.

Terrorism, which was most visible in the United States in the 9/11 attacks, remains a concern. The regular bombings, car attacks, and shootings across Europe and the United States demonstrate the vulnerability of large cities to the concerted efforts of a few terrorists. A great deal of the federal government's support for disaster planning is focused on terrorism. Part of the disaster planning of every urban community relates to terrorism response. Whole communities may be involved in disaster response drills, and people may be recruited to play the part of victims. A simulated disaster is staged, and all the plans of the various community agencies are activated. A disaster drill provides a mechanism to find out what works and to plan more effectively.

COMPLEMENTARY AND ALTERNATIVE HEALTHCARE

The National Center for Complementary and Integrative Health (NCCIH) states that "If a non-mainstream practice is used together with conventional medicine, it's considered complementary" and if the "non-mainstream practice is used in place of conventional medicine, it's considered alternative" (NCCIH, 2016, para. 1). Conventional medicine may also be referred to as allopathy, Western, mainstream, orthodox, regular medicine, and biomedicine. This definition of complementary and alternative medicine (CAM) focuses more on what alternative care is *not* than what it *is*, because of the broad range of healthcare practices included in this category. Common among these practices are acupuncture, homeopathy, naturopathy, music therapy, and herbal medicine. NCCIH includes prayer for health reasons as a therapy practice.

The list of healthcare practices considered complementary and alternative shifts constantly as some are proven safe and effective, others are proven of little value or even harmful and fade from use, and still others emerge. According to a 2012 survey by the CDC (2015), 36.8% of adults aged 45 to 64 years in the United States use some form of CAM. Overall, CAM use is greater among women and people with higher education levels. Survey results indicated that CAM is most often used to treat and/or prevent musculoskeletal conditions or other conditions that involve chronic or recurring pain.

These healthcare approaches are considered **alternative** when they are used in place of conventional medical care. The same approaches are considered **complementary** when they are used along with conventional medicine. **Integrative medicine**, as defined by NCCIH, "combines mainstream medical therapies and CAM therapies for which there is some high-quality scientific evidence of safety and effectiveness" (NCCIH, 2016). Thus, integrative medicine supports the higher standard of research evidence for effectiveness.

NCCIH provides training for researchers in the area of CAM, funds grants for research into the effectiveness of all types of alternative care, and disseminates research findings about CAM to both professionals and the public. The National Library of Medicine maintains a database, CAM on PubMed, which allows for research in relationship to specific diseases, conditions, and therapies (see end of chapter websites).

CAM takes place almost entirely within the community, and the client often serves as its primary controlling factor, as opposed to conventional medicine, in which the official healthcare provider controls access to care through ordering diagnostics, prescribing treatments, and determining admission to and discharge from a care facility. As complementary and alternative healthcare practices remain popular with the public, healthcare providers are challenged to understand these diverse approaches and to work effectively with clients who choose those resources. There is also a need to assist in client education so that choices are made wisely and with sound information.

Major Types of Complementary and Alternative Medicine

NCCAM has categorized CAM into four domains for the purpose of discussion and study. These domains include mind–body medicine, biologically based practices, manipulative and body-based practices, and energy medicine (Tables 10.1 and 10.2). Additionally, CAM studies alternative whole medical systems that cut across many of the domains.

Table 10.1 Alternative Whole Medical Systems

System	Examples
Traditional indigenous systems	Traditional oriental medicine Qi gong Acupuncture Herbal medicine Oriental massage Ayurvedic medicine Native American medicine Other folk medicine systems (Mexican, South American, etc.)
Unconventional Western systems	Homeopathy Naturopathy

Table 10.2   Types of Complementary and Alternative Practices

Classifications	Specific Therapies
Mind–body medicine	Relaxation exercises Hypnosis Meditation Dance Prayer Visualization Biofeedback
Biologically based practices	Herbal medicines Special diets Food supplements Vitamin therapy Biologic substances, such as bovine and shark cartilage
Manipulative and body-based practices	Chiropractic Massage therapy Reflexology
Energy medicine	BEM applications to the body Radiofrequency hyperthermia Radiofrequency diathermy Magnets Nerve stimulators Biofields—manipulations of energy fields originating within the body: Reiki, therapeutic touch

Specific alternative care providers may use more than one type of treatment in their practice. Additionally, there are many areas of overlap between conventional medical practice and CAM. The major types of alternative care available are described briefly in the following sections.

Whole Medical Systems

Whole medical systems represent complete systems of theory and practice that approach healthcare differently than the traditional Western biomedical approach. NCCIH has identified two approaches to entire systems of healthcare that differ from Western medicine: traditional indigenous systems and unconventional Western systems of medicine (NCCIH, 2016). Each system uses a variety of specific therapies.

Traditional Indigenous Systems

In indigenous medicine, there are complete systems of explanation for health and illness, and therapies are chosen based on these theoretic systems of belief. Some indigenous systems are quite formal in approach, with individuals studying and serving apprenticeships before practice. These include traditional Asian medicine and Ayurvedic medicine from India. Traditional Asian medicine may include the use of qi gong (a form of energy therapy), oriental massage, acupuncture, and herbs. Ayurvedic medicine, a traditional system from India, has existed for more than 5,000 years and has a specific theoretic and therapeutic focus on imbalance in the individual's consciousness. Lifestyle interventions are the major form of Ayurvedic preventive and therapeutic treatment. As the popularity of Ayurvedic treatment has grown, a number of medical centers, retreats, and spas provide these treatments in the United States.

Informal approaches are often termed *folk medicine*; these traditions usually are handed down by word of mouth and are used by individuals and families to treat common health problems. Indigenous medicine practitioners use a variety of approaches to healthcare, often combining herbs, food, and traditional ceremonies. Little is understood about many of the herbs used, but some have demonstrated therapeutic effects while others may be questionable.

In a given ethnic group, certain people may be designated as healers or as having special knowledge and ability regarding illness. They may have had a period of apprenticeship, but it is informal in nature and not mandated by any outside authority. The advice of the indigenous healer may be sought instead of the advice of a physician. Native American cultures may use a *shaman*, or medicine man/woman. Mexican Americans may use the services of a *curandero*, or healer. A system of understanding hot and cold disorders and foods that help to balance heat and cold in the body is part of many of these folk traditions. NCCIH points out that in addition to natural products and mind and body practices (like yoga or tai chi), there are other forms of traditional healing such as Ayurvedic medicine and traditional Chinese Medicine (NCCIH, 2016), although there are many other types of traditional medicine . To work most effectively with a client who uses folk medicine, you need to learn about the specific beliefs and resources that the client is using.

Unconventional Western Systems of Medicine
Unconventional Western systems of medicine originated in Western society but did not find general support. Some individuals continue to practice in the theoretic precepts of these systems and have re-emerged as the public looks for alternatives to conventional medical care. Perhaps the most common of these unconventional Western systems is homeopathy. **Homeopathy** is based on the belief that exposure to extremely small quantities of either the substance causing an illness or a related substance will stimulate a cure. Of course, this principle is also the basis for immunization and allergy desensitization. The application of this principle to other diseases, however, has not been accepted by the medical community. The dilutions used in many homeopathic remedies are so great that a dosage may contain only a few molecules of a substance. Homeopathy was popular in the early 20th century but fell into disrepute as standard medical research advanced. There is currently a resurgence of interest in this approach to therapy, and new research is being done. Homeopathic practitioners once again are offering an alternative to standard medical care.

Naturopathy gets its name from the natural agents used in treating disease, such as food, exercise, air, water, and sunshine. The naturopathic physician treats people by recommending changes in lifestyle, diet, and exercise and promoting the use of vitamins and herbs. For many, lifestyle and dietary changes are a successful form of treatment. Naturopathic physicians follow a prescribed course of study that includes clinical experiences with clients and results in the doctor of naturopathy degree. Currently, 19 states, the District of Columbia, and the US territories of Puerto Rico and the U.S. Virgin Islands have licensing laws for naturopathic doctors (The National Association of Naturopathic Physicians, 2017). However, questions have been raised about the use of naturopathic physicians in primary care, especially regarding the adequacy of their training in the recognition and treatment of more serious illnesses and the concern that many of the herbal remedies prescribed by naturopathic physicians are untested and unregulated.

Mind–Body Medicine

Mind–body medicine seeks to control physical processes through the mind's capacities. In addition, it treats emotional concerns. Increasingly, mind–body interventions are being incorporated into standard healthcare practice. Traditional psychotherapy, a well-established part of standard healthcare, is a mind–body approach to health. The use of prayer, support groups, yoga, meditation, relaxation, biofeedback, and visualization is all mind–body therapies.

Relaxation exercises, breathing techniques, meditation, and visualization are used to reduce anxiety, reduce blood pressure, and lessen the body's response to stressors. Yoga and other forms of controlled exercise also focus on breathing and mind-calming processes for these same purposes. While yoga originated in Hindu religious practices, most yoga in the United States keeps the techniques but does not include the religious philosophy. These techniques also are designed to prevent stress-related problems from developing; for many people, they are part of a plan to increase health and well-being. These techniques may be suggested for the management of specific health problems such as those causing pain or those related to cardiovascular responses and may be used in conjunction with traditional medical treatment.

Every major religion of the world responds in particular ways to those who are ill. A well-established way for supporting an ill person is through the prayers of others who care. Nurses recognize that spiritual distress has a significant impact on a client's ability to move toward wellness. Supporting the individual's quest for spiritual solace and healing has been a part of the mission of many healthcare agencies that were established by religious bodies. Healthcare providers frequently feel poorly equipped to deal with spirituality. There are assessment tools available to assist in opening conversations on spirituality. Interdisciplinary team members such as chaplains can also help in providing holistic care.

Visualization may be used to help children manage painful medical procedures. Suggestions regarding healing and postoperative recovery are used in the operating room by some anesthesiologists and surgeons. The anesthesiologist may talk to the client who is still anesthetized, suggesting that pain will be minimal, nausea will not occur, and recovery will be rapid. This is similar to posthypnotic suggestion. Hypnosis has been used in other illnesses for symptom relief (Fig. 10.3).

Biofeedback is a specific mechanism used to assist individuals by altering physiologic responses through mental processes. The machines used for biofeedback provide visual or auditory feedback of physiologic parameters such as blood pressure or galvanic skin response. By observing these parameters, the individual learns to change the underlying physiologic process. Some individuals with migraine headaches use biofeedback control over circulation to abort migraine attacks rather than take medications. Biofeedback is recognized as effective for a variety of processes that are under autonomic nervous system control.

Mind–body interventions in general allow people to participate actively in their own care. People often are changed emotionally and psychologically in the process of treating illness or disease. A big advantage of the mind–body therapies is that they are safe and economical and can be used easily in conjunction with other therapies.

Biologically Based Practices

Biologically based practices include herbal medicine, special diets, food supplements, vitamins, and specific biologic substances such as bovine and shark cartilage. Nonvitamin,

Figure 10.3. Alternative healthcare is moving more and more into mainstream practice.

nonmineral natural products such as fish oil and flaxseed are the most commonly used alternative medicine (NCCIH, 2016).

Herbal medicines are plant products that are used to treat illnesses. As research into plant products continues, our understanding of the efficacy of herbs increases. Many in the United States who describe themselves as herbalists received their training in herbs during an apprenticeship with an experienced herbalist. There are educational programs for herbalists, but they are not regulated in every state.

Potential problems in the use of herbs and supplements include unreliable dosage and bioavailability, safety and efficacy, and interactions with prescribed medications. The bioavailability of various herbal preparations may vary widely, making it difficult to stabilize dosage. And because plants grow under different circumstances and with different soil and other conditions, the proportion of active ingredient within the plant may vary considerably. This makes accurate and stable dosage of herbs difficult.

While herbal products are available in tablet form with doses listed on the label, at present, there are no laws regulating the potency or purity of herbs sold in the United States. Many herbs are imported from around the world where accurate labeling and content purity may not be monitored. Because herbs are not considered drugs, there are no regulations regarding testing for efficacy or safety, as there are with products that must be approved by the Food and Drug Administration (FDA). This means that some herbs that are sold may contain contaminants. Serious illnesses and even deaths have been traced to contaminants in herbal medicines.

Some countries, such as Germany, have regulated herbal medications for many years. Canada has a system of regulating "natural health products" that includes regulations for herbal and homeopathic remedies. The Canadian system is based on a phased-in process that addresses products with the highest risk potential first (Natural and Non-prescription Health Products Directorate, 2016).

Sometimes the active ingredient in an herb may have potent side effects or interact with medications prescribed. One event that left many people with permanent damage was the herb ephedra. The FDA took action to remove ephedra from the market in 2004 after severe illness, including stroke and cardiac effects, and death were associated with its use (FDA, 2004). In September 2016, the FDA issued a warning about homeopathic teething tablets and gels that were potentially harmful to children and infants (FDA, 2016). The FDA monitors a variety of products and issues regular press releases when a problem is detected or new treatments are released. Go to https://www.fda.gov/NewsEvents/Newsroom/PressAnnouncements/default.htm for more information.

When nurses interview clients regarding their medication history, asking specific questions about vitamins, herbs, supplements, and other therapeutic agents is critical. Clients may not consider these to be medication and so may not provide information about taking these substances. The result may be that the source of an adverse response is missed or a harmful interaction with prescribed medications occurs. With increasing frequency, medical clinics and physicians' offices are asking clients to list on medical histories all over-the-counter medications, vitamins, and herbs as well as those requiring prescriptions.

Biologic treatments include a variety of substances not approved as medical treatment by the FDA. These products have been developed by individuals and organizations and are often sold as food supplements rather than as medicines. Cartilage products from sharks, cattle, sheep, and chickens are being used to treat both cancer and arthritis. Peptide fractions derived from human blood and urine, called antineoplastons, are being used to treat cancer. Coley's toxins are killed cultures of bacteria that have been used for treating cancer. Apitherapy is the use of honeybee venom to treat rheumatic diseases, dermatologic conditions, chronic pain, and cancer. Research on the efficacy of these treatments is costly, and sponsors willing to bear that cost are hard to find. Some small studies are being funded with federal grants.

Daily Ethical Dilemma 10.1: Culturally Competent Care

You are taking care of Nancy, a 62-year-old Ojibwe (Native American) woman with gangrene of her right foot. She has been receiving treatment for the better part of a year with no success. The doctor has recommended amputation of the foot and states that she will die without surgery. However, Nancy and her husband are adamant about returning to the reservation to treat her foot with boiled bark. You have developed a great working relationship with Nancy and her husband and they remind you of your grandparents. What are the ethical principles that are in conflict? What would you say to Nancy and her husband? How would you document the conversation?
(Source: Silva & Ludwick, 2001, in part.)

Communication in Action 10.2: *Assisting With Complete Reporting*

Serena Johnson works in an ambulatory clinic. She is reviewing Mabel Wilson's written new client information. As she speaks with Mrs. Wilson, she says, "I see that you wrote here that you take supplements. Would you please tell me exactly what supplements you are taking?" Mrs. Wilson says, "Oh, I figured those didn't make any difference; they aren't like real medicine or anything, just like food." Serena replies, "Supplements need to be considered along with medicines because they all have some effect. Sometimes that is a benefit to you, but sometimes they could interfere with drugs that might be prescribed. Whenever you see a doctor, you need to be sure to let the doctor know all the prescribed medicines, over-the-counter medicines, and supplements that you use. Please tell me what you take so I can add them to your record."

Medical research is beginning to identify some benefits of using food and vitamins in therapeutic ways. We have long known that many individuals who develop type 2 diabetes may be able to manage their blood sugar through dietary control. The role of antioxidants in decreasing cell damage and the effect of certain phytochemicals contained in cruciferous vegetables in preventing bowel cancer are just two examples of the theoretic benefits of nutrients. Some parents have used strict dietary regulation as a management tool for children with attention deficit hyperactivity disorder.

There are hazards in this approach to healthcare, however. Megadoses of vitamins may prove toxic such as liver toxicity from excessive vitamin A. Some nutrients interact with medications, decreasing their effectiveness. Individuals who choose to avoid all traditional medical care and rely on unsubstantiated claims about the therapeutic effects of nutrients may suffer deterioration in health.

All healthcare professionals need to support and encourage healthy dietary practices. Often, it is possible to assist clients who rely on the use of nutrients for healthcare by becoming knowledgeable about the research regarding nutrition, accepting what clients believe helps them (as long as it is not detrimental to their well-being), and keeping an open mind. When we are willing to acknowledge the validity of some aspects of their preferred approach to healthcare, these clients may be willing to combine more conventional medical care along with their nutritional approaches.

Manipulative and Body-Based Practices

Manipulative and body-based practices include the physical manipulation of the body to achieve health goals. Some authors refer to these as *manual healing*. Manipulative therapy is found in massage therapy and reflexology. Massage therapy uses both fixed and movable pressure and holding by the hands and sometimes the forearms, elbows, or feet. There is evidence that these techniques affect the musculoskeletal, circulatory–lymphatic, and nervous systems. Reflexology is massage of the feet to activate points on the feet that correspond to other body parts or systems.

Perhaps the most commonly known type of manipulative practice is chiropractic. Chiropractic care is based on the theory that disease is caused by interference with nerve function. It uses manipulation of the body joints, especially the spinal vertebrae, in seeking to restore normal function. The chiropractor also may use other treatments commonly associated with physical therapy, such as massage and exercise. There are definite differences among chiropractors. Some state that there are illnesses that cannot be treated through manual healing and do recommend that certain clients seek conventional medical care. Others believe that all illnesses may be treated by chiropractic methods and do not refer clients for conventional medical care. A major concern is that some clients may have more serious illnesses that may be missed altogether or not recognized in time to be given optimal medical attention. Another problem with chiropractic care is the use of chiropractic treatments on infants and young children in place of immunizations and other well-child services. Many people with joint and muscle strain and tension find that chiropractic treatments relieve discomfort and support effective functioning.

Acupuncture, which is a part of traditional Chinese medicine, is growing in popularity as an alternative care practice. While primarily used for managing musculoskeletal pain where evidence of efficacy is accumulating, acupuncture has also been used to control appetite for weight loss. There are few adverse effects; most, including infection from nonsterile needles and penetration of organs, are associated with unskilled practitioners.

Energy Medicine

The use of **energy medicine** (sometimes referred to as bioelectromagnetic [BEM] therapies) is based on the understanding that electrical phenomena are found in all living organisms. There are magnetic fields that extend from the body, which can be measured and may be affected by external forces. The mechanisms by which the electromagnetic fields occur in the body, how these can be changed, and the effects of such changes are under study. Many modalities have been used for years without clear studies of their effectiveness. Some believe that BEM may be a unifying theory explaining why such widely diverse therapies as acupuncture and homeopathy produce results.

Some energy medicine is based on applying external energy to the body. There are thermal applications of BEM therapy in the form of radiofrequency hyperthermia and radiofrequency diathermy. Nonthermal applications include magnets and nerve stimulation. One common application is the use of magnets to relieve musculoskeletal problems. Magnetic insoles for shoes and magnets to be worn on the body are widely available.

There are also methods used to manipulate the interior biofields of the individual. These include therapeutic touch and Reiki. Both of these practices are based on a system of changing the energy fields without applying external energy forces to the body. In therapeutic touch, the practitioner moves his/her hands above the body or touches lightly, perceives energy fields, and modifies them through hand movements. While the originator of therapeutic touch (Krieger, 1979) and some practitioners claim that their research supports this practice, others studying therapeutic touch have not been able to discern either the energy fields or methods of change and find the methodology of those studies reporting effectiveness to be flawed (Bullough & Bullough, 1998; Coursey, n.d.). Therapeutic touch has found acceptance by some within the nursing community, and a nursing diagnosis titled "energy field disturbance" has been included in the NANDA-I taxonomy. This is a matter of controversy, and there are strong objections by some to its inclusion without replicable research support. Nurses interested in therapeutic touch should research it further.

Understanding the Use of Complementary and Alternative Healthcare

According to the 2012 survey by the CDC (2015), the use of alternative and complementary therapies is increasing. For many clients with chronic conditions, mainstream medical care offers few options. Long-term treatments with medications often produce their own iatrogenic (treatment-caused) health problems, some of which are as troubling to the individual as the original disease process. A common response of conventional medicine to these problems has been to add more medications and more treatments, each with its own potential adverse effects. Mainstream healthcare providers often give little attention to the problems of daily living that are of greatest concern to the individual. Stress and anxiety also add to the burden of these clients. For clients with acute health conditions, certain treatments or medications may produce unpleasant or harmful side effects. Clients often are looking for alternative treatment methods that do not appear to have the same potential for harm.

Some alternative therapies have been available for many years, and there are people who believe that they have been helped significantly by these approaches. Unfortunately, traditional healthcare providers often have dismissed these therapies without investigating them thoroughly. On the other hand, few alternative therapies have been formally researched, and proponents often rely on undocumented reports of effectiveness.

Research into alternative therapies now is supported by the federal government but only in a small way compared with other research. The federal government has a National Center for Complementary and Integrative Health, the NCCIH, and a Web page of references (see list of websites). More attention is being paid to the responses of individuals. Concern about the role of stress in illness has prompted an increased openness to nonmedical methods of managing stress. The possibility of alternative care practices working in a complementary fashion with traditional medical care is gaining wider acceptance. Often, these complementary therapies are used to address the whole person and not simply the disease.

Part of the appeal of alternative healthcare is the caring and personalized response that clients often receive. People who have been intimidated by businesslike clinics and made to feel unimportant by impersonal professionals may find that the warm, concerned, accepting atmosphere of the nonconventional setting meets many personal needs. The fact that stress and anxiety play a major role in any health problem may help explain why many people are helped by therapies that may not be based on sound scientific knowledge. Because of the trust placed in nurses, they are in a unique position to relate with people about the issues that surround alternative and complementary therapy. Gallup's polls continue to identify nurses as the most trusted professionals when ethics are considered (Gallup Poll, 2016).

To learn more about any specific therapy, or to research alternative and complementary therapies for any condition, use the CAM Citation Index found on the website of the NCCIH (see References). You may also search MEDLINE, the database of the National Library of Medicine, or the literature review through the NCCIH website (https://nccih.nih.gov/health/providers/litreviews.htm) to research various therapies.

Assisting Clients Who Choose Alternative Healthcare

Many people who support conventional methods of healthcare have long ignored or repudiated the value of unorthodox healthcare traditions. We must recognize that complementary and alternative healthcare practices persist because people find them to be valuable. Acknowledging healthcare alternatives and working cooperatively with them is usually much more productive than trying to oppose them.

NCCIH suggests a five-step process for the consumer considering a particular complementary or alternative therapy. This process has a heavy emphasis on careful information gathering.

Assess Safety and Effectiveness

The first step is for the individual to assess the safety and effectiveness of the therapy in relationship to his or her own condition. One of the difficulties is finding accurate safety and efficacy data. Websites and other sources of information require close scrutiny to determine the qualifications and bias of the sponsoring individual or group. The NCCIH website (https://nccih.nih.gov/) contains fact sheets regarding specific therapies and additional links to research reports and scientific papers. Research reports may also be found through PubMed, the National Library of Medicine's online access (www.ncbi.nlm.nih.gov/PubMed). All complementary and alternative therapies are classified there under the Medical Subject Heading of "complementary therapies."

Examine the Expertise of the Therapy Practitioner

The second step is to examine the expertise of any therapy practitioner. Whether this person is a physician or another type of provider, determine whether there is appropriate education and licensing if that is required. Consumers should be encouraged to ask directly about education and credentials for practice. Some consumer organizations will direct individuals to reliable practitioners in the community. Clients who may be reluctant to ask directly about credentials can check whether credentials are available on a website or in printed information from the practitioner.

Investigate Service Delivery

Service delivery is the third aspect the client should investigate. How many clients are seen per day? Where can the therapy be available and what barriers do that pose? Are standards for safety, privacy, and confidentiality in place? Remember that alternative providers are not included in the federal Health Insurance Portability and Accountability Act (HIPAA) of 1996 legislation that mandates confidentiality in conventional healthcare settings unless they are eligible for reimbursement through Medicare or Medicaid. Most alternative providers are responsible for establishing their own standards and policies without outside oversight.

Research the Cost of Therapy

A fourth consideration is the cost of the therapy. Part of this is investigating what coverage may be obtained from an insurance carrier or whether any is available. Are the costs clear? How are payments made? Some unscrupulous practitioners collect large sums of money before any service and then may not provide what was promised. Some types of alternative care (eg, chiropractic care for an acute back injury) may be reimbursable under a traditional health plan.

Discuss the Treatment With Your Regular Healthcare Provider

The fifth step is to discuss this proposed treatment with a regular healthcare provider. The interaction of any traditional treatment and a complementary or alternative treatment may or may not pose a problem. Many healthcare providers support the use of various complementary therapies.

Things that the healthcare provider must also consider are such issues as client choice, informed consent, and the ethical principles of beneficence and nonmaleficence (see Chapter 8). As complementary and alternative therapies move into the mainstream, greater accountability to the public is essential.

Evidence-Based Practice 10.1: Complementary Medicine and Pain Management

Nahin, R. L., Boineau R., Khalsa, P. S., Stussman, B. J., & Weber, W. J. (2016). Evidence-based evaluation of complementary health approaches for pain management in the United States. *Mayo Clin Proceeding, 91*(9), 1292–1306.

A literature review of several research studies on complementary approaches to five different painful conditions found that most of the approaches had more positive results than negative. Acupuncture helped with back pain and osteoarthritis of the knee, while yoga helped with back pain. Massage worked well for neck pain, although only temporarily, and relaxation techniques were helpful for severe headaches and migraines. This literature review illustrates the success, even if limited, of several complementary treatments to help clients deal with pain.

Critical Thinking Activity: What Does the Research Say?
Identify a specific form of complementary or alternative therapy. Search the health literature regarding this therapy. Review the information available in other sources. Analyze the information to determine whether the data supporting the use of this therapy are weak, moderate, or strong. Provide a rationale for your determination.

Stegen & Sowerby Stories: Part 2

Ms. Jeffrey has been home for 1 week and Jared calls to check on her. She reports that her legs are a little more swollen today. Jared makes sure she knows the time and date for her follow-up appointment with her primary care physician. He also takes time to review some of the teaching that he did prior to her discharge from the hospital. Ms. Jeffrey suddenly exclaims, "Oh, I know where I went wrong!"

What do you suspect the problem might be? What are other ways that we, as healthcare providers, can improve continuity of care to improve outcomes for people? Read the rest of the story at www.thePoint.com.

Want to Know More?

A variety of resources are available on thePoint® to enhance your learning and understanding of this chapter, such as:

- Full Stegen & Sowerby Stories
- NCLEX-Style Student Review Questions
- Journal Articles
- Case Studies
- Learning Objectives
- Relevant Websites
- And more...

KEY CONCEPTS

- Community-based nursing emphasizes advocating for clients, promoting self-care, focusing on health promotion and disease prevention, and recognizing the importance of the family, culture, and community.
- Health promotion and prevention of illness and disease are a part of nursing practice in all settings.
- Client empowerment through teaching, explaining options, and supporting decision-making is a foundation for community-based care.
- Primary prevention focuses on preventing disease; secondary prevention focuses on early diagnosis through screening and preventing complications; tertiary prevention focuses on preventing long-term disability and restoring functional capacity.
- Disease management strives to promote health through effective treatment of targeted diseases and health conditions.
- *Healthy People 2020* is a federal effort that includes overall goals, priority areas, and leading indicators to measure progress in developing healthier communities.
- Maintaining continuity of care requires transition planning, with special emphasis on reconciling medication records from one setting to another.
- Ensuring that healthcare records are available wherever the client seeks care is becoming a possibility through computerization of medical records and the development of transportable records that contain essential information.
- Alternative healthcare encompasses those types of care outside of conventional Western medicine and includes mind–body medicine, biologically based practices, manipulative and body-based practices, and energy medicine as well as alternative whole medical systems.
- Alternative care therapies are considered complementary therapies when used along with traditional medical care. Integrative medicine involves the deliberative planning for using both traditional medical care and alternative care in a coordinated manner.
- Understanding the different types of alternative healthcare services, why people choose alternative healthcare, and how nurses may assist people who seek this care will form a foundation for more effective relationships with clients.
- Alternative and complementary therapies can be evaluated based on a five-step process that includes safety and effectiveness of the therapy, credentials of the provider, service delivery, cost of services, and consultation with the regular healthcare provider.

NCLEX-STYLE PRACTICE QUESTIONS

1. What is the purpose of medication reconciliation?

   A. To ensure the best care
   B. To prevent overdosing
   C. To create standardization
   D. To comply with The Joint Commission

2. The doctor orders physical therapy for an older client experiencing knee pain. This is an example of what type of prevention?

   A. Primary
   B. Secondary
   C. Tertiary
   D. Disease

3. What are the reasons for disease management? (Select all that apply.)

   A. Improve cost savings
   B. Improve quality of life
   C. Increased life span
   D. Decreased staffing

4. You are teaching a student nurse about complementary medicine. What are some points that you would want to make regarding the subject? (Select all that apply.)

   A. Mechanism of action is not always understood.
   B. More effective than conventional medicine.
   C. Tends to be cost-effective or low cost.
   D. May not be compatible with other treatments.

5. A client asks you how to figure out if a complementary treatment is right for them. What would you advise?

   A. Try it and see if it works for you.
   B. Research it and talk to your doctor.
   C. Don't do it. It may be dangerous.
   D. Tell them about your cousin's experience.

REFERENCES

American Red Cross. (2017). *Anyone can be Red Cross ready*. Retrieved June 4, 2017, from http://www.redcross.org/

ASTM International. (2005). *ASTM Standard E2369-051. Continuity of care record (CCR)*. West Conshohocken, PA: Author. Retrieved January 7, 2011, from www.astm.org/Standards/E2369.htm

Bullough, V. L., & Bullough, B. (1998). Should nurses practice therapeutic touch? Should nursing schools teach therapeutic touch? *Journal of Professional Nursing, 14*(4), 254–257.

CDC. (2015). Trends in the use of complementary health approaches among adults: United States, 2002-2012. *National Health Statistics Reports, 79*. https://www.cdc.gov/nchs/data/nhsr/nhsr079.pdf

Coursey, K. (n.d.). Further notes on therapeutic touch. *Quackwatch*. Retrieved January 4, 2011, from http://www.quackwatch.org/01QuackeryRelatedTopics/tt2.html

Food and Drug Administration. (2004). *FDA acts to remove ephedra containing dietary supplements from market.* Retrieved January 6, 2011, from http://www.fda.gov/NewsEvents/Newsroom/PressAnnouncements/2004/ucm108379.htm

Food and Drug Administration. (2016). *FDA warns against the use of homeopathic teething tablets and gels.* Retrieved June 4, 2017, from https://www.fda.gov/newsevents/newsroom/pressannouncements/ucm523468.htm

Gallup Poll. (2016). *Americans rate healthcare providers high on honesty, ethics.* Retrieved June 4, 2017, from http://www.gallup.com/poll/200057/americans-rate-healthcare-providers-high-honesty-ethics.aspx

Krieger, D. (1979). *Therapeutic touch.* New York, NY: Prentice-Hall.

Nahin, R. L., Boineau R., Khalsa, P. S., Stussman, B. J., & Weber, W. J. (2016). Evidence-based evaluation of complementary health approaches for pain management in the United States. *Mayo Clin Proceeding, 91*(9), 1292–1306.

National Association of Naturopathic Physicians. (2017). *Licensed states & licensing authorities.* Retrieved June 4, 2017, from http://www.naturopathic.org/content.asp?contentid=57

National Center for Complementary and Integrative Health. (2016). *Complementary, alternative, or integrative health: What's in a name?* Retrieved June 4, 2017, from https://nccih.nih.gov/health/integrative-health

Natural and Non-prescription Health Products Directorate. (2016). *Government of Canada.* Retrieved June 4, 2017, from https://www.canada.ca/en/health-canada/services/drugs-health-products/natural-non-prescription/regulation.html

Office of Disease Prevention and Health Promotion (DPHP). (2014). *Healthy People 2020 leading health indicators: Progress update.* Retrieved June 4, 2017, from https://www.healthypeople.gov/2020/leading-health-indicators/Healthy-People-2020-Leading-Health-Indicators%3A-Progress-Update

Pennic, J. (2016). Medscape EHR report: Top 5 most widely used EHRs by physicians. *Hit Consultant.* http://hitconsultant.net/2016/08/29/medscape-ehr-report-2016-10-things-know/

Silva, M. C., & Ludwick, R. (2001). Ethics: Ethical issues in complementary/alternative therapies. *Online Journal of Issues in Nursing, 7*(1). http://www.nursingworld.org/MainMenuCategories/ANAMarketplace/ANAPeriodicals/OJIN/Columns/Ethics/EthicalIssues.html#Leonard

The Joint Commission. (2017). *National client safety goal on using medicines safely.* Retrieved June 4, 2017, from https://www.jointcommission.org/assets/1/6/2017_NPSG_OME_ER.pdf

U.S. Department of Health and Human Services (US-DHHS). (2010, January). *About Healthy People.* Washington, DC. Retrieved April 19, 2011, from http://www.healthypeople.gov/2020/about/default.aspx

■ Accepting Greater Responsibility for Nursing Practice

T he third and final unit in this textbook is devoted to topics that will assist you to move into the world of employment as a registered nurse (RN). The major goal is to prepare you for the leadership role that you will one day execute as an RN.

Chapter 11 begins with a discussion of leadership, management, accountability, and authority and includes a brief review of theories of leadership. Information is provided about the various leadership and management roles nurses may perform as they fulfill their responsibilities in regard to leading and managing others. You will find helpful information on the distribution and use of power in the healthcare system, a discussion of emotional intelligence, a section on using communication skills effectively, and content related to performance evaluation and time management.

As leaders in the healthcare system, nurses have specific responsibilities regarding delegation within the nursing team and interacting with the interdisciplinary team. Leading requires the ability to build teams and to motivate others. It also requires the ability to bring about change and to manage conflict situations. These topics are explored in Chapter 12.

Chapter 13 helps to prepare you for the challenges you will face in today's workplace. Beginning with a discussion of reality shock and burnout, the chapter goes on to emphasize the importance of workplace safety and its effect on the health of nurses. It concludes with an exploration of the topic of sexual harassment and violence in the workplace.

A discussion of the political process—how it affects nursing and how nurses can affect it—follows in Chapter 14. An understanding of how politics can and does have an effect on the healthcare delivery system can be relevant to your professional experience.

Chapter 15, the final chapter of the unit and the text, emphasizes your role in a healthcare system where nurses are accountable for the development of nursing as a profession. A brief explanation of terms and processes involved in nursing research provides a foundation for fulfilling your responsibilities in this important work. Understanding evidence-based practice and its implementation is essential to providing quality care. The use of technology in healthcare now and for the future is discussed.

CHAPTER 11

Initiating the Leadership and Management Role

LEARNING OUTCOMES

After completing this chapter, you should be able to:

1. Compare and contrast the concepts of leadership and management and make a distinction in the skills involved.
2. Differentiate between the terms *authority* and *accountability*.
3. Discuss the major theories regarding leadership.
4. Compare and contrast three prevailing leadership styles.
5. Analyze the factors that have resulted in the development of transformational leadership.
6. Describe the relationship of power and empowerment and identify ways by which one individual can empower another.
7. Explain emotional intelligence and why it is an important quality of a leader.
8. Analyze methods by which the development of leadership style can be enhanced.
9. Describe the basic characteristics of effective communication.
10. Analyze the communication strategies that are essential for effective leadership, identifying the critical role of each.
11. Describe the elements of an effective performance appraisal system, including the conducting of the interview.
12. Analyze the importance of time management and evaluate methods that will help overcome major time wasters and procrastination.

KEY TERMS

Accountability
Authority
Autocratic/authoritarian leadership
   style
Charisma
Coercive power
Communication
Connection power
Democratic/participative leadership
   style
Emotional intelligence
Empowerment

Expert power
Informational power
Job descriptions
Laissez-faire/permissive leadership
   style
Leadership/management style
Legitimate power
Mentor
Mindfulness
Motivational power
Multicratic leadership
Performance appraisal

(continued on page 383)

Stegen & Sowerby Stories: Part 1

J ack is a 57-year-old computer programmer. He went to the clinic for his annual exam, and it was determined that it was time for his pneumonia vaccination. His provider, Karen (a nurse practitioner), was accompanied that day, by a medical student named Alice. Karen indicated that this was a routine injection and that if Jack had no objections, Alice would be giving the injection. Jack did not object and rolled up his sleeve. Karen began charting the visit on the computer in the exam room. Jack commented that there was some discomfort during the injection but was assured by Karen that this was normal and Jack left the clinic.

Two weeks later the pain in Jacks shoulder had increased to the point that it restricted his movement making it difficult to work and disturbing his sleep.

- What concerns do you have regarding the information given here?
- Who is responsible for the care provided by the medical student?
- What could have happened to cause the patients discomfort?
- What action should be taken now?

The novice in the area of managing a healthcare team can easily be dazzled by the many terms populating the literature that are devoted to the topics of leadership and management. Words such as authority, responsibility, accountability, team building, empowerment, coaching, mentoring, motivating, and collective power are but a few of those incorporated into articles, monographs, and books addressing the topic of successful leadership and management. In this chapter, we define those terms and discuss their application to the healthcare environment. This will make them useful to you as you begin your career as a staff nurse and later as you assume a leadership role in client care.

COMPARING LEADERSHIP AND MANAGEMENT

Although the terms *leadership* and *management* are often used interchangeably, differences exist in how each is practiced in the work situation. At some point in your nursing career, you likely will fill both roles: leader and manager. Understanding the uniqueness of each will help you be effective in either position. Let us explore the differences and how they are applied in the work situation.

Leadership refers to the ability to guide, motivate, and inspire and to instill vision and purpose. As you read this, you probably can think of individuals you know who possess strong leadership abilities—your class president or the person who arranges and guides your study sessions, for example. To provide leadership, you must be able to influence the beliefs, opinions, or behaviors of others and to persuade others to follow your direction. This can be accomplished in a number of ways, referred to as leadership styles, which we will discuss later.

Management refers to activities such as planning, organizing, directing, and controlling with the purpose of accomplishing specific goals and objectives within an organization. Essentially, management involves coordination and integration of resources to accomplish specific tasks. Often, management positions are roles to which one is appointed or hired after a competitive job application and interview. This appointment grants the manager the power to direct others and the responsibility for ensuring that certain tasks within the organization are completed effectively and efficiently.

The very best managers are also leaders, although this may not always happen. Conversely, not all leaders are officially managers in the sense we have defined it. A foremost authority on leadership and organizational management, Warren Bennis (2009), has stated that managers are people who do things right, while leaders are people who do the right thing. Individuals may become leaders because of the way in which they inspire others to follow them.

Critical Thinking Activity: Leader or Manager?

Can you think of a situation in which an individual was a leader but did not have the role of manager? Similarly, can you think of any situations in which the manager lacked the ability to lead a group of people? Can you recall situations in which the manager also was a leader?

DIFFERENTIATING BETWEEN ACCOUNTABILITY AND AUTHORITY

Three terms are frequently associated with leadership and management roles: accountability, responsibility, and authority. Are you clear about the definitions of each of these terms?

Accountability and **responsibility** are terms with similar meanings. They refer to the obligation to answer for one's actions and to accomplish what you have agreed to do. For example, the team leader assigns you the care of four clients and you agree to that assignment; therefore, the clients' care is your responsibility. You have an obligation to provide timely care to that group of clients and to achieve the desired outcome regarding that care.

By virtue of the state nurse practice acts, nurses are held responsible or accountable for their actions. This means they must provide the necessary care competently and in compliance with accepted standards, using sound judgment, thinking critically, and delegating wisely. Failure to perform in a responsible manner could result in legal action being taken against the nurse if harm occurs to the client (see Chapter 7).

Daily Ethical Dilemma 11.1: Medical Errors

A 10-year-old boy is brought to the clinic for a school physical. He has recently arrived in the United States from India and will be attending the local public school. The child has no relevant medical history. He is in excellent health, and his medical records brought to the appointment indicate that he is current on all his immunizations except the hepatitis B

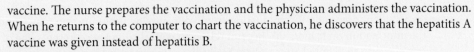

vaccine. The nurse prepares the vaccination and the physician administers the vaccination. When he returns to the computer to chart the vaccination, he discovers that the hepatitis A vaccine was given instead of hepatitis B.

- What is the primary dilemma in this situation?
- Is any harm likely to come from this error?
- Who is liable the doctor or the nurse?
- How could this error have been prevented?

Nurses have always been accountable for the care they give from both a personal and a professional standpoint. However, as we have witnessed the rapid technologic, fiscal, and operational changes occurring within the healthcare system, the term *accountable* now carries stronger legal implications. Nurses face greater legal vulnerability because of consumer rights, greater access of the public to information regarding health issues, the public availability of records, and increased client involvement in healthcare decision-making. This intensifies the necessity for nurses to be aware of the legal aspects of nursing and of the laws that protect the client. Individuals are accountable for their own actions and also for some of the actions of those they supervise. We understand that tasks can be delegated, but accountability cannot; nurses who delegate tasks to assistive personnel continue to be accountable for that care (see Chapter 12). For example, if you ask the nursing assistant to check the vital signs of four of your clients, you are asking the assistant to act in your place. You are still accountable for that activity (ie, that the vital signs are accurately measured, reported, and documented). This accountability has become a sensitive issue for nurses as, in an effort to contain costs, more unlicensed assistive personnel are hired to replace licensed staff.

Authority can be defined as the power to influence, give directions, command, take action, and make decisions. Traditionally, we have considered it the manager's job to command or make decisions. In this sense, the manager authored all critical decisions. As you read further, you will note that in today's work environment, authority is more often shared. Accompanying this shared authority and decision-making is a mutual responsibility for outcomes. We will discuss this concept in greater detail after we have talked about leadership.

In the ideal work situation, workers are given the amount of authority needed to carry out the responsibilities expected of them. However, many nurses experience frustration because they must be accountable for activities without the authority to affect the situation or create change. For example, a nurse has the responsibility of ensuring that all clients receive competent care, but the nurse may have no input into the staffing of the unit or the performance appraisal of nursing assistants working on that shift. Therefore, the nursing assistants may not be as responsive to the nurse's instructions as they should be. Or perhaps a nurse has the responsibility for seeing that there are adequate supplies on a unit but has no opportunity to affect the unit's budget.

Critical Thinking Activity: Authority and Responsibility
Think for a moment of behaviors you noted in your recent clinical experiences. What behavior did you observe that was a clear demonstration of authority? What were the characteristics that made it so? Can you recall a situation in which an RN accepted responsibility for an action that had been taken? How was this done?

THEORIES OF LEADERSHIP

As a student preparing for graduation from your nursing program, you may wonder how all the information on leadership theories relates to you. Healthcare represents one of the largest businesses in the United States. Historically, the administrative structure in hospitals has been predominantly bureaucratic, with a few decision-makers and many followers. That situation is changing as more hospitals adopt different organizational patterns. Having basic knowledge of the various approaches to leadership will help you understand the environments in which you work and will help you determine the leadership approach you wish to develop. The **theories of leadership** listed in Table 11.1 are those most frequently cited as helpful in understanding specific situations.

Today's healthcare work environment relies on teamwork and shared decision-making. Many believe that in this environment, the goals of the organization are most likely to be met if transformational leadership is employed. As you study the attributes of transformational leadership in Table 11.1, you will note that the differences in the role of the leader and the followers are de-emphasized. When effectively implemented, transformational leadership can

Table 11.1   Major Theories of Leadership

General Classification, Theory, and Theorist(s)	Essential Characteristics and Comments
Trait	Focuses on certain characteristics of the leader.
Great Man theory	Promotes the concept that certain people were born to be leaders because they inherited a set of special characteristics qualifying them for such responsibilities. Because leaders are "born," this theory suggests that leadership cannot be developed.
Attribution theory	Suggests that leadership relates to personal attributes people tend to characterize leaders as having, such as height, social background, creativity, assertiveness, initiative, integrity, ability, intelligence, etc.
Charismatic theory	Often listed as a quality of other theories, this theory relates to a special charm or allure possessed by the leader that inspires others to follow and give allegiance. Sometimes, this type of leadership is said to emerge in times of crisis and change.
Contemporary Theories	Includes theories most commonly in use at the present time.
Transformational leadership (Bass, 1985)	Places emphasis on the collective purpose and mutual growth of both the leader and the follower and deemphasizes differences in the roles of the leader and followers.
	Leader activities include creating a vision, building relationships, developing trust, and building self-esteem. Leader makes subordinates aware of how important their jobs are, helps them build skills, and motivates them to work for the good of the organization.
	Has four major components: idealized influence (attributes and behaviors), individualized consideration, inspirational motivation, and intellectual stimulation.
Transactional leadership (Bass, 1985; Burns, 1978)	Examines leadership in terms of striking a bargain in which there is a mutual exchange between leaders and followers of benefits for work sometimes referred to as a reward and punishment approach. Maintains stability of organization while offering rewards to employees for performance and met goals.
(Senge, Kleiner, Roberts, et al., 1994)	Identifies the role of the leader as that of a strategic visionary; promotes "learning" organizations in which the leader is the teacher who builds a shared vision.

result in agreements about priorities, shared values, perceived common goals, and meaningful purposes. You can see how this would be desirable in a healthcare environment.

Additionally, because of the demographics of the profession, a greater percentage of positions of leadership in nursing are held by women. A study conducted by Wilkes, Cross, Jackson, et al. (2015) found that nurse leaders need a wide variety of attributes, among which are being flexible, consistent, equitable, nurturing, resourceful, and courageous. Serving as a role model, both for clients and for coworkers, is one attribute of a good leader. This modeling behavior is key to Helen Erickson's theory of Modeling and Role Modeling (Theory Alert).

Theory Alert   Helen Erickson

Helen Erickson's theory of nursing focuses on the nurse acting as a role model for healthy behavior. Erickson was born in 1936 and she earned her graduate nursing degree from the University of Michigan in 1970. She has worked in leadership and management positions for much of her career, including Associate Dean of Academic Affairs at the University of South Carolina, and she is a professor emeritus at the University of Texas.

Dr. Erickson is the principal author of the Modeling and Role Modeling theory of nursing. According to this theory, modeling is the method by which the nurse comes to understand the client's perspective. This enables the nurse to role-model behaviors and develop a plan that can assist the client to return to optimal health. This model lists five goals of nursing intervention, Build trust, promote positive attitude, advocate for client control, validate client strengths, and assist with goal setting. This process is facilitated by examining the similarities and differences among clients. This theory also has applications in leadership. The five goals are applicable, as is understanding the perspective of others and facilitating progress toward a goal. (Source: http://www.nursing-theory.org)

Leadership/Management Styles

Lewin (1951), a theorist who has been mentioned previously, described three prevailing styles of behavior observed in leaders/managers that we refer to as **leadership** or **management styles** (Box 11.1), which sometimes are listed among the behavioral theories of leadership. They are autocratic or authoritarian leadership, laissez-faire or permissive leadership, and participative or democratic leadership. The focus of these three styles is on the amount of control the manager assumes over the actions of the workers and the beliefs of the leader/manager about the nature of workers (which is why they may be referred to as behavioral theories). The extremes extend from situations in which the manager makes all the decisions to situations in which virtually no direction is given to workers. In addition to the individual characteristics of the leader, several other variables will determine the type of manager a nurse might be. How authority is centralized or dispersed throughout the organization also affects leadership styles. The communication patterns, which are directly tied to organizational structure, also influence leadership styles. Equally important is the situation at hand.

A fourth leadership style, not identified by Lewin, is probably the one that is most frequently used in healthcare. **Multicratic leadership** combines the most favorable aspects of all styles as mediated by the circumstances at hand. A multicratic leader provides maximum

BOX 11.1 LEADERSHIP/MANAGEMENT STYLES

Autocratic/Authoritative
- Majority of decisions determined by the manager
- Dictates work to be done and who will do it
- Provides little opportunity for input or suggestions from followers
- Gives little feedback or recognition for accomplishments
- Communication flows downward, with emphasis on completing the task
- Works well in emergency situations where time is of the essence
- May be preferred style when working with unskilled or uneducated employees

Democratic/Participative
- Input to decision-making encouraged among workers
- Leaders see themselves as coworkers
- Communication, consensus, and teamwork stressed
- Leader leads by providing information, suggesting direction, supporting coworkers
- Communication flows both up and down
- Human relationships important
- Considered the preferred style in the majority of work situations

Laissez-faire/Permissive
- Little or no direction or guidance provided
- Coworkers develop their own goals, make their own decisions, and take responsibility
- Decision-making dispersed throughout the group
- Provides maximum freedom for individuals and motivates workers to perform at high levels
- If used inappropriately, a leadership vacuum may occur, in which an informal leader may arise

Multicratic
- Combines the positive features of authoritative, participative leadership styles
- Leader provides a maximum of structure when the situation requires it
- Leader provides maximum group participation when needed
- Support and encouragement provided to subordinates at all times

---

structure and direction when the situation calls for it and provides for maximum group input into decision-making when conditions are conducive to such an approach. Support, encouragement, and recognition of subordinates and their contributions are always present. Learning when to use each of the various approaches is something that a new graduate will need to study and to practice, just as with other nursing skills.

Critical Thinking Activity: Leadership Styles
In addition to the examples provided in the text, identify a healthcare-related situation in which each of the leadership styles would be appropriately employed. Provide the rationale for choosing that particular leadership style in the situation. What are the advantages of that leadership style? What are its limitations?

Changes in Approaches to Leadership

Nothing operates in isolation or in a vacuum; approaches to leadership are no exception. As you may surmise from the information in Table 11.1 and Box 11.1, the leadership systems have changed as societal values and norms changed.

As a society, we have experienced tremendous growth in information systems and technology. As a result, individuals at all levels within an organization have access to data, which is no longer reserved for a few selected individuals at the top of an organizational chart. Employees at all levels within an organization are knowledgeable about goals, operations, rewards, and critical areas. The information explosion also has brought a more intelligent and informed customer to the healthcare arena.

Today, more informed workers are developing into self-directed teams. This has resulted in managers spending time developing the abilities of others rather than directing them. Approaches to leadership have moved from authoritarian styles to a more collaborative leadership style, with the individuals closest to the problem helping to find solutions to it. The strategies used for developing human resources have undergone significant changes. Many organizations, healthcare facilities included, are encouraging employees to be involved in decision-making. The leadership required for this type of organization must be much different from that seen in the 1950s, when the manager instructed and directed and the worker acted and followed. Business leaders today would suggest that leadership needs to be visionary, ethical, supportive, facilitative, motivational, and open to new ideas. It also needs to provide for shared decision-making and be responsive to the needs of those it serves. The effective leader must be able to communicate clearly and effectively, build consensus and inspire people to do their best, deal well with ambiguity, and maintain diplomatic and productive relationships (Evidence-Based Practice 11.1).

Evidence-Based Practice 11.1: Leadership

Foli, K. J., Braswell, M., Kirkpatrick, J., & Lim, E. (2014). Development of leadership behaviors in undergraduate nursing students: A service-learning approach. *Nursing Education Perspectives (National League for Nursing)*, 35(2), 76–82. doi 10.5480/11-578.1.

Leadership behaviors are important across all healthcare settings. As many of the current nurse leaders approach retirement age, younger nurses are called on to fill leadership roles. This study focused on the development of leadership skills through service learning opportunities. Nursing education programs need to place emphasis on preparing new nurses for leadership roles.

As more leadership opportunities arise, nurses with less experience will be thrust into leadership roles. Nursing education programs can help prepare students to successfully fill those roles by providing opportunities to practice leadership skills in the educational environment. These opportunities have demonstrated effectiveness at developing leadership skills through practice.

THE CONCEPT OF POWER

Power, as we refer to it in a leadership sense, is the ability to do, act, or produce; the ability to control others. Power connotes having control, influence, or domination; in other words, the ability an individual has to get things done. The concept of power forms a basis for action in transformational leadership.

Types of Power

French and Raven (1959) identified five types of power based on the source of that power (Box 11.2). You can find all of these types of power at work in nursing: legitimate power, referent power, reward power, coercive power, and expert power.

Legitimate power that occurs by virtue of the position held in the institution is based on a specific job description. The most obvious of these forms can be seen in such positions as clinical director of nursing or director of coordinated care management.

Referent power is gained by an individual because others like and admire that person or what the person symbolizes. This can be observed when one selects a mentor or an individual after whom he or she wants to model behavior. The mentor has referent power that translates into the ability to change the behavior of those being mentored. Mentoring has gained much popularity in the past few years, and new graduates are encouraged to find a mentor when they begin their careers. We will discuss mentors in more detail later in this chapter. Referent power is often associated with charisma. **Charisma** is a combination of characteristics that makes a person appealing and that attracts others. Charisma includes the way the leader acts, talks, walks, and relates to others. It is sometimes listed separately as a theory of leadership and also is included often in the list of traits in the trait theory.

Reward power can be seen anytime one individual rewards another with positive statements, compliments, or other ego-boosting comments. It is also seen in promotions, salary

---

BOX 11.2 TYPES OF POWER

Legitimate power: Power based on an official position within the organization. Often referred to as authority, in which the manager has the right to direct others and workers are obligated to respond. Activities typically include making decisions on behalf of the organization and acquiring or controlling human and material resources.

Referent power: Power an individual has because others identify with the leader or what that leader symbolizes or represents. It also exists because others see the leader as powerful, as in the case of political figures.

Reward power: Power achieved by having the ability to grant favors or give rewards to others. Rewards might be in the form of praise, commendation, respect, or support.

Coercive power: Power that occurs because of the ability to place sanctions on another individual in the form of verbal threats, withholding pay increases, undesired assignments, or warnings. The opposite of reward power, it is based on the fear of punishment.

Expert power: Power gained through the possession of special knowledge, skills, or abilities that are respected by others.

Informational power: Power gained by having information or data that are important to others.

Connection power: Power that represents the cumulative effect of more than one person working toward a goal; for example, people working together to bring about a change or influence legislation.

Motivational power: The ability of the leader to stimulate the interest, enthusiasm, or participation of others with regard to a common goal.

Communication in Action 11.1: Using Reward Power

Jessica Brown was a new RN on the surgical unit. She worked with a charge nurse who had worked at the hospital for many years. After the end of the shift, Jessica stopped to talk with the charge nurse. "I just wanted to take a couple of minutes to thank you for the great job you did as charge this evening. I cannot believe how many details you kept straight and how you were still able to take the time to help me with that difficult IV start. It has really made a difference for me that you are willing to help me learn. Thanks a lot!"

Although Jessica was the newest person on the shift, she found that she could use reward power. Because Jessica was a willing learner and expressed her appreciation for learning opportunities, the charge nurse was very willing to help and felt rewarded for her efforts.

---

increases, and awards. Even beginning nurses will find reward power available to them if they focus on giving recognition to others' strengths and accomplishments.

Coercive power involves using threats of punishment to enforce desired behaviors. Coercive power also has its place in nursing. If you fail to practice safe, competent nursing after you are licensed, the board of nursing has the power to compel you to change behavior by the threat of revoking your license to practice (see Chapter 7). **Expert power** involves having specialized skills and abilities that serve to accomplish desired goals or influence others to follow one's leadership. Expert power is observed every day on hospital units. As nursing becomes more specialized, the individual with particular skills, knowledge, and ability will have power in the area where these skills are important.

Two other forms of power other than those originally identified by French and Raven have been described: informational power and connection power. **Informational power** exists when an individual possesses information that others need or want to accomplish a goal. An individual who has access to information about the unit's budget or one who is more informed about policies that guide behavior of others is an example of someone with informational power. **Connection power** is the cumulative effect of more than one individual working toward a goal. Connection power is responsible for the effectiveness seen in networking. Nurses who work collaboratively develop connection power. Connection power also can occur by working with persons who command power, respect, or access to desired positions or places. Nurses use connection power as they work with other professionals in the healthcare system or become politically involved. **Motivational power** is a new term. It refers to one's ability to arouse in others an excitement and enthusiasm for what they are doing. Because of its inherent or internal nature, motivation must be generated by the individual as opposed to being provided from outside. Motivational power, therefore, refers to the ability of the leader to stimulate the interest, enthusiasm, or participation of others with regard to a common goal. It involves recognizing the elements that drive individuals or creates satisfaction for them. McGregor's (1966) Theory X and Theory Y, Ouchi's (1981) Theory Z, Herzberg's (Herzberg, 1966; Herzberg, Mausner, & Snyderman, 1959) Satisfiers and Dissatisfiers, and Maslow's (1954) Hierarchy of Needs are all examples of approaches to motivation (see Chapter 12). In transformational leadership, motivational power is seen when the leader shares information, involves others in decision-making, recognizes accomplishments, and rewards behavior (Fig. 11.1).

Figure 11.1. Motivational power is seen when the leader recognizes the accomplishments of others.

Empowerment

The concept of empowerment has received a great deal of discussion over the past 30 years. **Empowerment** refers to the process of increasing the capacity of individuals or groups to make choices and to transform those choices into desired actions and outcomes. It transforms others to partners in the decision-making process by providing them with necessary knowledge and reinforcement (Fig. 11.2).

Numerous studies have demonstrated the benefits of an empowered nursing workforce including such factors as increased job satisfaction and intent to remain in the organization. We see empowerment at work where transformational leadership is practiced; transformational

Figure 11.2. Empowerment increases job satisfaction.

leaders seek to empower their followers and thus transform the work environment. Transformational leaders openly share information with workers so that everyone is aware of problems and the need for action. The leader provides a vision of what is to be accomplished and helps workers to understand that they are an integral part of the group. Workers are delegated authority for decision-making and for helping to find solutions to problems. Empowered workers have a greater sense of satisfaction derived from goal achievement (Evidence-Based Practice 11.2).

Evidence-Based Practice 11.2: Job Satisfaction

Roberts-Turner, R., Hinds, P. S., Nelson, J., Pryor, J., Robinson, N. C., & Jichuan, W. (2014). Effects of leadership characteristics on pediatric registered nurses' job satisfaction. *Pediatric Nursing, 40*(5), 236–256.

Autonomy is one aspect of job satisfaction that is associated with transformational leadership. This article examines the relationship of leadership style and job satisfaction. The study surveyed 935 pediatric hospital RNs who answered questions regarding job satisfaction and the impact of leadership characteristics.

Job satisfaction is an important factor for hospital management as employee turnover is costly and can have a negative impact on client care. Researching what influences RNs to stay in their current position relative to leadership is applicable information for many facilities. The biggest predictor of job satisfaction was autonomy, a key factor in the transformational leadership style.

Some organizations do not support empowerment of employees. Supervisors themselves may not be empowered within the organization. Some supervisors lack the self-confidence necessary to empower others and fear loss of control if workers assume greater responsibility in decision-making. In other instances, the supervisors may have moved into their roles while working in hierarchical organizations and may find it difficult to shift their approach to management in a new setting. Some employees do not want the accountability and responsibility that are required of the empowered individual.

Empowering Others

Nurses are expected to practice according to professional standards. However, nurses function within the constraints of their employment settings, and this affects their ability to engage in true professional practice. As we indicated earlier, if the organization does not support the empowerment of people, it is much more difficult to accomplish. If you want to work in an organization that empowers its employees, you will want to set this as one of your goals when seeking employment following graduation (see Chapter 4). An organization that is involved in transformational leadership styles also will support (and require) the empowerment of employees. The two are intricately interwoven. Manojlovich and Ketefian (2016) found that the organizational environment was a key factor in the development of nursing professional practice.

Empowering others can be accomplished through a variety of strategies that are appropriate for any situation in which the goal is to give others power and control over a situation. For a person to gain more control over a situation, that individual must be knowledgeable. So, a first step in empowering is often the open sharing of information. Sharing information with others is an important aspect of gaining the trust of your followers. Without information, others cannot act responsibly.

Once individuals are aware of the problems and situations being faced, they can be involved in setting the goal or developing a vision of what is to be accomplished. Through this process, the employee becomes more vested in achieving the desired outcome and buys into the excellence expected and the productivity needed to accomplish it.

Another characteristic of empowering others is involving them in finding solutions to the problems once they are aware of the problems being encountered. This is where the collective intelligence of the group is useful. Rather than support the belief that only the leader can propose workable solutions, empowered employees are respected for their contributions and first-hand knowledge of a situation. Ideally, employees will become involved in the development of strategies to accomplish the goal or vision.

Reaching this point in any organization requires that the leader has been able to help workers develop their skills. It involves teaching, team building, and coaching abilities on the part of the leader (see Chapter 12). Workers must gain confidence in their ability to make correct decisions and take appropriate action. Employees need to be able to see themselves as members of influential teams, with the ability to discover new resources. Recognizing the accomplishments of others, sharing credit, valuing honesty and openness, and rewarding behavior are important aspects of this development.

As you move into positions of responsibility, what are the behaviors and characteristics that you must possess to empower others? How can you motivate others to assume more responsibility and accountability for their actions? Box 11.3 provides a list of personal characteristics that are critical to being able to empower others and identifies some behaviors that help to create those characteristics. How many of those characteristics do you currently possess? Which ones will you need to develop?

Like many other endeavors, empowering others has no straight line to success; do not expect too much success early on. Being successful requires that you maintain an optimistic attitude, persevere in your goals and activities, and remain steadfast in your commitment to them. Continual assessment of yourself and the situation is essential. Be honest with yourself, and at the same time avoid being overly critical of your own behavior. Remember that the art of empowering others, like other skills you have mastered, can be learned.

Critical Thinking Activity: Empowerment

Think of a situation you have experienced or observed in which an individual was empowered. What were the factors that resulted in the individual being empowered? How did that individual respond? What additional actions might have made the empowerment even greater? Which of the behaviors that helped empower the person would you want to use? Which ones would you not use? Why did you choose these behaviors?

BOX 11.3 PERSONAL ATTRIBUTES THAT SUPPORT EMPOWERING OTHERS

Trustworthiness
- Honest in relationships with others
- Honors commitments, follows through on promises
- Can be relied upon
- Is predictable with regard to responses to others

Integrity
- Accepts responsibility for own actions
- Gives credit to others for things done well
- Is fair and just in relationships with others
- Is sincere
- Possesses sound moral values

Self-Confidence
- Knows one's abilities and limitations
- Models the values and behaviors desired of others
- Maintains a confident body language
- Is able to control one's own feelings and behavior
- Is not arrogant, conceited, or boastful

Sensitivity
- Is kind and thoughtful in interactions with others
- Actively listens to others
- Recognizes things that are important to others
- Is free of cultural and racial biases

Intelligence
- Is reasonable in decision-making
- Learns from experience
- Able to respond quickly and successfully to new situations
- Maintains keen approach to problem-solving
- Seeks new information regularly

Skill in Communicating
- Communicates clearly and concisely
- Listens to others
- Knows when not to talk
- Maintains positive body language
- Is sensitive to nonverbal cues
- Does not interrupt others when they are speaking

ENHANCING YOUR EMOTIONAL INTELLIGENCE

With increasing frequency, we hear the term "emotional intelligence," which is sometimes referred to as emotional quotient. **Emotional intelligence** refers to the essential quality of understanding how emotions function within oneself and others and the ability to use emotions effectively. It is considered by some to be as critical to high performance as is basic intelligence. As a result, a number of large businesses are now assessing an individual's emotional intelligence before hiring that person into an important position in the organization or before making promotions. Interest in emotional intelligence grew when leaders on the topic found that traditional types of intelligence, such as intelligence quotient (IQ), fail to fully explain cognitive ability. In 1995, Daniel Goleman wrote a best seller titled "Emotional Intelligence: Why it can matter more than I.Q." and the topic became a part of the approaches to leadership. As you read more about emotional intelligence, you will find that descriptions will vary among authors.

Self-Awareness

Self-awareness involves recognizing and understanding your own moods and feelings and includes appreciating how your emotional behaviors affect others. When this skill is well developed, individuals typically see themselves realistically and are able to act confidently. Developing self-awareness requires an ongoing commitment to examining your own feelings and behavior and noting their effects on yourself and on others. It may be likened to holding up a mirror to yourself and inspecting yourself very critically.

Self-Regulation

According to *yourdictionary.com* (2017), self-regulation refers to the ability to control one's own behavior without external control or monitoring. Research on mindfulness training indicates it is a positive strategy for managing emotionally charged situations (Grecucci, Pappaianni, Siugzdaite, et al., 2015). **Mindfulness** is a process of being aware of the present while keeping distressful thoughts away. Persons who have developed skill in this area continue to respond to human emotions such as anxiety, anger, and sadness, but they do not overreact to them and are able to direct them in positive ways.

To increase your ability to self-regulate, try to develop the ability to not take things personally. You might begin by using stress-management techniques. Deep-breathing exercises, stress relief through physical exercise, and meditation may all help. Using such techniques as deep breathing when faced with an emotional situation may give you time to decide how to react rather than simply reacting from immediate feelings. However, you may still find yourself in a situation where you cannot control your emotions. In such cases, you need to exit the situation. Simply saying "Please give me a few minutes" may be adequate. Another important point is that you should not put into writing anything that you would not want to say before a large group of people. This includes writing in e-mail, on social networking sites (Twitter, Facebook, LinkedIn), or on personal blogs. These are not private and may be shared widely, thereby creating many other problems for you in the work environment.

Motivation

Motivation relates to the desire to achieve or get things done. The motivated individual is optimistic and works in self-directed ways toward positive goals (see Chapter 12 for more discussion of motivation). The motivation discussed here is self-motivation, the ability to set goals, standards, and expectations for yourself and meet them. As a new graduate, seeking new learning experiences is an example of self-motivation. Volunteering to serve on committees and accepting a challenging assignment are other activities that demonstrate self-motivation.

Empathy

You are well acquainted with the meaning of empathy from your other nursing courses. Empathy involves the ability to observe accurately and respond appropriately to the emotions of others. Expressing empathy for others is important for effective functioning in groups or teams. Individuals who have developed this skill listen carefully to what others say and react in effective ways to this information. When responsible for directing the activities of others, do not control unpleasant situations by talking. Listen carefully to what is being said. Maintain eye contact when listening to others; it helps assure them that they have your attention.

Social Skills

Social skills, also referred to as people skills, center on being able to relate to many different types of people and groups. Greeting people when you meet them, remembering and using preferred names, listening with interest, and using the common courtesies of "please" and "thank you" are all a part of social skills. Individuals who possess people skills initiate conversations with others, look for opportunities to interact, and respond positively to the communications of others. Being a pleasant and courteous member of the healthcare team demonstrates social skills.

Developing Your Own Emotional Intelligence

Although emotional intelligence may be learned from life experience, it does not improve greatly without sustained effort and attention. A number of techniques have been suggested to enhance one's emotional intelligence and can be reviewed by browsing the topic on your computer and following the links. As we frequently have suggested in this book, emotional intelligence begins with a thorough self-assessment. Table 11.2 contains statements that will assist you in this exercise.

Table 11.2 Self-Assessment of Emotional Intelligence

Item	Always	Usually	Seldom	Never
I am able to recognize my emotions and I know what they are.				
I consistently think before I act and do not act rashly.				
I am aware of my own behavior and can describe how it affects others.				
I am able to manage my own feelings in a wide variety of situations.				
I consistently express my negative emotions in an acceptable manner.				
I am able to remain calm and collected when interacting with people who are angry or verbally abusive.				
I am self-motivating and do not require someone else to get me going.				
I find it easy to empathize with others and they frequently share feelings with me.				
I can identify when emotions can be used effectively and when not.				
Others would describe me as an optimistic person.				

> **Critical Thinking Activity: Emotional Intelligence**
> Review the self-assessment you just completed. How did you do on the self-assessment? Did you have many areas where you answered "seldom"? Were most of your responses "usually"? What would you like to improve? Which techniques will help? Improving your ability to identify your own emotions and how they are perceived by others is critical.

DEVELOPING YOUR LEADERSHIP STYLE

In today's healthcare environment, all professional nurses will find themselves involved in working conditions that require some leadership skills. Both acute and long-term care facilities use assistive personnel who have less educational preparation and who require direction from RNs. It is anticipated that this trend will increase. As you move into the world of employment, think about your own leadership style. What approach will you use when directing others? How will you develop those skills? The following suggestions may help to enhance this process:

- *Continue to learn and to grow.* Subscribe to a nursing journal that focuses on content related to your area of practice so that your clinical knowledge continues to grow. Attend meetings and participate in committees so that you learn more about the organization in which you work. Complete continuing education programs, such as those found on nursing websites and in nursing magazines, and attend education events and workshops.
- *Seek out a role model or a mentor.* A **mentor** is a more experienced individual who is willing to support and guide an individual who is new to a work environment and who systematically develops a subordinate's abilities through tutoring, coaching, and guidance. It is a fortunate novice who has a good mentor (see additional content on mentors in Chapter 13).
- *Maintain your personal physical resources.* One of the significant criticisms directed at today's healthcare environment by those who are employed in it is the high level of stress encountered daily. This stress can best be managed when a person is physically and mentally fit. It is important to maintain outside interests and relationships that help to balance life and provide diversion from the stresses of work. As you move into the world of employment, be certain that your lifestyle includes a healthful diet, exercise, rest, and relaxation.
- *Retain an open mind and develop flexibility.* Individuals who are open to new ideas and who can cope with unpredictable circumstances have an advantage in the workplace. Remember that there is often more than one way to approach a problem. Learn as much about the organization in which you are employed as you can. Developing a broad view of how the organization functions will help you to see where you and your unit fit in. Be willing to compromise and to negotiate; these skills are critical to any good team player. Ask questions when you are not sure.
- *Demonstrate respect and consideration for others.* All individuals bring unique perspectives and contributions to the workplace that should be valued. Practice common courtesies and etiquette. Address people by the name by which they wish to be addressed. Be polite and considerate to others, and generally, you will find they will return this behavior. Be sensitive to things that may be distressful to those with whom you work.

- *Believe in yourself.* Develop your own self-confidence. Give yourself credit for the things you know you do well. Identify the things that you need to learn more about and do so. Develop a body language that inspires confidence in others; walk tall. Maintain good grooming and dress. Become articulate in your communication patterns and remember the importance of being a good listener. Review the language you use in reference to yourself. Don't discount your own skills and abilities or minimize your accomplishments.

COMMUNICATING EFFECTIVELY

In previous studies, you learned that **communication** involves the sending and receiving of a message from one person to another. Let's list some of the other things that you know about the communication process:

- Communication occurs in four settings: intrapersonal, interpersonal, group, and societal. Intrapersonal occurs when you talk to yourself. Interpersonal occurs between two or more individuals. Group communication takes place when a number of persons are involved. Societal communication relates to an entire society or culture.
- Communication takes several forms, notably, verbal, nonverbal, and written. Verbal communication occurs in the use of words. Nonverbal involves one's body language and dress and includes facial expressions, body positions, eye contact, boundaries, and body movements. Written communication is that which is recorded, as in charts, memos, letters, and the like.
- Verbal and nonverbal communication systems interrelate and may either complement each other or contradict each other. For example, if you say, "It doesn't matter to me" and at the same time shrug your shoulders, the messages complement each other. However, if you say, "Please tell me more" but look away, you have given two different messages. Looking away can suggest you do not really care.
- Certain skills can facilitate the communication process and result in therapeutic communication or communications that are goal directed. Therapeutic communication has a purpose and direction and employs processes to achieve established objectives. It focuses on the needs of the other person and involves active listening and observation.
- The words we use when communicating can mean different things to different individuals. Chief concerns include the use of figures of speech, jargon, slang, and idioms with which not everyone is familiar, such as "She heard it straight from the horse's mouth" (meaning from a reliable source) or "Up a creek without a paddle" (meaning in a difficult situation without a means of exiting). Another example is abstract messages that use vague terms, such as asking a client in an urgent care center, "What brings you here?" when inquiring about symptoms and receiving the reply, "I came in a car."
- Communication involves feedback that allows us to know which messages were received and understood as intended and which messages need correction. Feedback performs a regulatory function and helps us to evaluate the communication process.
- Communication is influenced by a variety of factors, including a person's perceptions and values. Words represent generalized symbols that may vary from individual to individual. Perceptions can be altered by crises and anxiety-producing situations.
- Blocks to communication occur when unhelpful responses are made, such as generalizing, labeling feelings, making judgmental statements, or changing the subject. Blocks to commu-

nication can involve such things as telling the individual how to do something that he or she has already learned. Belittling others' feelings, disagreeing, disapproving, refusing to admit that a problem exists, or being defensive are other examples of blocking communication.

- Communication is culturally sensitive and culture bound as a result of impressions formed at an early age about how the world is structured. This applies to both verbal and nonverbal communication. For example, not all cultures maintain eye contact during communication in the manner of those in the Western culture. In some cultures, it is not acceptable to make eye contact when talking because it is a sign of disrespect (Michigan Nurse, 2015). Touch, which is a nonverbal form of communication, may be viewed differently by different cultures. Although it may be comforting to some, others may see it as an invasion of personal space.

In the past few decades, electronic devices have significantly affected our communication systems. The computer, e-mail, faxes, the Internet, and smartphones have greatly increased the ease and speed with which we can communicate with one another. At the same time, they have resulted in ethical concerns about the sharing of information, how it is stored, and who has access to it. Be careful with these methods of communication, always think about client privacy and recognize that brief comments are more easily misinterpreted than are more complete interactions. What may be intended to be matter of fact may be misunderstood as being rude.

Communication in Action 11.2: *Determining Understanding*

Alice McAdams worked as the evening charge nurse in a local long-term care facility. Her nursing team was composed mostly of nursing assistants from an Asian culture. Hardworking and eager to please, they struggled with English as a second language. During care planning time, Alice said to two of them, "I would like you to do range of motion exercise on Mrs. Howard and then get her up in a chair for 30 minutes." Both assistants smiled and looked at one another, but Alice was not sure her instructions were clearly understood. She then said, "Now, can either of you tell me how you are going to do that? How will you know it is okay to get Mrs. Howard up?" The assistants rather shyly smiled and one volunteered, "We move her joints and then put Mrs. Howard into chair." "That is correct," said Alice. "And how will you know if it is okay to get her up?" "If she says no, we don't get her up," replied the other. "Well, it is important that she get out of her bed, so if that happens, please come get me so that I can talk with her and explain. But if she says she is dizzy or not feeling well, check with me before getting her up. I will check with you later to see how things are going."

In this situation, Alice clarified that the nursing assistants knew what they were to do and also that they understood the importance of getting the resident out of bed and did so without demeaning them. She also offered her help should it be needed.

USING COMMUNICATION SKILLS IN THE LEADERSHIP ROLE

The importance of being able to use communication skills effectively in a leadership role cannot be overemphasized. To be an effective leader, one must possess an adequate understanding and application of communication techniques. The following are some basic guidelines for skillful communications (Fig. 11.3):

Figure 11.3. Communication takes many forms.

- *Communications should be clear.* A message being given to others should be free of ambiguities, and the person receiving the message should have no difficulty interpreting what is meant. If messages are not understood, the individual being addressed should ask for clarification. Sometimes, individuals do not want to acknowledge that they do not understand because they fear it will cost them their job. Instead, they may nod, smile, or give other nonverbal cues that suggest understanding.
- *Communications should be concise.* This applies to both verbal and written messages. We should work at stating the necessary information as briefly as possible while still providing enough data to be clear. The longer messages become, the more extraneous information is included, and the longer it takes for someone to receive the communication. This is particularly important when using e-mail messaging. Learning to communicate in a concise and clear manner is another learned skill that will improve as we become more proficient.
- *Communications should maintain a positive approach or perspective.* When problems arise, individuals respond better to communications that give positive direction and that focus on finding a solution rather than on fault finding or the problem itself. When people become defensive, their energy is diverted to self-protection rather than to problem resolution, and they become stressed. This detracts from accomplishing the goals.
- *Communication should recognize and accommodate diversity.* Any work environment presents a variety of personalities, cultures, educational experience and capabilities, and gender differences. Maintaining an open mind and being willing to listen to others will help in difficult situations. While being sensitive to cultural values, it is equally important not to stereotype. Recognize and acknowledge that differences often occur in communication patterns.
- *Communicating effectively involves active listening.* Active listening tells others that you value both what they have to say and their membership in the team. Active listening involves hearing the facts in the verbal message but also listening for feelings, values, and opinions and observing the nonverbal cues. A busy work situation may not lend itself to this type of communication. You may need to assess the situation as to its urgency. When time is available, remember to use the communication skills you have learned earlier: accepting, focusing, reflecting, clarifying, questioning, paraphrasing or restating, and summarizing. Listen

for vocal cues such as pressured speech or slow, hesitant responses. This will assist you to understand the context of the situation. A major deterrent to active listening is the fact that we often begin to formulate a response to the individual with whom we are communicating before that person has finished talking. This prevents us from listening to all the cues in an individual's message to us.

Communication in Action 11.3: *A Slippery Floor*

John Brice worked in a busy urgent care center. After a hectic afternoon of seeing an unusually large number of clients, John noticed a puddle of water on the floor. In the next room, two staff LPNs were relaxing over a cup of coffee. Both would have had to go past the puddle of water to get to the room. John walked into the room and said, "I notice there is a puddle of water in the hall. We can't leave things like that because falls and injuries can result. I need to get to the client in Room C, but would one of you please see that the water is cleaned up? It is important to maintain a safe environment." Both got up to get a rag to mop up the spill.

In this instance, John did not focus on the fact that the spill had been overlooked in favor of a coffee break, nor did he overlook the hazard because he did not have time to address it personally. He was courteous in his request and explained why it was important.

PERFORMANCE APPRAISAL

Performance appraisal represents a formal process by which an individual's performance is reviewed and evaluated against established standards, most commonly a job description. It might also be appropriately referred to as performance evaluation, performance review, or performance assessment. At all times, the focus should be on the performance and not on personality characteristics of the individual being evaluated. At one time, it was not uncommon for statements on evaluations to include "cheerful," "smart," "likeable," and "attractive," which, unless critical to the job description, should not be a part of the appraisal. Regular performance appraisal represents one of the standards for approval for many private, federal, and state accrediting agencies.

The primary objectives of performance appraisal are to maintain or improve employee performance and to enhance the development of employees. As a result of the performance appraisal, the employee should know how he or she has been performing and what he or she can expect in the coming months. Performance appraisals also can be a part of identifying individuals for special assignments or for advancement within the organization. Properly conducted, they can also provide the institution with information regarding the effectiveness of its recruiting and hiring processes.

Guidelines exist for conducting good performance appraisals. Box 11.4 outlines these standards. Please review them carefully.

Often, those responsible for conducting the performance appraisal as well as those being evaluated have an aversion to the process. Some of the reasons managers dislike the process

---

BOX 11.4 CHARACTERISTICS OF AN EFFECTIVE PERFORMANCE
APPRAISAL SYSTEM

- The appraisal system has administrative support
- Evaluation is based on standards such as job description or other well-defined criteria
- Clear and objective criteria exist for the evaluation used
- Employees know the evaluation standards and who will be evaluating them
- Evaluation procedures are consistently applied
- Evaluations are conducted in a timely fashion at regular intervals
- Evaluators are well trained in the use of the appraisal system
- The appraisal interview is a two-way communication
- All individuals know the related rewards or disciplinary action
- The final disposition of the evaluation is known to the employee

---

relate to the amount of time it consumes, the fact that unpleasant messages may have to be transmitted (many persons are hesitant to criticize others), and fear of legal repercussions. Persons being evaluated may dislike the process because it feels much like receiving a report card or because the process is intimidating. Performance appraisals in the work situation should help you grow professionally.

Criteria for Evaluation

All performance evaluations, whether formal or informal, should be based on appropriate standards of performance. Standards of performance include job descriptions, policies and procedures, and professional standards of practice.

Job descriptions contain statements that describe the duties for which the employee is responsible. These usually include reporting relationships and accountability. To be useful for evaluation, they should be up to date and clearly written to avoid ambiguous interpretation.

Policies and procedures education should be part of the employee orientation processes and relate to client care activities, as well as to timeliness, absenteeism, and participation in agency committees. More institutions are including customer relationship skills in their policies. By this, they usually are referring to what we think of as people skills or soft skills as they are sometimes called. For example, in one facility, the customer relationship procedures include that when meeting a person who looks lost or confused, any employee must stop, ask if there is a concern, offer assistance, and even escort the person to the correct place if that is necessary. The goal is that the institution will become known as friendly, helpful, and a place where one would like to receive healthcare.

Professional standards are written statements that describe a minimum level of performance common to the profession and that reflect the values of that profession. In nursing, standards of practice reflect expectations for the behaviors of professionals in relationship to specific areas of practice. Standards of care, which reflect expected processes and outcomes that should occur for individual clients, may be developed by healthcare agencies or by regulatory groups.

Table 11.3   Commonly Used Performance Appraisal Systems

System	Description
Rating scales	Comprises a list of behaviors or characteristics to be evaluated and a rating scale to indicate the degree to which the criterion is met. Rating scales may be numeric (1–5), lettered (A–E), graphic (always, frequently, seldom, never), or descriptive. Rating scales are a widely used type of evaluation instrument in nursing.
Checklist	Describes the standard of performance; the evaluator puts a checkmark in a column (usually yes or no) as to whether the employee demonstrates the behavior. Behaviors can be weighted based on importance.
Essay or narrative	Calls for evaluator to write several paragraphs outlining the employee's strengths, weaknesses, and potential. The evaluator may be provided with a guide for development of the narrative.
Critical incident	Requires that the evaluator observe, collect, and record specific instances of the employee carrying out responsibilities critical to the job. Incidents must be recorded regularly.
Group appraisal methods	May take one of two forms. The first involves using multiple judges. Several people form an appraisal team, typically the immediate supervisor and three or four other supervisors who have knowledge of the work being evaluated. Each person does an independent evaluation and then the results are combined. The second form may be used as a supplement to a supervisor's evaluation. Members of a team evaluate one another and team members' evaluations are included in the final evaluation. All persons use exactly the same job-based criteria for their evaluations.

Instruments Used in Performance Appraisal

Instruments are the forms and tools used in the performance appraisal process. They should be designed around the predetermined standards described above. A number of different instruments can be used for the performance appraisal. Table 11.3 identifies some of the more commonly used approaches. In nursing, a rating scale is frequently employed. It has the advantage of being easy to use and does not require a great deal of time to complete. The most critical aspect is that the assessment methods and the instruments used should focus on what the person actually does as opposed to personal characteristics of the individual. In many organizations, the appraisal process may also include a self-evaluation. In such instances, the employee and the manager would use the same instrument to guide the evaluative process and would compare ratings during the appraisal interview. Some organizations add peer evaluations to their process for professional employees.

The Appraisal Interview

As pointed out above, the primary objective of performance appraisal from the organization's perspective is to maintain or improve performance. However, the manner in which it is accomplished can make a significant difference. The interview associated with the performance evaluation should occur in a timely fashion, be held in a setting that provides for privacy, and have a constructive focus. The dialogue may include both positive and negative feedback. Positive feedback is information that communicates to others what they have done correctly. Negative feedback, sometimes referred to as "areas of opportunity," is more difficult because it identifies areas of unsatisfactory performance. Areas for improvement and growth may be included as well.

Negative feedback is best provided at the time the incident occurs and should be objective and accurate. For example, if you see a nursing assistant moving from client to client without washing her hands in between contacts, do not wait until the formal evaluation conference to correct the behavior.

As a new graduate, you are more likely to be the one being evaluated as opposed to being the one doing the evaluation, although you may be provided an opportunity to evaluate your supervisor. There are some steps you can take to assist with the interview aspects of this performance appraisal session.

Preparing for the Performance Interview

Effective performance appraisal is a two-way street. Think about your current role in terms of purpose, skills, and past performance. Assess your past performance evaluating what has gone well and what has not. Think about the goals you set the last time and your career pathways. Before the interview, prepare three or four questions that you can ask during the interview session. These might be as simple as "How do you think I am doing given the time I have been here?" or "Are there ways that you think I might organize my work more efficiently?" "What areas do you recommend I focus on for growth?" These questions would indicate that you are eager to try to improve your performance and meet the demands of the job.

Dealing With Negative Feedback

It is possible that your performance will include some negative feedback or criticism of your behavior. The purpose of criticism should be to help you perform better on the job. Nonetheless, it is often difficult to face. When it occurs, you should strive to listen coolly and without interruption. Remain composed and do not offer excuses. If there is a reasonable explanation to address the shortcoming, offer it in a calm manner. If you believe that some of the statements made by your manager are not accurate or are broad generalizations, it is appropriate to challenge the statements. Of course, you will want to do so in a polite and constructive manner. Ask your manager to talk about the specifics of your behavior and performance. For example, if the manager says, "You seem to have difficulty completing tasks on time," ask for an example of a particular task that should have been done more efficiently. This will bring the conversation back to specifics rather than dealing in generalities. Be prepared for the fact that this could result in more negative feedback than might have otherwise occurred. If you receive negative feedback, it should be accompanied with some constructive suggestions for improvement. If the suggestions are not provided, ask for guidance, such as "Okay, what can I do to work more effectively?" Then set a time frame with your manager for the improvement. If you receive ratings that you believe are inaccurate, negotiate with the manager about the rating. If you can convince the manager that specific aspects were overlooked, he or she may be willing to change the score. These behaviors will be ones you will want to work at improving. Box 11.5 identifies some of the aspects of a performance interview that we all desire. Be certain that you consider these when you are being evaluated or if you are responsible for evaluating others.

BOX 11.5 EMPLOYEE EXPECTATIONS OF THE APPRAISAL INTERVIEW

- A feeling that they were dealt with fairly
- An appreciation for their contribution to the organization and its goals
- Recognition of special accomplishments, efforts, or endeavors
- Some indication of how their performance can be improved, with specific recommendations on how it can be achieved
- An honest appraisal of future potential or prospects
- A sense of being fairly rewarded financially relative to others who are in the same position
- A sense that they have been allowed to contribute to the appraisal session and discussion and that the evaluator actively listened to the comments

Adapted from McConnell, C. R. (1993). *The health manager's guide to performance appraisal.* Gaithersburg, MD: Aspen Publishers, Inc.

Communication in Action 11.4: Providing Negative Feedback

Patricia Black, unit manager, was not looking forward to the performance interview she had to conduct with Richard Wilson, a new graduate who has just completed his first 3 months of employment. Although obviously trying hard while on the job, Richard was consistently late to work, and his tardiness upset the operation of the entire unit. When Richard arrived at her office, she offered him a beverage and invited him to sit down at the table across from her. Using the standard evaluation form developed by a nursing committee in the hospital, Patricia reviewed Richard's strengths as a new employee. He seemed pleased that his efforts have been recognized. Then she discussed his habitual lateness. She said, "I do have a concern, Richard. You arrive on the unit 20 to 30 minutes late on an average of 2 days a week. For example, this week you were 25 minutes late on Monday and 20 minutes late on Thursday. This disrupts the start of the day for the unit because we count on everyone being here at the start of the shift. Can you explain to me why you believe it occurs?" Richard took a sip of his beverage. "Well," he said, "I know it is a problem. You see, I never was an early riser. Most of my jobs in the past have started in the afternoon. As a student, I always tried to get into the afternoon clinicals. Perhaps I am not cut out for a 7:00 AM shift."

"That may be true," agreed Patricia. "Nonetheless, the hospital has a policy that all new graduates spend a 6-month orientation on the day shift so that they best can learn the policies and procedures of the hospital. When you have completed that period, we could think about rotating you to the later shift. For now, you need to develop some strategies for correcting your tardiness. Do you have any ideas?"

"Well," replied Richard, "I guess I could begin by setting my alarm clock 30 minutes earlier."

This manager recognized the strengths of the employee but did not neglect discussing areas of concern. While acknowledging Richard's statement of the problem, the nurse manager placed the responsibility for solving it on Richard and did not try to solve the problem for him. The employee, when directly asked to develop a plan, responded with a concrete proposal.

Behaviors to Avoid in the Interview

If you are responsible for evaluating the performance of another, the following lists some of the behaviors that should be avoided.

- Avoid letting the interview deteriorate into an argument. Arguments are counterproductive and destroy communication.
- Steer clear of discussion of personal characteristic or traits other than those that affect or relate to job performance.
- Do not scold or reprimand the employee. Behavior needing a reprimand or correction should have been dealt with when it occurred.
- Do not dispense personally referenced advice. Providing constructive instructions is part of the evaluation and is often considered advice from the supervisor. It should not be confused with advice that has a personal reference rather than advice of a professional nature. Making statements such as "If I were you, I would …" possess a personal reference and should not be a part of the appraisal process.
- Do not wield your authority by making statements designed to coerce, intimidate, or demonstrate your power. The employee already understands your role, and wielding authority in this way will destroy the two-way nature of the process.

Common Problems With Performance Appraisal

In the best of circumstances, performance appraisal probably falls somewhat short of accomplishing the goals for which it is intended. Often, managers find the process to be unpleasant and time consuming. Evaluations will be done late, hurriedly, or not at all. Training in the use of the evaluation instruments and the process helps to decrease variations in rating from manager to manager and will reduce inconsistencies in application of the process. The discomfort sometimes felt by the evaluators may also present a problem to the appraisal system. Many people dislike giving feedback to others when it is aimed at correcting shortcomings or weaknesses. Criticism, when given, needs to be assertive, constructive, and specific and relate to a particular behavior required in the job (Fig. 11.4).

Another problem area relates to fear of legal repercussions. As employee organizations have gained strength and recognition, managers have concerns that actions may be taken against them either in a legal form or in the nature of complaints, grievances, or appeals. When assessments are completed using specific criteria and definable measures, unsupportable judgments are less likely to occur. Maintaining consistency is as important as avoiding surprises. Evaluations should focus on what an employee does, not who the employee is.

> **Critical Thinking Activity: Performance Evaluation Interviews**
> Think back to the last time you were evaluated. What were the positive aspects of that evaluation interview? Were there any negative aspects? How did you feel throughout the interview? How could the interview have been made more productive?

Evaluating Your Manager

Most organizations supportive of personnel evaluation will provide an opportunity for you to evaluate your supervisor. Be certain to adhere to all the principles that you would want

Figure 11.4. Criticism should be constructive and related to job performance.

observed in your own evaluation. Work from clearly stated job expectations, a job description, or other document outlining the standards to be observed. Deal with aspects of the position, not the personality. Word any negative comments as positively as possible. Try to form the comments into constructive criticism. Avoid the use of words like "always" and "never." Rarely are statements that include these words completely true. If you can think of some corrective action or constructive suggestion that would make the situation better, include it. Do not attempt to address areas about which you have no knowledge—just indicate that you cannot respond to those criteria. Be fair, kind, and honest.

TIME MANAGEMENT

As a new graduate, one of the biggest challenges you may face in your first position is **organizing** and using your time efficiently—a process known as **time management**. The number of clients assigned to your care will be greater than you had as a student, and you have not had time to become efficient in many of the technical procedures required in your job. Time management can be learned.

Principles of Time Management

As you work at learning to manage time more effectively, some general principles will be of assistance to you. The following general guidelines can be applied in every setting and will facilitate your work in any role:

- Plan your activities. This will help you feel more in control as well as help you accomplish more. Keep a schedule. Developing a time schedule or a plan for how you use your time helps you to stay focused and to avoid interruptions.

- Prioritize your list of activities to ensure that you spend your time and energy on things that are important.
- Delegate those tasks that can be passed on to someone else.
- Take time to do things right the first time. Errors result in time spent making corrections.
- Limit distractions. This might involve closing your door or turning off the phone, pager, or e-mail. Some activities, such as developing a client's plan of care, require thoughtful attention. Seeking a quiet place where you are least likely to be disturbed will increase your efficiency in completing the plan. Some hospitals now structure units with a room located away from the major area of activity where such tasks can be carried out.
- Take needed breaks. Stress prevents attempts to get organized so take a break from activity and re-energize.

In addition to these strategies, we offer these further suggestions. Do an assessment of yourself. This includes a review of your lifestyle: your eating, sleeping, and recreational patterns. Identify things that restore and enhance your level of energy. Analyze your body rhythms and determine when your energy is at its peak. Plan activities requiring the greatest energy output and concentration to coincide with these peaks whenever possible. Take control of your own life. This may mean saying "no" when others ask for assistance. Offering assistance often means we have to interrupt what we are doing. Interruptions rob us of valuable time. In addition to stopping an action in process, we often have to restart or reorient ourselves to the task at hand before starting again—all lengthening the time it takes for completion. You may need to be assertive with those who have a tendency to interrupt you frequently; explain as kindly as possible that you cannot be interrupted. Sometimes, it is easier to refuse assistance. One instance is being asked to do something for which you lack the required skills; for example, being asked by a seasoned nurse to watch a critical client while she takes a break, and you lack the needed knowledge to safely evaluate that client. Another example would be assisting another when doing so means you cannot complete your own assignment.

Dealing With Procrastination and Time Wasters

Two final behaviors that help manage time are related to avoiding time wasters and managing the tendency to procrastinate. We all experience time wasters. Certain occurrences in our day-to-day existence are sure to rob us of valuable time. Perhaps the greatest time waster is social chitchat. Nurses typically are a gregarious group, and while no one intends to waste time, it just happens. Although it is fun and interesting to learn what other team members are doing, it is easy to lose 15 to 30 minutes in such an exchange. If you find yourself frequently involved in such conversation, excuse yourself by saying, "I need to check my client now, but can we discuss it during break time or over lunch?" If your message is communicated in a kind and genuine manner, feelings will not be hurt and people will not feel put off.

In his classic book on time management, Mackenzie (1997) has identified a list of 20 common time wasters that include telephone interruptions, drop-in visitors, ineffective delegation, personal disorganization, socializing, attempting to do too much, poor communication, and lack of self-discipline. To some extent, time wasters are unique to each individual. One individual spends too much time on the telephone, another makes too many trips to the water fountain, while another only manages by crisis. When you complete your personal analysis suggested earlier, look at ways in which you spend your time and decide which of those activities represent time wasters. Once identified, make plans for eliminating or decreasing the time spent in such activity.

Procrastination is defined intentionally and habitually putting off doing something that should be done (Merriam-Webster.com, 2017). Some individuals are more inclined to procrastinate than others. If procrastination has been a big part of your life, avoiding it may be the most difficult of the tasks we have outlined. Delaying a task can result in it seeming to be much larger, more time consuming, or more difficult than it actually is. Perhaps you have experienced these feelings in the past when you have put off writing a paper due for class or postponed starting an important assignment. Researchers include fear of failure, lack of interest, and feelings of anger or hostility among the many explanations for procrastination. Regardless of the basis of the behavior, an important step in correcting it lies in making a personal commitment to complete tasks on time. This involves establishing realistic deadlines and adhering to them. Determine the time of day when you are most productive. When you have determined what works best for you, use this time to initiate projects. This will make the task seem less overwhelming.

Barriers to Effective Time Management

The modern healthcare environment poses many barriers to the individual's ability to manage time effectively. These barriers may be either within the system or within the individual. One of these barriers is a system in which more is expected of the individual that can be accomplished in the workday. For many nurses, client care loads have increased both in numbers of clients and in terms of the acuity of clients. Bragadóttir, Kalisch, and Tryggvadóttir (2017) studied the reason for omission of care. Routine omissions included basic care measures such as ambulation, turning, feeding, and hygiene, as well as the more professional behaviors of client teaching and surveillance. Appropriate staffing considering both number of clients and acuity is key to addressing this issue. Examining the work environment before accepting a position may help you guard against this problem.

Another system barrier lies in whether the nurse truly has any control over the personal practice. Those who do not perceive that they have control often give up on planning because they feel it does not change the situation. The work done in Magnet hospitals to give nurses greater control over their practice has been a big step in offsetting this obstacle.

Personal issues that may interfere with time management include both physical and mental health problems. For those with physical health problems, it may not be possible to move at the consistent speed required in many direct care nursing positions. The nurse facing physical health problems may need to consult with the human resources department or with a career counselor to identify positions that mesh with their health status. When a nurse finds that he or she cannot complete work, a self-appraisal in terms of mental health and possible discussion with a counselor may be needed. Successful treatment of mental health problems will enable the person to function effectively.

Critical Thinking Activity: Procrastination
Identify one activity about which you procrastinated. Using the material discussed above, determine why you delayed completing the task. Does this occur frequently? What steps can you take in the future to avoid such behavior? In what ways will you benefit from avoiding procrastination?

Stegen & Sowerby Stories: Part 2

R emember Jack, the client who experienced increasing pain at injection site after receiving his pneumonia vaccine by a medical student? He made an appointment to see the doctor at the clinic and was found to have subacromial bursitis and a frozen shoulder. He discussed with the doctor his feeling that this pain was related to the pneumonia shot he received. He went on to file a claim against the clinic stating that the student was not adequately supervised. Read the rest of the story at www.thePoint.com.

Want to Know More?

A variety of resources are available on thePoint° to enhance your learning and understanding of this chapter, such as:

- Full Stegen & Sowerby Stories
- NCLEX-Style Student Review Questions
- Journal Articles
- Case Studies
- Learning Objectives
- Relevant Websites
- And more...

KEY CONCEPTS

- Differences exist in how leadership and management are practiced. Leadership refers to the ability to persuade others to follow your direction, to motivate, to inspire, and to instill vision and purpose, while management refers to activities such as planning, organizing, directing, and controlling resources.
- Accountability and responsibility often are used synonymously and refer to the obligation to answer for one's actions and to do what is promised. Authority can be defined as the power or right to give directions, take action, and make decisions.
- A number of theories exist regarding leadership. The theories can generally be classified as trait theories, attitudinal theories, situational theories, and contemporary theories.
- Three major leadership styles prevail: autocratic or authoritarian leadership, laissez-faire or permissive leadership, and democratic or participative leadership. Each is appropriate in a particular situation or setting.
- A multicratic leadership style that combines the most favorable aspects of all styles is probably most frequently used in healthcare.
- Theories of leadership evolve with social cultures, a leadership approach referred to as *transformational leadership* is advocated by many theorists. A transformational leader shares information and decision-making with all employees.

- Power refers to the ability an individual has to get things done. Empowerment refers to the process by which one individual who has power is able to share it with another. Both are essential components of effective leadership.

- For individuals to realize their full potential, they must be empowered. Empowerment occurs when information is shared, when individuals are involved in goal setting and finding solutions to problems and decision-making, and when efforts are recognized.

- Emotional intelligence refers to the ability to use emotions effectively. This involves recognizing one's emotions and how they affect others. Emotional intelligence is a critical quality in high-performance areas.

- Emotional intelligence has five components: self-awareness, self-regulation, motivation, empathy, and social skill.

- Leadership is a skill that can be developed. You can enhance the development of your leadership skill by continuing to learn and grow, seeking a role model or a mentor, maintaining your personal physical resources, retaining an open mind and developing flexibility, demonstrating respect and consideration for others, and believing in yourself.

- Communication is a critical part of everything we do. It occurs in intrapersonal, interpersonal, and group settings and is experienced in verbal, nonverbal, and written forms that may complement or contradict one another. Therapeutic communication has purpose and direction, focuses on the needs of others, and involves active listening. Words mean different things to different individuals, and feedback allows us to know which messages are received and how they are understood. Communication is influenced by a variety of factors, and blocks to communication occur when unhelpful responses are made. Communication is culturally sensitive and culture bound.

- In the leadership role, communications should be clear and concise, should maintain a positive approach or perspective, should recognize and accommodate diversity, and should involve active listening.

- Performance appraisal represents a formal process by which an individual's performance is evaluated. Employees should know who will be conducting the evaluation and where the records will be placed. Good performance evaluation systems are based on appropriate standards of performance, have top management support, are conducted in a timely fashion, involve a two-way communication, and assist the employee to grow in his or her position. Evaluators should have training for this responsibility.

- Effective performance appraisal interviews are a two-way communication system that recognizes an employee's accomplishments and provides direction and motivation for further growth. The interviews are conducted in a setting where privacy can be ensured.

- Time management involves learning to use your time more effectively and efficiently. To accomplish this, you must understand yourself, take control of your own time, develop a time schedule, avoid procrastinating, and avoid time wasters.

- You can avoid time wasters by examining the ways in which you spend your time and then deciding which of those activities were time wasters. Once identified, they can be decreased or eliminated. Making a game of tasks that you want to delay doing can help prevent procrastination. Breaking tasks into smaller, more manageable units can also help.

- When inability to complete required job components is due to system problems, a system change is required. If physical or mental health inhibits individual functioning, that must be addressed in order to manage time effectively.

NCLEX-STYLE PRACTICE QUESTIONS

1. The medical–surgical unit of a community hospital has experienced a 15% increase in client load over the past 6 months. In addition, they are understaffed by 1 RN and 2 aides. As the leader of that unit, you know that which of the following is an example of shared leadership?

   A. Encourage the formation of self-directed work teams.
   B. Offer professional development opportunities to those who have exemplary charting.
   C. Offer constructive criticism to help the unit achieve goals.
   D. Assign a staff member to provide evidence-based ideas for improvement.

2. You are organizing a support group for clients who are coping with grief related to the death of a loved one. To meet the needs of this group what action would be effective?

   A. Evaluate the impact of such a program on the community.
   B. Develop a list of goals and objectives for the group.
   C. Assess the needs of all areas of the community.
   D. Involve potential members of the group in the planning process.

3. A client on the orthopedic floor collapses while walking in the hallway with an aide. The nurse at the nurse's station sees this happen and rushes to the client's side. She determines that the client is not breathing and calls a code. She begins resuscitation protocol and assigns other assistive personnel to tasks. Which of the following leadership styles would be most effective during an emergency situation?

   A. Democratic
   B. Autocratic
   C. Laissez-faire
   D. Multicratic

REFERENCES

Bass, B. M. (1985). *Leadership and performance*. New York: Free Press.

Bennis, W. (2009). *On becoming a leader: The leadership classic—Updated and expanded*. Cambridge, MA: Perseus Books Group.

Bragadóttir, H., Kalisch, B. J., & Tryggvadóttir, G. B. (2017). Correlates and predictors of missed nursing care in hospitals. *Journal of Clinical Nursing, 26*(11/12), 1524–1534. doi:10.1111/jocn.13449

Burns, J. M. (1978). *Leadership*. New York: Harper & Row.

Culturally competent nursing care and promoting diversity in our nursing workforce. (2015). *Michigan Nurse, 88*(3), 7–11.

Foli, K. J., Braswell, M., Kirkpatrick, J., & Lim, E. (2014) Development of leadership behaviors in undergraduate nursing students: A service-learning approach. *Nursing Education Perspectives (National League for Nursing), 35*(2), 76–82. doi 10.5480/11-578.1

French, J., & Raven, B. (1959). The basis of social power. In D. Cartwright & A. Lander (Eds.), *Studies in social power* (pp. 150–167). Ann Arbor, MI: University of Michigan, Institute for Social Research.

Goleman, D. (1995). *Emotional intelligence: Why it can matter more than I.Q.* New York: Bantam Books.

Grecucci, A., Pappaianni, E., Siugzdaite, R., Theuninck, A., & Job, R. (2015). Mindful emotion regulation: Exploring the neurocognitive mechanisms behind mindfulness. *Biomed Research International, 2015*, 1–9. doi:10.1155/2015/670724

Herzberg, F. (1966). *Works and the nature of man.* New York: World Publishing.

Herzberg, F., Mausner, B., & Snyderman, B. B. (1959). *The motivation to work.* New York: John Wiley.

Lewin, K. (1951). *Field theory in social sciences.* New York: Harper & Row.

Mackenzie, A. (1997). *The time trap* (3rd ed.). New York: American Management Association.

Manojlovich, M., & Ketefian, S. (2016). The effects of organizational culture on nursing professionalism: Implications for health resource planning. *Canadian Journal of Nursing Research Archive, 33*(4). Retrieved from http://cjnr.archive.mcgill.ca/article/view/1656/1656

Maslow, A. (1954). *Motivation and personality.* New York: Harper & Row.

McConnell, C. R. (1993). *The health manager's guide to performance appraisal.* Gaithersburg, MD: Aspen Publishers, Inc.

McGregor, D. (1966). *Leadership and motivation.* Cambridge, MA: MIT Press.

Merriam-Webster.com. (2017). *Procrastination.* Retrieved June 7, 2018, from https://www.merriam-webster.com/

Ouchi, W. G. (1981). *Theory Z: How American business can meet the Japanese challenge.* Reading, MA: Addison-Wesley.

Roberts-Turner, R., Hinds, P. S., Nelson, J., Pryor, J., Robinson, N. C., & Jichuan, W. (2014). Effects of leadership characteristics on pediatric registered nurses' job satisfaction. *Pediatric Nursing, 40*(5), 236–256.

Senge, P. M., Kleiner, A., Roberts, C., Ross, R. B., & Smith, B. J. (1994). *The fifth discipline fieldbook: Strategies and tools for building a learning organization.* New York, NY: Doubleday, a Division of Bantam Doubleday Dell Publishing Group, Inc.

Wilkes, L., Cross, W., Jackson, D., & Daly, J. (2015). A repertoire of leadership attributes: An international study of deans of nursing. *Journal of Nursing Management, 23*(3), 279–286. doi:10.1111/jonm.12144

yourdictionary.com. (2017). *Self-regulation.* Retrieved June 7, 2018, from http://www.yourdictionary.com/

CHAPTER 12

Working With Others in a Leadership Role

After completing this chapter, you should be able to:

1. Discuss why teams are essential in healthcare settings and identify key factors in effective team function.
2. Describe the various roles a nurse may occupy on a healthcare team and discuss why each is important.
3. Describe the team-building process and identify behaviors that will strengthen a team.
4. Discuss the concept of motivation and outline actions that will motivate others.
5. Explain the process of effective delegation explaining why it is necessary in today's healthcare environment.
6. List the five rights of delegation and discuss why each is important.
7. Discuss situations that create a need for change and discuss effective change as it occurs in today's healthcare environment.
8. Discuss how Lewin's theory of change can be applied to situations on a nursing unit.
9. Describe the role of the change agent.
10. Identify strategies that will facilitate change.
11. Outline ways in which a novice nurse can respond positively to change.
12. Identify various sources and types of conflict in a healthcare setting.
13. Discuss the positive outcomes of conflict and strategies of managing conflict.

Champion
Change agent
Conflict
Conflict management
Conflict resolution
Delegation
Dissatisfiers
Driving forces
Hygiene factors
Motivation
Motivators
Motives

Movement stage
Normative–reeducative approach
Organizational conflicts
Reactive change
Refreezing stage
Restraining forces
Role ambiguity
Role conflict
Satisfiers
Stakeholders
Team building
Unfreezing stage

Stegen & Sowerby Stories: Part 1

R ose sustained a burn to her lower left leg when she leaned against the open oven door. The wound was slow to heal, and she had required daily dressing changes by the nurse practitioner (NP). Finally, after 3 weeks of treatment, her wound had improved enough for her to only be seen three times a week. Rose was delighted with the progress and looking forward to only visiting the clinic three times a week. Because of the progress, the dressing changes were delegated to the health-care assistant (HCA).

Care continued with the HCA doing dressing changes for 3 weeks. The 4th week, the HCA was on vacation so the NP did the dressing change and noticed an odor and drainage that had not been present 3 weeks earlier.

- What concerns do you have regarding the wound care of this client?
- What could have been done to improve delegation of this client's wound care?
- What do you think has happened?
- Who is responsible?

All healthcare settings require a variety of workers with differing skills in order to meet client needs. The role of the nurse among these workers is critical and challenging as it is that individual who carries much of the responsibility for organizing and coordinating the activities of the team. This chapter explores and explains some of the challenges of leadership.

TEAMS AND HEALTHCARE

The very nature of healthcare requires the development of healthcare teams and collaboration among all the variously prepared individuals caring for a particular client or within a given setting. A client care team could include a nurse, a physician, a pharmacist, a nutritionist, a social worker, clergy, a physical therapist, a speech therapist, a respiratory therapist, and housekeeping staff members, just to name a few. Sometimes their roles overlap. For example, both the social worker and the registered nurse (RN) may see discharge planning as an important part of their work.

Teams enable us to capture the skills, abilities, and creativity of all persons who work with the group, a factor that can be used to measure the strength of a team. Teams make things happen and create solutions to problems. What one person may not think of, another person very well might. When a team functions as it should, it generates a kind of synergy that makes the work of all members greater than the sum of the contributions of the individuals comprising the group. Teams may be led by facilitators or coaches; have members who share responsibility for decisions, setting goals, and achieving outcomes; use communication patterns that flow both up and down; and have members who share responsibility for decisions and outcomes. Thus, we can define a team as a group of people working toward a shared goal in ways that maximize the individual skills of each member and for which they all share responsibility.

Nurses are in a pivotal position to affect how the team functions because they contact all the various individuals who are involved in the team. The nurse, with input from other disciplines, develops the client's plan of care. This role requires finely tuned interpersonal and coordinating skills as well as excellent communication proficiency.

> **Critical Thinking Activity: Building a Healthcare Team**
> Review the number and background of caregivers in the clinical area to which you are currently assigned. How many health careers are represented? What are the primary responsibilities of each area? If responsibilities overlap, what are they? Who is responsible for bringing the individuals together as a team? Who is responsible for coordinating all the various client care activities, such as x-rays, lab work, treatments, and the like?

Communication Within the Healthcare Team

To be successful in this team environment, the importance and contribution of each person needs to be recognized. Respect should be the hallmark of all relationships within healthcare. Although their education differs significantly, nursing assistants should receive the same respect as a team member as does the physician or the pharmacist. You have many opportunities to demonstrate respect for others; use their preferred names when you address individuals, avoid intrusion upon privacy, and use language that reflects courtesy and consideration (such as saying "please" when making a request).

Along with respect for all team members, trust in the integrity and purpose of all individuals with whom you work creates the foundation for successful interaction and problem solving, as well as for team building. Others must be able to trust that you will fulfill your obligations and carry through on responsibilities, regardless of the role you play on the team. Conversely, you must be able to trust that they will fulfill their responsibilities.

Sharing information is central to building trust and responsibility among team members. When we share information, there is an implied element of trust that the information will be handled appropriately. There is also the indirect message to the person to whom the message is communicated that he or she is valued and is important enough in the scheme of things to have the information. Nurse theorist Imogene King proposed a nursing theory called Goal Attainment. This theory is centered on communication as the method to achieving goals. See the Theory Alert that follows.

Theory Alert   Imogene King

Imogene King was born in Iowa in 1923 and received her nursing diploma from St. John's Hospital School of Nursing in 1945. King went on to earn both bachelor's and master's degrees from St Louis University and a doctorate from Teacher's College at Columbia University in 1961. She died in 2007.

Her nursing theory, introduced in the 1960s, was called the theory of Goal Attainment, which promoted the concept that the client and the nurse are a team communicating and acting together to help the client work toward getting healthy. In the healthcare field, nurses and clients work together in much the same way that nurses and nurse leaders work together. By using the process of communication, goal setting, and action, to achieve goals outlined by the Goal Attainment Theory, clients can regain health and nurses can progress toward career objectives.

(Source: www.nursingtheory.org)

Relationships Within the Healthcare Team

In healthcare settings, there has been a pervasive tendency for individuals to align relationships into a hierarchical system (see Chapter 1). Those in lesser-paid jobs frequently are assigned lower status and typically have less power. Often, they accept this as the expected way the system will operate. Some are even content with this because they do not want the added responsibility that often accompanies a higher-level position.

The approach to working with teams has changed significantly over the past century, with the quality improvement movement having a major effect. In the early 1950s, interest grew in the area of quality-improvement initiatives. The work of leaders in this movement led to many changes in approaches to management, especially with regard to respect for everyone in the system and trust among various members of the team. Trust and respect, as mentioned earlier, are considered vital factors in creating a work environment that will result in quality products, including quality healthcare.

Nursing Teams

Nursing teams focus on the provision of nursing care (Fig. 12.1). RNs, licensed practical nurses (LPNs) (known as licensed vocational nurses, or LVNs, in Texas and California), nursing assistants (with various titles), and nursing students may all be members of a nursing team. In most situations, it is anticipated that the RN will lead the nursing team. However, in some long-term care facilities, LPNs lead nursing teams. In that situation, however, an RN must be available for oversight of the nursing care. There are a wide variety of nursing teams in different settings, some small, composed of two or three persons, others quite large.

The Many Roles of the Nurse

Traditionally, the public and even some nurses have thought of the nursing role as being one of providing care. While that certainly remains true in today's healthcare environment, the role

Figure 12.1. Successful teamwork is essential in nursing.

of the nurse has expanded to include many other responsibilities and obligations. Nurses often find themselves simultaneously carrying out several responsibilities: educator, client advocate, counselor/coach, manager and team leader, and worker in nursing informatics and research.

The Nurse as Educator

An important role filled by the nurse is that of educator. As a client educator, the nurse is responsible for ensuring that clients and their families have a clear understanding of managing personal healthcare and medications when returning home from the clinic, the hospital, or the long-term care facility. As a leader of the nursing team, the RN plays a key role in the ongoing education of team members with lesser educational preparation. RNs improve client care through coaching and teaching staff on a day-to-day basis. As a member of the community, the nurse is an informal educator who can provide important information related to health issues for friends and others within the community. In an era when health promotion and health maintenance are emphasized, this role takes on new dimensions.

Daily Ethical Dilemma 12.1: Client Nonadherence

Jane Allard, an 87-year-old female, was being seen as an outclient in a large health maintenance organization. After a routine physical with blood work, the physician placed Jane on 3 mg of warfarin daily, told her to discontinue taking the 325 mg of aspirin she took each day, and asked her to return for more blood work in 2 weeks. He then hurried on to the next waiting client. Mary Beth, the nurse in the clinic, talked with Jane following her examination. She learned that Jane had taken aspirin for many years and was convinced that the cause of her blood being "too thick" was related to the fact that she ate too much raw spinach in salads because she liked it so much. Mary Beth realized that Jane planned to adjust the dosage of the warfarin on her own and without the knowledge of the physician. Jane also stated that she really did not want to quit taking her aspirin daily. She planned to treat her condition by not eating any more spinach.

- What is the primary dilemma in this situation?
- How might Jane's health be affected by her resistance to the physician's new treatment plan?
- What should Mary Beth say to the client?
- What should be communicated to the physician?

The Nurse as Client Advocate

The need for advocacy can originate from a number of causes, including clients' lack of knowledge and understanding of the health problem, confusion about the way the healthcare system operates because of the complexity of the system, ethical and legal concerns, frailty or disabling conditions that will not allow clients to speak for themselves, or perhaps inadequate care. When serving in an advocacy role, the nurse can assist the client to be involved in informed decisions that affect that individual's healthcare. Since 1991, advocacy has been included in the ethical standards of clinical practice prepared by the American Nurses Association (ANA).

Because nurses spend more time with clients than do other healthcare workers, they are in a prime position to fill this role, may have a keener understanding of the client's desires and values, and have an established trust relationship.

The Nurse as Counselor/Coach

Tied closely to the role of advocate is that of counselor or coach. In their educational programs, nurses are provided with interpersonal knowledge and skills that allow them to assist others to express their concerns, seek alternative approaches and second opinions, and ask questions. Through such activities, the nurse is able to empower the client and family. Assisting those with less experience to move into effective roles within the organization is an important aspect of the responsibility of more senior individuals (see Chapter 13 on mentoring).

The Nurse as Manager and Team Leader

Manager and leader of healthcare teams are other important roles nurses occupy. Often, these involve serving as a change agent within the healthcare environment. Leadership and management were discussed in Chapter 11, and we will discuss the change process later in this chapter.

The Nurse in Nursing Informatics and Research

RNs fill a wide variety of other roles in healthcare. Two roles that are increasing in importance relate to nursing informatics and nursing research (see Chapter 15). The need for information management in healthcare has never been greater, and nurses are in a unique position to take a key role in data management for decision making. Similarly, the demand for nurses who will manage and participate in research increases.

Critical Thinking Activity: Staff Education
You have just moved into a new position in the long-term care facility where you have been employed for 6 months. The position requires that you do more teaching and counseling of staff than you have done in the past. What resources will you seek to gain information to increase your skill in these areas? Who might you contact? How will you assess your new competencies? How can you be alert to personal biases?

Nurse–Physician Relationships

Nurses work more closely with physicians in the acute care or long-term care setting than any other group. Throughout the 1990s, much was written about the importance of "good" nurse–physician relationships. The relationships of nurses with physicians may be very positive, but they also result in some of the most stressful encounters for nurses. Because this stress plays a key role in client care, job satisfaction, and retention of nurses, studies were done focusing on nurse–physician relationships (Baggs, Ryan, Phelps, et al., 1992; Larsen, 1999; Nelson, 2008; Rosenstein, 2002). The studies indicated that when these relationships lack respect and trust, the result is a taxing working environment and potential for ineffective client care. These same issues are still present in the work environment of today. As stated by Siedlecki and Hixson (2015), simply focusing on elimination of bad behavior is not enough. Old habits of behavior continue if they are not replaced with other, more desirable behaviors.

Disruptive behavior is discussed in detail in Chapter 13. As a manager of nursing care, the nurse can reduce the incidence of disruptive behavior by being certain when placing calls to physicians that you have all necessary information available before placing the call. Be certain that assessments are complete and that you have all needed vital signs and other information. This is doubly important if that call is made in the middle of the night. None of us appreciates being wakened from a sound sleep, especially if we know we have a busy day ahead. A physician might be distressed if the call were made without adequate assessment data to allow a decision to be made. Using a standardized approach to communicating in such situations such as SBAR (Situation, Background, Assessment, Recommendation) will assist you in planning your interaction to facilitate an effective response (see Chapter 9). Some settings require that the nurse consults with a supervisor for verification of the situation and consultation regarding options before making a middle-of-the-night call.

Communication in Action 12.1: The Client With a Changing Condition

Patricia White worked the 11 PM to 7 AM shift in a small community hospital. She cared for a client admitted to the unit during the evening shift who had been involved in a serious motorcycle accident that resulted in multiple injuries. Although morphine sulfate 1 mg had been administered intravenously (IV) every hour, the client continued to complain of pain, particularly in the abdomen. Patricia knew Dr. Whittle, the client's physician, did not like to be disturbed during the night; however, she was concerned that the medication had not helped relieve the pain. She called Dr. Whittle and said, "This is Patricia White on 3-South at Mercy Hospital. (**S**) I am calling about your client Jim Short who was admitted this evening following a motorcycle accident and is experiencing severe pain. Despite the fact that I have given him morphine sulfate 1 mg IV every hour, he continues to complain of pain, particularly in his abdomen, rating it as an 8 on a scale of 1 to 10. (**B**) As you recall, he has a fractured left leg and multiple contusions and abrasions. His leg was set in surgery after admission and is currently casted and elevated. (**A**) His vital signs show some change with a slight drop in blood pressure from 130/80 to 122/72 in the past 3 hours. His pulse is slightly increased from 80 to 88 over that same time period. His abdomen is tense and is the site of the majority of his pain. His neuro signs remain normal. He is alert and complaining. (**R**) I believe that his condition urgently requires a medical assessment of the abdomen." Dr. Whittle replied, "Make him as comfortable as you can, and I will be there in 30 minutes. There may be more injury than we first believed. Please, tell him I am on my way and prefer that he not have more medication until I see him."

In the preceding communication example, the nurse carried out the responsibility of alerting the physician to the needs of the client. Recognizing that the phone call would awaken the physician, she used the SBAR format, reviewing the situation and providing background status about the client to assist with orientation. She provided the physician with assessment data and a clear recommendation of the action she was requesting.

Because nurses are held legally accountable if they make medication errors, the nurse must follow through with appropriate communication with the prescriber (most commonly the physician) if there is a lack of clarity about a medication order or if the order does not conform to documented expectations. Communication should be conducted in a collaborative and polite manner. Often it is not what is said, but the manner in which it is said, that will determine the emotional content of the response. Keep in mind that the prescriber also desires that no errors occur and that appropriate care is provided. Provide information such as reference or resource about the medication or assessment data to help substantiate your concern. In some settings, the pharmacist may assist with this process.

When receiving communication from the physician or another leader of the healthcare team, recognize and allow for situations in which the emergency nature of what occurs with the client may affect the nature of communication. Direct orders for action are appropriate in these situations. The tenseness of a crisis may make individuals abrupt, and they may appear somewhat rude. Responding calmly and confidently in your role may relieve tension and help to ensure that care is rendered quickly and efficiently. A difference exists between meeting the demands of the situation and disruptive behavior.

The importance of interdisciplinary interactions and collaboration can't be overemphasized. This can be fostered by regularly scheduled interdisciplinary rounds in which everyone's participation is encouraged and nurses have the opportunity to share information they have regarding the client's response to treatment. Nurses must be mindful that they work and communicate within the scope of practice of nursing and remain in the realm of nursing practice when initiating suggestions for care.

Ensuring competence and possessing excellent nursing skills fosters positive nurse–physician relationships. If procedures are not carried out correctly, if medication errors occur, or if the nurse appears inept in a particular situation, client care is jeopardized, and it can be anticipated that the physician will be critical of the behavior. Nurses are empowered when they feel secure in their knowledge and expertise. Fortunately, the number of physicians who display inappropriate behavior is small.

Critical Thinking Activity: Communication With Physician
It is 2:00 AM on a busy surgical unit. A new surgery client, who had a nephrectomy late the previous afternoon, is experiencing a high level of pain. You have administered all the medication for which orders were left without alleviating the pain. You have decided that the client situation requires that you call the attending surgeon. What should you consider before calling? What information should you have? Are there other persons with whom you should discuss this before making the call?

TEAM BUILDING

In the late 1980s and 1990s, the concept of team building began to receive a great deal of attention in business environments as well as in healthcare. As managers responded to recommendations designed to improve quality, changes occurred in management strategies. In implementing a quality improvement process, satisfaction of staff and respect for their abilities should be taken into consideration. Without these attributes, team building will not be successful. Today, we see the concept of team building, especially with interdisciplinary (interprofessional) staff, being added to the curricula of helping professions.

Team building itself sometimes seems rather nebulous. People are not quite sure what it is. For purposes of our discussion, we will refer to our earlier definition of a team: a group of people working together toward a shared goal in ways that maximize the individual skills of each member and for which they all share responsibility. The goal of team building is to create a type of synergy, in which the effect of everyone working together toward the shared goal results in a greater total effect than could be achieved by the sum of the efforts of everyone working individually.

One of the most obvious forms of team building that exists in today's world can be found in the sports arena, where teams and team functions are integral to the activities that take place. Much of the literature about team building comes from the area of athletics. Through the process of goal setting, members of the team recognize their contribution and its importance in the work of the team. All members of the team have an ownership in the process and the product.

Teams are composed of a diverse membership, with a variety of skills and abilities represented. Each has a special role to play on the team. On the interdisciplinary healthcare team, some have special knowledge of pharmacy, some of medicine, some of respiratory therapy, some of nursing, with each member contributing to the client's recovery. These are considered formal roles. The informal roles are defined by natural skills and talents. For example, some have natural abilities to smooth over potentially volatile situations, some individuals are good at detail, others have a bent for creative ideas, and some are able to energize a team. Team members need to recognize both the formal and informal roles of each of the members.

Many of our life experiences have not encouraged team behaviors. Our early schooling may have emphasized individual achievement, recognizing those who excelled over others. Many of our work experiences may have occurred in environments where decisions were made by a few and passed down to others who were expected to follow though without questioning. Work was accomplished by a group directed by a supervisor. As we move into a work environment that requires greater teamwork, we need to make mental shifts that place more value on working together and less on personal triumphs.

Central to building effective teams is the belief that those who are closest to problems may best be able to provide the sound solutions to address the concern. All share in the problems that occur; all should share in the success that is achieved. One benefit of this approach is that it helps each team member to feel necessary and included in the team and that the member's contribution is important. They become engaged, feel valued, and take pride in the activities of the team.

Another part of team building relates to celebrating successes. As we look at building healthcare teams, we need to look for opportunities to celebrate the good things that happen. This will help members appreciate one another and the effort that has been made as a group.

Leaders focus on how problems can be corrected rather than on how they occurred. If one approach to treatment does not provide the outcome desired, a conference is held, and other strategies are discussed and decided upon. The focus centers on how things can be made better rather than on what was not working right.

Team building works to eliminate individual faultfinding. Instead of spending valuable time discussing with a nursing assistant why the dinner trays were not promptly delivered for the evening meal, helping that individual develop an organized approach to tray distribution would have more long-lasting and better results. The role of the manager often becomes more one of coach than that of boss.

Critical Thinking Activity: Staff Morale

As a new graduate, you have accepted a position on the medical unit of a community hospital. After working for 1 month, you have determined that the morale among the nurses and nursing assistants on the unit is low, that they do not function as a team, and that they do not have much team spirit. What can you do about this situation? Where would you begin? What are your limitations?

BECOMING A GOOD TEAM MEMBER

Although you eventually may be responsible for leading a nursing team, when you initially move into a staff nurse position, you will likely be a member of a team rather than its leader. How can you best fulfill that role?

Once again, we suggest a self-assessment. How well do you listen to others' opinions and ideas? Sometimes we forget that listening is just as important to effective communication, sometimes more important, than talking. People who are good listeners learn things that others may miss. Good listeners communicate a message to others that they are interested in what is being said and value the individual who is speaking.

Do you communicate your ideas clearly in an open and honest manner? It is important to team effort that you contribute ideas and concerns when appropriate. Contributions should be constructive and should be expressed in positive language that does not imply a lack of respect for previous ideas or approaches.

Can you accept constructive criticism? Part of growing and improving involves having one's actions evaluated. Evaluation should involve feedback, and it may not always be glowing. Pouting, clamming up, withdrawing, or having an emotional outburst are not appropriate emotionally mature responses. Feedback and recommendations can be used as steps toward professional growth. Analyze your performance honestly and make changes where needed.

Do you support others? Just as you want support in the role you play in a group, others need support also. When someone does a task well, let him or her know you noticed. Give credit where credit is due. Simple statements such as, "I think Warren has a good idea" or "I'd like to try Wendy's approach" are supportive in nature. And when things are going poorly for another, be helpful and encouraging. Offer your assistance if it is appropriate to do so.

Do you ask good questions and contribute? One of the reasons why teams succeed is because they use the collective intelligence of all members. If you fail to share your ideas or ask pertinent questions that could lead to new approaches or prevent poor ones, you are letting down other members of your team.

Are you a team player? Are you willing to give a little to accomplish the goals of the team? This means making team goals your goals and, in some cases, giving up a little of the spotlight.

BOX 12.1 QUESTIONS TO ASSESS YOUR COMPETENCE AS A TEAM MEMBER

- Are you a good listener?
- Do you communicate ideas clearly?
- Can you accept criticism?
- Do you support others?
- Do you ask good questions and contribute?
- Are you a team player?
- Can you deal with change and conflict?
- Are you self-motivating?

There may be more than one effective path to the goal. Team players are willing to take the path that someone else prefers rather than insisting on their own preference.

Can you deal with conflict? Conflict is a natural part of our lives. When we are unable to deal with conflict, we may become frustrated, jealous, or angry or may withdraw from the situation. Conflict must be dealt with in ways that are constructive and positive rather than negative (discussed later in this chapter).

Are you self-motivating? Being able to set your own time lines and commitments and meet them are indications of self-motivation. Demonstrating ability and confidence to manage what you do are important behaviors to nurture. Box 12.1 summarizes these questions you can use to assess your competence as a team member.

THE COACHING ROLE

The activities of the team leader often involve one of coaching less experienced members of the team as we strive to involve all team members in decision making and team effort. Schaubroeck et al. (2016) found that coaching can improve team effectiveness, task learning, and performance. The learning may be associated with job skills, understanding the operation of the organization, meeting new challenges, increasing efficiency and productivity, or other issues specific to the organization. The goal is to help the individuals who are being coached to fulfill their potential, thus building a stronger team.

In a coaching role, a more senior nurse supports and nurtures the learner, providing positive reinforcement as well as information. Rather than telling less experienced nurses what to do, the coach might ask how they plan to approach a problem and then help refine the plan so that success will be realized and the team members learn to handle situations on their own. Coaching involves asking reflective questions and providing feedback. It may be consultative, educational, motivational, or a combination of all three.

An individual who accepts the coaching role must possess certain qualities. This individual must be competent and emotionally stable. He or she must be willing to take risks, be honest and credible, communicate clearly, and possess energy and enthusiasm.

In some ways, the coaching role is a style of management. The unit manager who can coach teams to efficient and effective performance will have a much happier and more motivated group of workers than the manager who tells them what to do. The coaching role is further discussed in Chapter 12.

MOTIVATING OTHERS

Team building and motivating are closely related. What team building is to a group, motivating is to an individual. Motivating others to perform at their best for the benefit of the organization is a huge task. It requires strong people skills, leadership, clear personal goals, and participatory supervision.

Understanding Motivation

Motivation encompasses the sum of all those individual factors that cause or impel an individual to do something. Individual factors, called **motives**, are generally referred to as extrinsic or intrinsic.

Extrinsic motives include things such as salary, the work environment, and recognition by others—in other words, factors outside the individual. As far back as we can remember, society has relied on a combination of threats and rewards (considered external **motivators**) to get people to do what it wants them to do. Much of our early history saw a predominance of the threat or punishment as a motivator. As time went on, rewards were introduced and those who performed well were rewarded for their action. Today, the use of punishment or threat is considered less effective in motivating individuals than are rewards for work well done. Sometimes, these awards are financial in the form of increased pay, bonuses, or promotions. However, there are times when the organization cannot afford to continue to increase financial rewards. Managers and leaders must then find other types of rewards to motivate workers.

Intrinsic motives are more difficult to work with than extrinsic motives because they arise from within the individual. Some would argue that all motives are intrinsic and that the most we can do is try to foster within the individual the desire to act in a certain way, to perform certain activities, or to strive for certain goals, because the motivation to do so originates from within the person who will be doing the acting. Those who adhere to that approach state that when we talk about motivating others, it is limited to those acts of persuasion that will fire the inner desire within another individual to take the desired action.

When it comes to grades, why do some individuals strive for As, while others are satisfied with Cs? Why do some seek leadership roles within organizations, while others prefer positions that may capture a lower salary but be less stressful? Why do some people seek doctorate degrees, while others believe a high school diploma will provide them with all the education they need? A lot of study and a number of theories have been set forth to explain why people make the choices they do from among a variety of possible behaviors.

You may already have learned about human needs as motivation and that needs appear in a hierarchy, with unmet needs creating motivation. People engage in actions that help them to meet their needs (Maslow, 1954). Abraham Maslow, an American psychologist whose work has been popular since the 1950s, established the highest level of functioning as self-actualization. The needs for food, shelter, belonging, esteem, and self-esteem (in approximately that order) provide motivation for behavior. Self-actualization, the highest level, occurs when esteem needs are met and the individual is no longer driven by the need to prove himself or herself.

Herzberg, Mausner, and Snyderman (1959) and Herzberg (1966) discussed **dissatisfiers** or hygiene factors and satisfiers or motivators, which were essentially independent of one another in his Motivation-Hygiene theory. Herzberg's theory stated that people focused on the environment in which they were working when dissatisfied with the job. His **hygiene factors** related to conditions under which the job is performed and include such things as organizational policies, working conditions, salaries, status, and job security. These factors could be considered quite applicable today as nurses leave the profession because they are unhappy with work situations (see Chapter 13). When satisfied with working conditions, they focused on the job. **Satisfiers** referred to feelings regarding the work itself and included such items as achievement, professional growth, recognition, responsibility, and advancement. When workers are satisfied, work performance increases.

Another approach to motivation suggests that some people are motivated by a desire for affiliation, the desire for power, or the desire for achievement (McClelland, 1953, 1961). Affiliation referred to the desire for friendly, close social relationships—to be liked. Power referred to the need to be in control—to manage things. Achievement related to the desire to excel, advance, succeed, and grow.

A central concept for you as a beginning nurse is that different factors motivate different people and that one individual might be motivated by one factor at one point in life but by another factor at a different time. Keeping a broad view of what might motivate others will enable you to work more effectively to motivate nursing staff. Table 12.1 summarizes the theories mentioned above and describes how they may be used to motivate people.

Developing Your Ability to Motivate Others

As a team leader, how will you motivate others? What behaviors on your part will encourage others to perform at their best? What people skills can you develop that will assist you in working with others? A key aspect of being successful in this area relates to your ability to develop the kind and quality of relationships with others that will positively influence the way they perform. You will want to know your team members well enough to know what things you can do that will bring out the best in them: personal praise may result in outstanding performance in one individual; another may respond best when given new responsibilities or challenging assignments. Some motivating behaviors are discussed below and are summarized in Box 12.2.

Table 12.1 Application of Theories of Motivation

Theorist and Theory	Description	Application
Maslow Hierarchy of Needs	Established a pyramid of human needs ordered from simple to complex. The needs at the base of the pyramid are physiologic (food, shelter), then self-preservation, affiliation (love, belonging), esteem (confidence, recognition), and self-actualization (maximum achievement).	Facilitate opportunities for workers to meet as many basic needs as possible in the workplace, thus attracting more workers.
Herzberg Motivation-hygiene	Dissatisfiers/hygiene factors prevent job satisfaction and result in workers focusing on work conditions.	Provide enriching opportunities for workers in the work environment.
	Satisfiers/motivators promote work performance and work achievement.	Recognize performance and achievements.
McClelland Affiliation, power, achievement	Major motivators are the need to belong, the need to control, and the need to succeed.	Foster opportunities within the work environment for gratification of needs.

BOX 12.2 PERSONAL BEHAVIORS THAT MOTIVATE OTHERS

- Inspire trust and confidence from others
- Role model the behaviors you want to see in others
- Treat others with respect
- Give recognition for things done well
- Maintain a positive attitude

Inspire Trust and Confidence

As you examine the personal behaviors that will help you motivate others, give serious consideration to the things that people do to inspire trust and confidence in others. What helps build credibility—the assurance that people can count on you to do what you say you are going to do when you say you will do it? Behaviors that lend credibility to actions include exercising good judgment and being knowledgeable about procedures, policies, and protocols. Performing in a timely fashion is also critical. You will want to be even-tempered and patient, even in stressful situations. As a result of developing these qualities, others will view you as a person from whom they can seek answers and directions.

Role Model Behaviors

You will want to model the behaviors you want to see in others. In doing so, you set the pace for your team. When you are energized, others also will be energized. When you respond to others in a positive way, it becomes contagious and others respond positively. Avoid any behaviors that would undermine a team member's motivation, such as being arrogant, showing favoritism, telling jokes that put down others, making racist statements, or issuing threats.

Treat Others With Respect

Foster all opportunities to take pride in the accomplishments of the team and share ideas for improvement. Get to know your team members and show a genuine interest in things that are important to them. Be sensitive to problems they may encounter away from the workplace as well as within. Learn what their personal goals and aspirations are and encourage activities that will help them to reach those goals. Avoid gossip or humor that makes someone else the object of the joke. Do not talk about one person with another. When you need to speak to someone about a problem, do so privately.

Communication in Action 12.2: Avoiding Gossip

One evening at dinner, Sarah, a new graduate, ate with an LPN and a nursing assistant from her unit. The nursing assistant said, "I get so tired of Jennie [another LPN] always showing how smart she is!" The LPN replied, "I know just what you mean—you would think she was the nurse manager or something. Sarah, haven't you noticed how bossy and controlling Jennie is?" Sarah replied, "I feel really uncomfortable discussing Jennie behind her back. It seems unfair. I guess if it is a problem for you, maybe you should try to talk to Jennie about it." She then introduced a new topic of conversation. Sarah has not labeled the others but has indicated she will not participate in gossip and laid the framework for others to expect that she will not gossip about them.

Recognize Achievements

Receiving recognition for things done well helps motivate many people. Giving praise for accomplishments means that you will be working closely with individuals, so that you know when they have done something well. Praise and recognition, even in the form of a thank you, serve as great reinforcers and encourage people to keep trying. Most individuals seek to please others by their performance and need to know when that has been achieved. If you can offer this praise in public, it will reap even greater rewards. Praise publicly and correct privately. This is certainly true when trying to motivate others to do their best **(Fig. 12.2)**.

Another aspect of encouraging individuals to perform at their best focuses on having them know that their opinion is wanted and valued. This means involving them in decision making. We talked earlier in this chapter and in Chapter 11 about involving those closest to the action in the decision-making process. You can provide the opportunity for others to have input into decisions and to articulate their thoughts and opinions. When you initially try this, you may run into resistance. When encouraging others to participate in decision making, you may get the response, "That's what they pay *you* for." If this occurs, continue to offer opportunities for input. If this is a new experience for the team member, that individual may doubt your sincerity. Developing a genuine approach when working with others creates the basis of trust and respect as mentioned at the beginning of this chapter.

Maintain a Positive Attitude

Maintaining a positive attitude will help both you and those with whom you work. If you avoid becoming upset and angry, you can respond to problems or errors more effectively. This may

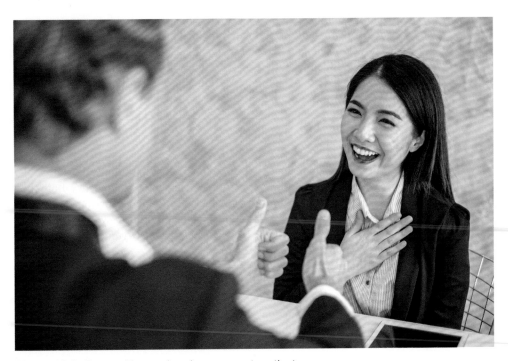

Figure 12.2. Recognition and praise are great motivators.

require using your sense of humor when things go awry. The discomfort of many situations can be decreased by being able to laugh at things that fail to meet our expectations. In contrast, becoming upset or angry if something is done incorrectly will only cause your team members to avoid you. They will consider you unapproachable, and communication will decrease. The opportunity to build the strength of the team will be missed.

A final word should be said about redirecting the efforts of others. Especially when working with unlicensed assistive personnel (UAPs), you may identify techniques that are incorrect or approaches to client care that need improvement. When this occurs, always focus your comments on the observed behavior you believe needs to be changed, not on the individual's personal characteristics. You will find it useful to ask personnel for their own commitment to make the needed change in behavior or performance. This places the responsibility for correct performance on the individual. Then, when you observe the corrected behavior, be certain to positively comment about it. More discussion related to supervising the actions of others follows later in this chapter.

Communication in Action 12.3: Lost Privacy

John Wilson was making rounds of the clients in a long-term care facility when he noticed a nursing assistant with an older resident. The assistant was preparing to move the resident onto a commode, but the curtain was not pulled. John moved to the bedside and simply said, "Here, let me get that curtain for you," and pulled the curtain around to protect the resident's privacy. When the nursing assistant was finished, John approached her privately and said, "I am concerned that you did not pull the curtain when you were assisting the resident to the commode. You must always remember to pull the curtain before providing care to assure that our residents are provided privacy. Will you agree to work on that?" He avoided making general statements such as, "You are inconsiderate and careless of the modesty of our residents," but was specific about the incorrect behavior and the rationale for the correct behavior. Also, John asked the nursing assistant to make a commitment to changing her own behavior.

Learning to Delegate

In today's healthcare environment, the need for all RNs to skillfully delegate, assign, and supervise those with less educational preparation is an essential competency. Both the ANA and the National Council of State Boards of Nursing (NCSBN) have developed resources designed to make the delegation process easier to understand and utilize. Two such resources are the *ANA Principles of Delegation* and NCSBN's *Decision Tree on Delegation* that reflects the four phases of the delegation process (NCSBN, 2016).

Delegation may be defined as "allowing a delegatee to perform a specific nursing activity, skill, or procedure that is beyond the delegatee's traditional role and not routinely performed" (NCSBN, 2016). An example would be an RN asking that a nursing assistant help a client ambulate in the hall. The nursing assistant assists the client to walk; the RN is still responsible for seeing that the client ambulates and that it is completed safely and documented in the client's record.

In today's healthcare environment, which uses variously prepared caregivers, the importance of being able to effectively delegate responsibilities is critical. Nurses would not be able to complete their duties, tasks, and responsibilities without the ability to delegate some nursing activities. Delegating effectively requires that you have skill in the ability to guide, teach, and direct others. Like other skills you have mastered, it can be learned.

Reasons to Delegate

There are a number of reasons that we delegate certain tasks to others. Primary among these is the current trend in healthcare facilities to allow the RN more time for critical aspects of care by hiring UAPs to perform those tasks that they can perform safely. This also results in cost cuts, as a UAP commands a much lower salary than does an RN. Individuals with less educational preparation can carry out certain aspects of care such as taking vital signs, ambulating, transporting clients, and performing basic procedures. This allows the RN to focus on activities such as client assessment, care coordination, and teaching. In this way, delegating provides for effective time management.

Another reason to delegate relates to the positive effect it can have on building team spirit. As team members are able to effectively perform the tasks delegated to them, a sense of satisfaction is created and self-esteem is increased. Thus, teams function more effectively.

Critical Aspects of Effective Delegation

It is critical to remember that although you have asked someone else to carry out a nursing task, you are still accountable for the care that is given. You need to be able to ensure that the task will be completed in compliance with accepted standards, in a timely fashion, and that the activity, along with the client's response, if appropriate, is adequately documented. Review these factors before you begin delegating tasks to others (Evidence-Based Practice 12.1).

Evidence-Based Practice 12.1: Delegation and Accountability

Taylor, K. (2015). Principles of delegation and accountability. *Practice Nurse, 45*(7), 40–43.

Because of the increasing demands of the nursing role, it is necessary to delegate some of the work of nursing to those assistive personnel who are able to carry out the tasks. In addition, clients expect the same level of care from all caregivers. It is important that delegated tasks be within the scope of practice and the capability of the person to whom they are delegated.

There are regulations in place to guide decision making in delegation. The NCSBN has established the five rights of delegation to guide nurses in appropriate delegation process. The most important thing to remember about delegation is that regardless of who the task is delegated to, the ultimate responsibility for accomplishment of the task stays with the nurse who has delegated it to assistive personnel, and the delegating nurse is therefore liable for the outcome.

Knowing When Not to Delegate

Are there tasks that should not be delegated? When should I not delegate a task? What are the situations in which I should retain responsibility for doing the task? How will I know the difference? These are questions frequently asked by the nurse who is just moving into the role of managing the activities of others.

Certain tasks cannot be delegated. The most obvious of these are activities that are not within the scope of practice of the individual to whom you might delegate the task. Any activity that requires knowledge and judgment that is unique to the function of an RN cannot be delegated to others (Fig. 12.3).

You may not delegate responsibilities that call for professional judgment, skill, or decision-making ability such as asking the UAP to do assessments or evaluations. An RN must complete all assessments of the client and attend to client needs. Information from the assessment that is important to the client's care then needs to be communicated to any person to whom care is delegated. The ability to do a thorough assessment and to not overlook some critical need is part of the nursing judgment acquired through your education. Someone with lesser preparation might overlook that need. For example, if you admit a client with head trauma to your unit, the assessment of that client cannot be delegated.

You may not delegate roles that are limited to licensed individuals under the nursing licensure laws. For example, giving medications cannot be delegated in most settings, because medication administration involves assessment, understanding of appropriate procedural safeguards, knowledge of pharmacology, and the ability to evaluate the effectiveness of the medication. Because of this, the law limits who may administer medications. In some states, routine medication administration can be delegated to specially trained medication aides in long-term care or to home care aides in community settings. In these instances, the task is delegated, but an RN retains accountability for the assessment and decision-making surrounding

Figure 12.3. Knowing when *not* to delegate.

BOX 12.3 SITUATIONS IN WHICH DELEGATION IS INAPPROPRIATE

When Delegation Is Inappropriate	Rationale
When the activities to be delegated fall outside the scope of practice of the person to whom they would be delegated.	You cannot delegate something the individual is not allowed to do.
When the activities to be delegated require independent, specialized nursing knowledge and judgment.	This protects the safety of the client.
When the activities to be delegated fall within job description and role of the RN and delegating it would erode that role.	This would apply to situations in which the nurse is responsible for evaluating the performance of others.
When the work situation will not allow time for adequate supervision of those to whom tasks are delegated.	Delegated tasks must be supported and supervised at all times.

medication administration and for assuring that the task is carried out correctly. Box 12.3 summarizes information on what should not be delegated and provides the reason why.

Identifying to Whom to Delegate

You can delegate only to a person who is competent to perform the task delegated. The nurse who is delegating tasks must know and understand the level of care that can be performed by the person to whom the task is being delegated. In other words, you need to understand staff members' competency level or, if they are licensed, their scope of practice—what activities a person with a particular license may legally perform. The scope of practice for RNs and for LPNs is outlined in state nurse practice acts and may vary from state to state (see Chapter 3). You will want to be familiar with the nurse practice acts of the state in which you are employed. When working with someone who is not licensed, you will want to be knowledgeable about that individual's skill level, job descriptions, specific competencies, and agency policies and protocols.

Determining What to Delegate

The tasks delegated to UAPs should not require nursing judgment while being carried out. This implies that the tasks should be routine in nature, ones that can be performed according to certain exact standards, and that the client's condition be relatively stable. We have said it before, but it bears repeating—activities that require specialized nursing skill, knowledge, or experience cannot be delegated. It is the use of this specialized nursing judgment that constitutes the heart of professional nursing.

The anticipated outcome of the care that is being delegated should be reasonably predictable. For example, if the responsibility for checking the vital signs of a client is assigned to an LPN, the result will be the accurate assessment and recording of the client's vital signs.

Tasks associated with any situation requiring ongoing assessment, complex observations, additional instructions, or critical decisions should not be delegated. Again, these activities require the use of nursing judgment and, therefore, should be completed by the RN. This would apply to any situation in which a client's condition is unstable, changing, or whose acuity level is high.

Matching the Task to the Person to Whom It Is Delegated

When delegating, you have the responsibility for ensuring that a match exists between what care the client needs to have performed and the level of competence and understanding of the person being asked to provide that care. In this way, you are assured that the tasks that are delegated are not beyond the ability of the individual asked to do them. This requires that you know the members of your team, their abilities, and their legal scope of practice. This can be an important consideration in situations in which an RN is floated into a special care unit to assist during especially busy times. Aspects of care in that unit that are specialized should not be delegated to someone who has not had the additional training and education required to render safe care, even if that person has the RN license. Rather, the floated nurse should be asked to perform only those aspects of care with which he or she is familiar.

Supervising Delegated Tasks

The supervision of delegated activities is essential. Supervision is defined as "the act of watching a person or activity and making certain that everything is done correctly and safely" (dictionary.cambridge.org, 2017). This means that an individual with greater skill and education is available, usually in person, but occasionally through alternate means, such as written or verbal communications, to give directions and ensure that activities are carried out properly. For delegation to be successful, there must be sufficient personnel and adequate time to provide the needed supervision and follow-up. If either of these is missing, problems may result.

The Five Rights of Successful Delegation

If you have followed all these guidelines when delegating responsibilities to others, in all likelihood you will have also followed the five rights of successful delegation. The NCSBN issued these five rights in 1995, when changes in delivery of client care first included use of UAP and similar care providers (NCSBN, 1995). (Examples of UAP include positions with job titles such as nurse aides, certified nurse assistants, nurse technicians, client care technicians, personal care attendant, or unit assistants.) The five rights as identified by the NCSBN are found in Box 12.4.

Suggestions for Successful Delegation

A number of elements can result in delegation either enhancing or compromising client care. Following the steps in the nursing process will help ensure the best outcomes.

Assess the Situation

Before you decide which aspects of care you can ask others to do and which you should complete yourself, be certain that a complete assessment of the client has been done. You will want

---

BOX 12.4 THE NCSBN'S FIVE RIGHTS OF DELEGATION

- Right Task
- Right Circumstances
- Right Person
- Right Direction/Communication
- Right Supervision/Evaluation

to know what that individual's needs involve, what priorities have been set, the goals of care, the time you have to accomplish the care, and other factors that impinge on the situation.

If you are to make a good match between the skills of the person to whom you delegate responsibilities and the complexity of the task, you must know the abilities of the person to whom you will delegate tasks. This can sometimes be determined through hospital protocols that establish the competencies of various levels of caregivers or via job descriptions that define what an individual in a certain job category is capable of performing. If the individual is licensed, you can be guided by what that category of worker can legally do. The length of time he or she has worked in that position or on that unit can also give some guidance. The best way to understand what individuals can and cannot do is to have worked with them for a sufficient period of time. If you are unfamiliar with the skills of a particular worker, you will need to provide greater supervision as you begin working with that person.

Initially, you will want to delegate only those tasks that have the highest level of predictive outcome, that is, those that are routine and standard. In so doing, you also are considering the potential for harm to the client and how difficult a particular task is to perform. You will note that your process of assessment has broadened to include the client, members of your team, and the work situation.

Plan Your Actions

You will need to compare, in your mind, the information you have about the skill level of your team and the nursing care activities to be accomplished. Using the information you have gleaned in your assessment, you will then identify the specific persons to whom you may delegate the various tasks. Plan the time to give them their assignments to ensure that you have adequate opportunity to clearly communicate your expectations. Also plan time for them to ask any questions they may have regarding the assignment.

Implement Your Plan

As you begin to direct the activities of others, your instructions should be complete, easily understood, and able to be followed correctly. What activities need to be completed immediately? Which ones can be done later in the shift? What are the expected outcomes? If you are working with an individual whose primary language is not English, this may take more time (see "Communicating Effectively" in Chapter 11). Be certain that the assistants know what to report back to you and when you want to receive that information. Listening carefully to their response to your instructions will help you to know that they have understood what you want accomplished. Watch for both verbal and nonverbal cues to their comprehension of your expectations. Ask them to repeat back to you what they plan to do and when. Ask whether they have any questions before beginning their work. Tell them where you will be if they need assistance.

Supervising care constitutes an essential part of delegation; it means that you know what is occurring with the clients and the staff, what has been accomplished, what remains to be done, and what problems may have occurred in the process. This requires that you check with individuals throughout the day to determine how they are progressing, what problems they may be having, or what assistance or instruction they may need. Asking questions such as, "How are you progressing with your task?" or "Are you having any difficulties with care?" or "Is there anything with which you need help?" will provide opportunity for feedback.

Sometimes the individual who is a novice in the supervising role finds it difficult to know when to step in and assist and when to step back. Initially, you may be so concerned about doing a good job that you micromanage the situation. When you delegate responsibilities, provide an appropriate amount of autonomy for the person to decide how to accomplish the work. Generally speaking, once you delegate a task you should not take it back. This is a good opportunity for you to use your skills as a coach. Ask questions that will help people to whom tasks are delegated find the answer for themselves. Cueing questions such as, "What did you do the last time you had this to do?" or "What do you think will work best?" stimulate individuals to begin to solve problems for themselves, elevates their self-confidence, and builds stronger teams. If your assistance is required, provide just that—assistance—rather than taking over the situation. You want to develop team members who have confidence in their own abilities and who feel they are valued members of the team.

Evaluate the Results

When you are responsible for the activities of others, evaluating the outcomes of care is more important than ever. Remember, the fact that you have delegated part of it to another person does not absolve you of the responsibility of seeing that it is completed according to established standards and in a timely manner. You will want to evaluate all clients in your care and determine that their needs have been met to the highest degree possible. Be certain that all documentation is complete and done according to standards. Talk with members of your team to obtain needed information about the care they gave and any observations they made in the process of providing that care. Asking questions such as, "Did any problems arise while care was being given?" or "How did Mr. Drummer respond to the range of motion you performed?" or "Did Mrs. Winston seem comfortable when you finished?" or "How much apple juice did Julie drink?" will help elicit responses.

If, in your evaluation, you believe there is some aspect of care that has been done well, comment on it. We all like to know our efforts are appreciated and to receive recognition for a job well done. If corrections need to be made in the care, be certain that such conversations occur in a private, supportive manner. Box 12.5 summarizes suggestions for delegating successfully.

BOX 12.5 SUGGESTIONS FOR EFFECTIVE DELEGATION

- Know what your team members are able to do, including their scope of practice and educational preparation.
- Plan ahead to avoid problems, decide what tasks to delegate.
- Match the task to be accomplished with the abilities of the individual to whom you are assigning the task.
- Communicate clearly the task you are delegating and your expected outcomes.
- Provide the necessary authority and responsibility to accomplish the task to the individual to whom you are delegating.
- Monitor and assess the performance of the task.
- Provide positive feedback as is appropriate; take corrective action when necessary.

Blocks to Effective Delegation

Situations exist in today's healthcare environment that result in blocks or barriers to effective delegation. If these blocks can be eliminated or reduced, delegation will be more satisfying to all who are involved.

Lack of Job Descriptions

The first serious block to good delegation is the lack of current and complete job descriptions for all employees within the institution. As mentioned earlier, the RN must know the abilities and competency of members of the nursing team. These are most commonly found in the job descriptions of the institution. As new positions are created, management should distribute up-to-date job descriptions. This will help ensure that the individual responsible for delegating tasks has access to the information and can use it for decision making. Similar to this problem is that of jobs being changed and tasks redistributed but job descriptions reflecting these changes may not be completed. Thus, those needing the information find themselves having to make decisions without being fully informed.

Time Required to Delegate and Supervise

A second concern rests with the time required to effectively delegate and supervise. Many nurses believe they do not have enough time to spend with their clients. Time that is taken to plan, implement, supervise, teach, coach, and evaluate activities delegated to others may be viewed as taking even more time away from that spent at the bedside. This is especially true when working with inexperienced UAPs, who may require a lot of teaching and support. The high rate of turnover in UAP positions heightens the frustration. There are no simple answers to this problem. To some extent, these are system problems that need to be addressed at a level higher than the individual nursing unit. The best action you can take in such situations may be to let your supervisor know that the problem exists. Perhaps longer periods of orientation can be planned for the assistants or better screening in the hiring process.

Inadequate Training

A final block to effective delegation rests with inadequate training both for those who will be involved in client care and for those who are moving into management positions. Formal orientations to the facility and to on-the-job-type skills for the position the employee will fill help ease new employees into their roles. This is also true for those who will be responsible for supervising the new employees or who are new to the management role. It is one thing to know how to provide quality care to a small group of clients and quite another to oversee the activities of a team that is caring for a large group of clients. As with other situations in nursing, you will develop greater skill with experience.

LEADING CHANGE

When referring to change, we generally think about something that is altered or made to be different, something transformed or modified. As an individual who will have the responsibility for managing others, you need to know how to deal with change yourself and how to help others deal with the change process.

Origins of Change

Typically, change occurs because of **driving forces** that push individuals and organizations to change and may be internal or external. Internal forces may come from within the individual organization or the individual. External forces originate outside the entity experiencing the change.

Internal changes within healthcare organizations can result from new ideas about the system of nursing care delivery, changes in the way pharmacies dispense medications, the opening of new units, or the implementation of a new computerized system for charting. All of these might be initiated to improve the quality of client care and/or client satisfaction. A shared governance structure could be initiated to improve the work environment, thus creating greater employee satisfaction. Change might also be required to reduce costs due to economic constraints.

Internal forces within the individual that create the need for change may include the desire to advance oneself, to retire, to marry, to find a more challenging job, and so forth. Other internal factors, such as a desire for more efficiency, greater competence, and additional education that would give individuals greater knowledge, also create change.

Some external factors that create the need for change in the healthcare field include technology, healthcare legislation, medical and nursing research, new standards, and changing population demographics. How many specific examples of each of these can you cite? What would you add to the list? Regardless of the reason for the change, you can anticipate that things will not remain the same. And whether the change is internal or external, whether it is within the individual or the organization, you will want to be able to work with the change and, if in the position of providing leadership, be able to assist others in the process.

Planned and Unplanned Change

Change has been defined as "to make or become different" (Cambridge Dictionary, 2017). Thus, planned change has a definite design and structure established to facilitate the process, including time lines, identification of stakeholders, goals, plans for implementation, and processes for evaluation. Thoughtful planning often results in more effective and efficient change processes and is essential for projects that are complex or large in scope and that require greater time, resources, or skills.

Change also may be unplanned and occur as a reaction to another issue. This is referred to as **reactive change**. Reactive change occurs when some problem or event arises that requires a different way of doing things. There are many theorists who have developed theories about change. See Table 12.2 for a list and description of various theories of change.

Lewin's Theory of Change

Kurt Lewin's (1951) force field theory of change is one of the most widely accepted theories and remains in current use today, particularly with planned change. This theorist was discussed in Chapter 5, and more information on his theory is provided in Box 12.6.

Selecting the Change Agent

Once the decision has been made to implement a change, some person or group must be responsible for leading that change. A **change agent** may initiate change, assist others in understanding

Table 12.2 Additional Theories of Change

Theory and Author(s)	Important Terms	Summary
Phases of Change Theory Lippitt, Watson, and Westly (1958)	• Recognizing and diagnosing the problem • Determining the ability to change • Selecting the change • Planning, implementing, and evaluating the change • Stabilizing afterward	This presents a logical method of approaching change and may sound very much like the problem-solving methods with which you already are familiar.
Diffusion of Innovations Theory Rogers and Shoemaker (1971)	• Relative advantage compatibility • Complexity • Divisibility • Communicability	Compatibility refers to the change possessing values that are similar or compatible with the existing values held by the individual or group. Complexity suggests that simple techniques are more readily adopted than more complex ones. Divisibility states that changes attempted on a trial basis will have a greater chance of succeeding. Communicability implies that the easier the change is to describe, the more likely it will grow. The proper balance of all factors would result in achieving the desired change.
Theory of Change Asprec (1975)	• Active resistance through frustration and aggression • Organized passive resistance or resisting change as a group • Indifference by ignoring or attempting to divert attention elsewhere • Acceptance on the surface or by not openly opposing change	This writer emphasized the importance of decreasing the resistance in order to reach the goal set forth in the change process.
The 10 Stages of Change Perlman and Takacs (1990)	• Equilibrium—there is a sense of peace or balance before the change occurs • Denial—the reality of a change is denied, thus draining energy from the process • Bargaining—effort and energy go into attempting to eliminate the change • Chaos—energy is diffused with an accompanying loss of identity and direction • Depression—no energy remains to produce results • Resignation—energy is used to passively accept the change • Openness—renewed energy becomes available • Readiness—energy is used to explore new events • Reemergence—energy is rechanneled, resulting in feelings of empowerment	This theory focuses on the strong feelings most people have about the change process. As you work with change, explore some of the ideas described by these authors more fully.

BOX 12.6 KURT LEWIN'S FORCE FIELD THEORY OF CHANGE

Lewin's (1951) force field theory of change is one of the most widely accepted theories and remains in current use today, particularly with planned change. In order for change to occur, an imbalance must exist between the forces that call for change—the driving forces, which push the system toward change and the **restraining forces** that pull the system away from change. These may include economic factors that make the change too expensive. It might be the lack of staff who have the knowledge and skills to make the change. In some instances, it may be that the change dramatically affects one group more than others and the group strongly resists the change. Systems may maintain equilibrium through the interaction of the two forces. Equilibrium is reached when the sum of the driving forces equals the sum of the restraining forces.

For change to occur, the balance between the driving forces and restraining forces must be altered so that the driving forces outweigh the restraining forces. Lewin's change theory identified that change has three stages: unfreezing, movement, and refreezing.

Unfreezing Stage	Movement Stage	Refreezing Stage
According to Lewin, the **unfreezing stage** occurs when an individual is motivated by the need to create a change. This person becomes a change agent, the person who seeks to create the change and is responsible for facilitating the change process with others. Having gathered data, identified the problem, and decided that change is needed, the change agent sets about making others aware of the need for change. The change agent attempts to "unfreeze" or lessen the resistance to change or selects someone else who can help to unfreeze the current position by notifying those who will be affected of the need for change and garnering their support and cooperation.	The second phase of Lewin's theory is called the **movement stage**. During the movement stage, a knowledgeable and respected person responsible for initiating the change identifies strategies that will facilitate the change and then plans and implements them. The process of facilitating change is described below.	In the final phase, the **refreezing stage**, the changes are integrated and stabilized and become part of the value system of the organization. The change agent helps to stabilize the change that has been made in the organization so that it becomes part of everyday operation. This step is necessary to prevent the system from reverting to old patterns of behavior. Refreezing occurs when the new behaviors have occurred frequently enough that people are comfortable with them and feel rewarded because of them. Most changes need between 3 and 6 months before being totally accepted. During this time, the change agent supports those affected by the change and helps them adapt to it.

why the change is needed and what it involves, recruit support, manage the change process, and/or assist in resolving conflict (Cambridge Dictionary, 2017). This may be an individual within the organization who is particularly knowledgeable about theories of change and skilled in assisting people in the process of change, or it may be someone hired from outside the organization who has the skills needed to bring about the process. On occasion, teams are established to bring about a change. To be effective, the change agent must be able to affect the attitudes of others through interpersonal influence, power, or control. In organizations that have adopted continuous quality improvement, the change agent is often referred to as the **champion**. Within that system, anyone could have an idea for improvement of the organization.

Facilitating Change

As with many other management and leadership skills, facilitating change can be learned. One of the first aspects that must be recognized and dealt with relates to overcoming the resistance to the change.

Understanding Resistance to Change

Because making a change will require that we alter the way we have been doing things, most people are initially resistant to change. We become comfortable with the way that things have been done and may be apprehensive of new approaches that require us to change established patterns of behavior. The new approaches may take additional time to learn or may be threatening to us if they involve skills with which we are not entirely familiar. Resistance to change may be the basis of sayings such as, if it's not broken, don't fix it. In some instances, resistance to change occurs because of fear for job security. Overcoming resistance to change is a major role of the change agent **(Fig. 12.4)**.

Most authorities on change agree that change is most easily implemented when it is the result of a collaborative process (the **normative–reeducative approach**, see Table 12.2). This means involving everyone who is going to be affected by the change or those referred to as **stakeholders**. All persons involved need a good understanding of the change, why it is necessary, what the benefits will be, and how it is to be accomplished. Suggestions from those affected by the change need to be built into the change model whenever possible. Mutual trust and respect must exist among all persons working with the change.

The Importance of Communication

One of the most valuable tools for facilitating change and overcoming resistance to it is communication. Communication should remain open throughout the entire process. When

Figure 12.4. Resistance to change.

BOX 12.7 COMMUNICATION SKILLS FOR FACILITATING CHANGE

- Communicate openly, frequently, and honestly
- Provide as much information as possible
- Allow for questions and suggestions
- Accept feedback constructively
- Address rumors quickly
- Supply facts when perceptions are incorrect
- Listen actively to people's concerns, feelings, and objections
- Remain matter-of-fact and avoid being argumentative or defensive

---

questions regarding the whys and hows of the change arise, answer them in an honest and straightforward manner. Often during the change process, rumors will begin to circulate. Address these rumors as quickly as possible and supply facts where perceptions are incorrect. Listen to and address the concerns of those affected by the change to the best of your ability. People need the opportunity to express their fears and possible losses they believe will occur when the situation is changed. They need time to grieve those losses. Their feelings need to be accepted, not disputed. Provide opportunity for input and suggestions and implement these when possible. Box 12.7 identifies some of the communication skills to be used in facilitating change.

Communication in Action 12.4: Resistance to Developing New Processes

A hospital nursing staff meeting is called. Janet Chasey, a unit manager on the medical floor, announces, "Hi folks! Thanks for taking the time to come to this staff meeting. I'll be very brief because I know you all have things to do and places to go. The only agenda item is to inform you that a committee is being formed by nursing administration to develop and implement a standardized approach to communication between caregivers when clients are moved from one department to another within the hospital." One nurse responds, "It really isn't fair to ask us to take on a committee when we are already overworked." Another says, "It just sounds like more paperwork to me! We don't need that!" A third speaks up, "I think the forms and taped messages we currently use are more than adequate. Why change what isn't broken?" Janet explains, "There is a new standard set by The Joint Commission. It requires that we have a standardized process to ensure that all information about the client's condition is shared, including allergies, potential problems, medications, and stability of vital signs." She further explains, "The whole purpose of this is to make client handoff safer, and I know that is your concern too. Maybe one or two of you might like to be involved in developing the process and help shape the direction it takes." Elsa, who had graduated from her nursing program the previous year, notes, "I have never been involved in setting up a policy or procedure. It would probably be a good thing to learn. You can put me down for that committee."

By respecting the concerns of the nursing staff, explaining carefully, and pointing out shared goals, Janet is able to achieve her objective of having a unit member participate.

Assessing the Setting

Before beginning the change process, it is important to have a good understanding of the existing power structure within the setting where the change is to occur. Who within that area gets things done and makes things happen? Where is support typically found? Where—or with whom—can obstacles be anticipated? Are there values one must be sensitive to? Are there factors present that could prevent the change from taking place?

Thinking and Planning

Successful change is well thought out and planned. A process similar to that of the nursing process provides good guidance. First of all, once a problem that might benefit from change has been identified, data need to be gathered that will assist with the diagnosis of the problem. Is it a problem? If so, why is it a problem? Who does it affect? How are they affected? Might there be a better way to approach the situation? What would the costs be in terms of time? What would be the personal cost to those affected? What would be the effects of not addressing the problem? Should we move forward with the change or look for other solutions? Early in this process, those who are going to be affected by the change need to be included. They need to be informed of intentions to make changes and be brought into the collaborative process for planning.

Once a reasonable amount of data have been gathered, begin to plan. Who needs to be involved? Who should be the key players? How might the change best be implemented? When would be the best timing? What resources will be needed? What needs to be done to help those affected to unfreeze? What needs to be built into the plan that will help to ensure that the changes remain in place? What additional training and education will be necessary? Box 12.8 highlights these questions.

BOX 12.8 QUESTIONS TO CONSIDER WHEN PLANNING FOR SUCCESSFUL CHANGE

Questions About the Situation

- Is the present situation a problem?
- Why is it a problem?
- Who is affected by the problem?
- How are they affected?
- Is there a better way to approach the situation?
- What would be the costs in terms of time?
- What would be the personal cost to those affected?
- What would be the effects of not addressing the problem?
- Should a change be initiated or should other solutions be sought?

Questions Related to Planning

- Who needs to be involved?
- Who should be the key players?
- How might the change best be implemented?
- What would be the best timing?
- What resources will be needed?
- What needs to be done to help those affected "unfreeze"?
- What additional training and education will be necessary?
- What needs to be built into the plan that will help to ensure that changes remain in place?

Implementing the Change

Once plans are well formulated and people who will be affected have full information as well as a role in the process, the change needs to be implemented. Establishing a timetable is often useful.

Generally, it is wise to implement change as quickly as possible. The slower the change process, the greater the opportunity for individuals affected by it to ruminate on how things were, to build up anger, and to develop fears and resentment. Once dates have been announced, it is unwise to change them or to postpone actions, because people will become suspicious and/or critical of the process. If delays are necessary, share the full explanation of the reason(s) for the delay. This is a continuation of the open communication process. Recognize and praise positive efforts toward making a change. Celebrating milestones of accomplishment throughout the entire process can generate team spirit. It helps create feelings of well-being about the change and builds a bond among those who are involved in it.

Evaluating the Change Process

Monitor the change process throughout its implementation and evaluate it after it is completed to determine whether the change is accomplishing the desired outcome. Evaluation provides information about how people are adjusting to the change and how satisfied they are with it—data that are crucial to sustaining the change. When implementing and evaluating change, remember that change does not occur instantly but rather over a period of time. Additionally, the pace of change is not regular. It tends to have periods when it slows down and other periods of rapid progress. The slower periods can be viewed as reflective time, when the individuals involved in the change have the opportunity to assimilate new facts, approaches, values, and other items involved in the change.

Standardizing and Refining the Change

For a change to be sustained, it must be standardized and refined. The change agent, if outside the usual staff, needs to transfer responsibility for the continuance of the project to the participants in the change. If the change requires modifications in policies or protocols, those need to be written and incorporated in organizational manuals. People who have made notable contributions need to be recognized for their efforts.

It is through careful planning, implementation, and follow-up that successful change occurs. Flexibility in addressing and adjusting problems that arise is important. Interpersonal relationships need to be given high priority during this time.

Responding to Change

As a new graduate, you most likely will be one of the individuals affected by change rather than the one trying to implement change. How will you react if a change must occur on the unit to which you are assigned? Will you drag your feet and be one of the last to accept the change, or will you be one of the first to join the change team? How can you be an effective participant?

Learn About the Change

Take all available opportunities to learn about any anticipated changes. Attend scheduled meetings and read all announcements that are circulated. If there are matters that seem unclear to you, ask questions at the appropriate time. Learn what the benefits will be for you and for others. Discuss your thoughts and findings with others and share any suggestions you have. Validate any information about which you may not be certain. Rumors often run rampant during the process of change. Be sure you are dealing with facts rather than rumors.

Express Your Concerns

As you learn about the anticipated changes, you may develop concerns about various aspects. If you have concerns, express them. If you are anxious, there are probably others who share your feelings. Remember that most often those who are closest to a situation are the individuals who understand it best. When setting forth your concerns, take a minute to organize your thoughts. Be clear, concise, and unemotional. Speak clearly in a well-modulated voice.

Actively Listen

We often are encouraged to actively listen when working with others. Active listening involves focusing entirely on what the other person is saying and refraining from other mental activities. This works well in many situations, including conflict, which we will discuss later in this chapter. The following behaviors are usually included in active listening:

- Always be respectful and courteous.
- Use constructive language, both in verbal and nonverbal (eg, body language) communication.
- Remain calm and unemotional.
- Maintain eye contact.
- Do not interrupt.
- Be serious but cheerful.
- Use nondirective techniques to encourage the person to share concerns.
- Ask for clarification as needed to facilitate your understanding.

Listen very carefully to the responses that are given to your concerns. If you are not clear about what has just been said, ask the other individual to please repeat it. Too often, people are so busy thinking about what they will say next that they do not hear the explanations that are being provided.

You will find that if you actively participate in the change, it will be much easier to move into the new behaviors it may require. Change can be energizing for some individuals. It often opens the door for new opportunities. It can provide empowerment and enjoyment if managed correctly.

Critical Thinking Activity: The Process of Change

You have just learned that a new form of charting is being initiated on your unit. As a new employee, you have just become comfortable with the current system, which was quite different from anything you used as a student. You are dismayed that you will now need to learn a new system. What steps can you take to participate effectively in this change? How can you develop a more positive attitude toward this change? What will facilitate the process for you? What role do you see for yourself in the change process? If you become really frustrated during the change process, to whom will you speak?

MANAGING CONFLICT

Conflict is not a new topic to you. You have dealt with it from the time you were a child. Like change, it is a part of everyday living. The very nature of conflict is what keeps attorneys, marriage counselors, mediators, and arbitrators in business. Our ability to work positively with conflict may determine our success in today's world, both in the work situation and outside of it.

Conflict and Nursing

Conflict, broadly defined, results when people with differing values, interests, goals, needs, or approaches come together to address a common concern. Because people view things from different perspectives and bring different values to the situation, incompatible ideas, or approaches. The settling of a conflict is known as **conflict resolution**. The process through which the conflict is recognized and resolved is called **conflict management**. The critical element is not that conflicts come about—but how we deal with them. What are some of the conflicts you may encounter in nursing?

Earlier in this chapter, we discussed the conflict that can occur between physicians and nurses. As nurses command a more independent role in client care, become involved in evidence-based practice, and accept responsibility and accountability for their actions, they may feel devalued if their suggestions for care are not acted upon, thus leading to anger and a breakdown of communications.

In Chapter 5, we discussed collective bargaining, a major area in which there can be discord. This can occur nurse to nurse and nurse to administration. Unfortunately, conflicts at the bargaining table may spill over into conflicts in the workplace.

As nurses exercise professional judgment, differences of opinion may arise regarding the best approach to treatment for a client. There may be disagreements about staffing patterns, particularly during the holidays. Overlapping roles can result in conflict, and not having sufficient resources, either monetary or physical, can cause discord. Often, the utilization of space in the healthcare environment leads to conflict.

These represent just a few of the many situations in nursing in which disagreements can happen. Conflict leads to stress and the disruption of professional relationships. As you will see in Chapter 13, the consequence of all this conflict, between coworkers or among client family members, can be burnout (Evidence-Based Practice 12.2).

Evidence-Based Practice 12.2: Conflict Mediation

Fung Kei, C. (2015). Mediation skills for conflict resolution in nursing education. *Nurse Education in Practice, 15*(4), 310–313. doi:10.1016/j.nepr.2015.02.005

In nursing education, students are taught therapeutic communication skills used to counsel clients, but there is little or no education about conflict mediation. Increasingly, in our culturally diverse world, nurses encounter clients and families that do not agree on the best course of action during a crisis. Because the situation is already stressful, disagreements can escalate quickly. The stress created by constant conflict can lead to burnout.

This study proposes that mediation, as a tool for conflict resolution, can assist nurses to reduce stress in the workplace and in their personal lives as well. The ability to effectively assist others to come to an agreement is a skill that could benefit all those employed in helping professions. It is suggested that mediation training be part of nursing education curricula.

The Positive Side of Conflict

Conflict can have positive aspects; not all conflict is serious, ominous, or intimidating. Conflict can result in personal growth and development. We learn by contrasting our values and beliefs with those of others. As we learn about others, we learn about ourselves.

Conflict can provide the impetus for change and it can contribute to innovation and creativity. When conflict is a major part of any operation, reasons for its presence must be identified and alternatives set forth. Conflict also helps employees of an organization to have a better understanding of one another's jobs and responsibilities. As healthcare becomes more specialized, differences become greater and give rise to conflict. Conflict may result in people from different areas sitting down and talking to resolve the problem. As talk continues, a greater appreciation for others can develop, thus creating unification within the organization.

Conflict can also open new channels of communication. As efforts are made to eliminate sources of conflict, new approaches and avenues may evolve. Similarly, conflict can be a positive source of energy and creativity. It may serve to invigorate people. A good disagreement has the potential to sharpen people's awareness, to get them thinking, and to put new spark into their work.

Types of Conflict

Conflict can be looked at from a number of perspectives and broken into several categories. Your approach to dealing with the conflict may vary depending on the type of conflict that exists.

Intrapersonal, Interpersonal, and Intergroup Conflict

Intrapersonal conflict occurs within one's self in circumstances in which a choice must be made between two alternatives. Choosing one alternative means that you cannot have the other. An example would be a situation in which the nurse must decide whether to participate in a committee on nursing practice that will take time away from direct client care or decline the opportunity in order to spend more time with clients. Either choice carries benefits and drawbacks. The conflict occurs within the nurse who must decide which is more important personally.

Interpersonal conflict occurs between or among individuals with differing values, ideas, perceptions, and goals. If nurses disagree on which is the most important aspect of care for a client, interpersonal conflict results. Ethical issues such as abortion, gene therapy, stem cell research, do-not-resuscitate orders, and decisions to withdraw or withhold treatment can result in conflict among those responsible for delivery of care. Different leadership styles and organizational climates can also result in interpersonal conflict.

Critical Thinking Activity: Interpersonal Conflict

Think of an interpersonal conflict that you recently observed or in which you were involved. What was the basis of the disagreement? How did the individuals conduct themselves during the heat of the conflict? How were the issues resolved? How might the conflict have been avoided?

Intergroup conflict is seen when two or more groups of people or departments struggle for power, authority, territory, or resources. Each group operates within its own value system, attributing negative stereotypes to the other group. This can be especially true if the group includes racial minorities who feel discriminated against. Intergroup conflicts also occur between those who work on different shifts of a nursing unit—the evening shift personnel critical of the day shift and the day shift people believing that their job is harder than that of the evening shift. Intergroup conflicts might also occur between the nursing staff and another department in the hospital, such as housekeeping, over priorities related to work responsibilities. Intergroup conflicts can increase in both number and perception when those in one group spend time recounting to others within their group all the perceived inadequacies of the other group. As they do this, they may gather additional anecdotes to support their own perceptions. Thus, the conflict is maintained and spread.

Organizational Conflict

Some conflicts originate within the structure and function of an organization. Typically, when conflict is generated, it relates to policies, procedures, channels of communication, and style of management. These are termed **organizational conflicts**. In organizational conflict, the leader's role and behavior are particularly important to both the origin and resolution of the conflict.

Role ambiguity and role conflict are major causes of organizational conflict. **Role ambiguity** refers to a situation in which the role is not clearly defined. **Role conflict** occurs when two or more individuals have role descriptions that overlap. This frequently occurs because of the lack of good job descriptions and clear communications regarding what is expected. An example of role conflict might be seen in the provision of discharge planning. Both the RN and the social worker clearly may view this as an important aspect of their professional responsibilities, and the job descriptions of both may include this aspect of client care.

The structure of the organization may also lead to conflict. The term *turf* refers to the territory that one or one's group controls. Turf battles are not uncommon in organizations, with various individuals within the system attempting to protect, expand, or advance the area for which they are responsible. Again, good job descriptions, organizational charts, chains of command, channels of communication, and the like will minimize the advent of this type of problem (see Chapter 5).

Conflict within an organization also can arise when a scarcity of resources exists. Scarcity of resources refers not only to money but also to supplies, equipment, space, personnel, and similar necessities. When the budget for the organization is developed, not all requests are likely to be funded. Competition occurs as various departments vie for the resources that are available. When nursing shortages occur, conflicts related to securing and retaining adequate nurse staffing can be anticipated.

Conflict Outcomes

Filley (1975) was the first to write about the three positions or outcomes of conflict that have become so well known that they are often included in our everyday language: lose–lose, win–lose, and win–win.

One type of outcome addressed by Filley (1975) is the lose–lose outcome, in which there are no winners because the resolution of the conflict is unsatisfactory to both parties.

An example can be seen in collective bargaining relationships that stalemate and go to arbitration where a decision is made that neither side finds totally acceptable.

A second type of outcome is referred to as win–lose outcomes, in which one person obtains desired goals in the situation and the other individual fails to receive what is desired. The most obvious example of this would be elections for public office, in which decisions are made by majority rule with only one winner possible. An example in a hospital environment might be one unit receiving all the money available for new equipment, while the other areas receive none. Although this may have been the most prudent approach if the budget for new equipment was very small, it remains an example of a win–lose situation with one department actually getting what it needed (winning) and others receiving none (losing).

The most desirable type of outcome is the win–win outcome. In such situations, both parties walk away from the conflict feeling they have achieved most of the things that were important to them. For example, if we are working on a project and everyone feels good about it when it is done and each individual reaps some rewards, it is a win–win situation for all. If both units received an equal amount for equipment from a constrained budget, both might feel they had won in the situation that existed. In collective bargaining, a collaborative approach may result in both employer and employee feeling that they achieved desired goals—a *win–win* outcome.

Strategies for Coping With Conflict

The approach that you use to deal with conflict will depend on a number of factors. The nature of the conflict, the individuals who are involved, your ability to influence the outcome, and the possibility of retribution are all elements that will affect the situation. On occasion, conflicts occur that are not worth the effort of resolving. Thus, a wide variety of approaches to the management of conflict exist. They tend to fall into one of five categories: withdrawing from or avoiding conflict; smoothing or accommodating; forcing the issue or competing; negotiating and compromising; and problem solving and collaborating.

Withdrawing From or Avoiding Conflict

You employ the strategy of avoiding or withdrawing from the conflict when you choose not to address the issue at hand. Some would also refer to this as denying the existence of the conflict, sometimes with the hope that if it is ignored it will go away. There are many times when this approach is appropriate. This may be appropriate when the conflict clearly is not your problem, when there is little or nothing that you can do about it, when there is more to lose than to be gained by becoming involved, when you lack sufficient information about the conflict and its cause, or when the problem will straighten itself out if given time. It is also a good approach to use if the situation is volatile and individuals need some time to regain composure. For example, one of two staff nurses who are becoming distressed about an issue might say, "You may be right, let's find a time to talk about it later." The issue may never be discussed later, or the parties involved in the disagreement may gain new understandings that change their perspectives.

Although appropriate at times, avoiding conflict is often preferred by people who are very uncomfortable with conflict situations, and it may not be the best approach. In a competitive society, individuals who will back away from a conflict can be taken advantage of. It is important to learn to advocate for yourself as well as for your clients. An example might be a situation in which both you and another nurse want to be off duty on Halloween evening so that you can participate in your children's trick-or-treat activities. Although the other nurse enjoyed that evening off last year, you again concede to her request because you do not want to deal with her comments and criticisms if you are awarded the evening off.

Smoothing or Accommodating

Smoothing or accommodating conflict involves trying to relieve feelings associated with conflict without solving the underlying problem. It may involve apologizing for something that is not one's fault, stating agreement with a position with which one does not truly agree, or taking action that one does not really support to stop the feelings of conflict from occurring. Similar to avoidance of the issue, smoothing or accommodating also may be referred to as surrendering to the conflict. In such situations, it is easier not to address the issue and to deal with feelings of anger than it is to deal with the conflict.

This approach may be used by individuals with a strong need to be liked, or those who are overly concerned with the welfare of others. They tend to take a self-sacrificing approach that will result in a peaceful environment. An individual who wishes to preserve harmony or build up social credits may employ this technique.

Smoothing or accommodating may be appropriate and the best approach if the conflict and anger that accompanies it disrupts the work situation or interferes with the immediate needs of the clients. In such situations, harmony and constancy are important. If the outcome does not matter to you, or if you obviously are wrong, this is a good approach. If you have little chance to win, or if this represents a situation in which you can lose the battle but win the war, it is appropriate. Consistently using this approach may make one feel *put upon* and as if you don't count in the organization.

Forcing the Issue or Competing

Competing or forcing the issue in a conflict situation means you are working exclusively for your own solution to the problem. You may have taken this approach because you believe you know more about the issues involved than others or when your values will allow no other compromise. Typically, individuals who use this approach are accustomed to being the winner and often fail to consider the needs and opinions of others. This strategy can prevent good problem solving and innovative approaches. This would be considered a win–lose outcome—one person wins, others lose. It is an aggressive approach that could result in retaliation at another time. However, it might be the best approach if you observe a violation of ethical or legal standards.

Negotiating and Compromising

Compromising and negotiating involve give-and-take; one factor is balanced against another. It is the approach to the conflict seen in collective bargaining—one factor in the situation is balanced against another. It serves to minimize the losses for all parties while allowing each to realize some gains. It may be the approach of choice if the opposing goals are so incompatible that no resolution can be reached and discussion has stalled. It would also be appropriate if an immediate settlement to the issue were needed because of time constraints or other factors.

Problem Solving and Collaborating

Although problem solving or collaborating to achieve a mutually agreed-upon plan of action may be the most difficult to achieve, many believe this to be the best approach to conflict. It encourages participants in the conflict to work toward common goals and to work toward consensus. The process can be time-consuming and requires that all persons involved come to the table willing to examine and discuss issues openly and honestly. When effective in resolving the conflict, it is viewed as a win–win situation for everyone.

Personal Preparation for Conflict

If you find yourself in a conflict situation, try to be as prepared as possible to deal with the conditions at hand. This is often hard to do at the time the conflict occurs. One of the best techniques is to practice for the situation. Rehearse what you will say. Think about the tone of your voice, the speed with which to talk, and your body language. Think positively about yourself. Be confident. Visualize what a successful interaction would be like.

When engaged in the confrontation, do not interrupt others. Give them an opportunity to express their position. When they talk, practice the good listening skills discussed earlier in this chapter. Insist that you are given the same courtesy of uninterrupted explanation. Politely saying, "Please let me finish" usually ensures that you can continue presenting your position. Be clear and concise in presenting your point of view. Long, complicated presentations lose everyone's interest. Be assertive but considerate of others.

If you find that you are involved in conflict situations more frequently than most other individuals, a personal inventory is appropriate. Questions you should ask yourself might include the following:

- Do I have good relationships with most of my coworkers?
- How do I manage stress in other situations?
- Do I have the proper balance between work and relaxation?
- Do I feel competent in this situation?
- Do I hold personal biases that are interfering with my interactions with others?
- What else is going on in my life?

If after completing this inventory you find there are areas that give you concern, they can be addressed in an appropriate manner. If you are experiencing high levels of stress in any area of life, you may find yourself more easily in conflict with others and less able to manage conflict effectively. If there is a lack of opportunity for relaxation in your life, you can adjust your schedule so that you maximize the time you spend on things that result in leisure and rest. If you feel less than competent regarding the expectations of your job, some continuing education, reading, or research may be helpful. Seeking and working with a mentor may also bring positive results. If relationships with other coworkers or in your private life are lacking, seeking the help of a qualified counselor may be the best approach.

Stegen & Sowerby Stories: Part 2

Remember Rose, the burn client whose wound care had been delegated to the HCA? On removing the dressing completely, the NP discovered that the wound had deteriorated considerably and was probably infected. She took a culture of the wound for analysis, and the client was prescribed broad-spectrum antibiotics. The NP redressed the wound and told the client that she would have to come for daily dressing changes until an improvement was noted. Read the rest of the story at www.thePoint.com.

Want to Know More?

A variety of resources are available on thePoint® **to enhance your learning and understanding of this chapter, such as:**

- Full Stegen & Sowerby Stories
- NCLEX-Style Student Review Questions
- Journal Articles
- Case Studies
- Learning Objectives
- Relevant Websites
- And more...

KEY CONCEPTS

- A team is a group of people working together for a common goal. Because of the diverse disciplines that are now involved in healthcare, the effective functioning of the healthcare team is critical to the provision of quality healthcare. Trust and respect of others are key aspects of team function.
- Nurses have key roles on the team and have a number of roles other than that of provider of care. They may serve as an educator, a client advocate, a counselor/coach, or a manager, and a leader for the nursing team. They also might work in nursing informatics or in nursing research.
- Because they fill key positions on the healthcare team, the relationship between nurses and physicians must be symbolized by mutual respect and consideration. Nurses can take positive actions to help assure that this occurs.
- Many leaders in healthcare are using team-building techniques to strengthen the functioning of their teams. Team building involves setting common goals, recognizing the contribution each person makes to the team, involving others in decision making, focusing on problems rather than on individuals associated with the problem, and sharing in accomplishments.
- Being a good team member is as important as being a team leader. Most new graduates begin in the role of team member. You need to be able to assess your abilities as a team member.
- The coaching role is being seen more frequently in healthcare. Rather than telling a younger nurse what to do, an individual serving as a coach helps him or her search for answers, providing necessary support, encouragement, and information.
- Motivation encompasses the sum of all the factors that cause an individual to do something. To motivate individuals, the leader must understand personal behaviors and role model those that are desired in others.
- In nursing, delegation is the process by which a nurse directs another person to perform nursing tasks and activities. Nurses remain accountable for all nursing care that is provided. It is important to follow the guidelines for effective delegation and know which aspects of care can never be delegated.
- The five rights of successful delegation include the right task, the right circumstances, the right person, the right direction and communication, and the right supervision and evaluation.

- Nurses cannot delegate aspects of care that require nursing judgment, including such activities as client assessment.
- Change is inevitable in today's healthcare environment. Individuals tend to resist change, and leaders must become familiar with the steps that will facilitate the change process.
- A number of theories of change have been developed. Many of them describe processes to facilitate change, including helping others see the need for change, involving those who will be affected by the change in the process, and stabilizing the change once it is in place.
- Three major strategies for change include the empirical–rational strategy, the power–coercive strategy, and the normative–reeducative strategy. Each one might be the appropriate strategy to use in a particular situation.
- Changes often are led by a change agent who may come from within the organization or might be hired from outside to assist with the change. Sometimes groups or teams can serve as change agents.
- A number of activities facilitate change. Good communication is primary. In addition, the environment where change is to occur should be assessed, thinking and planning need to occur, the change must be implemented, and the process evaluated. Finally, the change should be standardized and refined in order for it to persist.
- As you experience change as a new employee, you can make the process more positive by learning all that you can about the anticipated changes, understanding the benefits, asking appropriate questions of the right individuals, and respectfully expressing any concerns you may have to the right people.
- Conflict occurs in all aspects of our lives; it can be intrapersonal, interpersonal, intergroup, or organizational.
- Filley (1975) has identified three possible outcomes of conflict: the lose–lose outcome, in which both parties leave the situation feeling defeated; the win–lose outcome, in which one party wins and the other loses; and the win–win outcome, in which both parties have positive feelings about the end results.
- Strategies for dealing with conflict include withdrawing or avoiding the conflict; smoothing, suppressing, or accommodating to the conflict; forcing, fighting, or competing; negotiating or compromising; and problem solving or collaborating. There is a proper time and circumstance for the use of each strategy.
- Conflict can have positive aspects. It can provide an impetus for change, it can energize individuals, it can help persons in different roles better understand one another, and it can facilitate communication.
- If you find yourself in conflict more than is desirable, a self-inventory can be helpful. Asking yourself a variety of questions may help identify the actions you will want to take.

NCLEX-STYLE PRACTICE QUESTIONS

1. One of the aides on your unit is struggling to get her work done. As her supervisor, you need to coach her on her performance. Which statement reflects effective coaching?

    A. You never chart vital signs on time.
    B. Your prompt response to call lights is exemplary.
    C. You always forget morning blood glucose checks.
    D. It may be helpful to restock gloves when you are filling water containers.

2. You and an aide are giving a bed bath to an incontinent client. Which action requires you to intervene?

    A. The aide log rolls the client toward herself.
    B. The aide places an incontinence pad under the client.
    C. The aide answers the phone while wearing gloves.
    D. The aide leaves the client laying on his or her left side with the head elevated.

3. Which client would you, the RN, delegate to an LPN/LVN under your supervision?

    A. A 25-year-old client admitted yesterday after sustaining a concussion in a motorcycle accident
    B. A 76-year-old client with chronic obstructive pulmonary disease and emphysema admitted 24 hours ago
    C. A 40-year-old client with a new diagnosis of diabetes who will be discharged today
    D. A 62-year-old client newly admitted with congestive heart failure exacerbation

4. You are a pediatric nurse floated to a medical–surgical floor. Which client would be an appropriate assignment for you?

    A. A 59-year-old client newly diagnosed diabetic that needs teaching related to disease management
    B. A 62-year-old man who had a transurethral resection of the prostate (TURP) this morning
    C. A 90-year-old client recovering from pneumonia who has dementia and will be transferred to a long-term care facility today
    D. A 23-year-old client with severe leg weakness and a tentative diagnosis of Guillain–Barré syndrome

REFERENCES

Asprec, E (1975). The process of change. *Supervisor Nurse, 6*, 15–24.
Baggs, J. G., Ryan, S. A., Phelps, C. E., Richeson, J. F., & Johnson, J. E. (1992). The association between interdisciplinary collaboration and client outcomes in a medical intensive care unit. *Heart Lung, 32*(1), 18–24.
Cambridge Dictionary. (2017). Retrieved July 27, 2017, from http://dictionary.cambridge.org
Filley, A. (1975). *Interpersonal conflict resolution*. Glenview, IL: Scott, Foresman.
Fung Kei, C. (2015). Mediation skills for conflict resolution in nursing education. *Nurse Education in Practice, 15*(4), 310–313. doi:10.1016/j.nepr.2015.02.005
Herzberg, F (1966). *Works and the nature of man*. New York: World Publishing Co.
Herzberg, F., Mausner, B., & Snyderman, B. B. (1959). *The motivation to work*. New York: John Wiley.
Larsen, E. (1999). The impact of physician-nurse interaction on client care. *Holistic Nursing Practice, 3*(2), 38–46.
Lewin, K. (1951). *Field theory in social service: Selected theoretical papers*. New York: Harper Brothers.
Lippitt, R., Watson, J., & Westley, B. (1958). *The dynamics of planned change*. New York, NY: Harcourt, Brace, & World.
Maslow, A. (1954). *Motivation and personality*. New York: Harper & Row.
McClelland, D. (1953). *The achievement motive*. Norwalk, CT: Appleton-Century-Crofts.
McClelland, D. (1961). *The achieving society*. Princeton, NJ: Van Nostrand.

National Council of State Boards of Nursing. (1995). *Delegation: Concepts and decision-making process.* Chicago, IL: Author.

National Council of State Boards of Nursing (NCSBN). (2016). *National guidelines for nursing delegation.* Retrieved July 27, 2017, from https://www.ncsbn.org/NCSBN_Delegation_Guidelines.pdf

Nelson, G. A. (2008). Nurse-physician collaboration on medical-surgical units. *Medsurg Nursing, 17*(1), 35–40.

Perlman, D., & Takacs, G. J. (1990). The ten stages of change. *Nursing Management, 212*(4), 33–38.

Rogers, E., & Shoemaker, F. (1971). *Communication of innovations: A cross cultural approach.* New York: Free Press.

Rosenstein, A. H. (2002). Nurse–physician relationships: Impact on nurse satisfaction and retention. *American Journal of Nursing, 102*(6), 26–34.

Schaubroeck, J., Carmeli, A., Bhatia, S., & Paz, E. (2016). Enabling team learning when members are prone to contentious communication: The role of team leader coaching. *Human Relations, 69*(8), 1709–1727. doi:10.1177/0018726715622673

Siedlecki, S. L., & Hixson, E. D. (2015). Relationships between nurses and physicians matter. *Online Journal of Issues in Nursing, 20*(3), 1. doi:10.3912/OJIN.Vol20No03PPT03

CHAPTER 13

Facing the Challenges of Today's Workplace

After completing this chapter, you should be able to:

1. Compare the skills and abilities in each stage of "novice to expert" with the expectations of employers regarding new graduates.
2. Construct personal strategies to prevent or alleviate reality shock.
3. Analyze your own values and life situation and relate those to your personal risk for burnout.
4. Adapt personal stress management techniques to use in controlling your work stress.
5. Identify the relationships between staffing levels, reality shock, burnout, and client safety.
6. Describe the physical hazards in the workplace and identify the strategies to protect yourself from each.
7. Discuss how nursing has been affected by racial, ethnic, and sex discrimination.
8. Describe appropriate techniques to manage sexual harassment in the workplace.
9. Explain how to respond effectively to disruptive behavior in the workplace.
10. Describe approaches to managing physical violence in the healthcare workplace.

KEY TERMS

Burnout	Novice to expert
Coaching	Occupational hazard
Discrimination	Preceptor
Ergonomics	Reality shock
Mentee	Sexual harassment
Mentor	Stereotype

Stegen & Sowerby Stories: Part 1

Sally is a new nurse who just started working on the medical unit at a local hospital. She feels overwhelmed but excited, as she has always wanted to be a nurse. Shortly after completing orientation, she is working a 12-hour night shift when she realizes she forgot to check a blood glucose on one of her clients. Another nurse who has been there for a couple of years says to her, "Wow, you'd think that they would have taught you how to organize your care in nursing school so you wouldn't forget the basics!" Sally feels sad and unsupported by the comment and begins to wonder if maybe nursing was a bad choice for her.

What would you say to Sally? Is making a medication error or forgetting to get a blood glucose a reflection on your nursing skills? How do we as nurses contribute to the feelings of dissatisfaction of those around us? What are ways that we as nurses can support each other to improve the nursing profession?

For many of you, graduating from a nursing program and becoming a registered nurse (RN) are the realization of a long-cherished goal. You have put a great deal of effort into preparing for this status, and now it is almost here! What you have viewed as an ideal state, freed from financial pressures that you have felt as a student and liberated from the tyranny of assignments and examinations, may prove to be quite different from what you expect. Let us consider some of the problems that may emerge as you make this transition from student to professional.

MOVING FROM "NOVICE TO EXPERT"

The path from **novice to expert** is a challenging one. Benner's (1984) classic research in this area provides a basis for an understanding of the process. Based on the work from Dreyfus and Dreyfus (1980), she examined nursing and described five stages through which an individual moves as a professional: from *novice* to *advanced beginner* to *competent* to *proficient* to *expert*. Table 13.1 presents the characteristics of these skill levels.

Table 13.1   Benner's Levels of Function

Level	Characteristics
1. Novice	No experience of the situations. Have context-free rules to guide behavior. Relatively inflexible.
2. Advanced beginner	Marginally acceptable performance. Have some experiences with real situations. Can identify "aspects of the situation" (p. 22). May formulate principles or guidelines for action.
3. Competent	Begins to see current situation in terms of long-range goals. Is able to prioritize among clients and base actions on conscious deliberate planning. May still lack speed and flexibility.
4. Proficient	Perceives situations as wholes rather than as a collection of parts. This perception is not thought out but is unconscious. Experience has given this nurse a "web of perspectives" (p. 28). Responds to nuances of the situation using maxims.
5. Expert	Has an intuitive grasp of the whole situation and does not rely on rules, guidelines, or maxims. Focuses immediately on the most critical elements of the situation. May have difficulty articulating the thought processes that resulted in decisions.

Benner, P. (1984). *From novice to expert: Excellence and power in clinical nursing practice.* Upper Saddle River, NJ: Prentice Hall.

The first role Benner identified is the *helping role*. This role encompasses planning and implementing all the basic nursing skills used to assist clients. The second, the *teaching–coaching role*, pertains to teaching clients and their families to manage their own health status and adaptations in living. The third, the *diagnostic and monitoring role*, relates to assessment and evaluation of the client's health status and various needs. Responding to changing situations is rooted in critical thinking and a comprehensive knowledge base. While all of these roles differ between the novice and the expert category, it is in the fourth role of *responding to changing situations* that outsiders more clearly see the differences between the novice and the expert nurse. The fifth role of *administering and monitoring the therapeutic interventions and regimens* relates to the medical plan of care. The final role is the *leadership and management role* that all nurses must perform but differs for the nurse in each stage. All nurses in all stages must be concerned about quality improvement and ensuring the best healthcare practices for the client, but expert nurses can influence changes for the system as well as changes for the individual client.

Through interviews with nurses, Benner described the depth of nursing skills and abilities found in the expert nurse. This expertise is forged over time and results from personal experience and personal knowledge. One of the challenges for beginning nurses is pressure to function as a competent, proficient, or even expert nurse without this background of growth. Competent in the Benner context reflects an ability to work independently and be responsible for decision-making. This is different from the use of the term "competent" in many other contexts where competent means that you have the skills for your current state—that is, you can be a competent novice. The transition from novice to advanced beginner to competent in Benner's categorization usually happens within the initial months of employment during an orientation period.

It is estimated that almost 20% of new graduates leave nursing within the 1st year and 33% leave nursing after 3 years (Grote, 2015). These attrition rates are costly for hospitals and other healthcare organizations. Resources of the educational system are not well used when new graduates leave the profession soon after graduation. These writers suggest that employers should do more to manage this transition for new graduates. Strategies to support transition are being developed in many institutions. Some states have developed statewide initiatives to address this concern.

As you look for a first nursing position, learn about the mechanisms the employer has in place to facilitate your transition to the independent RN role. Is there an orientation program specially designed for new graduates? Will you have an individually assigned preceptor or mentor for support? How long will you be given support before being expected to function independently? If you feel you need more time to be independent, will the employer accommodate this need? As a new graduate, will you be expected to float to different units or will you be helped to become competent in one area before being asked to go to another? Is there assistance with and support for continuing education for nurses to help you develop beyond the level of competent to proficient and expert? As you answer these questions, you will begin to develop a broader picture of the employer and be able to evaluate whether this job is a fit for your personal journey from novice to expert. This, along with personal preparation, may protect you from the impact of issues that lead to early retreat from nursing (Evidence-Based Practice 13.1).

Evidence-Based Practice 13.1: Retention of New Nurses

McDonald, A. W., & Ward-Smith, P. (2012). A review of evidence-based strategies to retain graduate nurses in the profession. *Journal for Nurses in Staff Development, 28*(1), E16–E20. https://doi.org/10.1097/nnd.0b013e318240a740

This article is a literature review of six other articles that discuss research findings of methods and interventions that increase retention of new nurses. The interventions were transition programs, internship or preceptorship programs, residency programs, externship programs, and postorientation programs and each varied in time and expense. All of the programs were designed to help the new nurse acclimate to the profession either prior to taking NCLEX-RN, as with the externship program, or after completing NCLEX-RN and starting to work full time. Some of the programs were combined such as a preceptorship program combined with a postorientation buddy program. The main idea behind each program is to increase support of the new nurse as he or she transitions from novice to experienced nurse in order to "develop feelings of empowerment and clinical competence" (p. E19).

Critical Thinking Activity: What Level Are You?
Examine your own background and experience in light of the characteristics noted in Benner's levels of skill. In your analysis, identify areas where you might exhibit a particular level of skill. What do you believe is the general level of skill expected of the new graduate?

REALITY SHOCK

One problem confronted by the new graduate is the seeming impossibility of delivering quality care within the constraints of the system as it exists. You may feel powerless to effect any changes and be depressed over your lack of effectiveness in a given situation. Marlene Kramer (1979) was the first to call the feelings that result from such a situation **reality shock**. She noted that the new graduate often experiences considerable psychologic stress and that this may exacerbate the problem. The person undergoing such stress is less able to perceive the entire situation and to solve problems effectively **(Fig. 13.1)**.

Effects of Reality Shock

The person experiencing reality shock may feel discouraged and depressed over the conditions of work. There may be anger toward the system, and this may result in diffused anger that erupts over situations that in other circumstances might be met with a calm demeanor.

In an attempt to cope, some push themselves to the limit, trying to provide ideal care while criticizing the system. This may result in their being labeled nonconformists and troublemakers. Still others give up their values and standards for care and reject ideals as impossibly unrealistic expectations that cannot be fulfilled in the real world. These persons simply mesh with the current framework and become part of the system. When reality shock occurs, some nurses begin to job-hop or return to school, searching for the perfect place to practice

Figure 13.1. Some new graduates are disillusioned by the working conditions that they find on their first job.

perfect nursing as it was learned. Others become disillusioned and leave nursing altogether (Kramer, 1979).

Causes of Reality Shock

With all of the uncertain expectations and demands, the new graduate often feels caught in the middle. As a student, you may think that you are expected to learn a tremendous amount in an alarmingly short time. The expectations may seem high and in some ways unrealistic.

As a new graduate suddenly thrust into the real world, you may feel unsure of yourself without the security of the instructor's availability and the support of your fellow students. You may think that your education program did not adequately prepare you for what is expected of you. On one hand, you are expected to function like a nurse who has 10 years of experience, but on the other hand, your new ideas may not be considered because you have so little experience. You may become frustrated because you do not have time to provide the same type of care you gave as a student. For example, you may not have sufficient time to deal with a client's psychosocial problems or teaching needs.

As a student, you are taught that the good nurse never gives a medication without understanding its actions and side effects and that evaluating the effectiveness of the drug is essential. As a staff nurse, you may find that the priority is getting the medications passed correctly and on time and that there is little or no time to look up 15 new drugs. As for evaluation, that becomes a dream. How can you evaluate the subtle effects of a medication in the 2 minutes spent passing the medication to a client you do not know? The individually and meticulously planned care that was so important to you as a student may become a luxury when you are a graduate. Often the focus is on accomplishing the required tasks in the time allotted, and it is efficiency in tasks that may earn praise from a supervisor.

Pellico, Brewer, and Kovner (2009) investigated the experiences of newly licensed graduates. They identified that colliding expectations, the need for speed, expectations that are perceived as too great, and unacceptable communication patterns form the basis for serious reality shock and people leaving nursing. *Colliding expectations* describes conflicts between nurses' personal views of nursing and their lived experiences. The *need for speed* describes the pressure related to a variety of time management issues. *You want too much* expresses the pressure and stress that newly licensed RNs feel personally and professionally. *How dare you!* describes unacceptable communication patterns between providers. Hezaveh, Rafii, and Seyedfatemi (2014) echoed those findings in their research and labeled the same problems such as *functional disabilities* (lack of speed and accuracy), *communicative problems* (difficulty communicating with doctors, coworker, and clients), and *managerial challenges* (lack of experience planning and coordinating care).

In the healthcare environment of today, these problems should not be normalized because they hurt the work environment and contribute to high turnover, particularly of new graduates. Seeking an employer who recognizes the novice role and accommodates for it will help you to make a successful transition.

As a new graduate, you, yourself, can address the potential for reality shock. You will need to develop a realistic view of the RN's role in today's healthcare environment and a better understanding of reality shock and what its effects on you might be. Based on this you can plan your own strategies to manage the issues that will confront you as a new graduate.

Finding Solutions for Reality Shock

It is possible to create a role for yourself that blends the ideal with the possible—one in which you do not give up ideals but see them as goals toward which you will move, however slowly. To do this, you need to be realistically prepared for the demands of the real world.

Self-Appraisal and Personal Development

One way of meeting the challenge is to assess yourself as you approach the end of your education program. Evaluate your own competencies in relationship to the common expectations of employers of new graduates that were discussed in Chapter 4.

After you have done a self-appraisal and gained information about prospective employers, analyze your own ability to function in accordance with an employer's expectations. If you identify any shortcomings, try to remedy them before graduation. If you identify a lack in certain technical skills, register for extra time in the nursing practice laboratory to increase your proficiency. You could even time yourself and work to increase speed as well as skill. Consult with your clinical instructor to arrange for experiences that would help you gain increased competence, especially in procedures with which you have had little experience. If you recognize that you consistently have difficulty functioning within a time frame, you might obtain employment in a hospital or other healthcare facility while still in school; this will give you more experience in organizing work within the time limits that the employer sees as reasonable.

> **Critical Thinking Activity: Managing Reality Shock**
> With a group of nursing students, develop personal strategies for managing reality shock. Discuss your rationale for any strategy you propose.

Evaluating Employers

It is helpful to understand what prospective employers in the community in which you plan to seek employment expect of a new graduate. You can gain this information by talking with experienced nurses, meeting with faculty, and contacting recent graduates who are currently employed. Try to get specific information. If you have a nursing student organization, setting up a forum for speakers from various agencies might be one avenue to gaining this insight. Once you apply for a position, you could explore this issue in an employment interview.

When you are selecting a place of employment, there are many factors to consider. While the specific position is important to you, there are aspects of the overall setting that will make a great deal of difference to your success. You are not as likely to experience severe stress if the employment setting is a good match for you. The professional practice environment makes a difference in the problems of reality shock and of burnout, which we will discuss later.

All hospitals and other healthcare settings will have a general orientation for new employees. Some will also have mentoring or precepting models to assist new nurses during the orientation process. Nurse internships or residencies in some settings have been created to provide a planned and organized transition time during which the new graduate participates in a formal program, including classes, seminars, and rotations to various units of the hospital. In some settings, the new graduate is required to be more self-directed in identifying needs and the ways that those might be met within the constraints of the system. Regardless of the type of orientation provided, it is helpful to get to know the experienced nurses on the floor and determine if one (or several) are willing to answer questions and provide guidance through informal mentoring as you transition into your new role. Some hospitals provide an opportunity for nursing students to work during the summer before the last year of their undergraduate studies to become familiar with the hospital and the nursing role. In this case, the nursing student may be employed in a position that introduces the role of the RN to nursing students. In other instances, nursing students work as nursing assistants, and the orientation to the nursing role in the agency depends on the initiative the individual takes. You may wish to inquire whether hospitals in your area have developed any of these or other programs to assist you when you are a new graduate.

Preceptors, Coaches, and Mentors

In nursing, many new graduates are assigned to a preceptor as part of their orientation process. A **preceptor** is an officially assigned role in which an experienced and capable employee assists with the orientation and development of a new graduate. Some of you may have experience with preceptors as part of your educational program. The preceptor usually has responsibility for supervising and evaluating the work of the preceptee. Some preceptors may see the role as primarily one of supervising, teaching, and evaluating in relationship to the specific job and do not see it as a broader role of encouraging professional development. Some preceptors develop personal relationships with new nurses. They act in ways described as mentoring (discussed later).

If you are fortunate enough to have a preceptor who becomes your mentor, you will have additional support and guidance from the beginning of your career. If your individual preceptor does not view the role that way, then you may wish to develop relationships with other experienced nurses who might provide a mentoring relationship.

Coaching is an informal teaching/helping relationship. Coaches are experienced nurses who focus on a specific aspect of growth and development such as helping a nurse to master a more advanced skill or to understand how to work within the organization. A coach may help individuals at all stages of their work life. Coaches may help an individual navigate the stressful aspects of the job by sharing tips on how to manage organizational challenges and by simply providing a listening ear.

A **mentor** is an individual who actively supports the overall professional development and growth of another person (referred to as the **mentee** or protégé). Within a professional field, the mentor is usually an experienced professional who develops a supportive relationship with someone with less experience in the profession and provides advice and emotional support for that person. Mentor–mentee relationships typically begin when an experienced senior nurse takes an interest in a nurse with beginning experience who is pursuing a similar professional pathway as the senior nurse. It often works best when it occurs spontaneously as a relationship develops between a junior and a senior employee within an organization.

The mentor usually assists the mentee with career and personal development and provides personal support, acceptance, and counseling. The mentor may sponsor the mentee and often facilitates that person's advancement within the organization by helping to establish networks and organizational know-how. Any plans for the development of the mentee need to be discussed and reviewed with periodic feedback and debriefing sessions. While the mentor may provide some direct assistance in learning the specific skills of the nursing role, more importantly, the mentor provides help in learning how to work effectively within the system. The mentor is a role model of effective practice.

A good mentor is an experienced practitioner. Attributes that contribute to success for a mentor are a positive attitude, a caring approach toward others, and effective communication. Mentees or protégés also have significant responsibilities in the relationship. The mentee must be willing to accept feedback, to try new ways of functioning, and to communicate with the mentor regarding what is helpful and what is not. Honesty and trust must lie at the heart of the relationship. Guidelines for setting up mentoring programs are available, such as the Academy of Medical-Surgical Nurses (ASMN) Mentoring Program (AMSN, 2012).

Mentor–mentee relationships change over time and may become more collegial. As you progress in your career, you may need a new mentor in a new setting or in regard to a new field of practice. Once you are an experienced nurse, it is important that you help to mentor new nurses, as well as role model caring and professionalism.

Peer Support Groups

Understanding that you are not alone in your feelings of frustration in a new job is often helpful. It may be useful to form a peer support group of new graduates who meet regularly to discuss problems and concerns and seek solutions jointly. A peer support group is usually composed of new nurses at a particular facility and is often initiated by the new nurses themselves. The group meets regularly to share its experiences, offer support and advice, and help all the individuals to recognize that others are also experiencing stress during this time.

Some peer support groups are composed of individuals from a single graduating class who may be working in different settings. Although their settings differ, many of the individuals' concerns surrounding transition are similar, and their relationships with their educational program have created a bond that makes the group able to function effectively.

Personal Stress Management

Recognizing your own response to stress and identifying your personal stress management strategies will be significant. As a nursing student, you experienced stressful times and coped successfully or you would not have graduated. Remind yourself of your own successful coping and draw on the strategies you found successful in the past. As is always the case, personal health needs to be a part of those strategies. Attend to your diet, rest, and activity plan. Maintain time for family and friends in order to have balance in life. Life should never be all work.

When confronted with areas of practice in your work environment that you would like to see changed, weigh the importance of an issue. Use your energies wisely. The "politics of the possible" is important. Learn how the system in which you are employed functions and how to use that system for effective change. You are important to nursing, so it is essential that you neither burn yourself out nor abandon the quest for higher-quality nursing care. You should be able to continue to work toward improving nursing and bringing it closer to its ideals (see Chapter 12 for more information about change).

BURNOUT

Burnout is a form of chronic stress related to one's job. Burnout can occur to individuals in any occupation, and articles regarding burnout appear in the professional literature for almost all the helping or supporting professions.

This problem arises after you have been in practice for a period of time. It can be identified by feelings of hopelessness and powerlessness and is accompanied by a decreased ability to function both on the job and in personal life. Burnout occurs more frequently in nurses who work in particularly stressful areas of nursing, such as critical care, oncology, or burn units. Some writers explore burnout as "compassion fatigue," relating it to the high stress of managing personal feelings in the face of overwhelming crises experienced by others. Burnout also occurs when staffing is inadequate or interpersonal relationships are strained. The downsizing of nursing staff and the rapid changes in the healthcare environment have contributed to burnout in some settings.

Theory Alert *Rosemarie Rizzo Parse*

Rosemarie Rizzo Parse developed a theory of nursing that focuses of quality of life as the client sees it. Dr. Parse first graduated from Duquesne University and then earned both her master's and doctoral degrees from the University of Pittsburgh. She has served as faculty and dean of nursing during her career as well as working as a consultant and visiting scholar. From 1983 to 1993, she was a professor and the coordinator of the Center for Nursing Research at the City University of New York.

Her theory was originally called the man-living-health theory and was later renamed the Human Becoming theory. It is unique because it focuses on the quality of life more than on the biology of healing. The three themes associated with this theory are meaning, rhythmicity, and transcendence. *Meaning* refers to personal meaning or the reality of the experience for the client. *Rhythmicity* is a reference to the rhythmical patterns of the universe that the person and the environment create and *transcendence* indicates that human beings can reach beyond limits. Reaching beyond limits, finding meaning, and focusing on quality of life are important parts of facing challenges in today's world.
(Source: http://www.nursing-theory.org)

Symptoms of Burnout

Symptoms of burnout include both physical changes and psychologic distress. The items found in the Maslach Burnout Inventory (Maslach, Jackson, & Leiter, 1997) provide an overview of symptoms that may occur in burnout. These include exhaustion and fatigue, frequent colds, headaches, backaches, and insomnia. General disinterest in the job and dreading going to work may occur. There may be changes in disposition, such as being quick to anger or exhibiting all emotions excessively. Individuals experience a decreased ability to solve problems and make decisions as burnout progresses. This frequently results in an unwillingness to face change and a tendency to block new ideas. There may be feelings of guilt, anger, and depression because one cannot meet the expectations for doing a "perfect job." Burnout begins gradually and is more effectively managed early in its onset.

In response to these feelings, some nurses quit their jobs and move on to other settings that may be outside the nursing profession. Others remain in their jobs but develop a personal shell that tends to separate them from real contact with clients and coworkers; they may become cynical about the possibility of anyone doing a good job and may function at a minimal level. A few become increasingly unable to function and find themselves in jeopardy of losing their positions.

Causes of Burnout

Many causes of burnout have been discussed in the literature. Prominent among them is the conflict between ideals and reality. Just as this is a problem for the new graduate, it is also a problem for the experienced nurse. These nurses believe they are responsible for all things to all people and often take on more responsibility, thus increasing their own stress level.

Another cause of burnout is the high level of stress that results from practicing nursing in areas that have high mortality rates. Continually investing oneself in clients who die can take a tremendous toll on personal resources. In addition, the demand for optimal functioning is constant.

Inadequately staffed institutions also may place great stress on nurses. The clients are in need of care, the nurse has the skills to provide the care, and yet the clients do not receive good care. The nurse typically tries to accomplish more, putting in overtime, skipping breaks and lunch, and running throughout the shift. Despite this effort, there is little job satisfaction because the things that are left undone or that are not done well seem to be more apparent than all the good that is accomplished.

Daily Ethical Dilemma 13.1: Nurse Burnout

After delivering what the doctor said was a stillborn infant, the young couple was still trying to come to terms with the news. The young parents looked over to where the baby lay on the warmer and saw that the baby's heart was beating. Confused, they questioned the nurse who immediately wrapped up the infant and handed it to the mother. The physician knew that the infant had no chance of survival and so had elected not to tell the couple that the baby's heart was beating. He told the nurse to withhold the information as well. He felt that this would make it easier for them. A bereavement coordinator was called in to help resolve the conflict that resulted.

- What is the primary dilemma in this situation?
- Is any harm likely to come from this error?
- What could the nurse have done differently?
- How might this situation contribute to nurse burnout?

Preventing and Managing Burnout

As an individual nurse, you can take actions to prevent burnout. These are the same general actions that are designed to control stress in any aspect of life and may help you if you believe that you are beginning to experience burnout.

Paying attention to your own physical health is an important preventive measure; this includes maintaining a balanced program of rest, nutrition, and exercise. Another important point is not to subject yourself to excessive changes over short periods of time, because changes increase stress. You may decide, for example, not to relocate your living setting (apartment or house), and at the same time you can change to a different shift. A period of wind-down or decompression after work will help you to avoid carrying the stress of the workplace into your private life; this period may involve physical exercise, reading, meditation, or any different activity. This may seem like a daydream to individuals who are working full time and have responsibility for children and, perhaps, also for aging parents. Yet, it is important that some personally rewarding activity be incorporated into the daily routine. The activity you choose should not create more demands and increase stress. An important resource is someone who is willing to listen while you express your feelings and talk about your problems. Sometimes this is a family member or personal friend, but it may be more appropriate for this to be a coworker or counselor.

Rotating out of a high-stress area, such as a burn unit or pediatric oncology, before you begin to experience burnout or when you first identify that you are beginning to burn out may allow you to rebuild resources and return to the job with enthusiasm. This can be done only if there is no stigma or blame attached to the need to rotate and if other nurses are available for replacement.

Communication in Action 13.1: *Acting to Prevent Burnout*

Linda Wilson returned to employment after maternity leave when her baby was 3 months old. A new critical care unit was being opened in the hospital and she eagerly accepted the invitation to work there. However, after 2 months on the 3 PM to 11 PM shift, she found she was burning out, due in part to understaffing, lots of overtime, and the critical nature of the clients for whom she cared. With the demands of the baby, she seldom got more than 4 to 5 hours sleep. She approached the supervisor of the unit and asked for an appointment to meet with him prior to beginning her shift. During their meeting Linda explained, "I am very appreciative of the opportunity to work in this unit. However, I think it was not the right time in my life to undertake such a challenge. With the demands of a new baby at home, I just do not have the energy that this position demands. I get home late, often have trouble going to sleep, and the baby wakens during the night and is up early. I would like to request a transfer to a less intensive work unit." The supervisor was supportive of Linda and her request and agreed to follow through on the request for transfer.

In this communication, Linda did not blame others for the situation in which she found herself. She was honest and forthright in her explanations and clear in her request.

Another strategy is to focus on those positive aspects of nursing that drew you to it initially. Cognitively reframing your thoughts and focusing on positive feelings, such as gratitude, has been shown in research to improve job satisfaction (Derby-Davis, 2014) and improve coping (Lin, 2015). Spend time identifying those situations where you made a difference, where you demonstrated both the art and science of nursing, and focus on things for which you are grateful (ie, coworkers, supervisor, etc.) or did well. You then are able to recognize when you are focusing on the problems or being negative in the situation and blaming yourself for them. Instead, refocus your attention on the fact that you did not create the situation, but that you are a positive force in that milieu.

The most effective prevention of burnout is an institution-wide stress-reduction effort to prevent burnout involving the nursing staff, supervisory personnel, the hospital administration, and other healthcare workers. The most important objective seems to be bringing burnout into the open and acknowledging the existence of the problem. This alone helps the individual nurse move away from the feelings of separation and alienation that often accompany burnout. Whatever the problems, they seem less frightening if they are defined as normal and if the individual nurse does not see himself or herself as the only person not performing as the perfect nurse. Investigate the resources that a prospective employer has to assist nurses in preventing burnout.

Employers can offer resources to prevent and manage burnout. Having adequate staff and support for taking days off and vacation time are all ways employers can help fight burnout. In client care areas that are known to be stressful, it is helpful to have a counselor available for nurses. Consulting with this counselor should be viewed by the staff as a positive step and not as an admission of some lack or fault. The counselor needs to be someone who understands the setting and who has the skills to assist people in coping with stress.

Another approach may be initiated by individual nurses but requires the cooperation of the institution; this includes establishing group discussions during which nurses can share feelings and specific concerns in an accepting atmosphere. This sharing may lead to concrete plans to reduce the stress created by the setting. For example, if one source of stress is conflicting orders between two sets of physicians involved in care, a plan might be developed whereby the nurses no longer take responsibility for the conflict but refer the problem to some authority within the medical hierarchy. This type of resolution is possible only when the whole healthcare team addresses the problem of burnout. However, it also requires that nurses give up trying to control everything for which they feel responsible.

Giving nurses more control over their own practice often decreases stress. Although more control is limited by the constraints of the setting, it could involve flexible scheduling, volunteering for specific assignments, and participating in committees that determine policies and procedures.

> ### Critical Thinking Activity: Preventing Burnout
> Compare burnout with the stress response you have studied in relation to client care. Compare the strategies that you have taught clients with those suggested for preventing burnout. Discuss these with a classmate and see how many similarities you have.

WORKPLACE SAFETY AND HEALTH FOR NURSES

Nurses have expressed concern regarding safety in the working environment for many years. Employees have a right to expect their employers to provide the safest working environment possible. Some hospitals employ an occupational health nurse to examine the working environment and use employment practices to promote health and safety on the job. Nurses themselves, however, often have been lax in recognizing on-the-job hazards and acting for self-protection; this can be likened to the response of those who continue to smoke despite their knowledge of the health hazards of smoking or those who fail to wear seatbelts even though some state laws require it and statistics show fewer fatalities in automobile accidents when seatbelts are worn. Some people continue to do those things that they know are detrimental to their health and well-being. Unfortunately, nurses are no exception. Employers have a responsibility to provide a safe and healthy workplace, but employees also have an obligation to use protective equipment, follow policies and procedures, use proper body mechanics, and inform management of workplace violence or if policies and procedures are not being followed in order to protect self and others (Brent, 2016).

Nurse Staffing Levels

As acuity levels in hospitals have risen, concerns about the nurse to client ratio have become prominent. Inadequate staffing contributes to burnout because nurses are unable to meet all the needs of clients. An even more compelling concern regarding staffing involves the increased rate of errors when the staffing is inadequate.

Across the country nurses have begun to lobby for legislation that would control staffing levels. California was the first to pass such legislation. The results of this legislation are mixed in a situation in which there have been serious nursing shortages. Because of the wording in the law, both LPNs and RNs are included in "nurses" when calculating staffing ratios.

The American Nurses Association (ANA) has launched a major campaign titled *Safe Staffing Saves Lives* (n.d.). Research has demonstrated that inadequate staffing has a direct impact on risk of dying and increased risk "of failure to rescue" (Mensik, 2014). On the other hand, it has been found that when a higher proportion of hours of registered nursing care per day are available, there are positive client outcomes with lower rates of urinary tract infections, pneumonia, shock, and upper gastrointestinal bleeds with cost savings to the system (AHRQ, 2004). The ANA recommends that institutions be required to establish appropriate ratios at the unit level through negotiation rather than mandating absolute ratios for all settings. Other groups are seeking mandatory staffing levels through regulation or legislation.

In settings with limited staffing of RNs, other problems emerge. There may be difficulty in obtaining RN coverage for anyone who leaves the units and nurses may work an entire shift without a break. Overtime becomes more common when there are too few nurses to accomplish the needed tasks during the shift. When facilities mandate that unit staff provide their own coverage for sick days and all shifts, nurses may end up working many extra shifts. As these demands increase, the problem of nurse fatigue increases. Nurse fatigue is dangerous to both nurses and clients with errors due to fatigue costing billions of dollars annually (Reed, 2013).

Infection as an Occupational Hazard

An **occupational hazard** is a risk that is inherent with the job. For example, transmission of infection is a major concern when caring for infected clients. The presence of resistant organisms causes extra concern and makes treatment difficult. All hospitals have an infection control officer, usually an RN, who has the expertise to guide the staff in planning appropriate infection control procedures. Staff in other settings may not have access to such an expert.

The hidden danger for nurses lies in those clients who have not been diagnosed as having an infection and for whom specific infection control measures have therefore not been prescribed. Universal precautions have been mandated by the Occupational Safety and Health Administration (OSHA) for use with clients in all settings to protect staff members from blood-borne pathogens. These precautions prevent the spread of human immunodeficiency virus (HIV), hepatitis B, and other such blood-borne pathogens.

One of the first employer actions toward preventing blood-borne diseases was the provision of sharp containers wherever needles were used. Another important employer responsibility is the provision of a supply of gloves and protective eyewear for employee use. OSHA mandates these measures as part of universal precautions. However, not all cases of transmission of blood-borne pathogens can be prevented by universal precautions. Needlestick injuries—especially those with large-bore needles (eg, bone marrow aspiration needles)—continue to be the most frequent transmission source. Wearing gloves does not prevent these injuries.

More attention is now being given to designing needles and other sharp devices in ways that prevent needlestick injuries. For example, a needle with a protective plastic housing is available for injections. Even if these needles are not handled properly, they are unlikely to injure the individual. Needleless intravenous connections are also available. Syringes are available that have a protective cover into which the needle retracts immediately after use.

To participate knowledgeably in decisions regarding needle systems and devices, nurses need to seek information about what devices are available. OSHA does mandate that healthcare facilities have in place a plan to reduce the risk of needlestick injuries through using safe devices. The ANA has been active in workplace advocacy related to needlestick injuries and prevention of those injuries. Please go to http://www.nursingworld.org/safeneedles or https://www.osha.gov/SLTC/etools/hospital/hazards/univprec/univ.html for more information.

Blood-borne pathogens are not the only pathogens of concern in the healthcare environment. The Standard Precautions recommended by the Centers for Disease Control and Prevention (CDC) are used in all settings. These precautions protect clients and staff members from infections that might be transmitted by any bodily substance with the addition of transmission-based (contact, droplet, and airborne) precautions for known or suspected infections such as tuberculosis (TB), measles, clostridium difficile (C-Diff), etc. (CDC, 2017a).

The incidence of TB is again on the rise, with drug-resistant strains of the organism appearing. Although rooms with special ventilation and special masks that are impervious to the TB organism are available, individuals with the disease may be in contact with healthcare providers long before they are clearly diagnosed. Should nurses in high-risk areas, such as the emergency room, wear special masks during all client contact, or is this unrealistic? And what do we do about other antibiotic-resistant "superbugs" that are appearing? These are important questions to consider. Nurses are responsible for maintaining up-to-date knowledge about infection control measures and emerging diseases so that we can help in preventing the emergence and spread of new infections.

Although the details of infection control are beyond the scope of this text, we remind you that you hold the key to protecting yourself in many ways. Healthcare workers often become lax in their attention to the use of gloves or eye protection because these measures are inconvenient. It is your responsibility to use the very best techniques for self-protection, including diligent attention to hand hygiene. Nurses must assume responsibility for their own protection by conscientiously carrying out appropriate measures at all times (Fig. 13.2). Employers must be held accountable for providing the supplies and environment to make this possible.

Doing your own part in infection control also extends to maintaining your personal immunizations in order to not be a source of illness for clients or colleagues. During flu season, a healthy individual may carry a subclinical case of influenza and transmit it to vulnerable clients. All healthcare providers are urged to be immunized (CDC, 2017b) and you may be required to be immunized by employers. Employers may pay for immunizations that will protect everyone in the healthcare environment.

Hazardous Chemical Agents

Anesthetic gases can increase the risk of fetal malformation and spontaneous abortion in pregnant women who are exposed to them on a regular basis. Standards exist for waste gas retrieval systems and the allowable level of these gases in the air. Nurses working in operating rooms should seek information on the subject and expect hospitals to provide a safe work environment.

Chemotherapeutic agents used in the treatment of cancer are extremely toxic, and nurses who work in settings where such agents are prepared and administered should seek additional education regarding their administration, not only in relation to the client's safety but also in relation to personal safety. The employer is responsible for providing the equipment needed

Figure 13.2. Maintaining personal immunizations and wearing personal protective equipment are essential elements for infection control.

to maintain safety when handling these agents. In many settings, protocols now require the routine use of personal protective equipment when handling chemotherapeutic agents.

Contact with many medications, especially antibiotics, during preparation and administration may cause the nurse to develop sensitivity. This can create transitory problems (eg, a hand rash) and may be a threat if treatment for a serious infection is compromised later. Other medications are absorbed through the skin and may produce an undesirable effect. Nurses must take responsibility for their own safety regarding these agents. Nurses who understand these hazards handle all drugs with discretion and are careful not to expose themselves to these agents.

Communication in Action 13.2: *Speaking up Regarding Unsafe Practice*

Jose Morales, RN, worked in the medication administration area side-by-side with another RN. He noted that the RN spiked an antibiotic bag, hung the bag on a hanger, and proceeded to open the tubing to clear air but got fluid from the bag on the counter. Jose spoke up, "Hey, John, I don't mean to be overly critical, but I am concerned about antibiotics getting spilled around here. That contributes to the development of resistant organisms that are a danger to us as well as clients. Besides, you and I might get sensitized to that stuff. I learned a technique for backfilling from the primary bag so that there is never a danger of spilling. Are you familiar with that technique? I would be glad to show you."

Cleaning agents and disinfectants used in the hospital may also be hazardous if used improperly. Employers are now required by OSHA to maintain a list of all chemicals used in the work environment, along with information on their possible effects and the appropriate treatment if individuals are accidentally exposed to them. If you work with these agents, seek out this information, found in the Material Safety Data Sheets (MSDS), and be sure that you handle chemicals correctly.

Ergonomic Hazards in the Workplace

Ergonomics is the science of fitting a task to one's physical characteristics in order to enhance safety, efficiency, and well-being. When the task does not conform to one's physical characteristics, musculoskeletal stress and injuries may occur. Client handling and transfer require the movement of a weight load beyond that which most human bodies are designed to manage. In addition, the healthcare setting often requires that client movement and transfer be done in awkward positions and inadequate spaces. Nearly half of all reported injuries are musculoskeletal injuries resulting from lifting, reaching, or bending (OSHA, 2013).

Many employers have programs to prevent musculoskeletal injuries. Some institutions provide instruction in lifting, transfer, posture, body mechanics, and other back-saving strategies to help prevent injury. None of these strategies can protect an individual from repetitive stress injury from lifting more than is appropriate. Further, a client is, by definition, unstable when being helped, and a sudden move or change in the client can have a devastating effect on the caregiver. Mechanical lifting and transfer devices provide a means of moving clients without danger to staff members. More types of lifting and transfer devices are now available, and more employers are open to purchasing equipment to prevent these costly injuries.

The ANA, in cooperation with Johnson & Johnson, spearheaded a nationwide campaign titled "Handle With Care," aimed at safe client transfer (ANA, 2004). In its materials titled "Safe Client Handling" client, the ANA emphasized that that there is no safe way for caregivers to lift and transfer dependent clients. They advocated a no-lift policy, the use of mechanical devices for lifting and transfer, and the use of lift teams when lifting is essential. The goal for the ANA is that utilizing safe lifting techniques will become standard practice (AHC Media, 2013). The ANA is active in supporting the efforts of state constituent organizations to work for the enactment of safe client handling state legislation, which has now passed in over 11 states. Many nursing programs are using materials from the ANA Toolkit regarding safe client handling to teach students about this important issue.

An ergonomic concern for nurses relates to computer workstations. Those who work at computer workstations for long periods of time are subject to back, neck, wrist, and hand strain. While most nurses do not spend long periods of time at the computer, this is changing as nurses work in telephone care while sitting at computers and even spend long periods documenting care. When one individual uses the same computer station throughout the work day, that station can be adapted to the individual. However, in most nursing settings, the computer station is used by many people. Adjustability of the screen, keyboard, chair, and armrests becomes important in order to provide each person using it with an ergonomically safe workstation. In many settings, computer workstations were added to an existing desk area. This may or may not serve the users well. Be alert to the problems that may occur; help yourself by maintaining correct posture and using the adjustments available; report concerns to the appropriate manager.

Be aware of the potential for musculoskeletal injury and examine your work habits. Some nurses feel that they must accomplish certain tasks even if the necessary assistance is not available and therefore carry out actions that can cause harm to themselves. Nurses need to continue to work toward safer workplaces for all healthcare providers. They must learn to be assertive regarding their own safety.

> **Critical Thinking Activity: Workplace Hazards**
> Research the occupational health program offered by a local employer of nurses. Evaluate that program in relation to health hazards in the workplace of which you are aware.

Workers' Compensation

If you believe that you have a work-related injury or illness, follow the policies and procedures prescribed by your facility or by state regulation. This includes reporting the injury as soon as possible after it happens. In most institutions, this is done on an incident report or quality assurance report. A common error is to delay reporting in the belief that you should report something only if you know it will be serious or require medical care. By the time you know this, it may be much more difficult to prove that the problem was work related.

Employers may seek to have workers' compensation claims disallowed to limit their financial liability. Because back injuries are the most common work-related injuries and often have no clear objective evidence of damage even when pain is present, stigma is frequently attached to those who have back injuries. HIV and hepatitis B are transmitted through needlestick injuries, but they are also transmitted through other unsafe behaviors. These factors may underlie attempts by an employer to disallow claims for care and time lost from work due to these work-related illnesses or injuries. Prompt, thorough reporting is essential to future claims.

Have any injury assessed by an appropriate healthcare provider. If your agency has an occupational health nurse, you may be required to be seen by that individual for initial screening. One concern is whether you may receive care from the provider of your choice or whether you must receive care from a designated provider. This varies based on the regulations governing work-related injury and illness in your state. Ask this question of your employer and then research it through your state workers' compensation office. If the laws allow the employer or a state agency to designate the provider and you go to another of your choice, you may not be reimbursed for expenses incurred.

Compensation for time off work is another concern when a work-related problem occurs; you are usually required to use your sick leave, but additional time may be available through the workers' compensation program. In general, these programs do not match your working salary, so your income will be lessened. This is one reason why many individuals choose to have private disability insurance that provides replacement income when they cannot work because of illness or disability.

The Americans with Disabilities Act (ADA) of 1990 requires that employers seek ways to provide reasonable accommodation for individuals with disability so that they can continue to work. This might include transferring an individual to a different position or modifying the work environment to provide a setting in which the individual can function. Employers have been known to refuse to make accommodations and to try to terminate an individual who has an ongoing disability. Those with work-related illness and disability do have legal rights within the system. Sometimes it requires considerable effort to sustain those rights. There are both state and federal resources to assist an individual who does not receive reasonable accommodation for disability. The United States Department of Justice maintains a web page with links to many different resources about upholding the provisions of the ADA (https://www.ada.gov/).

Discrimination in Nursing

Discrimination relates to treating others differently based on **stereotype** (an oversimplified idea about a person/thing/group of people). Discrimination may occur regarding racial or ethnic background, gender or sex, sexual orientation, and/or age.

Racial/Ethnic Discrimination

Racial and ethnic discrimination remain problems in society as a whole, and unfortunately, healthcare systems are not immune to these problems. Although there are indications that nurses have moved into greater acceptance of all individuals in advance of some other portions of society, concerns about discrimination remain. Historically, the American Association of Colored Graduate Nurses united with the ANA in 1952, before the general civil rights movement in the United States. There have always been prominent nurses of color, such as the past president of the ANA (Beverly Malone) who is now the Chief Executive Officer of the National League for Nursing, former president of the National League for Nursing (Rhetaugh Dumas), and past president of Sigma Theta Tau (May Wykle), who are all African-American women who have been leaders for all of nursing throughout their long and distinguished careers. They are just three of the many ethnic/racial minority nurses who have made significant contributions to nursing.

However, the number of minorities in nursing does not reflect the number of minorities in the general population. A 2013 Sample Survey of the RN workforce by the National Council of State Boards of Nursing (NCSBN) revealed that 19% of nurses represent minority groups (AACN, 2015). This contrasts with a general population that had approximately 37% racial/ethnic minorities in 2012 (AACN, 2015). This difference in the composition of the nursing profession and the general population may stem from many causes but is of concern because a workforce that reflects the population is more likely to meet the healthcare needs of that population in a culturally sensitive manner. Some of the root causes of the lower participation of minorities in nursing have to do with access to education, support for high career goals, economic status, the image of nursing, institutionalized racism, and other general societal problems.

A survey of minority nurses published by the ANA indicated that many believe they have been adversely affected by discrimination in the nursing profession. Some concerns cited were the perception that others questioned their capabilities and that they were passed over for promotions. To combat these issues as well as to serve as a voice for care for ethnic minority clients, several organizations for ethnic nurses have joined together to create the National Coalition of Ethnic Minority Nurses Associations (http://www.ncemna.org/).

All nurses are challenged to examine this situation and be a part of the solution. All of us need to recognize and welcome diversity in the nursing profession. We need to acknowledge that a diversity of views and life experiences will enrich nursing as a profession and support excellence in client care. When we see discrimination occur, whether in education or in the workplace, we each need to speak up as agents for change. The National Student Nurses' Association has supported a program called Breakthrough to Nursing, in which nursing students mentor minority individuals in nursing education. These efforts and similar ones help nursing to move forward as a profession that welcomes and provides opportunities for all.

Discrimination Against Men

Men in nursing also have expressed concern about discrimination. Their concern is related to being allowed to practice in all areas of nursing and being accepted within the profession. Men continue to experience discrimination in nursing by clients, families, and other nurses. Wojciechowski (2016) shared the experiences of male nurses who talked about how people believed that they were gay because they were nurses, or thought that the nurse was the doctor, or simply refused to have a male nurse because of the belief that women are better nurses. It is important that as a profession we support each other (men and women) and continue to educate society, one person at a time in order to strengthen nursing as a whole. Anti-male sexism of nurses in the United States was brought to the forefront by the research of Kus (1985), who pointed out that society stereotypes men just as feminists have criticized that it stereotypes women. He made a strong case for the importance of nurses examining the stereotypes they hold about men. Stereotypes narrow our thinking and interfere with people being able to develop to their fullest potential. It is important for women in nursing to examine their own behavior and identify whether they have been guilty of perpetuating outmoded stereotypes of the nurse and supporting a type of discrimination toward men that they would fight to eliminate for women.

Stereotyping may have contributed to the low percentage of men in the nursing profession but changes in society are occurring. Men represent 9.6% of RNs and 8.1% of LPNs (US Census, 2013). This number remains low but has gradually risen since only 2.7% of RNs were men in 1970 (US Census, 2013).

In some facilities or areas, men are not allowed to care for women clients, or if they are allowed to care for women, restrictions are placed on them in terms of obtaining consent for care from each client. Those who support the limitations on the practice of men in nursing state that it is a matter of providing for the modesty and privacy of female clients. The argument is made that clients cannot freely choose a nurse but, rather, are assigned a nurse for care, and therefore restrictions are appropriate.

In an interview, Luther Christman, PhD, RN, discussed the discrimination that he encountered throughout a long and prestigious career in nursing. His career began with his graduation from a hospital-based diploma program in 1939 and extended through doctoral studies and a joint position as dean of Rush University and vice president of nursing for Rush-Presbyterian-St. Luke's Medical Center in Chicago. Dr. Christman identified overt acts that excluded him from positions and covert acts that tried to undermine his influence. He believed that this was an issue of power and control just as is sex discrimination against women (Sullivan, 2002).

Those who oppose limitations on the practice of men in nursing state that, as a professional, a nurse (whether a man or woman) should always consider the privacy and modesty of a client of either gender. This can be done without excluding anyone from providing care in any area. By careful assessment, the nurse can determine the true needs of the client and plan for appropriate avenues to deliver that care. Furthermore, the point has been made that male physicians have not been excluded from any branch of medicine and this has not created problems. The client does not always choose physicians either. Resident physicians are assigned, referrals are made to specialty physicians, and many group plans designate a physician to provide care. Female nurses care for male clients in all situations. This has been accepted because women are seen in a nurturing, mothering role that the public associates with nursing.

The American Association for Men in Nursing (AAMN) provides a forum for the concerns of men in nursing and those who are concerned about the problems of sex discrimination. This organization seeks to educate people and opposes any limitations on opportunities available to men. The AAMN website has information on scholarships, conferences, and a newsletter to support men in nursing. Further information is available at http://aamn.org/.

Critical Thinking Activity: Gender Bias
Review the advertisements for nursing positions in three current journals and analyze them for gender bias.

Sexual Harassment

Sexual harassment, disruptive behavior, and violence are often discussed together because they may be rooted in the same issues of the abuse of power. Disruptive behavior and violence are discussed as follows.

Sexual harassment is grouped into two sets of behavior. The first is the creation of a hostile work environment through behavior of a sexual nature. This type of sexual harassment may take the form of comments about an individual's body, persistent unwanted attempts to initiate a personal relationship, the ongoing use of suggestive or obscene language, unwanted touching, or direct sexual advances. Another type of sexual harassment is called *quid pro quo*. This involves the explicit offer of job-related benefits (working conditions, salary, privileges, or even simply the benefit of remaining employed) in return for sexual favors (Roberts & Mann, n.d.).

Both men and women may be the objects of sexual harassment. Because nurses are involved with personal care of individuals of the opposite sex, there is sometimes the unspoken assumption that nurses will not be offended by sexual comments, jokes, or innuendo.

Sexual harassment was the subject of a position paper by the ANA (1993), as nurses began to voice their concerns about its presence in nursing. This position paper provided background on the costs of the problem and identified areas of redress for nurses who were subjected to sexual harassment.

Harassers in the healthcare workplace may be clients, coworkers, or physicians. The general data show that sexual harassment is a demonstration of personal power over others. Traditionally, physicians have had the most power in healthcare environments and are the group most often identified as harassers. While recognizing the problem, it is important not to stereotype physicians, because the majority of physicians are professional and appropriate in their relationships.

Individuals should take steps to stop sexual harassment by giving clear, direct verbal messages indicating that the behavior in question is unwanted, unpleasant, and must stop. Sometimes this action alone stops inappropriate behavior. If clear, direct messages are not successful, the individual then should report the matter in writing to an immediate supervisor. Any individual who believes that he or she has been the victim of sexual harassment should keep personal records of the behavior and of all attempts to stop the behavior in question.

Most organizations and agencies have an individual designated to deal with issues related to sexual harassment. If you encounter problem behavior, discuss your concerns with this person. If you belong to a collective bargaining group, that group can serve as a resource to assist you. Unfortunately, some employers do not respond appropriately to sexual harassment. In some instances, it may be necessary to seek independent legal counsel familiar with workplace legal issues to force resolution of the problem. Employers are legally and ethically responsible for having clear policies that prohibit sexual harassment and for providing an appropriate work environment. If an employer fails to respond appropriately, the employer may be legally liable. These policies should be publicized so that everyone is aware of them. The courts support the responsibility of the employer to maintain a work environment free of sexual harassment (Equal Employment Opportunity Commission [EEOC], n.d.).

Communication in Action 13.3: A Clear Message About Sexual Harassment

Jean Wilson, RN, was new to the medical center where she worked. While sitting at the desk by herself in the evening, a male resident physician sat down beside her. He draped his arm around her shoulders, put his face close to hers and said, "Hi there, sweetie! How's it going for the prettiest nurse on 3-Southwest?" Jean was taken aback and very uncomfortable. She immediately stood and said, "We are virtual strangers. I don't like your touching me in that way or calling me 'Sweetie'. It is inappropriate. Don't do that again." He then said, "Hey, hey—don't get so upset. I was just being friendly." She replied, "We're not friends, we are colleagues, and that does not include touching me and calling me names like 'Sweetie.'" He muttered to himself and walked away. Jean felt nervous but glad she had stood her ground.

Disruptive Behavior

Disruptive behavior which includes incivility, verbal abuse, and bullying may occur in any setting (Scott, n.d.). Lateral worker-on-worker violence, also referred to as incivility or bullying, is one of the most common reasons that nurses give for leaving the profession. Incivility is defined as being rude or discourteous while bullying is an intentional effort to offend, intimidate, or humiliate a coworker and creates a hostile work environment (Rose, 2015). Bullying can "include hostile remarks, verbal attacks, taunting, verbal intimidation, and withholding support" (Rose, 2015, para. 4). In the past, these behaviors were often tolerated from physicians because other health professionals knew that they did not have the power to change them. The Institute for Safe Medication Practices (2013) has identified disrespectful behavior or incivility as contributing to errors in healthcare and client mortality. The person who fears being the subject of verbal abuse may delay communicating about a problem and the person who feels free to be disrespectful of a colleague may carry that disrespect into ignoring concerns about the client.

While disruptive behavior may occur from a person in a more powerful position, there is a lot of research demonstrating the destructive power of horizontal violence or nurse-to-nurse verbal abuse. As noted earlier in the chapter, it is a common reason for nurses to leave their job and/or the profession. There are many articles and resources available to help nurses learn how to effectively handle horizontal violence or incivility from coworkers.

Why do disruptive and uncivil behaviors continue? There are many contributing factors, including individual characteristics, healthcare and societal culture, and a stressful work environment (Institute for Safe Medication Practices, 2013). The bottom line must be that regardless of why it happens, disruptive and uncivil behaviors must be stopped.

Employers have a duty to create a safe and effective working environment. Establishing a culture of civility toward one another and a zero tolerance policy toward disruptive behavior are steps that employers and nurses must take (ANA, 2015). When such policies are established, education of all staff will be needed to underscore the components of civil and respectful behavior and to sensitize people to the problem. Everyone can be encouraged to be part of the solution. Familiarize yourself with your employer's policies; there may be policies regarding collegial behaviors and reporting mechanisms for disruptive behavior.

Scott (n.d.) suggests the following general strategies to establish a more equitable workplace initially. Nurses must assess themselves and identify their own feelings about self-worth. They must recognize their own potential for verbal abuse toward others and deal ethically with one another. She suggests that nurses must be willing to engage rather than avoid conflict when disruptive behaviors occur. The only person who benefits from silence and avoidance is the disruptor. Specific actions a nurse should take regarding disruptive behaviors are similar to those suggested above for sexual harassment. Address the behavior at the time it occurs in a clear, calm manner. Describe the behavior and its effect on you and your ability to function. Ask for that behavior to stop. Longo (2010) suggests that confronting an individual in private may yield better results. When personal efforts are not successful, you should talk with your manager about the situation. Managers also have responsibilities to work with disruptive behaviors. Making a plan and taking action are essential. The aggressor should be confronted and formal written complaints filed when appropriate. Legal action may be needed. Keep good personal records with details of the incident, the time, the circumstances, and a listing of any witnesses. Nurses need not remain powerless regarding situations of workplace abuse.

Nurses must work together to not succumb to intimidation. Some hospitals have initiated what they are calling a code white, which is a signal for others to come and be observers when an individual begins any type of verbal abuse. This verbal abuse might consist of insults, a personal attack, a temper tantrum, or a tirade. These people are witnesses and provide emotional support to the recipient of abuse. Administrators, nurses, and other employees (including physicians) must also learn not to turn their backs to abuse occurring in the environment. They have both ethical and legal (in the case of administrators) responsibilities for the workplace and for creating a civil, respectful culture **(Fig. 13.3)**.

Figure 13.3. Good manners and respectful behavior are important for a healthy work environment.

Violence in the Workplace

Most nursing students think of hospitals as places where victims of violence are helped. Rarely do they think of themselves as potential victims of violence in their own workplace. The CDC (n.d.) recognizes four types of workplace violence for nurses: (1) criminal intent where the nurse is assaulted or mugged while leaving work or while working in the community; (2) client-on-worker violence where the nurse is assaulted by a client, visitor, or family member; (3) lateral worker-on-worker violence; and (4) personal relationship violence when an acquaintance of the nurse comes into the work environment. The majority of workplace violence incidents are assaults by clients on nursing staff, and more client assaults occur in psychiatric mental health settings than in other settings. Assaults on staff members by visitors and outsiders also occur; most of these take place in emergency rooms. Violence is very costly when costs of treatment, lost work time, and even loss of an educated professional to healthcare are considered.

OSHA has issued guidelines for use by facilities trying to establish a safer workplace. These are not enforceable rules but may represent what is termed the "General Duty" clause (Section 5(a)(1) in the OSHA Act [OSHA, 1970]). The guidelines call for clear programs designed to protect workers. These programs would include an assessment and analysis of the workplace for hazards and a plan for prevention of problems.

One form of prevention is to train employees in the management of hostile and violent behavior. Ways of identifying hostile and assaultive clients should be developed so that staff can be warned to take extra personal safety precautions. The ANA released a position statement on

Incivility, Bullying, and Workplace Violence in 2015 that outlines the definitions, consequences, and recommended interventions that align with the CDC training on Workplace Violence Prevention for Nurses. There are many valuable resources available to nurses and healthcare providers to learn how to prevent and handle workplace violence.

Other important environmental safeguards include the use of such devices as metal detectors, panic buttons, and bulletproof glass, where appropriate. Adequate staff to manage potentially violent behavior is of particular concern in psychiatric/mental health settings. The addition of security personnel is important in some environments. There should be an attitude throughout the institution of zero tolerance for abusive or assaultive behavior.

In addition to preventing and managing problem situations, there should be clear guidelines for reporting both verbal and physical abuse and following through on all complaints. Healthcare institutions should work with law enforcement professionals when abusive or assaultive behavior occurs to ensure that legal procedures are carried out correctly.

Those who report incidents should receive support and assistance and be assured that there will be no reprisals or blaming. Some nurses have been reluctant to report verbal and physical abuse or assault because of personal and institutional beliefs that healthcare employees should be able to handle these behaviors independently. Another common belief in healthcare environments is that all behavior has meaning for the individual and that employees should accept inappropriate behaviors on the part of clients. Social constraints and adverse consequences related to inappropriate behavior are a valuable ally in redirecting the behaviors of those who are cognitively impaired, mentally ill, or developmentally delayed. Nurses need support from their work environments in accessing these avenues to protect themselves.

Critical Thinking Activity: Verbal Abuse in the Workplace
A client's family member is yelling at you for "providing poor care" and threatening legal action. Formulate an appropriate response to experiencing this type of verbal abuse in the workplace. Include specific statements you would use and each step you would take if the verbal abuse occurred again.

Stegen & Sowerby Stories: Part 2

Sally initially felt demoralized by her coworker's comment about not organizing her care appropriately, but after speaking with her mentor she decided to let those feelings go and concentrate on how she could learn from the experience and improve the care she provided. A few months later while Sally is giving report to the same nurse, Sally notices that she has forgotten to remove a catheter per the physician's orders because of more pressing multiple demands from other clients. When Sally points out to the nurse that she missed removing the catheter the nurse says, "Wow, you just can't seem to get this job figured out, can you?"

What should Sally's response be to this incivility? What are Sally's options in dealing with this coworker? Read the rest of the story at www.thePoint.com.

Want to Know More?

A variety of resources are available on thePoint° to enhance your learning and understanding of this chapter, such as:

- Full Stegen & Sowerby Stories
- NCLEX-Style Student Review Questions
- Journal Articles
- Case Studies
- Learning Objectives
- Relevant Websites
- And more...

KEY CONCEPTS

- The process of moving from novice to expert has been divided into five stages: novice, advanced beginner, competent, proficient, and expert.
- Reality shock occurs when an idealistic new graduate enters the real world of practice and has difficulty with the expectations and demands found there. You can prepare for the stress created by this transition through attending to your own expectations and developing personal strategies for coping including self-appraisal; evaluating employers; seeking mentors, preceptors, or coaches; joining a peer support group; and using personal stress management strategies.
- Burnout is a stress response experienced by nurses and others who work in occupations that make many emotional demands. Burnout may be alleviated by planned actions. In some instances, it may be necessary to change job settings when stress accumulates.
- Occupational safety and health are special concerns for nurses because of the infectious nature of the illnesses with which they come in contact, the toxicity of some chemicals in the nursing environment, and the potential for musculoskeletal injury and violence.
- Nurses who experience a work-related injury must carefully follow all relevant rules and regulations for reporting the injury, completing appropriate forms, and seeking care to ensure that they receive assistance for any medical care and lost wages.
- Nurses may see discrimination in the workplace manifested as racial/ethnic discrimination, wage discrimination against women, and job opportunity discrimination against men.
- Sexual harassment in the workplace is illegal. Understanding how to defend oneself against sexual harassment provides a greater feeling of personal power and control in the situation.
- Disruptive behavior contributes to client safety concerns as well as to an aversive workplace where individuals decide to leave nursing. Administrative authorities should act to stop all types of disruptive behavior, but nurses working collectively can also act to decrease the impact of disruptive behavior.
- Violence in the workplace is found in healthcare settings as well as the rest of society. Nurses working individually and collectively can develop strategies to combat this serious concern.

NCLEX-STYLE PRACTICE QUESTIONS

1. The symptoms of burnout include: (Select all that apply)

   A. Rashes
   B. Depression
   C. Anger
   D. Exhaustion

2. What makes a good mentee?

   A. Always be on time, honest, and hardworking
   B. Willing to accept feedback and make changes
   C. Be hardworking, caring, and work extra shifts
   D. Have a positive attitude and act in a caring manner

3. What are some potential workplace safety issues? (Select all that apply)

   A. Inadequate nurse staffing ratios
   B. Transmission of infection
   C. Musculoskeletal stress and injuries
   D. Inadequate food choices for meals

4. Place the following in the appropriate order for responding to sexual harassment.

   A. Speak to your supervisor _____
   B. Speak to human resources _____
   C. Ask the person to stop _____
   D. Make a written record _____

5. What are things you can do to create a civil work environment? (Select all that apply)

   A. Be respectful
   B. Don't gossip
   C. Mind your own business
   D. Take action when needed

REFERENCES

Academy of Medical-Surgical Nurses (AMSN). (2012). *AMSN mentoring program.* Retrieved from https://www.amsn.org/sites/default/files/documents/professional-development/mentoring/AMSN-Mentoring-Mentor-Guide.pdf

AHC Media. (2013). Safe lifting becomes standard practice. *Hospital Employee Health: The Practical Guide to Keeping Health Care Workers Healthy.* Retrieved from http://www.nursingworld.org/FunctionalMenuCategories/MediaResources/ANA-in-the-News/Archived-ANA-News/Safe-lifting-becomes-standard-practice.pdf

AHRQ. (2004). Hospital nurse staffing and quality care. *Research in Action: Agency for Healthcare Research and Quality,* 14. Retrieved from https://archive.ahrq.gov/research/findings/factsheets/services/nursestaffing/nursestaff.pdf

American Association of Colleges of Nursing (AACN). (2015). *Fact sheet: Enhancing diversity in the nursing workforce.* Retrieved July 23, 2017, from http://www.aacn.nche.edu/media-relations/diversityFS.pdf

American Nurses Association. (1993). *Position statement: Sexual harassment.* Retrieved March 23, 2010, from http://www.nursingworld.org/harassmentps.aspx

American Nurses Association. (2004). *Handle with care.* Retrieved from http://www.nursingworld.org/MainMenuCategories/OccupationalandEnvironmental/occupationalhealth/handlewithcare/hwc.aspx

American Nurses Association. (2015). *Position statement on incivility, bullying, and workplace violence.* Retrieved from https://www.nursingworld.org/~49baac/globalassets/practiceand-policy/nursing-excellence/official-policy-statements/ana-wpv-position-statement-2015.pdf

American Nurses Association. (n.d.). *Safe staffing saves lives.* Retrieved March 13, 2010, from http://www.safestaffingsaveslives.org

Benner, P. (1984). *From novice to expert: Excellence and power in clinical nursing practice* (Commemorative edition 2001). Upper Saddle River, NJ: Prentice Hall.

Brent, N. J. (2016). Workplace safety a must for nurses. *Nurse.com.* Retrieved from https://www.nurse.com/blog/2016/11/16/what-nurses-need-to-know-about-workplace-safety/

Centers for Disease Control and Prevention (CDC). (2017a). Get vaccinated. *Influenza (Flu).* Retrieved July 20, 2017, from https://www.cdc.gov/flu/consumer/vaccinations.htm

Centers for Disease Control and Prevention (CDC). (2017b). Transmission-based precautions. *Infection Control.* Retrieved July 20, 2017, from https://www.cdc.gov/infectioncontrol/basics/transmission-based-precautions.html

Centers for Disease Control and Prevention (CDC). (n.d.). *Workplace violence prevention of nurses.* Retrieved July 25, 2017, from https://wwwn.cdc.gov/wpvhc/Course.aspx/Slide/Unit1_5

Derby-Davis, M. J. (2014). Predictors of nursing faculty's job satisfaction and intent to stay in academe. *Journal of Professional Nursing, 30*(1), 19–25. http://dx.doi.org/10.1016/j.profnurs.2013.04.001

Dreyfus, S. E., & Dreyfus, H. L. (1980). *A five-stage model of the mental activities involved in directed skill acquisition.* Unpublished report supported by the Air Force Office of Scientific Research (AFSC), USAF (Contract F49620-79-C-0063), University of California at Berkeley, 1980 (as reported in P. Benner [1984], *From Novice to Expert*, Upper Saddle River, NJ: Prentice Hall).

Equal Employment Opportunity Commission (EEOC). (n.d.). *Sexual harassment.* Retrieved July 20, 2017, from https://www.eeoc.gov/laws/types/sexual_harassment.cfm

Grote, T. (2015). *Nursing turnover estimated to be 33% in the first three years.* American Association of International Healthcare Recruitment. http://www.aaihr.org/blogpost/1288345/227334/Nursing-turnover-estimated-to-be-33-in-the-first-three-years

Hezaveh, M. S., Rafii, F., & Seyedfatemi, N. (2014). Novice nurses' experiences of unpreparedness at the beginning of the work. *Global Journal of Health Science, 6*(1), 215–222. http://www.doi.org 10.5539/gjhs.v6n1p215

Institute for Safe Medication Practices. (2013). *Disrespectful behavior in healthcare...Have we made any progress in the last decade?* Retrieved July 25, 2017, from https://www.ismp.org/newsletters/acutecare/showarticle.aspx?id=52

Kramer, M. (1979). *Reality shock.* St. Louis, MO: CV Mosby.

Kus, R. J. (1985). Stages of coming out: An ethnographic approach. *Western Journal of Nursing Research, 7*(2), 177–194.

Lin, C. (2015). Impact of gratitude on resource development and emotional well-being. *Social Behavior and Personality, 43*(3), 493–504. http://dx.doi.org/10.2224/sbp.2015.43.3.493

Longo, J. (2010). Combating disruptive behaviors: Strategies to promote a healthy work environment. *OJIN: The Online Journal of Issues in Nursing, 15*(1), Manuscript 5. doi: 10.3912/OJIN.Vol15No01Man05. Retrieved from www.nursingworld.org/MainMenuCategories/ANAMarketplace/ANAPeriodicals/OJIN/TableofContents/Vol152010/No1Jan2010.aspx

Maslach, C., Jackson, S. E., & Leiter, M. P. (1997). Maslach burnout inventory manual. In Zalaquett, C. P., & Wood, R. J. (Eds). *Evaluating stress: A book of resources* (pp. 191–218). New York: Scarecrow Press.

Mensik, J. (2014). What every nurse should know about staffing. *American Nurse Today, 9*(2). Retrieved from https://www.americannursetoday.com/what-every-nurse-should-know-about-staffing/

Occupational Safety and Health Administration (OSHA). (2013). *Worker safety in your hospital.* Retrieved from https://www.osha.gov/dsg/hospitals/documents/1.1_Data_highlights_508.pdf

Pellico, H., Brewer, C. S., & Kovner, C. T. (2009, July). What newly licensed registered nurses have to say about their first experiences. *Nursing Outlook, 57*(4), 194–203.

Reed, K. (2013). Nursing fatigue and staffing costs: What's the connection? *Nursing Management, 44*(4), 47–50. https://doi.org/10.1097/01.numa.0000428198.52507.0a

Roberts, B. S., & Mann, R. A. (n.d.). *Sexual harassment in the workplace: A primer.* Retrieved March 21, 2010, from www3.uakron.edu/lawrev/robert1.html

Rose, J. F. (2015). *Nurse incivility and bullying: How to know the difference.* Retrieved from https://www.travel-nursing.com/news/features-and-profiles/nurse-incivility-and-bullying-how-to-know-the-difference/

Scott, D. (n.d.). *10 tips for addressing disruptive behavior at work.* Center for the American Nurse, Webinar. Retrieved from www.centerforamericannurses.org/displaycommon.cfm?an=1&subarticlenbr=195

Sullivan, E. (2002). In a women's world. *Reflections on Nursing Leadership, 28*(3), 10–17.

United States Bureau of the Census. (2013). *Men in nursing occupations: American community survey highlight report.* Retrieved from https://www.census.gov/people/io/files/Men_in_Nursing_Occupations.pdf

United States Department of Labor. Occupational Health and Safety Administration (OSHA). (1970). *Occupational Health and Safety Act (1970) Section 5 Duties.* Retrieved December 28, 2010, from http://www.osha.gov/pls/oshaweb/owadisp.show_document?p_table=OSHACT&p_id=3359

Wojciechowski, M. (2016, November 14). Male nurses confronting stereotypes and discrimination: Part 1, the issues. *Minority Nurse.* Retrieved from http://minoritynurse.com/male-nurses-confronting-stereotypes-and-discrimination-part-1-the-issues/

CHAPTER 14

Valuing the Political Process

After completing this chapter, you should be able to:

1. Explain why it is beneficial for nurses to have knowledge about and be involved in the political process.
2. Review seven ways an individual might influence the political process.
3. Summarize the various ways in which the United States federal government is involved in healthcare.
4. Outline common state legislative concerns.
5. Describe common local political concerns.
6. Explain why there are so many nursing organizations.
7. Report the major purpose of each nursing organization presented in the chapter.
8. Analyze the ways that nursing organizations seek to affect the healthcare delivery system and the political processes that control healthcare delivery.
9. Explain how politics is relevant to your participation in organizations.

Allocation of resources
Appropriations act
Authorization act
Conditions of participation
Department of Health and Human
    Services (DHHS)
Hatch Act
Lobbying

Nurses Strategic Action Team (N-STAT)
Occupational Safety and Health
    Act (OSHA)
Omnibus Budget Reconciliation Act
    (OBRA)
Political action committees (PACs)
Politics
Tri-Council for Nursing

Stegen & Sowerby Stories: Part 1

Kim has started working at a local hospital on the surgical unit since his graduation from nursing school. Recently, the hospital administration began discussing the need for mandatory overtime for nurses due to a shortage of staff. Kim is concerned as he already works more than 40 hours each week and has other responsibilities outside of work that he will not have time for if he has to work more hours. He wonders how and if he can have an influence on the decision by administration.

- Does the individual nurse have a voice?
- What are some possible ways for Kim to get involved with the discussion and potential decision on mandatory overtime by his hospital administration?
- What would you recommend?

Politics is the way in which people in any society try to influence decision-making and the **allocation of resources** (money, time, and personnel). Because resources are limited, it is necessary to make choices regarding their use. There is no perfect process for making optimum choices, because whenever one valuable option is chosen, some other option must be left out. Politics is a part of every organization and a part of government at every level. In a democratic society, all individuals can choose to be involved at some level in this decision-making process. This chapter presents the political process, discusses some of the current issues regarding political decisions, and describes how nurses can play a role in the political arena and in nursing organizations.

RELEVANCE OF THE POLITICAL PROCESS FOR NURSES

Nurses have always been involved in politics. Florence Nightingale used her contacts with powerful men in government to obtain support for traveling to the Crimea, including securing the supplies and the personnel she needed to care for wounded soldiers (Bostridge, 2008). Hannah Ropes was able to fight incompetence and obtain decent care for wounded Civil War soldiers because she understood who was influential in Washington and who would be receptive to her efforts on the soldiers' behalf (American Association for History of Nursing, Inc., 2007). Isabel Hampton used the buildup and excitement of the World's Fair and Columbian Exposition of 1893 to bring together nurse leaders to form the first nursing organization (ANA, 1996).

Modern times are no different. With many voices competing to be heard in the decision-making circles of any nation, the person who understands power and politics is the one most likely to obtain the resources needed to accomplish desired ends.

Decisions are made at federal, state, and local levels of government and with each healthcare agency. These decisions may be legislated or made by administrative bodies. Within organizations, these questions are answered by committees, managers, and governing boards.

Your practice as a nurse is controlled by a wide variety of governmental decisions. One of the most basic is the Nurse Practice Act of your state or province as discussed in Chapter 3. All of the philosophic discussions about the role of the nurse must return to the reality of the nurse's role as legally defined in the state's practice act. Do you care what that role is now or what changes are made in it? Does it make any difference to you what education that law requires, or if that law requires continuing education? Answering "yes" to any of these questions emphasizes the relevance of the political process for you.

Knowing where the decision-making occurs, who makes the decision, and being familiar with how you can influence that process is critical. Each governmental entity, agency, and organization has its own mechanism for operating. However, they share many similarities that can help you plan your activities.

Critical Thinking Activity: Investigate a Healthcare Issue
Identify a current healthcare issue in your state or province. Investigate that issue and form a position that you can support with data. Examine your position for personal biases.

INFLUENCING THE POLITICAL PROCESS

You can have an effect on such things as what healthcare legislation is submitted, the content of the legislation, and what legislation is passed. However, this does not happen without effort and action. As a result of a variety of societal factors, historically, women have been less active in politics than men. Gradually, women are assuming a more active role in politics: More are being appointed to the high offices within the government, more are running for and being elected to office, more work with policy-making bodies, and more vote. Because more than 90% of nurses are women (Rappleye, 2015), this changing social climate is important to nursing. It is vital that as nurses, we become aware of the issues so that we may have a positive influence on the political process.

Each person must determine his or her own level of personal involvement, but in the broad realm of the political process, there is room for everyone to find a suitable role. Some of these ways are outlined here and in Box 14.1.

Becoming Informed

To become informed about legislation and healthcare, you need to learn about the sources of available information. Each source of information is valuable to you but should be weighed

---

BOX 14.1 INFLUENCING THE POLITICAL PROCESS

- Become informed through a variety of sources.
- Vote for candidates or ballot issues that reflect your concerns.
- Vote for officers within professional or political organizations.
- Express your opinions through letters or in public forums.
- Communicate directly with legislators and public officials.
- Work for or contribute to nonlobbying nursing organizations or political action committees.
- Work for or contribute to candidates who represent your views.
- Testify before decision-making bodies.

based on its known biases. Even the most objective-sounding report can be biased, not only in what is reported but also in what is not reported. Identifying the groups that support or oppose a particular viewpoint might help you to recognize bias. Determine whether a group and its members would tend to gain or lose personally by the passage of proposed legislation. Are special interest groups voicing an opinion? When biases are evident, it is advisable to obtain information from groups with divergent viewpoints. Decisions based on firm factual data are more likely to benefit the entire group, organization, or society as a whole.

Once you are informed about the current issues in legislation or in an organization, you are better prepared to form personal opinions about them and try to influence the outcome of the political process. A wide variety of resources are available.

News Media

The daily newspaper, weekly newsmagazine, and online news reports can be excellent sources of information about significant legislation being proposed, about controversial issues, or about an issue that has attracted widespread interest.

Television and radio news reports are usually quite brief and give only an overview of a particular piece of legislation being introduced. This overview may be helpful in alerting you to something that you will want to study more intensively. Often radio commentators, network talk shows, and social media posts speak from a particular viewpoint or bias. Remember to weigh information in light of that viewpoint and seek information more broadly. Some television programs, such as those on public television, do discuss issues in depth with commentators who hold different positions on an issue. These programs usually make an attempt to present both sides of any issue.

Specialized Publications

Voters' pamphlets are prepared by many governmental jurisdictions. These pamphlets may introduce each candidate for office and contain a brief candidate statement regarding their platform. Endorsements by groups are often included to help the reader better understand the position taken by the candidate. When issues are on the ballot, both a "pro" statement and a "con" statement are provided. The individuals and groups supporting each position may be identified.

Professional journals usually devote some space to current legislative issues. This is done routinely in *American Journal of Nursing* and *The American Nurse* in the United States and in *Canadian Nurse* in Canada. When major issues are being debated, other nursing periodicals often contain articles of interest. The journals of other healthcare professions also may carry information regarding current nursing issues. Web sites such as the ANA's www.nursingworld.org will usually have pages devoted to any major healthcare issue. Newsletters and journals of organizations that have a political focus provide information on what they see as current issues. These organizations include consumer groups such as Common Cause, political groups such as the Young Democrats and Young Republicans, and nonpartisan groups such as the League of Women Voters. Magazines directed to special interest groups, such as *AARP The Magazine* for those over the age of 50 years, carry articles related to political issues that would be of particular interest to that group.

Copies of legislation are usually available through your congressional representatives (for federal matters) and your state or provincial representatives (for state/provincial matters).

They are also available online at your legislature's Web site. Along with copies of the legislation, a legislator may send other informational material. Government agencies affected by proposed legislation may also provide information about the legislation's potential effects, although they are not allowed to try to influence legislation. You will find it helpful to understand the process of how a bill becomes a law to recognize where and when communication with a legislator might influence the process. Project Vote Smart (n.d.) provides an overview of this process that you might wish to review (https://votesmart.org/education/how-a-bill-becomes-law#. WXkESYjyvIU).

Online Resources

Online resources are an increasingly useful source of information. Some common ones were mentioned in the discussion above. In addition, there are specialized sites that may be useful to you. Federal legislation can be found at http://thomas.loc.gov/, a site maintained in the public interest by Congress. In most states, the text of bills being introduced is available on a governmental Web site, where you can read the bill on the computer or print the document to read. You can access state sites by going to www.loc.gov/rr/news/stategov/stategov.html.

Nursing and healthcare organizations that maintain Web sites often have a site devoted to political issues affecting members of the organization or relevant issues that affect healthcare. The American Nurses Association (ANA), for example, maintains a legislative Web site at http://nursingworld.org/DocumentVault/GOVA/default.aspx. Many news organizations (television stations, newspapers, and magazines) maintain Web sites with information on current issues. Project Vote Smart provides data on candidates and issues for both federal and state elections. Any of these sites may provide links to still more sites that provide useful information. There are also individuals and organizations that maintain Web sites with information and opinion. Investigating bias in these resources is critical and requires careful analysis.

Organizational Meetings

Nursing organizations and other health-related organizations, as well as community groups, sometimes hold open meetings to present and discuss legislative issues. Often, knowledgeable speakers can help you to understand what is being proposed and the potential effects of a proposal. These organizations may also sponsor email networks to get out information on important pending legislation. Nursing organizations can be excellent sources of information because they often are in touch with legislators and legislative staff.

Voting

Your individual vote on a ballot issue is significant (Fig. 14.1). Recent major elections in the United States have demonstrated the importance of every vote. According to the United States Census Bureau Survey of Voting and Registration (2017), in the 2016 elections, only 64.1% of those eligible to vote were registered to vote and only 56% of those eligible to vote actually voted. Nurses, as a group, are thought to vote in higher percentages than the general population, which may relate to a higher educational level among nurses. Although you cannot vote directly on legislative issues, you can vote for candidates whose positions you support on initiatives and referendums and who share your values. Absentee ballots are always available for those who cannot be present at their polling place on the day of an election. These ballots must

Figure 14.1. Voting is one avenue of political involvement.

be requested well in advance of the election, however. In many jurisdictions, you may elect to vote by mail; in some, it is the only option.

Voting for officers in organizations may be ignored by a large majority of members. They look at the ballot, are unfamiliar with those running for office, and therefore do not vote. Most organizations do make an attempt to introduce members to the various candidates. If you do not know the candidates, you can seek information about them by reading their prepared statements of position and learning about their previous activities. Those elected to office usually determine the direction and priorities of an organization. If you are paying dues, you want to have a voice in choosing those who are entrusted with making the decisions.

Shaping Public Opinion

Public opinion does influence the actions of legislators and regulatory bodies. As an RN, you can help to shape public opinion; your judgment about matters that affect healthcare can help others make their own decisions. Share the knowledge you have gained through your personal experience and research. Do not be afraid to state your own position, although you must be prepared to support your position with evidence if you want to be considered a thoughtful healthcare professional. Certainly, you will not want to make every social occasion an opportunity to share political positions, but do take advantage of opportunities that arise to present your concerns to others

Another means of shaping public opinion is by writing a letter to the editor of a newspaper or newsmagazine. Editorial letters are read by many people. The suggestions in Box 14.2 will maximize your chances of appearing in print.

BOX 14.2 WRITING LETTERS TO THE EDITOR

- Carefully follow the instructions provided by the publication for letters to the editor. These usually will refer to length, signature, address, and telephone number. Typically, letters should be short and to the point, about 200 to 300 words.
- Clearly present your opinion with well-reasoned arguments. Make only one point per letter.
- Including personal experiences that illustrate healthcare concerns can be useful; however, be careful that healthcare examples do not violate the confidentiality of clients or divulge confidential information regarding your employer.
- Use a direct but respectful tone. Avoid personal attacks on others.
- Include your name, address, and phone number as well as your nursing credentials after your name.
- If responding to a particular article, give the title of the article and include the date of publication in parentheses.

Within an organization, you may also influence opinion and action by clearly presenting reasoned arguments. You can discuss issues with other members and present your opinion at meetings. Remember that a viewpoint supported by strong, reasoned judgment, facts, and rationale will be better received than a simple statement of opinion.

Communicating With Legislators and Officials

Legislators are affected by the views of their constituents. The legislator's staff reviews incoming letters, tabulates views, and directs letters with significant opinions or information to the legislator for individual consideration. Although some groups encourage members to sign form letters or postcards, personal letters have a greater impact. A carefully written personal letter reflecting thoughtful and informed opinions on an issue will receive the most attention from any governmental person or department. As an RN, your expertise can provide a valuable viewpoint. Identify yourself as an RN in your letter and outline why you are concerned about the issue in question. Legislators often appreciate personal anecdotes from your practice (with client/family privacy protected, of course) that underscore your point. The names and addresses of your congressional representatives are available on the Senate and House Web sites. Go to https://www.usa.gov/ and link to the House or Senate. These sites also explain who serves on which committees. Canada maintains a similar site at https://www.canada.ca/en.html.

Concern regarding the rules and regulations of a specific department of government can be addressed to the officials of that department. Communication from concerned citizens can be as important to them as it is to legislators. To be most effective, letters addressed to officials should reflect the same care and professional viewpoint as those addressed to legislators.

Many governmental agencies, both legislative and regulatory, accept letters in the form of email. Email has the advantage of being extremely timely. However, be aware of the rules for Internet usage at your facility. Although you may have email access at your place of work, your employer may not allow you to use it for political activity. If you are employed by a government entity, such as a public health department, the law prohibits you from using governmental resources such as email for political activity.

An email message should be composed as carefully as a letter. One important point is to include your full name and home address in your message. Staff members review the address, forwarding only those messages that are personally identifiable and noting those from a congressperson's district. Do remember that email is public. Do not state things in an email that would make you feel uncomfortable to present in public. See Box 14.3 for an example.

You may make a telephone call to a legislator's office. Staff members keep a record of all calls, and the positions of callers are noted. To call a member of Congress, contact the United States Capitol Switchboard at (202) 224-3121 and ask for the individual's office. In some states, a toll-free number is maintained for calls to state legislators during the legislative session. You will be asked to leave a message. Be sure to identify yourself fully, including both your name and address. State the bill or issue about which you are calling and clearly state your position.

Visiting congressional or state representatives is also an effective means of expressing your concerns. One of the best ways to arrange to speak with congressional representatives and senators is to contact their local offices. Through these offices, you may receive assistance in arranging your visit. Staff members may help you to arrange other interesting and valuable activities, such as attending committee hearings, taking tours, and observing Congress in session. Make appointments well in advance, as representatives and senators have busy schedules. If your time is limited, you may have to modify your expectations and meet with a staff member who will relay your concerns. Plan your visit carefully; it is helpful to write out concerns and questions. Be sure to leave time for answers to the questions that you pose. Even when you disagree with the position taken by your legislator, be polite and present your concerns calmly. Rudeness could result in the legislator's unwillingness to listen to what you have to say.

BOX 14.3 A CAREFULLY WRITTEN EMAIL

Subject: House Bill 1458 Safe Client Handling

Dear Representative Smith:

As an RN constituent in your legislative district, I urge you to support passage of this important legislation. As a nurse in a hospital, I am familiar with the care needs of dependent individuals. Unfortunately, the current solution to care has been to urge care providers to lift and move clients, resulting in injuries, lost work, and even lost careers for the caregivers. I personally know two RNs who have become unable to work as nurses after sustaining back injuries in moving incapacitated clients. In addition to the human cost, the community cannot sustain the loss of needed RNs when there is such a shortage. There are now many effective lifting and transfer devices available for purchase. This legislation will provide the impetus for healthcare agencies to purchase them and implement their use. Thank you for your attention to this important matter.

Mary K. Winslow, RN
2314 12th Ave.
Seattle, WA 98201
Phone: (206) 981-1234

Some legislators hold public meetings (often referred to as town hall meetings) in their legislative districts for the purpose of hearing from their constituents. These meetings can be an opportunity both to learn about issues and the legislator's current position and to give input regarding issues of concern to you. If you bring written materials to support your viewpoint, these may be given to the legislator and further reinforce your position. These same activities may be useful in working within an organization. Those elected to office do not know the views of members unless communication occurs. For communication to be effective, you must know when and where boards meet, how to get information to board members, and the names of those responsible for specific aspects of the organization's operations.

Critical Thinking Activity: Lend Your Support!
Identify a current political issue about which you feel strongly. Write a letter or an email to a governmental official (local, state, or federal) that provides a sound rationale in support of your position. Ask someone else to review it for you and then send it.

Group Action

The political process in the nursing profession takes many forms. Nurses can be involved as individuals, but they are far more effective when they work in groups (**Fig. 14.2**). Because nursing is the largest single healthcare occupation, nurses have many votes. For this reason, legislators pay attention to positions held by groups of nurses.

Nonlobbying Nursing Organization Efforts

Most traditional nursing organizations are nonprofit groups and therefore are limited in their political activity. The major role of nonprofit groups in politics involves testifying to facts, organizational positions, and concerns in the healthcare arena. The ANA has an office in Washington, DC and tries to keep the nursing profession informed about legislative matters of importance in healthcare. The ANA also provides experts in the nursing profession who testify before congressional and regulatory groups about proposed legislation.

The **Tri-Council for Nursing** is a collaborative effort of four organizations: the ANA, the National League for Nursing (NLN), the American Organization of Nurse Executives (AONE), and the American Association of Colleges of Nursing (AACN) joined in support of nursing practice, education, and research. By working collaboratively, these organizations have strengthened the voice of nursing and its visibility in Washington, DC. This coalition has become the trusted representation for nursing. Legislators rely on the information it provides and recognize it as a united voice for the nursing profession.

The ANA organized the **Nurses Strategic Action Team (N-STAT)** to provide nurses with a means to mobilize quickly to influence legislative policy. This organization promotes grassroots involvement in legislative issues, meets with members of Congress, and organizes letter writing and telephone campaigns. Interested nurses can sign up to be a part of N-STAT on the http://www.nursingworld.org Web site. Those registered with N-STAT receive a message about an issue of importance along with information and resources on how to contact legislators. N-STAT includes thousands of nurses. You can imagine that receiving thousands of letters about a single topic might get the attention of a legislator.

Together we are a force to be reckoned with!

Figure 14.2. Nurses have more power in a group than as an individual.

Many specialty nursing organizations have a political action interest as well. Their Web sites and publications often provide information about issues of concern, and the organization may provide expert testimony for legislators.

Most state and district nurses' associations have legislative committees that monitor legislative and regulatory actions in their areas. They may provide educational events for nurses regarding current issues and testify at hearings concerning health-related issues. They also may seek to mobilize letter writing or telephone campaigns.

Political Action Committees

Lobbying is the process of attempting to influence legislators to take a particular action. The law differentiates lobbying from providing general information and places restrictions on who can lobby. Nonprofit groups such as the ANA can provide information but cannot take direct action on behalf of specific candidates or partisan issues. To take a more active role in seeking the passage of desired legislation, the defeat of undesired measures, and the election of particular candidates, groups form organizations called **political action committees (PACs)**. These organizations are registered as political action groups and are free to try to affect the political process. They are not considered nonprofit organizations because their funds are used for political purposes; therefore, donations to them are not tax deductible.

The ANA political action organization is titled the ANA-Political Action Committee (ANA-PAC). ANA-PAC actually lobbies for the passage or defeat of bills and supports candidates for public office. Since the 1976 federal elections, ANA-PAC has raised funds to support candidates for the Senate and the House of Representatives based on their expressed and demonstrated stands on key health issues, such as funding for nursing and biomedical research, funding for nursing education, and third-party reimbursement for nurses. Not all candidates endorsed by ANA-PAC were supported financially because of the limited funds available. Candidates' successes are attributable to many factors, but the effect of nursing support has been demonstrated. Many state nursing associations also have political action organizations. These groups serve the same function on the state level as ANA-PAC does on the national level. Many candidates actively seek the endorsement of nursing organizations that are perceived as influential with voters.

Although these nursing political action groups have not grown rapidly, growth has been steady. In addition, nurses are gaining more sophistication in their approach to the political process. The power of nurses in the political sphere is increasing.

Critical Thinking Activity: What Are the Issues in Your State?
Locate your state nurses' association Web site. Identify the issues that the organization believes are important to nurses in the state. Investigate those issues and identify ways you could support one of the issues presented.

Other Politically Important Groups

Many organizations, in addition to those specifically related to nursing, are concerned about health and social issues. Some are official lobbying groups; others provide information resources. Groups such as Common Cause (a consumer lobbying group), AARP, the League of Women Voters, and even church organizations often act to affect the political process. You may support these groups by donating money for their needs or by being actively involved in their work.

Testifying for Decision-Making Bodies

Many decisions affecting nursing and healthcare are made by committees and commissions at various levels of government. These decision-making bodies often hold hearings to gather information before decisions are made. Your testimony as a nurse may have particular value in certain areas of healthcare. A nurse may testify either as an official representative of an organization or as an independent individual.

You may learn of opportunities to testify through announcements in the newspaper and professional publications. In general, you must register in advance to testify. In some instances, there is registration at the door before a meeting begins, but for more formal situations, you will need to notify the committee in advance that you wish to testify. Increasingly, you can sign up online to testify.

If you have an opportunity to testify, be sure to make your position clear so that the decision-makers know whether you speak for yourself or for a larger group. Keep your testimony brief and concise. Prepare your testimony ahead of time (with copies for committee members), but do not simply read a statement. A less-formal presentation is usually more interesting for the listener. Be prepared with sources for any facts or figures you present and explain any technical terms you use. Find out whether there is a time limit for each testimony. If you are given a time limit, make sure that you present your most important arguments and facts first. Most committees will accept written testimony if you cannot be there in person, but the personal presentation is usually more effective (Evidence-Based Practice 14.1).

Evidence-Based Practice 14.1: *Research and Its Effect on Government Policy*

McAuley, A., Best, D., Taylor, A., Hunter, C., & Robertson, R. (2012). From evidence to policy: The Scottish national naloxone programme. *Drugs: Education, Prevention & Policy*, *19*(4), 309–319. http://dx.doi.org/10.3109/09687637.2012.682232

This is a study that demonstrates how research can affect policy. This research can also be used in conjunction with studies from the United States and other countries to have an impact on local policy. In this study, the aim was to reduce the number of drug-related deaths to opiates in one small region of Scotland. This is a problem globally with Scotland having one of the highest drug-related death rates in Europe. The researchers wanted to know if providing naloxone, with training to friends and family would reduce drug-related deaths. The study results showed that by distributing naloxone and providing training on its use to family and friends of opiate users the drug-related death rate dropped from 20, prior to the study, to two after. Reference was made to other studies with similar results and discussion of how programs across Europe and America are being implemented to address this current health crisis.

Individual Support for Legislation and Candidates

You may choose to personally support a specific piece of legislation by contributing money for publicity and campaigning, posting political signs, visiting door-to-door, sponsoring coffee hours, or working on a committee that is striving for the passage of a proposal. Both time and money are valuable to every candidate. Funds are needed for newspaper ads, television and radio announcements, and printing and distributing literature. Workers may be needed to perform secretarial tasks, contact people in a door-to-door campaign, and speak on behalf of the issue.

Supporting a candidate for public office is accomplished in the same way. In our political system, the reality is that those who have actively supported a candidate during an election campaign are listened to more closely when decisions are being made. Working for a candidate is one way to make your view known. It is also an excellent way to gain firsthand knowledge of the political process.

Working in Policy-Making Agencies

Nurses have been appointed to major administrative positions in state and federal health agencies and to the staffs of several senators and representatives. In these roles, they have major policy-making responsibilities. Knowledgeable nurses may be appointed to task forces that study healthcare concerns and recommend regulatory or legislative action. The Robert Wood Johnson Foundation has provided 1-year fellowships for nurses to study policy in Washington, DC. Nurses who complete these fellowships have the skills and abilities to be effective in influencing healthcare policy. All of this points to nurses having a promising future in the health policy arena.

Theory Alert   Martha Rogers

Martha Rogers' nursing theory considered that clients were whole people and should not be divided into narrow definitions of illness or parts. Rogers was born in Texas in 1914. She received her diploma from a hospital diploma program in 1936. She went on to earn a degree in public health nursing from George Peabody College in 1937. She studied for her master's degree at Teachers College at Columbia University and received her degree in 1945. She earned a doctorate in nursing at Johns Hopkins University in Baltimore in 1954. She died in 1994.

Rogers' theory is called the Science of Unitary Human Beings. She defined health as an outward expression of the life process and believed that illness and health were part of a continuum with the client moving through life on that continuum. Rogers proposed that nursing was part science and part art and that the nurse could serve her clients using both the art and science of nursing. A big part of her teaching was that the client always be treated as a whole person and not just an illness. This focus on the bigger picture is valuable when considering the political process in nursing.

(Source: http://www.nursing-theory.org)

Seeking Election to an Office

Those elected or appointed to an office, whether in a local nursing organization or the United States Congress, have the power to affect outcomes considerably. Leaders in nursing organizations help to shape the direction and efforts of those organizations. Legislators have power to affect significant regulations and spending plans. Nurses in several states have been effective in shaping health policy by being elected to office as members of their state legislatures. Eddie Bernice Johnson, elected as a congresswoman from Texas in 1994, was the first nurse to hold an elective federal office and still serves in that role. The 115th Congress of 2016 has three nurses serving. As women in general become more politically visible, nursing as a whole feels the impact.

Limitations on Your Political Activity

If you are an employee of any government agency, such as a public health department or the Veterans Administration, your political activity is subject to restrictions that do not apply to the general public. Restrictions applying to federal government employees are defined in the **Hatch Act** (5 USCA 7324) revision of 1993 (Hatch Act, 1993). Prohibited activities are mainly those that have to do with supporting a particular political party by being an officer or party spokesperson. The Hatch Act also prohibits any political activity on the part of a government employee, on behalf of a party, or in support of legislation, which could be construed as representing his or her government agency.

The Hatch Act does not interfere with a private citizen's right to support parties and candidates financially, to join political parties, to work for or against measures that will appear on a ballot, or to participate in nonpartisan (ie, not connected with a political party) elections as a candidate.

Each state has its own version of the Hatch Act. If you are employed by a government agency of any kind, investigate the limitations that your employment may place on your political activity.

THE FEDERAL GOVERNMENT'S ROLE IN HEALTHCARE

Federal legislation affects nursing and healthcare in important ways. If you understand key concepts of the federal government's involvement in healthcare and how federal legislation affects healthcare delivery, you will be more effective in the political arena.

Federal Agencies Related to Healthcare

The federal government operates in the healthcare field in complex ways. Literally, dozens of federal agencies are involved with healthcare in some way. The **Department of Health and Human Services (DHHS)** is a cabinet-level administrative unit of the federal government with four major service divisions and many different sections. The Public Health Service, which includes the Centers for Disease Control and Prevention (CDC), is one agency with which you should already be familiar. The National Institutes of Health (NIH), the Food and Drug Administration (FDA), the Health Resources Administration (HRA), and the Center for Medical & Medicare Services (CMS) are all part of DHHS. This agency has tremendous impact through its rules and regulations and the projects it funds.

The Federal Budget Process

Because funding is a driving force in all decision-making, you will find it useful to understand something of the federal budget process. The availability of government funding for each federal program depends on two legislative actions: the **authorization act** (which outlines the actions to be taken) and the **appropriations act** (which provides the funding). Both the House and the Senate pass a budget appropriations act. Then, a joint House and Senate committee meet to achieve a compromise that both will accept. The final result is called the **Omnibus Budget Reconciliation Act (OBRA)**, and it includes the compromises the budget committee has worked out between the House and Senate versions of the budget. Each budget act—for example, OBRA 2004—is identified by the year in the title. This is sometimes confusing because two monetary amounts, the authorized amount and the final budgeted (or appropriated) amount, may be reported in connection with the same act.

The budget act may also place restrictions on the people and organizations receiving federal funds. It is under this authority that the federal government sets standards for nursing homes that receive reimbursement through Medicaid and Medicare. The rules and regulations for nursing homes, called the **conditions of participation** (COPs), included in OBRA 1987, were extensive and included such issues as restraint reduction, nursing assistant training, and resident privacy. These rules and regulations did not take effect until October 1, 1990. This allowed the affected organizations to begin the process of change to meet the new requirements. Conditions of participation for Medicare continue to have great effects on healthcare systems as they are revised.

Historically, a third factor has affected the amount of money available for a specific federal program: the participation of the executive branch of government in decisions regarding how and when available funds will be spent. If money that has been authorized and appropriated has not been spent by the end of a budget period, it is lost. This money then must be reauthorized and reappropriated. The executive branch has used this mechanism to withdraw support for programs it opposes.

Funding for Nursing Education and Research

Beginning in 1964, the federal government provided funding to support nursing education through the Nurse Training Act, later called the Nurse Education Act, signed by President Bush in 2002 as the Nurse Reinvestment Act. The most recent is the Title VIII Nursing Workforce Reauthorization Act of 2017. In the 1960s and early 1970s, the funding was generous and included money for buildings, classroom renovation, equipment, faculty education and development, and student scholarships and traineeships. The current nurse shortage has once again resulted in political pressure by nursing organizations for increased funds for nursing education.

A major advance for nursing research in the 1980s was the addition of a National Institute for Nursing Research (NINR) to the other major divisions of the NIH. It is now a major financial source of nursing research dollars. Nursing groups continue to lobby for increases in the appropriation for the NINR. However, even the existence of the NINR is not guaranteed. Proposals for reorganizing the work and research conducted in all areas of healthcare have included the elimination of many specialty institutes and a different method of focusing research. Many nurses view this proposal with alarm because nursing research does not claim the high profile of disease-specific research.

Occupational Safety and Health

The **Occupational Safety and Health Act (OSHA)** mandates actions and prescribes safety equipment to improve the health and safety of the working environment. Many people think that the rules and regulations created by OSHA are too cumbersome. Nevertheless, concern for the safety of the working person is of considerable importance to nurses. Occupational injuries create major health problems for the adult population. They are costly not only in terms of health and personal loss but also in terms of lost productivity. Nurses are also affected by the provisions of OSHA in their own work environments. They, too, are subject to injury and accident on the job. The safety concerns of nurses in the workplace are discussed in Chapter 13.

Nurses in occupational health nursing are involved in OSHA through educating workers about job safety. In some situations, using safety precautions may be time consuming and physically uncomfortable, and workers may be tempted to ignore them. Nurses may be able to curb this by helping workers understand the importance of following health and safety regulations. Occupational health nurses also assist management in planning to make the environment safe and in establishing appropriate procedures for treating injuries. OSHA regulations have required healthcare employers to provide the equipment, supplies, immunizations, and education to enable the implementation of CDC recommendations for universal precautions.

There is a general duty clause in the OSHA regulations stating that employers "must provide each employee a place of employment which is free from recognized hazards that are causing or likely to cause death or serious physical harm to his employees" (OSHA, n.d., Section 5A). Under this clause, if the hazard is recognized, if it can cause serious harm, and if there are reasonable methods to avoid that hazard, the employer may be cited for failure to maintain safety. This general duty clause is now being directed toward healthcare workplace concerns such as repetitive strain injuries and infection.

OSHA has been investigating the effects of repetitive strain injuries, among which are back injuries in healthcare workers. In 2003, the ANA launched *Handle With Care*, a campaign focusing on solutions to the problem of musculoskeletal injuries among caregivers. Since that time, some states have passed legislation regarding safe client handling in hospitals and nursing homes. Manufacturers are providing a greater variety of lifting and moving equipment, and many facilities are developing policies that promote greater safety in client handling. The National Institute for Occupational Safety and Health has information and programs available titled *Safe Client Handling* (NIOSH, n.d.) for teaching safe client handling. The ANA supports all of these different efforts with information and resources (http://nursingworld.org/handlewithcare).

Another serious occupational concern to nurses that was politically addressed was needlestick injuries. Based on control of blood-borne pathogens, the FY1999 appropriations bill required employers to record all injuries from potentially contaminated needles and other sharp instruments, and in 2000, legislation was passed to require hospitals to provide safer devices to prevent injury (NIOSH, 2014).

Another safety concern of healthcare workers is violence in the workplace. Nurses in psychiatric settings have long recognized the hazards they face in working with aggressive, violent, and sometimes out-of-control clients. Emergency rooms are sites where the violence of society spills over into the healthcare setting. Even obstetric units may encounter violence by family members. OSHA provides guidelines and tools to help prevent workplace violence by educating and helping to create a "culture of safety" (OSHA, n.d.). See Chapter 13 for a further discussion of violence in the workplace.

Communication in Action 14.1: *Mobilizing Support for Safety Measures in the Workplace*

Irma Gunderson was an RN in the emergency room of a large urban hospital. There had been several instances when friends of clients had become belligerent and threatening to the staff, but there were no plans in place for managing staff safety. Irma began talking with her nurse manager. She said, "I was here the two evenings when those visitors threatened doctors, nurses, and others on the staff. I believe that we need to develop policies of how to manage such instances." Her manager replied, "What is the problem? I wasn't here those evenings, but I think the staff did fine—no one was hurt and the client was cared for." Irma then said, "I was really afraid, and it is affecting my work. I have talked to some of the others on the evening shift and some of them even have nightmares. Millie the receptionist said she is going to ask for a transfer because she doesn't want to be here the next time it happens. We don't have a clear plan of how to call security, what people are supposed to do, and what our rights are in terms of protecting ourselves." The manager said, "No one else has said anything." Irma said, "I think they believe that nothing can be done. I have done some reading and I have learned that other hospitals have extensive plans in place. Could we get a committee together to investigate some of those and make some recommendations?" The manager said, "I appreciate your talking with me. I will talk with the management team tomorrow and maybe we can get something started here." By speaking directly to the person in charge who had the authority to initiate change, by having specific instances and concerns, Irma had facilitated improving the workplace climate.

Nursing Home Regulations

OBRA 1987 contained regulations that for the first time mandated a national standard for quality of care in nursing homes receiving federal money through Medicare or Medicaid with the provisions of this act set to take effect in October 1990. Because some of the requirements required additional time for implementation, some of the provisions of OBRA 1987 took effect as late as 1994. Despite earlier concerns, it is now clear that these regulations have positively affected the care environment in nursing homes. The use of restraints has decreased, resident rights are more effectively supported, and basic care needs are identified and met.

THE STATE GOVERNMENT'S ROLE IN HEALTHCARE

Many issues that vitally affect the healthcare arena are decided at the state level. Because the healthcare issues in each state are different, only some general areas of concern are outlined here.

State Agencies and Healthcare

State institutions range from those that care for the mentally challenged and the mentally ill to penal systems and institutions of higher education. Healthcare is a consideration in all of these settings. When budgets are planned, topics as diverse as immunization and contraception may be part of the debate. Nurses often can advocate for those who are unable to speak for themselves about their own healthcare needs. Sometimes nurses who work in state institutions are unable to deliver quality care because of severe budgetary deficiencies. All nurses can support efforts to provide quality healthcare in such settings.

State Legislative Concerns

Some of the major workplace concerns of nurses are emerging as topics of state legislation. The passage of any revision to the nurse practice act is an important state-level issue for nurses. See Chapter 3 for a discussion of nurse practice acts. The ANA has identified nine major state-level legislative issues of importance to nurses (Box 14.4). In some states, legislation has already been passed regarding some of these issues.

BOX 14.4 STATE-LEVEL LEGISLATIVE CONCERNS IDENTIFIED BY THE AMERICAN NURSES ASSOCIATION

- Prohibition of mandatory overtime
- Nurse staffing systems and ratios
- Nursing workforce data collection
- Nursing education incentives
- Ergonomics
- Needlestick injury prevention
- Nursing quality indicators
- Violence in the workplace
- Whistleblower protection

Concerns about the nurse's vulnerability when unsafe care is part of an institution's practice have led to efforts toward achieving whistleblower protection through legislation. Whistleblowing was discussed in Chapter 8. The state of New Jersey was the first to pass legislation that protects from retaliation healthcare employees who refuse to participate in or who report unsafe practices. A major whistleblowing event took place in Texas in 2009. The nurse lost her job and faced criminal charges. She was ultimately acquitted and the hospital administrator and several county officials received jail time for retaliation (Lowes, 2011). The result of this case was a national conversation about how whistle-blowers are protected and brought about changes within the state (Lowes, 2011).

Many of the state-level issues, such as prohibition of mandatory overtime, nursing staffing systems and ratios, and safety in the workplace, relate to increasing workplace satisfaction. Improving working conditions is an important aspect of addressing the nursing shortage. These issues are discussed in greater detail in Chapter 13.

LOCAL POLITICAL CONCERNS

In most communities, budgets for public health departments, school nurses, and so forth are developed over a period of several months. Hearings are often held, at which members of the public may ask questions and address issues. Nurses often have found that involvement at this planning stage is most rewarding. Determining priorities for healthcare is essential, and nurses can speak with authority on these matters. Nurses actually employed in a public department undergoing review may be limited in making their views known because of regulations governing their action in the political sphere. For this reason, it is significant that nurses outside of government institutions recognize the importance of community health. It is not only the practice of the public health nurse that is affected by the priorities of the agency. For example, a nurse who is employed in a hospital may wish to refer a discharged client to a public health nurse for follow-up, only to find that, owing to changes in the ordering of priorities, home visits for the identified purpose are no longer being made.

In many communities, decisions about the allocation of federal money are made at the local level. Recent congressional actions have leaned toward enhancing state and local control through creating large block grants where priorities would be decided locally. Support for alternative healthcare centers, blood pressure screening, and senior citizen centers may depend on whether those who are knowledgeable about the benefits of these services are willing to voice their advocacy in local decision-making bodies.

Daily Ethical Dilemma 14.1: Helping the Community or Self?

Monte is a nurse and he is the administrator for ABC Home Health. Monte also serves on the board at the local hospital. The CEO of the hospital approaches Monte after a board meeting to discuss the possibility of setting up a contract with ABC Home Health to provide follow-up care to heart failure clients in an attempt to reduce readmission rates to the hospital. Monte thinks this sounds like a great service to the community. However, the CEO would like Monte to reduce the charge of those visits to a rate that will cause ABC Home

Health to make very little money on each visit but in return for signing the contract the CEO will give Monte a substantial payment for the contract.

- What are the ethical principles involved in this scenario and why did you chose those principles? Why is this an ethical dilemma?
- Is Monte hurting anyone if he agrees to the contract? Who would he be helping if he takes the contract?
- What are some alternatives that Monte could propose to the hospital CEO that could remove the appearance of a conflict of interest for Monte?

FEDERAL HEALTHCARE REFORM LEGISLATION

Financing healthcare for all citizens has been the focus of many efforts for healthcare reform going back as far as the Franklin Roosevelt administration during World War II. In 1965, legislation instituted Medicare and provided health insurance for those over 65 years, the disabled, and special groups. Many saw this as the beginning of a drive toward universal healthcare. Through many administrations and congresses, the subject of healthcare reform continued to be raised and continued to be set aside.

In the 2010 landmark and controversial federal legislation, the Patient Protection and Affordable Care Act (also known as the ACA or Obamacare) was passed, which began the process of providing health coverage for all legal residents of the United States. While including many reforms to healthcare insurance and how it is administered and made available, the legislation also makes changes in both Medicare and Medicaid to increase availability and affordability within these two programs. In 2017, the debate over healthcare began again. The changes have not been decided as of the writing of this textbook.

The law currently provides opportunities for nurses and nursing. Funding for nursing workforce development was reauthorized with incentives for nurses to seek advanced education. Nursing faculty in associate and baccalaureate programs are eligible for support to continue their education. The law supports, among other provisions, an increased scope of practice, encouraging the expansion of nurse-run clinics, home visits for high-risk populations, and increasing reimbursement for nurse midwives (Robert Wood Johnson Foundation, 2010).

Current healthcare law will require modification and compromise as time proceeds. There will always be some people not covered by the provisions established in legislation. Costs will continue to be a major concern.

> **Critical Thinking Activity: What Would You Propose?**
> Identify an aspect of the healthcare reform legislation that concerns you. Analyze the various proposals currently before Congress or your state legislature regarding that specific concern. Rank the proposals in order of your preference, providing rationales for your decision-making. In a small group, hold a discussion in which you share your analysis of the various proposals.

THE DEVELOPMENT OF NURSING ORGANIZATIONS

Nursing organizations have political processes similar to those found in governmental institutions. What is the role of the organization and how should its resources be spent? Where is authority for decision-making? How can individual members affect decision-making? What is the individual's role as a nurse in the organization?

When you first learn about the great number of nursing and nursing-related organizations, it may seem confusing, and their purposes and functions may seem duplicative. Here, we will try to clarify some of that information.

Understanding the genesis of nursing organizations can help you to understand their current focus and activities. By the end of the 19th century, changes were accomplished most effectively through organizations. Nursing pioneers saw this as an opportunity to bring about transformation in nursing practice and nursing education and began forming nursing organizations.

Nursing Organizations in England

In England, the establishment of an organization for nursing was driven by the energies of Mrs. Bedford Fenwick (Ethel Gordon Manson), a prominent leader who, in 1887, campaigned for nurse registration. She believed that standards were necessary to improve nursing. Although her ideas for nurse registration were not well accepted, she founded the British Nurses' Association in 1888. It grew rapidly to 1,000 members by the end of the first year. It later became the Royal British Nurses' Association.

The American Society of Superintendents of Training Schools for Nurses

In 1893, the World's Fair and Columbian Exposition was held in Chicago to celebrate the 400th anniversary of Columbus' arrival in the United States. The Fair provided the meeting place for many professions and artisans. The first nurses' meeting was held in the Hall of Columbus, June 15–17, 1893, as part of the International Congress of Charities, Corrections, and Philanthropy. The nursing meeting was chaired by Isabel Hampton and was attended by American and Canadian nurses. Attendees included such individuals as Lavinia Dock—suffragist, nurse activist, historian, and educator—who spoke about the relation of training schools to hospitals. An address sent by Florence Nightingale was presented to the group. The papers presented were later compiled in a publication, *Nursing the Sick, 1893*. The day after the meeting, Isabel Hampton arranged a meeting of a small group of leaders to discuss the possibility of starting a nursing organization. This meeting resulted in the formation in 1896 of the American Society of Superintendents of Training Schools for Nurses, so named because most of the attendees were directors of nursing schools and the membership was restricted to those nurses associated with nurse training. Concern for the standards of nursing education was primary, and a committee to study nursing education was quickly appointed. In 1907, the Canadian members formed their own organization, the Canadian Society of Superintendents of Training Schools. The American organization changed its name in 1912 to the NLN Education (Donahue, 1996, p. 326).

In 1952, the NLN Education became the NLN when six organizations merged into one. The organizations involved in the merger were the National Organization for Public Health Nursing (est. 1912), the Association of Collegiate Schools of Nursing (est. 1933), the Joint

Committee on Practical Nurses and Auxiliary Workers in Nursing Services (est. 1945), the Joint Committee on Careers in Nursing (est. 1946), the National Committee for the Improvement of Nursing Services (est. 1949), and the National Nursing Accrediting Service (est. 1949).

Nurses' Associated Alumnae of the United States and Canada

As the number of nurses increased throughout the United States and hospitals formed individual alumnae groups, the need arose for an organization of trained nurses. At the third meeting of the American Society of Superintendents of Training Schools in 1896, a committee prepared a constitution and bylaws for such an organization with the delegates representing the various alumnae associations. The constitution was accepted a year later, and the Nurses' Associated Alumnae of the United States and Canada was formed. The first president was Isabel Hampton Robb. The group had three purposes:

1. To establish and maintain a code of ethics
2. To elevate the standards of nursing education
3. To promote the usefulness and honor, the financial and other interests of the nursing profession (ANA, 1996, p. 2)

When it was discovered that New York law would not permit foreign membership in an incorporated association, the words "and Canada" were dropped from the title in 1901, and Canadian participation was prohibited. In 1911, the name of the organization in the United States became the ANA.

The Provisional Organization of the Canadian National Association of Trained Nurses was formed in 1908 and renamed the Canadian Nurses Association in 1924. This group also had as its primary concerns the education of nursing students, the improvement of nursing care, the amelioration of conditions for nurses, and state registration of nurses to protect the public.

NURSING ORGANIZATIONS OF TODAY

The existence of a large number of diverse organizations for nurses is, in many ways, a reflection of nursing itself. The profession offers a wide variety of employment opportunities to its members, with distinct and varied contributions and interests in healthcare. When nurses become committed to a particular specialty group, they have a tendency to want to advance the purposes and interests of the people working in that area. For example, operating room nurses have more in common with other operating room nurses, in terms of interests and concerns, than they have with nurses working in hospice care. Likewise, nurses involved in hospice care would probably prefer to share concerns with one another than to discuss them with critical care nurses. With more than 4.1 million nurses in the United States (Henry J. Kaiser Family Foundation), it is understandable that there are many different areas of nursing interest and therefore many different nursing organizations.

The formation of so many nursing organizations has resulted in concern regarding the overlapping of function and interrelationships among some of the organizations. Unfortunately, there has been a spirit of competition rather than cooperation among these groups in the past. Because nurses traditionally have not had high incomes, joining more than one organization has not been a desirable option for economic as well as philosophic reasons. Different nursing organizations can be found at http://nurse.org/orgs.shtml. The links provided at this Web site can help you to research individual organizations that may be of interest to you. As you review that list, you can understand why some critics suggest that nursing has too many organizations working in too many different directions.

Nursing organizations recently have made a concerted effort to promote cooperation. Nurses are better informed about the various organizations and receive better salaries than in the past. However, these facts have not resulted in significantly greater participation by professional nurses in their organizations. Some people specifically do not join because of philosophical differences, but many nurses seem to be apathetic and do not recognize the importance of nurses acting together. Some, because they are combining a job with family and home responsibilities, feel they do not have the time or energy to become involved. Nurses need to recognize the potential for power that they possess as a group. As the nation moves toward healthcare reform, this has never been a more critical issue.

The International Council of Nurses

The International Council of Nurses (ICN), the oldest of all international nursing organizations, was formed in 1899. Founded by Mrs. Bedford Fenwick, it held its first meeting in Buffalo, New York, at the World Exposition in 1901. Mrs. Fenwick was the first president of the organization. The membership originally was composed of self-governing national nurses' associations rather than individual members, although, until 1904, individual members could belong because few countries had organized nursing associations. Its purpose was to encourage communication among nurses of all nations and to provide opportunities for nurses from all over the world to meet and discuss concerns about the profession and about client care. At the present time, the ICN meets every 4 years.

The ICN is the international organization for professional nursing, with membership consisting of national nursing organizations. The ANA, as a constituent member of the ICN, sends delegates to its convention and participates in its activities. The ICN is interested in healthcare in general and nursing care in particular throughout the world. It works with the United Nations, when appropriate, and with other international health-related groups, such as the International Red Cross.

The ICN concerns itself with such issues as the social and economic welfare of nurses, the role of the nurse in healthcare, and the roles of national nursing organizations throughout the world and their relationships to their governing bodies. The primary governing body of the organization is the Council of National Representatives, which meets biennially.

The ICN has representatives from more than 120 national nurses' organizations. The Council of National Representatives governs the organization, which consists of all the presidents of the member organizations. Activities of the organization are carried out by its Board of Directors, the officers, volunteer nurse members of constituent organizations, and employed staff, including an executive director. The ICN maintains headquarters in Geneva, Switzerland.

Every 4 years, a quadrennial congress is held. This meeting is open to all nurses and to delegates from the national organizations. Information about the organization, its efforts, and how to belong may be found on the ICN Web site www.icn.ch.

American Nurses Association

The ANA has been identified as the professional organization for all RNs. As such, it has always had as its primary interest the concerns of the nurses it represents. Throughout history, the

Figure 14.3. Isabel Hampton Robb was the first president of the American Nurses Association from 1897 to 1901. Accreditation is designed to help ensure that the desired outcomes of education are achieved. (From the United States National Library of Medicine.)

organization has been active in issues relating to nursing education (see Chapter 2), licensure (see Chapter 3), collective bargaining (see Chapter 5), and a host of other concerns facing nurses and nursing. The ANA is referred to many times throughout this book. As a professional association, it has been involved in all the issues that nursing has confronted (Fig. 14.3).

Membership

The ANA membership comprises 49 state nurses' associations and the three territorial constituent units. In most cases, the individual nurse belongs to the ANA through the state nursing association. Since the organization has been restructured, individuals may now join the ANA directly. There are also opportunities for affiliate memberships.

While the reported number of professionally active RNs is 4.1 million (Henry J. Kaiser Family Foundation, 2017), the membership in the constituent associations of the ANA is a fraction of that (http://www.nursingworld.org). Those who do participate are often the leaders in the nursing profession. Individuals who do not join give a variety of reasons, such as cost, a lack of time to participate in activities, and a lack of interest in the issues put forth. Some nurses do not join because they do not agree with the position of the ANA on major issues such as collective bargaining, nursing education, and political involvement.

Strategic Imperatives

The ANA has identified a set of strategic imperatives that structure its efforts. These include championing professional practice and excellence, formulating healthcare and public policy as they affect the profession and the public, providing accurate and comprehensive health policy information based on knowledge from research, advocating for nurses in the workforce and through workplace rights, facilitating unification and advancement of the profession, and improving its own organizational structure and resources. In order to work on these, the ANA has a wide-ranging set of activities. For the most comprehensive and up-to-date information, go to www.nursingworld.org and examine the information under each of the main menu headings. An overview is provided as follows.

The ANA supports work on policies related to the profession as a whole, such as the Code of Ethics for Nurses update in 2015. The ANA also supports research on topics related to the profession itself. By serving as the coordinating body for the various affiliate organizations, the ANA helps to ensure its ongoing effectiveness. In its efforts to support the profession of nursing, the ANA has developed the Bill of Rights for Registered Nurses. This tool addresses the workplace environment needed for effective nursing practice. While not a legal document, this Bill of Rights serves as a guide to nurses as they seek to influence policy in organizations where they are employed (Box 14.5). A discussion of how this Bill of Rights might be used and the foundations underlying the rights are available on the ANA Web site (http://nursingworld.org/MainMenuCategories/WorkplaceSafety/Healthy-Work-Environment/Work-Environment).

The ANA researches and promotes information on a variety of workplace issues for nurses especially those relating to occupational health for nurses. Some of the major issues currently being promoted were discussed previously.

The ANA is extensively involved in legislative activity and healthcare policy. The organization often represents the profession in testimony before Congress on numerous issues affecting nursing. The need to be geographically closer to legislators to have greater participation in legislative and policy efforts was the major reason for the relocation of the ANA offices to

---

BOX 14.5 AMERICAN NURSES ASSOCIATION'S BILL OF RIGHTS FOR REGISTERED NURSES

1. Nurses have the right to practice in a manner that fulfills their obligations to society and to those who receive nursing care.
2. Nurses have the right to practice in environments that allow them to act in accordance with professional standards and legally authorized scopes of practice.
3. Nurses have the right to a work environment that supports and facilitates ethical practice, in accordance with the *Code of Ethics for Nurses with Interpretive Statements.*
4. Nurses have the right to freely and openly advocate for themselves and their clients, without fear of retribution.
5. Nurses have the right to fair compensation for their work, consistent with their knowledge, experience, and professional responsibilities.
6. Nurses have the right to a work environment that is safe for themselves and for their clients.
7. Nurses have the right to negotiate the conditions of their employment, either as individuals or collectively, in all practice settings.

Adopted by the ANA Board of Directors June 26, 2001. http://www.nursingworld.org/EspeciallyForYou/staffnurses/FAQs.aspx.

Washington, DC, in 1992. The organization provides testimony for or against legislation that will affect the profession, either directly or indirectly; legislative topics include funds for nursing education, collective bargaining issues, concerns for higher education, and human rights issues. It also testifies on health-related policy issues affecting the general public, such as the quality of care in nursing homes and healthcare reform.

Through its educational services, the ANA produces and distributes a wide variety of nursing materials, such as email updates, journals, films, and monographs. Reports of committees and commissions and special studies supported by the ANA are published. The ANA also publishes many pamphlets and informational resources of value to nurses. A complete list of publications is available at the ANA Web site and in print from the organization. The ANA Web site continues to expand the content available and includes the *Online Journal of Issues in Nursing* and the many documents and position statements produced by the ANA. *American Nurse Today* is the official publication of the ANA; official announcements of ANA business are published in this journal. ANA also publishes a newspaper, *American Nurse*, that contains current news relevant to nursing and healthcare, editorials, letters, and classified advertisements.

In addition to its activities on behalf of the profession as a whole, the ANA provides direct services to members. These services include online continuing education, access to a group professional liability insurance plan, and group insurance for health, disability, and accident coverage. The ANA also provides access to group travel arrangements and a variety of purchasing discounts.

American Nurses Credentialing Center

The ANA in collaboration with specialty nursing organizations established the American Nurses Credentialing Center (ANCC) as an autonomous organization to manage the process of specialty credentialing. The ANCC also operates the magnet hospital recognition program for hospitals that demonstrate excellence in nursing practice and the environment for nursing. The ANCC remains an affiliated organization for the ANA.

American Nurses Foundation

In 1955, the ANA established the American Nurses Foundation (ANF), an affiliate of the ANA, as a tax-exempt, nonprofit corporation for the purpose of supporting research related to nursing. It is independently financed and self-governing. Its board of trustees is composed of members of the board of directors of the ANA, other nurse members, and nonnurse members from other health-related fields and from the public. To accomplish its varied objectives, the ANF solicits gifts and contributions from individuals and organizations. These gifts are tax deductible.

The ANF maintains a three-pronged approach to supporting research. The first objective is to conduct policy analyses to provide nursing leaders and public policy makers with the information they need for decision-making. The second objective is related to developing nurse scholars, individuals who engage in study of such areas as journalism and public policy. Support is directed toward independent study, research, and doctoral and postdoctoral work for these nurse scholars. The third objective is to facilitate the research and educational activities of ANA. This includes providing consultation and funding for groups in the ANA that wish to initiate projects.

American Academy of Nursing

The ANA established the American Academy of Nursing (AAN) in 1973 as an honorary association in the ANA. The ANA's board of directors chose the original members. The AAN is now an independent organization that is an affiliate of ANA, and new members are selected by those currently in the AAN. Those elected to the AAN are considered fellows and may use the title Fellow of the American Academy of Nursing (FAAN). The purpose of this organization is to recognize nurses who have made significant contributions to the profession of nursing.

National League for Nursing

The mission for the NLN states, "The National League for Nursing promotes excellence in nursing education to build a strong and diverse nursing workforce to advance the health of our nation and the global community" (NLN, 2017). The goals of the organization focus on four areas: (1) being a leader in nursing education, (2) having a commitment to members, (3) acting as a champion for nurse educators, and (4) advancing the science of nursing education.

Membership

The NLN offers membership to individuals and agencies. It is unique among nursing organizations in that it also offers membership and participation to consumers, nonnursing members of healthcare teams, and institutions concerned with nursing service and nursing education.

Activities and Services

The NLN works in a complementary, rather than competitive, manner with the ANA. Whereas the ANA speaks as the official voice of nurses, the NLN seeks to unite the interests of nursing with those of the community in support of excellence in nursing education.

The NLN sponsors continuing education workshops and conferences related to nursing education throughout the country, often repeating a workshop in different locations to spare participants the expense of travel. Subjects are determined in consultation with members and are geared to current needs and interests. Curriculum, research, accreditation, testing and evaluation, student recruitment and retention, political awareness and healthcare legislation, and a nurse executive series are regular subjects for continuing education. The constituent leagues, which are grouped by regional assemblies, also offer workshops designed to meet the interests of particular areas of the country.

Through its journal, *Nursing Education Perspectives*, and a newsletter, *NLN Update* (both available on the Internet), members are kept informed about current issues. *Reflection and Dialogue* is an online publication that presents timely information regarding major topics relevant to nursing. Sometimes NLN spokespersons offer testimony on legislation or rulings significant to the organization. The NLN publishes many texts and references about curriculum, ethics, public policy, nursing administration, long-term care, and other topics of interest to nursing. It also produces educational videos.

The Centers for Excellence (nursing programs designated for their achievements) and documents such as *Hallmarks of Excellence in Nursing Education* and *Resources for Excellence* are all part of the Excellence Initiatives. Another excellence initiative, the Academy of Nursing Education honors nurses who have made significant contributions in nursing education. Members use the title Academy of Nursing Education Fellow (ANEF).

The NLN has developed a certification program for nurse educators. This includes educational materials and a testing program that recognizes those who meet these high standards for certification.

NLN serves as a resource for data regarding nursing education such as enrollments, admissions, and graduations. Other data such as the numbers of men and minorities in schools of nursing and faculty shortages are also gathered through their annual surveys of nursing programs.

Through its testing service, the NLN produces standardized assessment tests to be used in the nursing program admission process, achievement tests for various levels in a program that can be used by a program for evaluation, the NLN mobility examinations (which are used to provide advanced placement credit), and diagnostic examinations for those preparing for the National Council Licensure Examination, or NCLEX Exam.

Accrediting Organizations

The Accreditation Commission for Education in Nursing (ACEN), the National League for Nursing Commission for Nursing Education Accreditation (CNEA), and the Commission on Collegiate Nursing Education (CCNE) are the three nursing organizations that accredit nursing education programs. These organizations were discussed in detail in Chapter 3.

American Association of Colleges of Nursing

The AACN was formed to assist baccalaureate and higher degree schools of nursing in working cooperatively to improve higher education for professional nursing. Membership is limited to programs that offer a baccalaureate degree or higher in nursing, with an upper-division nursing major, and that are part of a regionally accredited college or university. The AACN focuses on the quality of nursing education in baccalaureate and higher degree programs and support and assistance to deans and programs in providing excellence in education. The organization also provides data regarding these programs and is active in public advocacy for nursing and nursing education both independently and through the Tri-Council.

National Council of State Boards of Nursing

Although it is not a nursing organization like those previously discussed, our discussion would not be complete without mention of the National Council of State Boards of Nursing, Inc. (NCSBN). This organization was formed in 1978 to replace the Council of State Boards that had been part of the ANA. The purpose of this organization is to provide a forum for the legal regulatory bodies (whatever their particular state titles might be) of all states, the District of Columbia, and United States territories to act together in the regulation of nursing practice for the protection of the public. There is one delegate to this council from each state agency. The actions of this council are particularly important because its membership represents the legal authority for the control of nursing education and nursing practice.

Although each state agency must operate within its own laws, it does have authority to establish many specific rules and regulations. Working together, the state boards hope to promote uniform standards for the nursing profession. One of the agenda items they have addressed is the development of a Model Nurse Practice Act, which serves to guide states as they work on licensure laws. Much energy has gone into the development, validation, and establishment of computerized testing for the licensing examination for both registered

(NCLEX-RN) and practical/vocational (NCLEX-PN) nursing. Currently, the organization is addressing the issues related to approving and licensing advanced practice nurses and the concerns associated with multistate practice.

Organizations Representing Licensed Practical/Vocational Nurses

Two nursing organizations are concerned primarily with advancing the interests of licensed practical/vocational nurses (LPN/LVNs). These two organizations are the National Association of Licensed Practical Nurses (NALPN) and the National Association for Practical Nurse Education and Service (NAPNES).

The NALPN is the professional organization for LPN/LVNs. It was founded in 1949 and was known as the National Federation of Licensed Practical Nurses until 2018. Its membership is limited to LPN/LVNs and students in practical nursing programs. This organization has developed a set of practice standards for the LPN/LVN and, through the NALPN Educational Foundation, offers an IV Therapy and Gerontology Certification by exam program for LPN/LVNs possessing the knowledge and skills necessary to complete client care tasks associated with these specialties. State and local groups of the NALPN are active in educational issues affecting the LPN/LVN and have supported the associate degree as the appropriate educational preparation for the responsibilities of the LPN/LVN in the current healthcare system. Further information is available on the NALPN Web site http://nalpn.org/.

The NAPNES was organized as the Association of Practical Nurse Schools in 1941. Its purpose was to address the needs of practical nursing education. The name was changed in 1942 to the National Association for Practical Nurse Education; in 1959, it added "and Service" to that title. The official publication of the organization is *The Journal of Practical Nursing*, which has been published since 1951. Membership is open to LPN/LVNs, LPN/LVN nursing students, faculty, directors, physicians, organizations, the lay community, and other individuals who are interested in promoting the professional practice and education of practical nurses. It was the first organization to provide accreditation for practical nursing programs, although that role now rests with the ACEN and CNEA. You can learn more about NAPNES and their three councils at www.napnes.org.

NANDA-I

In 2002, NANDA, originally established in 1982 as the North American Nursing Diagnosis Association, became NANDA-International (NANDA-I) to reflect the increasing worldwide interest in the field of nursing diagnosis terminology. It is open to individuals as well as group members. The purpose of this group is to work toward uniform terminology and definitions to be used in nursing diagnosis and to share ideas and information regarding this topic. The general outline of the taxonomy (classification system) was established by a group of nursing theorists and then accepted by the organization. NANDA-I is organized into a taxonomy that includes 13 domains (categories) of nursing practice: Health Promotion, Nutrition, Elimination and Exchange, Activity/Rest, Perception/Cognition, Self-Perception, Role Relationships, Sexuality, Coping/Stress Tolerance, Life Principles, Safety/Protection, Comfort, and Growth/Development. Nursing diagnoses are clustered under each of these domains. Members identify and research problems that nurses manage, prepare documentation, and submit these to NANDA-I to be included in the consideration process. Committees then review the problems. Those that meet the basic criteria for nursing diagnoses are submitted to the membership. For each problem, defining characteristics are identified, conditions that form the etiology or are related to the development of the diagnosis are identified, and a place in the classification is established. An international convention held every 2 years is the final forum for the debate and discussion of proposed new nursing diagnoses. Two publications— *The International Journal of Nursing Terminologies and Classification* and *Nursing Diagnoses and Classifications*—are used to disseminate the work of the organization. See the Web site at www.nanda.org. More recently, this organization is coordinating its work with those working on the Nursing Interventions Classification and the Nursing Outcomes Classification to fulfill the goal of a coordinated system of nursing terminology.

American Organization of Nurse Executives

The AONE was established in 1967 and has a mission "to shape health care through innovative and expert nursing leadership" (AONE, 2017). This organization provides the forum for nurses with managerial and executive responsibility to work collaboratively, both with other nurses in similar roles and through the organization with other organizations. AONE is one of the members of the Tri-Council for Nursing, which serves as an information resource for legislative and governmental personnel.

Sigma Theta Tau International Honor Society for Nursing

Sigma Theta Tau International Honor Society for Nursing (STTI) was founded by six nurses at the Indiana University Training School for Nurses in 1922. STTI is an international organization established in collegiate schools of nursing to recognize those with superior ability and leadership potential and those who have made important contributions to nursing. Candidates may be asked to join during the senior year of a baccalaureate program or any time thereafter. Sigma Theta Tau has established a nursing library at its headquarters in Indianapolis that has reference abilities to support advanced scholarship; the organization also provides two print journals *Journal of Nursing Scholarship* and *Reflections on Nursing Leadership* (which is also available online). Local chapters may maintain funds to support individual research projects, hold research conferences, and recognize those who have made significant contributions to nursing.

Tri-Council for Nursing

Mentioned several times earlier, the Tri-Council for Nursing is a joint effort of the ANA, the NLN, AONE, and the AACN to work collaboratively in presenting a unified voice for nursing in the policy arena. Addressing the three major areas of education, practice, and research, the Tri-Council establishes positions on health issues, proposed legislation, and regulations. When individuals represent the Tri-Council while testifying before decision-making groups, they have great credibility in regard to the issues.

Clinical Organizations

Some of the earliest specialty organizations were related to specific clinical practice areas of nursing. A major focus of these organizations now is continuing education related to a particular nursing specialty. Most groups also have some mechanisms, such as certification, for recognizing achievement in the field. One of the earliest specialty organizations, founded in 1941, was the American Association of Nurse Anesthetists. Approximately 90% of certified nurse anesthetists in the United States are members (American Association of Nurse Anesthetists, 2017).

Specialty organizations also include groups that began as auxiliaries to specialty physicians' organizations, such as the Association of Women's Health, Obstetric and Neonatal Nurses. This organization was started for nurses affiliated with physicians who were "fellows" of the American College of Obstetricians and Gynecologists. As more members joined and nurses became more active, groups such as this one became autonomous. Most specialty organizations, such as the Critical Care Nurses Association, began as nurses sought forums to exchange information and obtain education in their specialty.

The Nursing Organizations Alliance (The Alliance) was formed in 2001 when two long-standing coalitions of nursing organizations, the National Federation for Specialty Nursing Organizations (NFSNO) and the Nursing Organizations Liaison Forum (NOLF), united. The purpose of the Alliance is to provide a forum for identification, education, and collaboration building on issues of common interest to the specialty organizations to advance the nursing profession (http://www.nursing-alliance.org/About-Us/Our-History).

The American Association of Nurse Practitioners (AANP) was organized in 2013. Two nurse practitioner organizations, the American Academy of Nurse Practitioners, founded in 1985 and the American College of Nurse Practitioners, founded in 1995, joined forces. The stated mission of AANP "is to empower all nurse practitioners to advance quality health care through practice, education, advocacy, research and leadership" (AANP, n.d.). Its activities focus on advancing the role of the nurse practitioner in the healthcare delivery system and providing education and research opportunities.

Groups Related to Ethnic Origin

As the movement for self-determination and preservation of identity arose within ethnic groups in the United States, nurses within various ethnic groups began to unite to achieve a greater voice in healthcare. Some ethnic groups are nationally organized; others are organized on a more local level. As these groups have become stronger and more organized, their interests have included the recruitment and support of nursing students from the particular ethnic groups they represent. These ethnic groups also encourage their members to become more politically involved in nursing and nursing leadership. To find a specific group, either nationally or locally, an internet search is recommended.

Religious Organizations

The National Council of Catholic Nurses and the Nurses' Christian Fellowship (primarily a nondenominational Protestant group) were organized to assist nurses in sharing concerns and integrating their work and their religious beliefs. These two organizations place special emphasis on meeting a client's spiritual needs and on dealing with ethical issues. Other religious organizations can be located through an Internet search.

National Student Nurses Association

The National Student Nurses Association (NSNA), started in 1952, is a professional organization for students in schools of nursing. Although it works with the ANA, it is a fully independent organization, run and financed by nursing students. It sponsors its own annual convention.

Although the NSNA is an autonomous organization, it has close ties with the ANA. Members of the NSNA serve on selected committees in the ANA speak to the House of Delegates at the ANA convention to provide a student viewpoint and work together with the ANA regarding current issues.

Each state has a nursing student association that operates in the same relationship to the state professional organization as the NSNA does to the ANA. State conventions and workshops are held in many states. State issues are addressed by the state association in the same way that national issues are addressed by the NSNA. Local nursing student organizations may or may not exist in individual schools of nursing. These local organizations may be closely tied to the state and national groups or they may be independent. It is possible for an individual student to join the state and national student nurses' organizations even if no local counterpart exists.

A major project of the NSNA is "Breakthrough into Nursing," organized in 1965. This project is designed to recruit and maintain the enrollment of minorities in schools of nursing through mentoring and to create a respect for the differences and similarities between people. The project has enlisted nursing students to speak to minority teenagers to interest them in nursing early in their scholastic careers and to act as preceptors and tutors to increase the retention of minority students when they enroll in schools of nursing. Other activities are directed at the image of nursing and disaster planning. They publish a magazine titled *Imprint* and *NSNA eNews,* an electronic newsletter.

The NSNA is often asked to testify before congressional committees when issues relevant to nursing education are being considered. In this role, the organization becomes the public voice for all nursing students.

The NSNA has developed a series of documents that support the role of the nursing student. These include a Code of Ethics for Students: Part I Code of professional conduct, Code of Ethics for Students: Part II Code of academic and clinical conduct, and the Bill of Rights and Responsibilities for Students of Nursing. These documents are all available from the NSNA Web site (www.nsna.org).

Educational and Research Organizations

Since the 1960s, there has been a great deal of change and development in nursing education as it has moved from the hospital into the educational setting. During this time, there has been an increased emphasis on educational methods, curriculum development, and research.

In several major geographic regions of the United States, education organizations extending membership to schools of nursing, members of the state boards of nursing, and other interested individuals were developed to promote interstate and interinstitutional cooperation in seeking ways to improve nursing education and scholarship. These organizations are the Western Institute of Nursing, the Council on Collegiate Education for Nursing of the Southern Regional Education Board, the New England Organization for Nursing, the Midwest Alliance in Nursing, and the Mid-Atlantic Regional Nursing Association.

The Organization for Associate Degree Nursing (OADN), founded in 1984, is dedicated to enhancing the quality of ADN education, strengthening the professional role of the ADN, and protecting the future of associate degree nursing in the midst of healthcare changes. OADN publishes a quarterly journal *Teaching and Learning in Nursing.* Membership is open to individuals, states, agencies, and organizations.

Miscellaneous Organizations

The American Assembly for Men in Nursing (AAMN) was formed in 1971 by Steve Miller, a nurse who believed that, as a minority in the profession, men needed to speak about issues with a united voice. The membership has expanded to include women who are concerned about gender issues in nursing. The organization has addressed the issue of discrimination toward men in nursing and seeks to present nursing as a profession in which both men and women can contribute and excel.

Nurses House, Inc. provides assistance for nurses in need. It originated from a bequest in 1922 from Emily Bourne, who donated $300,000 to establish a country home where nurses might find needed rest. As the need for this residence decreased, supporters of this endeavor sold the estate and invested the proceeds. Income from the investment and funds donated by nurses (and friends of nurses) are used to provide guidance and counseling for nurses with emotional and chemical dependency problems, encouragement to home-bound nurses, and temporary financial assistance to nurses who are ill, convalescing, or unemployed. Nurses House seeks members and donations to assist in continuing these activities.

The GLMA Nursing is a group of nurses working to advance LGBTQ health equality (GLMA, n.d.). This group holds an annual summit to discuss issues related to LGBTQ health.

Critical Thinking Activity: Membership in a Nursing Organization
As a new graduate, assume you have $400 per year to spend on membership in a nursing organization. In trying to decide which organization to join, how would you go about learning the focus of several groups that have attracted your interest? What process could you use to ensure that you are joining the group that best serves your needs? Which organization would you join? Provide a clear rationale based on both economic and professional reasons for your choice.

Stegen & Sowerby Story: Part 2

Kim decides to arrange a meeting with his supervisor and presents the views of the nurses on the unit, research on mandatory overtime, position papers from nursing organizations, and a plan that allows nurses to sign up for extra shifts with another plan to rotate through nurses on a schedule for those shifts that are not covered. His supervisor says that she will take it to administration and asks if he would come to the meeting to present it.

- What if Kim's supervisor was not willing to present the plan to administration?
- What would his other options (if any) be?

Read the rest of the story at www.thePoint.com.

Want to Know More?

A variety of resources are available on thePoint® to enhance your learning and understanding of this chapter, such as

- Full Stegen & Sowerby Stories
- NCLEX-Style Student Review Questions
- Journal Articles
- Case Studies
- Learning Objectives
- Relevant Web sites
- And more...

KEY CONCEPTS

- Because scarce resources are allocated through the political process, nurses will find that understanding this process is essential to influencing the healthcare system.
- Each nurse has many opportunities to affect the political process. This can be done simply by keeping informed, voting, or trying to shape public opinion. Communicating with legislators and officials can be done individually or as part of a group. Testifying presents issues of importance, and individual support can be given to those running for office. You may even decide to run for a public office.
- The federal government is active in healthcare through many existing agencies in the HHS and in other branches of government. The federal budget process affects the healthcare services available through the many legislative acts affecting healthcare such as Medicare, for the elderly and certain disabled individuals, and Medicaid, for the poor.
- A political process is part of any large organization, and nursing organizations are no exception. Understanding the political process can help you participate more effectively in a large organization.
- The variety of organizations in nursing is often confusing to the new nursing graduate and to the public. These organizations represent the nursing profession as a whole, as well as special interest groups within nursing.
- The ANA, whose membership is open to RNs through their state constituencies, provides the voice of professional nursing. Actions of the ANA are directed toward nursing practice issues, economic welfare of nurses, and broader issues of healthcare.
- Another major nursing organization is the NLN, which, historically, has championed better nursing education. Membership is open to individuals and agencies interested in nursing.
- The NLNAC and CCNE provide for the accreditation of nursing programs throughout the United States.
- The NCSBN coordinates the development of the licensure examinations used for both practical nurses and RNs. It also coordinates and supports the development of common licensure standards, licensure agreements between states, and an examination for certifying nursing assistants.

- Two nursing organizations exist expressly to serve the needs of LPN/LVNs. These groups are the NALPN and the NAPNES.
- Organizations also exist that represent specialty groups in nursing. Members are usually drawn together by their common interests and concerns. A very active and prominent organization is the AONE representing nurse administrators. Some of the specialty organizations provide continuing education and, in some instances, certification.
- Some organizations, such as Sigma Theta Tau, are honorary in their focus. These groups strive to bring recognition to nurses and nursing.
- The NSNA addresses the interests and needs of nursing students. As a fully autonomous organization, NSNA membership is open to nursing students only.
- A wide variety of other organizations meet the special needs of their membership. This may relate to social interests, ethnic background, or other common denominators.

NCLEX-STYLE PRACTICE QUESTIONS

1. Nurses can be more politically active by: (Select all that apply)

   A. Joining nursing organizations
   B. Writing letter to representatives
   C. Writing letters to the editor
   D. Reading political opinions

2. The Occupational Health and Safety Act (OSHA) is important to nurses for which reason?

   A. Mandates restraint reduction and nurse aid training
   B. Provides budget appropriations annually for nurses
   C. Mandates a hazard-free work environment
   D. Provides oversight for drug administration

3. What are some state level concerns of nurses? (Select all that apply)

   A. Funding appropriations for Medicare
   B. Violence in the workplace
   C. Nursing education incentives
   D. Research on new medications

4. What is the purpose of nursing organizations? (Select all that apply)

   A. Exert political power of nurses
   B. Expand regulatory opportunities
   C. Share knowledge with other nurses
   D. Promote nursing issues to create change

5. The Code of Ethics for Nurses was developed by which organization?

   A. American Academy of Nursing
   B. National League for Nursing
   C. Sigma Theta Tau International
   D. American Nurses Association

REFERENCES

American Association for History of Nursing. (2007). *Hannah A. Ropes*. Retrieved January 19, 2011, from www.aahn.org/gravesites/ropes.html

American Association of Nurse Anesthetists. (2017). *Who we are*. Retrieved July 29, 2017, from http:// www.aana.com/aboutus/Pages/Who-We-Are.aspx

American Association of Nurse Practitioners. (n.d.) *About AANP*. Retrieved June 6, 2018, from https:// aanp.org/about-aanp

American Nurses Association. (1996). *In the beginning*. Retrieved January 19, 2011, from www.nursing-world.org/FunctionalMenuCategories/AboutANA/WhoWeAre/History.aspx

American Organization of Nurse Executives. (2017). *About AONE*. Retrieved July 29, 2017, from http:// www.aone.org/about/overview.shtml

Bostridge, M. (2008). *Florence Nightingale: The woman and her legend*. London: Penguin-Viking.

Donahue, M. P. (1996). *Nursing: The finest art* (2nd ed.). St. Louis, MO: CV Mosby.

GLMA Nurses Advancing LGBTQ Health Equality. (n.d.). *History*. Retrieved July 29, 2017, from https:// glmanursing.org/about/history/

Hatch Act. (1993). Retrieved from https://osc.gov/Pages/HatchAct.aspx

Henry J. Kaiser Family Foundation. (2017). *Total number of professionally active nurses*. Retrieved July 28, 2017, from http://www.kff.org/other/state-indicator/total-registered-nurses/?currentTimeframe= 0&sortModel=%7B%22colId%22:%22Location%22,%22sort%22:%22asc%22%7D

Lowes, R. (2011, November 7). Texas physician pleads guilty in whistle-blowing nurses case. *Medscape*. Retrieved from http://www.medscape.com/viewarticle/753029

National Institutes for Occupational Safety and Health. (2014). *NIOSH alert: Preventing needlestick injuries in healthcare settings*. Pub #2000-108, Retrieved July 30, 2017, from www.cdc.gov/niosh/ docs/2000-108/

National Institutes for Occupational Safety and Health Administration. (n.d.). Safe client handling. *Worker safety in hospitals: Caring for our caregivers*. Retrieved July 30, 2017, from https://www.osha. gov/dsg/hospitals/client_handling.html

National League for Nursing. (2017). *Mission and strategic plan*. Retrieved July 28, 2017, from http:// www.nln.org/about/mission-goals

Occupational Safety and Health Administration. (n.d.). Preventing workplace violence in healthcare. *Worker safety in hospitals: Caring for our caregivers*. Retrieved July 30, 2017, from https://www.osha. gov/dsg/hospitals/workplace_violence.html

Project Vote Smart. (n.d.). Retrieved July 29, 2017, from https://votesmart.org/education/how-a-bill-becomes-law#.WX0EPIjyvIU

Rappleye, E. (2015). Gender ratio of nurses across 50 states. *Becker's Hospital Review*. Retrieved from http://www.beckershospitalreview.com/human-capital-and-risk/gender-ratio-of-nurses-across-50-states.html

Robert Wood Johnson Foundation. (2010). *Health care overhaul means more opportunities and demand for nurses*. Retrieved January 10, 2011, from www.rwjf.org/healthreform/product.jsp?id=62128

United States Bureau of the Census. (2017). *Voting and registration in the election of November 2016*. Retrieved from https://www.census.gov/data/tables/time-series/demo/voting-and-registration/p20-580.html

CHAPTER 15

Applying Research and Technology to Nursing Practice

LEARNING OUTCOMES

After completing this chapter, you should be able to:

1. Construct an effective strategy for evaluating information resources.
2. Discuss the value of the research in nursing.
3. Describe the role of the staff nurse in nursing research.
4. Explain the term *evidence-based practice* (EBP) and its application to nursing.
5. List the types of evidence that may be used for EBP, moving from the most reliable to the least reliable.
6. Outline a process for establishing an evidence-based nursing practice in an institutional setting or in your own personal practice.
7. Analyze the role of technology in nursing.
8. Assess your own competence in the realm of nursing technology.

KEY TERMS

Clinical significance
Computerized provider order entry (CPOE)
Control group
Electronic ICU (eICU)
Evidence-based practice (EBP)
Informatics
Institutional review board (IRB)
Level of significance

Participant/subject
Population
Probability
Qualitative research
Quantitative research
Randomized controlled trial (RCT)
Reliability
Sample
Validity

Stegen & Sowerby Stories: Part 1

Tara is in charge of a nursing program at a community college. A lack of clinical sites makes it challenging to schedule all of the students for the amount of clinical hours that are required to complete the program. The program turns away more than half of qualified applicants each year, and Tara is receiving pressure from the college president and state legislators to increase the size of the program in response to the nursing shortage. Tara recently found a study from the National Council of State Boards of Nursing that states that simulation could be increased up to 50% of clinicals while maintaining student outcomes (Hayden et al., 2014).

- What are possible options that Tara has to meet address the demands of the college president and legislators while still meeting clinical hour requirements?
- What does research on the topic of simulation in nursing education say?
- Based on your knowledge of leadership and change, how do you think Tara should go about bringing a change in clinical hours and program size?

As you look toward the future, you may find it hard to imagine what nursing will be like. What new insights will nursing research bring? What expectations for practice responsibilities will rest with each nurse? How will evidence-based practice (EBP) change nursing? What technology will be a part of nursing practice? These factors are shaping nursing as you will practice it.

VALUING NURSING RESEARCH

If you are in a baccalaureate nursing program, a course in statistics and one in understanding nursing research are usually requirements. While a course in nursing research is usually not an essential part of associate degree (AD) education, more AD programs are presenting a brief introduction to research as the emphasis on EBP increases in all settings. Many students come to AD nursing having taken courses related to statistics and/or research in other fields. Here, we provide a brief overview of the development of research for nursing practice along with some basic concepts and information to guide your reading and participation in EBP.

The Development of Nursing Research

Nursing research essentially began after World War II, when academic nursing programs expanded rapidly. Nurses began obtaining graduate degrees and learning how to conduct research. *Nursing Research*, which began in 1951, was the first nursing publication to focus on research. Gradually more journals, in the United States, the United Kingdom, and Canada, began to focus on nursing research. Table 15.1 provides an overview of the nursing research journals available and the dates they were first published. In addition to the journals, whose total content is research, many other nursing journals devote a significant number of their pages to research along with articles related to policy and current practice descriptions. This increase in nursing research publication has been a reflection of the increasing emphasis of the profession on scholarly work and the growing number of nurses academically prepared to conduct effective research.

Table 15.1 Initial Publication Dates for Nursing Research Journals*

Year of First Publication	Research Journal
1951	*Nursing Research*
1963	*International Journal of Nursing Studies*
1968	*Journal of Nursing Scholarship: International* (Sigma Theta Tau)
1969	*Canadian Journal of Nursing Research*
1976	*Journal of Advanced Nursing* (UK)
1979	*Western Journal of Nursing Research*
1988	*Applied Nursing Research*
1991	*Clinical Nursing Research* (Canadian editors)
1992	*Nurse Researcher: The International Journal of Research Methodology in Nursing and Health Care* (UK)
1993	*Online Journal of Knowledge Synthesis for Nursing*
1995	*International Journal of Psychiatric Nursing Research*
1995	*Journal of Nursing Research* (UK)
1998	*Evidence Based Nursing Online Journal* (UK)
2000	*BMC Nursing Online* (UK)
2000	*Southern Online Journal Of Nursing Research: Electronic Publication Of Research* (http://snrs.org/publications/journal.html)
2004	*World Views on Evidence Based Nursing* (www.blackwell-synergy.com/links/toc/wvn/1/1)
2010	*Nursing Research and Practice* (https://www.hindawi.com/journals/nrp/)

*This does not represent all of the research journals available.

For many individuals, a key landmark along the path toward a research-based profession was the authorization of the National Center for Nursing Research (NCNR) in 1986 (National Institute of Nursing Research [NINR], n.d.). Prior to this, nursing research was found in a variety of federal endeavors, such as the Division of Nursing within the Office of the Surgeon General and the various sections with the National Institutes of Health (NIH). While the NCNR was an important milestone for nursing research, it did not have the prestige or funding that was provided for the NIH. Based on an increasing recognition of the importance of nursing research, the NCNR was changed into a full-fledged NINR within the NIH in 1993 and celebrated its 30th anniversary in October 2015 (NINR, n.d.).

An Overview of the Nursing Research Process

A research study begins with one unanswered question. Literature is reviewed thoroughly to determine what is already known about the question. The question is then refined based on the knowledge available and identified *variables* (things in the setting that vary or change) and questions about how they are interrelated. In a traditional research study, a *hypothesis* (statement of the expected relationships) is established. A research study is designed to gather information that will help to answer the question. The study is carefully carried out, and the information collected is analyzed. Then, the researcher reaches a conclusion about what has

---

BOX 15.1 STEPS OF THE TRADITIONAL NURSING RESEARCH PROCESS

1. Developing the research question
2. Reviewing the literature
3. Developing the hypothesis
4. Designing the study
5. Carrying out the study
6. Analyzing the data
7. Identifying concerns about the study
8. Drawing conclusions and applications
9. Identifying future research needed

---

been learned from the study, discusses the application of the study to nursing, any concerns with the study are presented, and identifies further research needed (Box 15.1).

Individuals within an institution who have research expertise are appointed to review research proposals and assure that they conform to standardized guidelines. This group is usually titled the **institutional review board (IRB)**, and it oversees the entire research process in any organization. The IRB determines whether the question is appropriate, the means of study fit the question, the study is ethical, and most important, the rights of any subjects or participants are protected (see discussion of *participants* later). No research is allowed in an institution that has not been approved by the institution's review board. For research that occurs outside of institutions, private organizations serve as review boards to ensure the protection of the public.

While this greatly oversimplifies the research process, it provides a foundation to help you understand some of the important concepts and terms in nursing research we are about to discuss.

Basic Research Terminology

The *independent variable* in a research study can be controlled by the researcher and is applied, or manipulated, to determine its effect on the *dependent variable*. The dependent variable is the phenomenon being studied. In healthcare, the dependent variable is usually a health problem of some kind.

Validity refers to the ability of the research methods to actually measure or accurately describe the variables in the study. A physical measure, such as blood pressure (BP), is usually thought of as valid. However, the device used for measuring the BP must be checked for accuracy in order for the measure to be valid. Questionnaires must also be examined for validity. For example, a questionnaire that purports to measure depression (such as by numbering severity using a scale of 1 to 10 or by using words indicating severity: none, mild, moderate, and severe) must have evidence that it really is measuring depression and not some other related phenomenon. The concern also arises that a questionnaire may be valid in one group (such as college-educated students on whom it was tested) and not valid in another group (such as clients with limited education who may not understand the terminology used in the questionnaire). There are many different processes for establishing validity in the setting in which the research is conducted. An important role of the researcher is demonstrating the validity of the research method.

Reliability refers to the ability of the research instrument or tool consistently to yield the same results over repeated testing periods. Again, there are multiple methods for establishing the reliability of any instrument, and the researcher must establish the reliability of any instrument used. Reliability and validity are closely related and often are discussed together.

In a study, the **population** is the entire group of people affected by the problem under scrutiny. The **sample** is that group of people who will actually be studied. How representative the sample is of the entire population is one factor affecting whether the study will be useful. Selecting a *random sample* involves some type of nonbiased approach to selecting the individuals from the population that ensures that all persons in the population have an equal and independent chance of being chosen to be sampled. The use of a random sample increases the likelihood that the sample adequately represents the population. This often is not possible, and a *convenience sample* (a group that may be conveniently accessed) is used. The **participant** or **subject** is the individual person in the sample. Although the term *subject* has been traditionally used, many people now encourage the use of the term *participant* to emphasize the choice that is made to be in the study and the important partnership that occurs.

At least two groups of participants are usually formed. One group is considered the **control group**, sometimes also referred to as the comparison group. The control group will not receive any special treatment or procedure being studied. The *experimental group*, however, will receive the new treatment or procedure. Sometimes there are multiple experimental groups to test different treatments, but one group continues to be the control group that demonstrates the outcome if no treatment is given. In some instances, having no treatment is not possible. In such cases, two or more treatments might be compared. For example, if the focus of the study was the effectiveness of treatments of pressure ulcers, it would be unethical to not treat a pressure ulcer at all. Therefore, the study might compare different methods of treatment to determine the most effective one. Assigning individuals to the groups using a random method may be done even if the sample selected is not random.

An essential part of any research study is the provision for informed consent of the participants. Informed consent for research has the same attributes as informed consent for medical treatment. The individual must be informed of both potential risks and potential benefits of participating. The researcher must disclose that the participant may or may not receive the treatment under consideration. As part of the consent process, any restrictions on other types of healthcare that may occur while in the study must also be disclosed. Participation must be voluntary, with no adverse consequences occurring if subjects choose not to participate. Further, participants must be informed of their right to withdraw from the study at any time without needing a reason for doing so.

Quantitative Research

Quantitative research refers to a study in which items can be counted or measured and statistics can be used to analyze the results. There are many types of quantitative studies, but in experimental research, in which a new or different treatment is given to a sample group, it is important to demonstrate in an objective way the effectiveness of the treatment being studied.

The Randomized Controlled Trial

The type of experimental research emphasized most often in medicine is the double-blind, randomized controlled trial, often referred to more simply as the **randomized controlled trial (RCT)**. Double-blind means that neither the participant receiving the treatment nor the person administering the treatment knows whether the participant is receiving the real or active treatment or a placebo. Randomized indicates that the participants are assigned to either the treatment group or the control group by some type of random process. Controlled, as we have discussed, means that there is both a treatment group and a group that does not receive the treatment (**Fig. 15.1**, Box 15.2).

RCT research is valued for determining appropriate medical care. Although this might be the best evidence for choosing a medical therapy or drug, even within medicine, this emphasis is narrow. RCTs often cannot be used for testing nursing actions. One cannot hide from a client that he or she is receiving extra or different nursing care. Nursing activities such as special education, spending time on psychosocial interactions, or even monitoring more frequently are all highly visible to clients and providers. Further, an RCT would not be able to accurately capture individual settings for care, the skills of the practitioners, or the attributes of the individual client, which include cultural background, expectations, preferences, and abilities.

Figure 15.1. Double-blind random controlled trials are often not possible when researching nursing care.

BOX 15.2 A DOUBLE-BLIND RANDOMIZED CONTROLLED TRIAL

Pharmaceutical Company X is testing a new medication for joint pain. People asked to participate in the research study are informed about the study in detail and are told that there will be a random control group that will not receive any actual medication. Those agreeing to participate are told not to take any other medication for joint pain during the study. The researcher uses a random number table to assign the individuals to the two groups: one that receives the new medication and one that will not. Those not receiving the medication will receive an identical tablet that is an inert substance (a *placebo*). The knowledge of which persons are receiving the active medication is not shared with either the participants themselves or with those who distribute the medications to the clients. All participants are evaluated for joint pain on a regular schedule using the same pain assessment tools. Those assessing the participants do not know who has received the active medication. At the end of the trial, the pain scores over time will be analyzed statistically to determine whether the new medication had a significant effect on joint pain.

Other Types of Quantitative Research

There are a variety of other types of quantitative research that may be more useful for nursing. It is sometimes possible to have a treatment group and a control group to be studied that occur naturally (ie, existing by nature and without artificial aid), rather than assigned as randomized groups. Research may be done by studying the same sample of people across time—called a longitudinal study. Other types of quantitative research studies include descriptive studies that collect naturally occurring data such as infection rates or complication rates. Methodologic research is another type of quantitative research that is used to develop research instruments.

Analysis of Quantitative Research

Quantitative studies are analyzed using statistical techniques. In a statistical test, the aim is to determine whether any difference between the control group and the experimental group may be due to chance rather than a result of the treatment. There are many statistical tests, but most result in the determination of the **probability** of the result occurring by chance. The probability is expressed as a decimal fraction. For example, a probability of less than 0.10 means that there is less than a 0.10 or 10% possibility that the result was due to chance. A probability of less than 0.01 means that there is less than 0.01 or 1% possibility that the result was due to chance.

Often a researcher sets a level of significance ahead of time. The **level of significance** is the level at which the researcher believes that the study results most likely represent a nonchance event. A level of significance of less than 0.01 (less than a 1% probability that the result is due to chance) is commonly used. A result that meets the appropriate level of significance is often referred to as a significant result.

Statistical significance is not the same as clinical significance. **Clinical significance** relates to having an effect on actual client outcomes. While the effect of the treatment might have made a change that is statistically significant, this change may not make a difference in the outcome for the client and thus will not be clinically significant.

Qualitative Research

Qualitative research, frequently used to gain greater understanding of the experience of the client and family, involves studying phenomena as they naturally occur. Qualitative research strives to look at the whole picture and may include interviews, lengthy observations, and detailed case histories. Analysis of qualitative research attempts to find themes within the data.

Types of Qualitative Research

Specific types of qualitative research include phenomenology, ethnography, case studies, and life histories.

In *phenomenology*, extensive and unstructured interviews are conducted with a limited number of participants. The goal is to identify the themes and patterns within their discussions. Phenomenology frequently results in extensive descriptive discussions of the lived experience of persons with a certain health concern, while *ethnography* examines cultures and cultural phenomena. Understanding what clients experience helps the nurse to focus communication and support strategies to address important areas of life.

Case studies and *life histories* provide detailed information about a single individual. These may serve as an example that will present the various concerns and potential health professional responses. Case studies help the reader to see the specific and particular circumstances of the individual more clearly and then apply that same comprehensive inquiry to their clients. A life history helps the nurse to understand how a health problem might fit into an entire life.

Analysis of Qualitative Research

Analysis of qualitative research differs from analysis of quantitative research. No statistical tests are used, and there is no effort made to try to determine probability in regard to the information.

The analysis of the data gathered in a qualitative study involves an extensive immersion of the researcher into the data to begin to detect themes and patterns. The report is usually a lengthy narrative discussion with the liberal use of quotations from the data to illustrate the topic being presented. Some qualitative research results in the development of conceptual models of relationships. The results of a qualitative research study enable the reader to gain increased depth of understanding about the research topic.

A Staff Nurse's Role in the Research Process

For the results of nursing research to be successful, it must be carried out by an individual who has the educational background to thoroughly understand and direct the process. This may be a nurse with a master's degree; but for large studies, for funded research, and in large institutions, the principal researcher is usually a nurse with a doctorate. The research itself is most often conducted by a team that includes individuals who provide the treatment (if this is a part of the research design), those who collect the data, and specialists in statistics who assist with data analysis. The staff nurse may fulfill a treatment role or a data collection role in this process.

A major role for staff nurses is to identify questions or problems. Within an institution, there may be a specific method for a staff nurse to communicate questions to an individual or a committee that might plan research. If you believe a topic should be studied, do not be concerned if your question is not clearly formulated. Any question will need refinement and reconsideration as it goes through the process. Your question may just be the beginning of gathering important information.

Another role of the staff nurse is to guard the welfare of the clients for whom he or she cares. This means asking questions to be sure the research proposed has gone through the appropriate institutional processes before agreeing to participate as a data gatherer or the nurse providing the research intervention. There should be a formal consent process that is clear to the participants. Just as the staff nurse is not responsible for medical consent, the staff nurse is not responsible for research consent. If clients who have agreed to participate exhibit ambivalence or uncertainty about participating, do not try to convince them to participate. Ask the person from the research team who is managing consents to speak with concerned clients about the study. Clients do have the freedom to withdraw from a research study at any time. Additionally, nurses need to be sure that effective care can be provided to the client. For example, they need to be able to assess for possible side effects or adverse reactions. Protocols for managing such side effects must be in place for client protection.

Daily Ethical Dilemma 15.1: *Misunderstanding*

Debbie is taking care of Mr. Anderson who has stage 4 colon cancer that has spread to his spine. A research study is being done on a new treatment for colon cancer, and Mr. Anderson wants to participate. The researcher meets with Mr. Anderson and explains all the potential risks and benefits and that he will be in one of two groups, one group receives the new medicine and the other group receives the current standard treatment. Mr. Anderson signs the informed consent but after the researcher leaves, Mr. Anderson says to Debbie, "I know this new medicine is going to help me!"

- Based on Mr. Anderson's comments do you think he understands the process? Why or why not?
- What would you say to him?
- Why does this represent an ethical dilemma?

Using research in practice is perhaps the most important role of the staff nurse. The process of using research in practice is discussed below as part of evidence-based nursing.

EVIDENCE-BASED PRACTICE IN NURSING

One major thrust for the future of nursing revolves around the development of **evidence-based practice (EBP)**. EBP first began in medicine and is expanding to all of healthcare. EBP in nursing is being instituted in many healthcare organizations. All nurses need to develop a spirit of inquiry in regard to their practice and incorporate evidence into all that they do (Melnyk, Fineout-Overholt, Stillwell, et al., 2010).

Establishing a Definition of Evidence-Based Nursing

A variety of definitions of evidence-based nursing have been proposed. EBP uses current research to solve problems while integrating the use of nurse's clinical expertise and the client's preference and values (AMSN, 2017). This definition provides an excellent foundation both for the individual nurse and for the institution to establish evidence-based nursing practice.

Let us examine this definition carefully. The major focus is on problem solving. Nurses are accountable for decisions, and they need to base those decisions on supporting evidence, not custom or habit. Another significant part of this definition is the emphasis on clinical nursing expertise. The expertise of nurses in applying information to the care of specific clients is essential. Nurses have an obligation to continually work to improve their own knowledge base and ability to identify appropriate applications of information to specific client situations. An important aspect found in this definition is the autonomy of the client. This supports views set forth by Melnyk (2004), who suggests that client values and preferences should always be added to any discussion of the use of EBP. Although the definition states "client," this can be expanded to consider the client, whether that is the individual, family, or community.

An issue not included in this definition is the consideration of the available resources. This would include both human and material resources and is strongly related to the cost-effectiveness of an intervention. Cost-effectiveness constrains decisions that individual clients make, as well as the decisions made by healthcare providers. The individual client may decide that the marginal difference between a new brand-name wound therapy and the older therapy is not worth several hundreds of dollars a month in costs. A system itself may reject providing certain high-cost options that demonstrate marginal improvement in outcomes. The human resources needed for implementation of some therapies may critically change the cost-effectiveness data. For example, some expensive wound management products may so significantly reduce nursing time and shorten the days of hospitalization that they are, in fact, still cost-effective. Thus, considering cost-effectiveness is critical for nursing **(Fig. 15.2)**.

Figure 15.2. The lack of resources may be a barrier to evidence-based nursing practice.

Determining Adequate Evidence

This brings us to the question of what constitutes adequate evidence upon which to base practice. Melnyk and Fineout-Overholt (2011) provide a rating system for examining the hierarchy of evidence that might be used as a basis for evidence-based nursing practice (Box 15.3). RCTs stand at the top of this list, with types of research studies encompassing the first four levels of evidence. Qualitative studies and single descriptive studies, as well as reports of expert committees, are included at the end of the list. Qualitative studies are often used in nursing because they are more likely to reveal the client's perception of the problem or of the intervention. This attention to client preferences is impossible in the RCT.

While the Melnyk and Fineout-Overholt list (2011) provides a good starting point, nursing generally relies on a broader array of evidence for determining the best practice for a nursing situation. Box 15.4 provides a list of the types of evidence commonly used to support nursing practice. Although they are in an approximate order of reliability, there is not a clear-cut hierarchy. Research reports (the first on the list) include all the types of research that are listed in Box 15.3 as levels I to VI. Retrospective or concurrent chart reviews, quality improvement, risk management, and benchmarking data are all site specific and useful to nurses.

Guidelines for practice developed by groups of experts based upon the best available evidence are a useful tool for EBP. These panels of experts—whether international, national, or local—use a variety of evidence and information resources as they seek to determine best practices. Their guidelines may be an excellent source for nursing decision making. The Agency for Healthcare Research and Quality (AHRQ) convenes expert panels to develop guidelines for some situations of common concern. It also maintains a clearinghouse of guidelines that have been developed by other authoritative groups. These guidelines may be accessed on AHRQ's Web site at www.ahrq.gov and are an excellent resource for staff nurses seeking to use EBP.

BOX 15.3 COMMONLY USED RATING SYSTEM FOR THE HIERARCHY OF EVIDENCE

Level I: Evidence from a systematic review or meta-analysis of all relevant randomized controlled trails (RCTs), or evidence-based clinical practice guidelines based on systematic reviews of RCTs.

Level II: Evidence obtained from at least one well-designed RCT.

Level III: Evidence obtained from well-designed controlled trials without randomization.

Level IV: Evidence from well-designed case–control and cohort studies. Some infection control studies or quality assurance studies may fall into this category.

Level V: Evidence from systematic reviews of descriptive and qualitative studies. This would include multiple retrospective or chart reviews, quality assurance reviews, or infection control reviews that provide descriptive information.

Level VI: Evidence from a single descriptive or qualitative study. This would include a single retrospective or chart review, quality assurance review, or infection control review that provides descriptive information.

Level VII: Evidence from the opinion of authorities and/or reports of expert committees.

From Melnyk, B. M., & Fineout-Overholt, E. (2011). *Evidence based practice in nursing & healthcare. A guide to best practices* (3d ed.). Philadelphia, PA: Lippincott Williams & Wilkins.

Infection control data provide an important foundation for nursing decision making as well. For example, the infection control data of an individual setting may be stronger evidence for the effectiveness of a certain practice than a research study conducted in a very different setting. The infection control data reflect this individual setting with its providers, client population, and physical setup. In the same way, quality improvement data may help an institution to target its own processes in a way that a RCT might not.

The difference between the evidence supplied in a RCT and that found in a real-life situation may be subtle but very real and important. Real-life situations lack the controls of research studies. Both clients and healthcare settings are more varied than typical research subjects and settings. Clients often have multiple health problems and confounding interactions that make their situations unique. Issues such as the client's view of quality of life profoundly affect decisions about appropriate healthcare. Healthcare settings have differing resources, both material and human.

Nurses must also face the reality that there is no research evidence regarding some aspects of nursing practice. One cannot just delay making decisions and withhold care until data are forthcoming. That is why the list in Box 15.4 also contains the use of basic scientific information in regard to pathophysiology. However, this also highlights the need to remain open and actively seeking evidence for practice. Sometimes what seemed very appropriate when reasoned out from a pathophysiologic basis turns out not to be the best action.

Client values and preferences are unique to each client situation, although there may be trends across client populations treated in some settings. An understanding of these values and preferences may guide decisions about what interventions to investigate. In some situations, client preferences may rise to the top of the list of appropriate evidence when a decision must be made and may outweigh all other evidence.

The expertise of the staff is also a factor in determining the most appropriate practice. Expert staff members may attend conferences, read widely, and access resources that they may use when problem solving in regard to appropriate nursing interventions. Additionally, the expertise of the staff is a factor in deciding whether certain types of actions can be implemented.

When looking for evidence, many believe this to be an entirely scientific inquiry. However, there may be competing interests involved as well as simply the evidence. The evidence is rarely so clear that there is no room for differences of opinion in regard to the meaning of the evidence. When decisions involve competing values such as safety, quality of life, length of life, or

---

BOX 15.4 SOURCES USED FOR EVIDENCE-BASED NURSING PRACTICE

- Research reports of all types
- Retrospective or concurrent chart reviews
- Quality improvement, risk management, and benchmarking data
- International, national, and local standards or guidelines developed by expert panels evaluating a variety of information resources
- Infection control data
- Pathophysiology information
- Cost-effectiveness analysis
- Client preferences
- Clinical expertise of individuals

cost, the process of determining the appropriate path becomes complex. Managed care organizations, insurance providers, and hospitals may make some decisions based on their own best interests more than those of the client. Nurses need to be aware of these political factors and recognize that adopting a new EBP may require astute attention to the politics of the setting.

The Evidence-Based Practice Process

Many different models for evidence-based nursing practice have been developed. One of the first was the project at the University of Minnesota in the late 1970s, which was designed to encourage the translation of nursing research into practice. Later in the 1980s, the Stetler Model of Research Utilization was developed as a process for the individual to incorporate research into practice. The Iowa Model of Research in Practice, developed in the 1990s, grew out of the quality improvement process and was designed for institutions moving toward EBP. That model has been broadened into the Iowa Model of Evidence-Based Practice 2015 (Iowa Model Collaborative, 2017) **(Fig. 15.3)**. At the University of North Carolina (UNC), a simple rubric of "5 As" has been established to stimulate individuals to adopt EBP. The steps in this rubric are (1) Ask, (2) Acquire, (3) Analyze (or Appraise), (4) Apply, and (5) Assess (UNC, 2017, Box 15.5). They relate these words to a process first described by Flemming in 1998.

All of these models describe the same phenomenon but use different language and may be divided into different steps; all are useful. For the beginner, the UNC model is easy to understand and follow. You may use this process to improve your own practice, but, more important, a group of nurses may use it to establish an EBP protocol or procedure. The use of the UNC model is described in the following.

Asking Appropriate Questions

The first step, Ask, involves developing a clear, focused question. This is essential to obtaining the information needed for decision making. Thompson, Cullum, McCaughan, et al. (2004) identified a variety of decision-making questions that often face nurses. The effectiveness of the intervention may be the one that is thought of most often. Other questions relate to the timing of the intervention and to referral patterns. Questions regarding assessment strategies are important. Which assessments provide clinically relevant data and which are merely

UNC model

BOX 15.5 THE FIVE As OF THE EVIDENCE-BASED PRACTICE PROCESS

Ask: Convert information needs from practice into focused, structured questions.
Acquire: Use the focused questions as a basis for literature searching in order to identify relevant external evidence from research and to identify relevant internal data from quality improvement, risk management, or infection control data.
Analyze: Critically analyze the evidence found for validity and the ability to generalize it.
Apply: Use the best available evidence alongside clinical expertise, the client's perspective, and knowledge of available resources to plan care.
Assess: Evaluate performance through a process of self-reflection, audit, or peer assessment.

Adapted from University of North Carolina. (n.d.). *Evidence based nursing.* Retrieved July 28, 2010, from http://www.hsl.unc.edu/services/tutorials/ebn/practice.htm; Flemming, K. (1998). Asking answerable questions. *Evidence Based Nursing, 1*(2), 36–37.

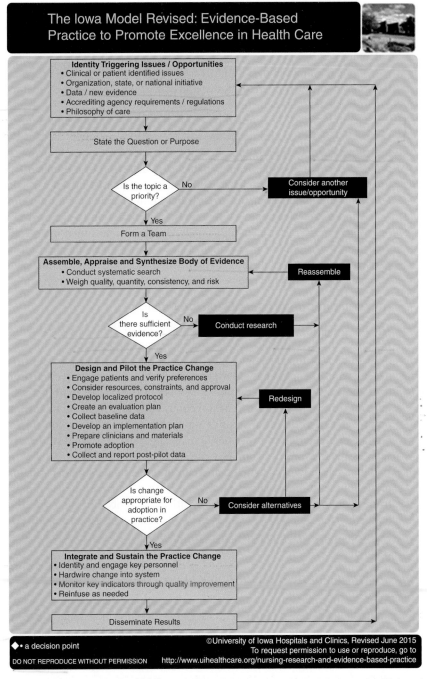

Figure 15.3. The Iowa Model, 2015. Used/Reprinted with permission from the University of Iowa Hospitals and Clinics. Copyright 2015. For permission to use or reproduce, please contact the University of Iowa Hospitals and Clinics at (319)384-9098.

custom? How frequently should assessments be done? Another category of questions are those that relate to communication and teaching strategies. Nurses must continually strive to find the most effective ways to communicate with and teach clients in order to achieve the desired outcomes.

Vague questions about "best care for [any given health problem]" are seldom helpful. The question should be framed to address a specific clinical problem in order to facilitate the literature search but at the same time remain focused on the client or the client population.

Flemming (1998) suggested that a good question has three parts: the *situation*, the *intervention/action* under consideration, and the *desired outcome*. The situation might be for an individual client or for a group of clients. The intervention might be one that will resolve the problem or an action that would enable early detection of a problem. The desired outcome focuses on the end result to be achieved such as decreased infection rate or decreased occurrence of some complication due to early detection of an incipient problem.

A more extensive approach to a question is based on the acronym PICOT—*population, intervention under consideration, comparison* (possible other interventions that might be used), *outcome*, and *time frame* (Polit & Beck, 2014). Thus, the question encourages the comparison of various possible interventions when those are known and includes the time needed to accomplish the desired outcome as an important aspect.

Acquiring Information for Decision Making

The next step is to Acquire information related to the concern. This requires a systematic review of the literature in your search for scientific evidence to answer the question. You need to be able to access and effectively use information resources in order to gather the needed data. The information might include research studies, practice guidelines produced by authoritative bodies, infection control data from one's own institution, benchmarking data regarding infection of central venous catheters from other institutions, information on processes used in other settings along with their infection control data, and costs (both human and material) of processes that are suggested. Original studies; syntheses of studies, such as those available from agencies such as the Cochrane Library (Cochrane Review); evidence-based journal articles; and computerized data support systems may all be appropriate sources of information. Gathering all this information may require the collaboration from many people and consultation with a reference librarian and those responsible for budgeting for supplies. A team approach often is set up to include relevant contributors to the data-gathering process. Accessing information for practice is discussed later in this chapter.

Analyzing Information for Application

After the information is acquired, it's time for Analysis. Analysis of a whole group of research studies is challenging. Often a clinical nurse specialist or other advanced practice nurse takes the lead in analyzing the research data. The reader must check that the research studied is valid, relevant, and can be appropriately applied to the given situation. Analysis does not end with traditional analysis of the research studies. There must be an integrative approach in which all the data are examined in relationship to other data. Consider resources, your own client population, and how this might fit with client preferences. The analysis results in a decision about a course of action. Again, a group discussion to analyze the data may be most productive. One result of analysis may be that no change is warranted. If that is the case, the analysis and report need to be written so that it can be accessed by others at a later time if a change is again contemplated.

Applying New Information

When the analysis has been completed and it has identified a need for a change in practice, preparations are made to Apply the new information. A protocol or procedure must be developed or adopted and a plan for implementation is needed. Will this plan be implemented for the entire facility, for a particular unit or units, or as a pilot project in one area with a decision about the entire facility made after results of the pilot are completed? How and when will this change in practice be introduced? What steps will be taken to ensure that the client's values and desires are considered? Are resources available? The application of a new intervention needs the thoughtful use of information related to change and its implementation (see Chapter 12). After this careful and thorough planning process, the intervention is initiated.

Assessing Outcomes of New Practices

Introducing the change by itself is not enough, however. The next step is to Assess the change using the quality improvement process in place in the institution. A detailed plan for assessing outcomes must be established and carried out. Documentation of all outcomes is essential to making decisions about the intervention. Assessment may involve assessing the response of a single client or of a group of clients. Is the desired outcome being achieved? What are the strengths as well as the drawbacks of the change in practice? What would be the challenges of expanding this change? Are nurses committed to the change in practice? Does the practice need modification or more education of staff to increase compliance with implementation?

Using Infection Control and Quality Improvement Data to Improve Care

In addition to specific questions that arise to care providers, most healthcare agencies are involved in processes of quality improvement. As part of these processes, ongoing data are collected and analyzed for problems or opportunities for improvement.

Using quality improvement processes requires that there be ongoing data collection regarding outcomes. When outcomes are known, then addressing areas for possible improvement in outcomes becomes possible. For example, if data collection reveals that the length of stay for a knee replacement varies from 3 to 6 days, the question might be raised as to how care processes might be improved to move toward a 3-day stay for the majority of clients. The process involved in making any changes would be the EBP described earlier.

Individual Accountability for Evidence-Based Practice

While this discussion has focused on the EBP process for an institution as a whole, individual nurses also have accountability for EBP. Nurses are obligated to adhere to evidenced-based guidelines developed by the institution. Nurses increasingly find the expectation that they must be critical decision makers in their own practice as well. This requires an ongoing commitment to asking questions and choosing paths.

The nurse as an employee, not an independent practitioner, has an obligation to identify how a change in personal practice will affect others and the system. Part of applying a new nursing intervention or assessment process may involve consulting with others, especially with the nurse manager. What may be needed is for the individual nurse to become the change agent to affect the practice within the system? (See Chapter 12 on leading change.)

Theory Alert   Katharine Kolcaba

Katharine Kolcaba's contribution to nursing theory was the comfort theory. Born in Ohio in 1944, Kolcaba earned her nursing diploma from St. Luke's Hospital School of Nursing in 1965. She went on to study at the Frances Payne Bolton School of Nursing at Case Western Reserve University and earned a doctorate in nursing in 1997.

Kolcaba's Comfort Theory of Nursing identifies three forms of comfort: relief, ease, and transcendence. Additionally, there are four areas that comfort can come from; physical, psychospiritual, environmental, and sociocultural. This theory proposes that when clients are comfortable, they are able to recover more quickly and with fewer complications. During her career, Kolcaba was involved in many different research opportunities and was a strong supporter of nursing research.
(Source: http://www.nursing-theory.org)

Barriers to Evidence-Based Nursing Practice

Although the development and production of nursing research has increased, the use of nursing research as well as other types of evidence to inform practice has not moved forward as quickly as some nursing leaders would like. This has its roots in many different issues.

Access to Information Resources

Factors affecting nurses are the availability of information resources and the access to search capabilities. Many people mistakenly believe that all needed information is available without charge online. While many government sources of information, such as guidelines through the AHRQ and the Medline database, are available at no charge, the majority of databases that provide full-text articles require subscriptions for online access. Subscribing to one or more journals in your field provides some information for practice, but most nurses will find that they need the resources of a good library to find and retrieve all the information they need.

Academic medical centers may have a wide array of resources; however, there are many hospitals and other employment settings with limited access. The libraries in smaller hospitals have historically focused on supporting medical practice rather than nursing practice. Some hospitals and nursing homes have blocked any Internet access in order to deter inappropriate use and create a stronger firewall against unauthorized entry into their own computer system. The side effect of this action is decreased access to online resources for staff.

Lack of Time for Seeking Information Resources

Within most employment settings for nurses, there is no time in the workday to seek new information for practice. While general reading in one's field may be appropriately expected to occur on one's own time, seeking specific information regarding a client currently receiving care or for establishing a policy or protocol would seem appropriate to the workplace. Integrating this need into a very busy workplace is a challenge. In facilities committed to EBP, individuals may be afforded time to meet in committees and to work on questions that need to be answered (Fig. 15.4).

Figure 15.4. Finding time for evidence-based practice is often daunting for nurses, who are pulled in every direction by competing needs.

Lack of Background in Understanding and Valuing Research

Another issue that may affect the utilization of all types of evidence is the fact that the largest number of currently practicing nurses received their nursing education in an AD or diploma program in which the research process was not emphasized. Without an academic background in research understanding and utilization, these nurses may find it challenging to effectively interpret research results and weigh that research against other evidence. This suggests that having nurses work in teams to evaluate evidence for practice might alleviate this concern as those with greater knowledge and expertise in research evaluation take a leadership role. Baccalaureate- and master's-prepared nurses who have a more in-depth background can be effective leaders for this process.

An ongoing concern is whether nurses are committed to supporting the use of research and other evidence to improve their practice. If nurses do not value and support the development of nursing research in their own settings, nursing as a profession will be hampered in its growth.

Critical Thinking Activity: Resources for Evidence-Based Practice

In the facility in which you have clinical experience, research the resources available for EBP. Is there a library? What resources for nursing in terms of databases, references, journals, and so forth are available? Can a nurse access the Internet? If so, what are the rules or restrictions? Does the institution have a committee or committees that have responsibilities in terms of evidence-based nursing practice? Are there nurse specialists who provide support and guidance for EBP? Analyze the resources and try to determine whether the resources are sufficient to meet the needs of the nursing staff for evidence-based nursing practice.

ACCESSING RESOURCES FOR EVIDENCE-BASED PRACTICE

With the rapid changes occurring in healthcare, all providers find themselves needing to access the most current information about specific illnesses, medications, and other treatments. Providers need strategies for finding information. Additionally, they need to be able to evaluate the information retrieved.

Strategies for Finding Information

When all bibliographic databases existed only in print form, the information lagged behind publication by many months. Additionally, searching databases was cumbersome and missing important information was not uncommon. With the development of electronic databases, the search function provides flexibility in the language used and the combination of terms that can be entered. This sets the framework for specifically targeted searches of the healthcare literature. Many nursing programs require that students learn to use bibliographic references to support their education, an important skill that will continue throughout your career.

The most comprehensive database is Medline, a resource of the National Library of Medicine (NLM), which may be searched through the PubMed search site. PubMed provides a thesaurus of specific terms that are used by the NLM librarians to index articles into relevant categories within the Medline database. Additionally, the Medline database can be searched in terms of key words that might appear in the title or in the abstract or even within the article itself. PubMed searches are free and available online. After the search has enabled the identification of appropriate references, a source for those references is needed. PubMed may also be used to identify resources and then the specific documents may be sought in a hospital, college, or medical center library.

Several databases include health-related publications to which libraries may subscribe. Access to these databases is restricted to those belonging to the agencies that subscribe to them, such as students and faculty of college and university libraries and employees of institutional subscribers. Many of these databases provide abstracts and some full-text articles.

The Cumulative Index of Nursing and Allied Health Literature (CINAHL) available through Ebsco Host is a bibliographic resource focused on nursing and allied health. Nursing content can be searched using nursing-related terms as well as broader health-related terms. The thesaurus for CINAHL includes nursing diagnoses and steps of the nursing process as well as terms related to common nursing interventions. CINAHL is available by subscription only and may be included in a library's subscription base. Some indexed articles (but not all) are available from the CINAHL with full-text subscription.

Cochrane Library is a database of systematic reviews available online (see discussion of systematic reviews below). It includes four databases: the Cochrane Database of Systematic Reviews, the Database of Abstracts of Reviews of Effectiveness, the Cochrane Controlled Trials Register, and the Cochrane Review Methodology Database.

Online journals are indexed in databases alongside print journals, but many online journals are also accessible through Internet search engines such as Google and Yahoo Search. Online journals typically require a paid subscription to access full-text articles. These Internet search engines may also reveal government and organization recommendations or standards, papers, conference proceedings, reports, and other resources that are available online.

After you choose a database to search, you will need to formulate your search strategy. The help of a librarian is invaluable in this process. A knowledgeable librarian will direct you toward the various indexed terms and categories that will tend to retrieve more specifically targeted results. While key words are useful, they often return many references that do not relate to your needs. Additionally, terms can be combined using connectors such as *and, or,* and *not.* Using such terms as "*clinical guidelines,*" "*systematic review,*" or "*meta-analysis*" will return articles that provide a broad base of information. A search may be limited to English language, a specified range of dates, populations studied, and others. These are usually available under an "advanced search" tab.

Critical Thinking Activity: Perform a Resource Search
Identify a nursing diagnosis with which you are not familiar. Using PubMed online, seek information on the nursing care needs of individuals with that particular nursing diagnosis. After using PubMed, use whatever databases (choose CINAHL if available) are in your school library to seek references about that topic. Then use an Internet search engine such as Google, MSN Search, or Yahoo Search to look up the same nursing diagnosis. Compare the resources you found from each of the different search techniques.

Evaluating Information Retrieved

Regardless of the resource used for accessing data, critical judgment regarding the reliability and validity of information retrieved is essential. You will need to ask a series of questions about the source and content of the material you have accessed. These same questions may be taught to clients who are often researching information about their health conditions using online references (Box 15.6).

BOX 15.6 KEY STRATEGIES FOR EVALUATING INFORMATION RESOURCES

1. Source of information:
   * Who controls the journal or Web site?
   * Is it peer reviewed?
2. The author or authors:
   * Are the authors or editors apparent in the resource?
   * What are the credentials of the authors or editors?
   * What are the affiliations of the authors or editors?
   * Who funded their research?
3. Context of the resource:
   * How closely does the resource speak to your situation or need?
   * Where was the provided information obtained? Consider the various sources for evidence-based care.
4. Consensus of multiple resources:
   * Are there other resources that agree with this one?
   * Is this resource suggesting actions that are outside the generally accepted standard?
5. Comparison of new information with previous information:
   * What are the differences from what you previously understood?
   * Are differences explained so that you can understand them?

The first question to ask is about the source of the information. If this is a journal, who publishes it? It may be a nursing or medical organization, an independent party, or a pharmaceutical company. What are the credentials of the individuals on the editorial board? Do you recognize any of the names? If this is a Web site, who controls the content on this site? Is it identified by a date? By an author? Examine the policies regarding publication. There is often a page or section of a Web site designed to give information to potential authors or contributors. This may provide you with information about how content is reviewed. Is there a process in which appropriate professionals peer review any manuscript before publication? Individuals are eligible to be peer reviewers when they have both subject matter expertise and an understanding of research. The journal selects appropriate peer reviewers, who read and critique the article and make recommendations as to whether it should be published. Peer review strengthens the reliability of the content. Consider the potential accuracy of the material and whether the source might be biased.

Look at the biographical material on the authors. What are their credentials for writing? If this is a report of a clinical practice in a particular institution, what is the author's role in that institution? If it is a research report, what are the author's credentials for research? Who funded the research?

As you read the material, consider the content from different perspectives. Consider how closely the basis of the report matches your situation or need. For example, a protocol used in a major medical center may be unrealistic for a small community hospital with fewer resources. Interventions that work well with a college-educated population may not work well for a low-income, low-educational-level group. An intervention that has limited study may be useful for an individual client for whom the standard interventions are not being successful. However, this same intervention might be inappropriate as a standard of care. Is the information anecdotal only or was there a planned method of measuring outcomes and results that are being reported?

When using references for practice, you will find it useful to look for multiple references. What worked in one small study may have been unsuccessful when a similar study was done. What might have contributed to this disparity in outcomes? If multiple sources all achieved the same outcome or made the same recommendation, this strengthens the recommendation. Consider how the recommendations fit in with prior standards of practice. While new standards will emerge, changing dramatically from known standards requires a higher level of proof than would be required when making a minor change.

For some problems, a systematic review may be available from a source such as the Cochrane Review or in an article. A systematic review examines a broad spectrum of research regarding a specific problem. The review presents the strengths and weaknesses of the various research studies and then provides an analysis of the meaning of all of them combined. Often this review is done by an expert panel providing excellent information on which to base decisions.

Always compare new information with old. Make sure that you clearly understand the similarities and differences. Sometimes the long-established practice is not based on research but rather is simply customary. If you do not understand the current practice, you will have difficulties making judgments about changing practices.

> **Critical Thinking Activity: Putting EBP Into Action**
> Working with a small group of students, identify a nursing care question that is of inter-
> est to you. Using the EBP process discussed, seek evidence for the best nursing prac-
> tices in relationship to this question. Be sure to document all references you used in
> your process. Based on the evidence you found, formulate a policy and/or protocol to
> address the nursing care question and present it to your class.

Sharing Information Retrieved

Information that has been retrieved and evaluated has value to other nurses as well as yourself. There are many ways to share information including bulletin boards, presentations at staff meet-ings, the designation of specific nurses as experts, posters on stands that can be moved about, and a cart or box containing information about a specific nursing care question. You and your colleagues may identify other effective strategies for your own work environment. Creating a climate of inquiry and responsiveness will support ongoing development of EBP. Make sure to give credit to sources and consult a librarian when in doubt to prevent violating Copyright Law.

TECHNOLOGY IN HEALTHCARE

Technology in healthcare is prolific and rapidly changing. It is found as an approach to man-aging general knowledge related to healthcare, as well as computerized client care data. It is widely recognized that nursing students must be appropriately prepared to practice in a tech-nologic environment.

From e-mail and Listservs to tablets and smartphones, nurses are using personal technol-ogy to support their practice. Both individuals and institutions rely on information technol-ogy to access resources and references. Institutions use computerized systems to gather data and manage the healthcare environment. The use of computerized systems in healthcare has increased steadily, and all information will eventually be managed by computer. This poses challenges to nursing to maintain a "high-touch" relationship with the client in the midst of the high-tech environment of healthcare.

Information technology is being used to store research data, disseminate research and practice information, and retrieve information for use. The study and management of infor-mation technology is often referred to as the field of **informatics**. The American Nursing Informatics Association (https://www.ania.org) is a national specialty group in nursing that focuses on nursing informatics.

Computerized Client Records

Computerization of client data began in most facilities with the computerization of payment and billing data. While forward-looking healthcare institutions began computerizing client care records beginning in the early 1980s, the beginning of the 21st century was characterized by directives from Medicare and Medicaid to computerize client records and communication. The Health Information Portability and Accountability Act of 1996 (HIPAA) mandated that all billing to the federal government be done electronically. In order to facilitate this, all providers submitting bills were required to use standardized documentation.

Early Computerization of Standardized Data

The *International Classification of Diseases* (ICD), published by the World Health Organization and currently in its 10th edition (11th edition anticipated in 2018), and the *Current Procedural Terminology*, published by the American Medical Association and currently in its 4th edition (a new CPT is published every October), both use a numbering system to enable the coding of diseases, treatment modalities, and procedures performed. Health information specialists became essential to manage these complex systems for data entry and retrieval. Billing of third-party payers is dependent on exact use of the correct codes. Deliberately using incorrect codes in order to generate increased income has been prosecuted as fraud. All statistical management became computerized with birth and death records, cancer registries, and other data-gathering requirements met by skilled coders taking each client's handwritten chart and extracting and coding the data into computer systems.

As health information specialists became responsible for reviewing client charts for billing purposes, they were given responsibility for monitoring charts for complete documentation. Their sphere of responsibility in most facilities also includes management of the client privacy mandates such as HIPAA and may involve quality monitoring processes.

Pharmacy and laboratory records usually followed billing data in the process of computerization. Computerized records could then be accessed more quickly by those who needed them. Pharmacy and laboratory records are, by their nature, specific, concrete, and objective, thus making them adaptable to and suitable for computerization.

Nurses are able to access laboratory data more quickly and respond by providing the appropriate intervention that is based on data. Many hospitals have made laboratory data available to providers who are not in the hospital to enable them to respond more effectively to information as it becomes available. The availability of data on the computer has freed the nursing department from a major collection, filing, and notification role. Although this was often delegated to a unit secretary, the nursing staff was responsible for ensuring that this was accomplished.

Computerized pharmacy records have decreased the nurses' need to process large volumes of paperwork related to medication administration. Information regarding allergies, drug interactions, and other concerns are often immediately available.

Computerized Nursing Care Records

Computerizing the nursing client care record has been a complex task. Many different people need to enter data into the record, and many need to extract it. Data that are nonstandardized and more qualitative in nature are more difficult to computerize. The increase in checklists and charting by exception paved the way for an easier entry into computerized data for some aspects of nursing care. The need for detailed narrative was lessened by these various tables, checklists, and charts. Many institutions are turning to the various nursing terminology systems such as the NANDA-I nursing diagnoses, Nursing Intervention Classification (NIC), Nursing Outcomes Classification (NOC), the Omaha system, and others to systematize the language used in documentation. By systematizing the language, uniform data can be extracted for quality improvement purposes as well as for research.

For nurses, there are still problems with computerized data systems. Some have been designed without the input of direct caregivers and are time consuming and cumbersome to use. The need for large numbers of computer entry stations for nursing units has been a problem in other settings. The move toward computerization of the nursing record will continue until all records are computerized. Learning a new computer system is a standard part of any orientation to a new facility.

Computerized Physician/Provider Order Entry

Computerized physician/provider order entry (CPOE) systems, sometimes referred to as computerized order entry (COE), are gaining in use. To institute CPOE, prescribers, whether physicians, dentists, nurse practitioners, or physician assistants, have had to change their practice patterns. One major advantage of CPOE is that errors based on handwriting difficulties are eliminated. Nurses do not have to decipher handwritten orders or spend time trying to contact the provider to clarify the order. Computer prompts may be used to indicate such items as default doses and a range of potential doses for each medication and to indicate a requirement to enter dosage, route, and frequency for each order. This has helped to eliminate the time-consuming process for nurses of contacting providers to obtain complete information when it was overlooked at the time of writing the order. There may also be prompts to suggest the need for laboratory monitoring, and the computer may be programmed to display values already in the client record. Most systems provide for a cross-check with client drug allergy data and drug–drug interactions for the medications already prescribed. The system may be set to reject the use of abbreviations that appear on a "do not use" list. All of these provide greater safety for the client and have the potential to decrease nursing workload in a time of nursing shortage.

CPOE can be used to facilitate the use of standard protocols for care. When the standard protocol with options for individualization is offered on the screen, it becomes easy for a physician to use the standard protocol. Institutions seeking to systematize best practices find this a valuable asset.

Some studies have shown a reduction in medication errors and mortality rates related to the use of CPOE, but other studies also show some negative effects, for example, so many alerts that healthcare providers stop responding appropriately (Khanna & Yen, 2014). Nurses need to be aware that CPOE does not eliminate all problems and should not become complacent. CPOE does not decrease the need for nursing knowledge and critical thinking in regard to the administration of medications.

Client Privacy and Computerized Records

Concerns about privacy become magnified when information is available to many people in many sites far removed from where the client is located. All systems require passwords for entry and contain tracking capabilities to determine who has accessed which record from which location. This is essential to enforce the restrictions that govern authorized access. Of even greater concern than the individual who violates confidentiality is the wholesale access to large databases for illegal purposes. As ambulatory care data are merged into overall systems with hospital data, the potential for misuse of information is expanded. HIPAA legislation has mandated that institutions using computerized records have safeguards for client privacy in place. Agencies that fail to implement appropriate privacy policies are subject to substantial fines.

Communication in Action 15.1: *Maintaining Integrity With Computerized Records*

Jose Martinez, an RN working on the evening shift, was approached by one of the nursing assistants who said, "My sister was admitted to the Birth Room just before I came on the shift. Would you check the computer and see if she has had the baby yet? I think it will appear on the new admissions." Jose replied, "I wish I could help you. I know how anxious you have been about your sister. But remember, none of us can access the computer for information if we are not involved in that person's care. But I can watch your clients for you so that you can go to the mother–baby area and see if you can talk with her or a family member there."

Advantages of Computerized Client Records

Computerized records have many advantages for clients and healthcare providers. Some of those were discussed in relationship to specific aspects of the record.

A major advantage of the computerized record is that it can be available at the point-of-care without the need to obtain a copy of the written record. Continuity of care is also facilitated when the information follows the client from setting to setting. Many health systems are integrating ambulatory care data with hospital data so that wherever the client is, the provider has access to the needed care information. Even when the records are not integrated, it is possible to send electronic forms of the record to the setting where it is required to facilitate continuity of care. Work continues to create a way to integrate different systems to create seamless access to client records for healthcare providers.

Computerizing Management of Client Care

The use of technology for direct care has increased gradually throughout the past 30 years. Within nursing, computerized devices initially became available in intensive care units as monitors for cardiac rhythms. Computerized pumps and controllers were introduced to monitor intravenous infusions. Automatic BP–measuring devices provide for frequent measurements accompanied by alarms for readings outside preset parameters. Small blood glucose monitors that allow for more precise control of blood sugar for the client with diabetes have become common. A wide variety of real-time client monitoring systems provide continuous readouts of physiologic measurements such as blood oxygen saturation and neurologic status. After beginning slowly in many places, the introduction of new technology for direct care has increased at a rapid pace. One of the trends for the future is wearable monitors that send information directly to the physician or other healthcare provider as telemedicine delivery and improve treatment of chronic illnesses (Health Data Management, 2016).

Distance Monitoring Using Technology

The ability for someone to monitor a critically ill client from another site has created the opportunity to develop what is being called the **electronic ICU (eICU)** or *tele-ICU*. The eICU includes both monitoring equipment and video cameras connected to a separate monitoring center. In the monitoring center, an expert ICU nurse assumes the role of overseeing the electronic monitoring of clients, analyzing data, and recognizing patterns. The eICU nurse uses the video monitor to view a client as well as review monitor information. The bedside nurse manages the direct care of two or three clients. The eICU nurse communicates with the bedside nurse to alert that individual to problems that occur and may initiate calling a physician if necessary. Working together, the bedside nurse and the eICU nurse form a strong team to ensure that the client receives optimum care.

Expert ICU nurses typically rotate through the eICU role as one of their assignments, but work as bedside nurses on other days. This ensures that the eICU nurse remains skilled in bedside care. A critical role of the eICU nurse is in mentoring beginning ICU nurses. The eICU nurse assists the new nurse in developing toward an expert role.

While in its infancy, the concept of the distance monitoring is expanding. Long-distance monitoring is one suggested expansion. An expert ICU nurse at a distant site also could assist by monitoring clients in a smaller hospital where there are fewer ICU experts. A meta-analysis of 25 studies of the eICU or tele-ICU found that implementation resulted in a decreased mortality, decreased costs, and decreased length of stay while in the ICU (Kumar, Merchant, & Reynolds, 2013). The studies also showed the largest barrier to implementation was the resistance by healthcare providers to accept the technology (Kumar et al., 2013).

Handheld Electronic Devices for Nurses

Personal digital assistants (PDAs) are used in all areas of life. Smartphones, and devices such as the iPod touch, are all small, handheld computers that provide the technology for nurses and physicians to have information resources immediately available. A personal electronic device may be loaded with a drug reference book, a laboratory reference book, a resource on diseases and their management, a medical dictionary, a calculator, and nursing references. The technologically proficient nurse can access information immediately when it is needed. Some nursing education programs have developed projects in which all students must have a PDA and, rather than purchasing print versions of reference books, purchase versions to be loaded on the PDA. Frequently assignments, papers, and quizzes are managed online and can be accessed from a PDA. All of these strategies help students prepare for the demand to use technology to support nursing practice.

Another nursing use for handheld computers is to manage assessment data as they are collected and to track nursing actions taken. For nursing students, this might include using the handheld to develop all of the paper work required for clinical experiences. The instructor may use a handheld to manage student data. There are Web sites that offer programs for organizing and managing assessment data.

When used in these ways, concerns arise about privacy and the protection of information for both clients (in accord with HIPAA) and students (who are protected under federal Family Educational Rights and Privacy Act). A healthcare agency will have specific rules regarding entering client data into a personal electronic device. The nurse who uses any such device to enter information has an obligation to use the available security provisions to protect the client. This includes setting up effective passwords to access the information and deleting information as soon as it is not needed for care. PDA loss prevention is another important responsibility. For students, personal identifiable health information about a client should not be entered into a handheld just as it should not be written on papers to be handed in. Please be aware of the policy at each healthcare agency that you go to for clinicals or employment to make sure that you are compliant.

Telehealth

Telehealth is the use of different types of technology to deliver medical, health, and education services virtually (Center for Connected Health policy, n.d.). There are four main categories of telehealth. **Figure 15.5** denotes the first category, which is a video conversation that can occur through phones, tablets, or computers. The second category is the transmission of health histories, x-rays, and photos to other providers instantaneously for consultations. The third category is remote client monitoring to collect and transmit from any location, which allows clients to receive individualized care and stay healthy with up-to-date information. Research has shown that this type of telehealth keeps people healthier, at home, and decreases hospital admissions (Center for Connected Health policy, n.d.). The fourth type is referred to as mobile health where text messages are sent to provide reminders to promote healthy behavior, alert people to disease outbreaks, or other message that contribute to health (Center for Connected Health policy, n.d.).

Telehealth has the potential for supporting effective care of rural populations that have difficulty accessing certain types of healthcare. Through online technology, nurses and physicians may be available to clients who reside far from the provider. Cameras can be used to facilitate long-distance assessment, and specific laboratory and physical assessment information can be communicated to the provider through the Internet. Telemedicine is another term that you may see in the literature that generally refers to services provided by physicians through technology while telehealth encompasses a wide range of healthcare services delivered through technology.

Figure 15.5. Telehealth is increasing accessibility for clients in remote locations and convenience for the public in general.

One area of practice for nurses in telehealth is in telephone triage. Clients and families call the telephone help line, and the nurse uses evidence-based protocols to assess and direct clients in self-care or in accessing medical care as needed. Telephone help lines are often supported by health plans to decrease the use of expensive emergency room care for less serious problems that could be managed in other ways. For clients, the consultation with the nurse provides expert advice and relieves anxiety over which steps appropriately may be taken.

Licensure and practice laws affect the practice of those in telehealth and telemedicine. One concern relates to the control of practice versus the control for client safety. If the client is in one legal jurisdiction and the provider is in another (which often occurs), to whom is the provider accountable for care? As telehealth and telemedicine continue to adapt and grow with changes in technology, the legislation and laws will also change. Information on specific states may be accessed through the Center for Telemedicine Law Web site (n.d.).

The value of technology for the education of healthcare professionals has become more apparent as opportunities arise. There are online degree programs, online continuing education for providers, and online conferences in which individuals may participate. Technology is overcoming the barriers to staying up to date that occur because of distance and funding for healthcare professionals living in smaller communities or rural areas.

Telehealth may also be used to facilitate improved screening and detection of illness, to improve client self-management of chronic conditions, for short- and long-term symptom monitoring, and for the delivery of appropriate health interventions (Evidence-Based Practice 15.1). To address all of these areas, many organizations are supporting research and projects that can be used to implement effective telemedicine and telehealth programs.

Evidence-Based Practice 15.1: *Telemedicine and Nursing Care*

Cryer, L., Shannon, S. B., Van Amsterdam, M., & Leff, B. (2012). Costs for 'Hospital At Home' clients were 19 percent lower, with equal or better outcomes compared to similar inpatients. *Health Affairs, 31*(6),1237–1243. http://www.doi:10.1377/hlthaff.2011.1132

This was a research study done in Albuquerque, New Mexico, where researchers adapted the Hospital at Home model to provide acute care to clients at home. The study showed that the clients at home had comparable or better outcomes to similar clients in the hospital and a 19% reduction in cost. Clients at home reported a higher satisfaction level, which means the study showed that with telemedicine, "clinical quality, affordability, and exceptional client experience" can be achieved.

Clinical Decision Support Systems

Clinical decision support systems are computer programs designed to integrate a medical knowledge base and client data and provide specific advice on how to manage the individual client case. The goal of clinical decision support systems is to provide the best of EBP to care providers in an efficient and cost-effective manner that maintains client safety. A wide variety of different computer systems have been developed for this purpose. A meta-analysis (integrative review of multiple resources) concluded that while computerized clinical decision support systems hold great promise, their benefits are yet to be realized (OpenClinical, n.d.).

Stegen & Sowerby Stories: Part 2

ara speaks with the nursing faculty and the college administration about her finding and presents a plan for increasing the program by 25% by increasing the use of simulation and hiring new faculty. The faculty questions if this is a good idea as they value working with "real" clients.

- How should Tara respond to these concerns?
- What additional resources will Tara need that she should consider?
- What else about the research would be important to know when contemplating the changes?

Read the rest of the story at www.thePoint.com.

Want to Know More?

A variety of resources are available on the Point® to enhance your learning and understanding of this chapter, such as:

- Full Stegen & Sowerby Stories
- NCLEX-Style Student Review Questions
- Journal Articles
- Case Studies
- Learning Objectives
- Relevant Web sites
- And more...

KEY CONCEPTS

- Nursing research has grown and developed since the middle of the 20th century and now is supported through the NINR, which is part of the NIH.
- Nursing research involves the development of a research question, a literature review, a plan for seeking answers, implementation of the plan, analysis of the data gathered, a discussion and evaluation of the results of the study, and recommendations for further research.
- Understanding research terminology and the types of research that can be conducted are essential to reading and using any nursing research.
- The staff nurse's role in relationship to conducting nursing research includes identifying research questions, safeguarding clients who participate in a study, and collecting data and performing treatments.
- "Evidence-based practice (EBP) is a problem-solving approach to the delivery of healthcare that integrates the best evidence from studies and client care data with clinician expertise and client preferences and values" (Fineout-Overholt et al., 2010). This definition provides an excellent foundation both for the individual nurse and for the institution to establish evidence-based nursing practice.
- A wide variety of evidence, including research reports, chart reviews, quality improvement, benchmarking, and data regarding risk management, infection control, pathophysiologic information, cost-effectiveness, and client preferences, may be used to support nursing practice.

- While many models for EBP exist, a simplified process is incorporated in the terms Ask, Acquire, Analyze, Apply, and Assess.
- Barriers to EBP include the availability of resources, time availability, educational preparation, and nursing commitment.
- Accessing information resources requires knowledge of information resources and the use of databases, as well as an understanding of data such as quality improvement and infection control data from the institution.
- Information must be evaluated in relationship to its source, the authors, its relevance to your own practice setting, support from multiple resources, and how this relates to current practice and then shared with colleagues.
- Information technology is dramatically changing how individual client care information and provider planning for care are entered into the record, stored, and retrieved. Personal electronic devices are allowing individual healthcare providers to manage large volumes of information more easily. Security and privacy of client information remain both an ethical and legal challenge.
- Computerized devices increasingly are used to manage the direct care of clients, from automatic blood pressure measuring devices to intravenous controllers to monitoring equipment both locally and from a distance. They are changing the way nursing is practiced.

NCLEX-STYLE PRACTICE QUESTIONS

1. What is one of the purposes of an institutional review board (IRB)?

    A. To decide what will be studied
    B. To protect the rights of the participants
    C. To review literature and other related data
    D. To protect the rights of the researchers

2. Which of the following is an example of a quantitative study?

    A. Perception of nursing students during finals
    B. Experiences of chemo clients with lymphoma
    C. Comparison of hepatitis B treatment regimens
    D. Views of healthcare politics by nurses and CNAs

3. Rank the following type of research evidence from (1) being the strongest evidence to (4) being the weakest evidence for use in evidence-based practice.

    A. Reports from expert committees ____1____
    B. Meta-analysis of all relevant studies ____4____
    C. Systematic review of qualitative studies ____2____
    D. Evidence from a randomized controlled trial ____3____

4. What are the barriers to evidence-based practice? (Select all that apply)

    A. Lack of available resources
    B. Lack of time for learning
    C. Lack of motivation
    D. Lack of nursing knowledge

5. What are some of the ways that technology has improved care? (Select all that apply)
   A. Better funding of vulnerable populations
   B. Ease of access to medical records
   C. Ability to receive care remotely or from home
   D. Instant access to reference materials

REFERENCES

Academy of Medical-Surgical Nurses (AMSN). (2017). *Evidence-based practice.* Retrieved August 2, 2017, from https://www.amsn.org/practice-resources/evidence-based-practice

Center for Connected Health Policy: The National Telehealth Policy Resource Center. (n.d.). *What is telehealth.* Retrieved July 31, 2017, from http://www.cchpca.org/what-is-telehealth

Center for Telemedicine and e-Health Law. (n.d). *Licensure.* Retrieved July 31, 2017, from http://ctel.org/

Connected Health Policy. (n.d). *Center for Connected Health Policy: The National Telehealth Policy Resource Center.* Retrieved June 25, 2018, from http://www.cchpca.org/what-is-telehealth

Fineout-Overholt, E., Melnyk, B. M., Stillwell, S. B., & Williamson, K. M. (2010). Evidence-based practice step by step: Critical appraisal of the evidence. *American Journal of Nursing, 110*(7), 47–52.

Fineout-Overholt, E., Melnyk, B. M., Stillwell, S. B., & Williamson, K. M. (2010). Evidence-based practice step by step: Critical appraisal of the evidence: Part I. *The American Journal of Nursing, 110*(7), 47–52. doi:10.1097/01.NAJ.0000383935.22721.9c

Flemming, K. (1998) Asking answerable questions. *Evidence-Based Nursing. 1*(2), 36–37.

Hayden, J. K., Smiley, R., Alexander, M., Kardong-Edgren, S., & Jeffries, P. R. (2014). The NCSBN national simulation study: A longitudinal, randomized, controlled study replacing clinical hours with simulation in prelicensure nursing education. *Journal of Nursing Regulation, 5*(2), S3–S64. https://doi.org/10.1016/s2155-8256(15)30062-4

Health Data Management. (2016). *Ten top healthcare information technology trends for 2017.* Retrieved August 2, 2017, from https://www.healthdatamanagement.com/list/10-top-healthcare-information-technology-trends-for-2017

Iowa Model Collaborative. (2017). Iowa model of evidence-based practice: Revisions and validation. *Worldviews on Evidence-Based Nursing, 14*(3), 175–182. doi:10.1111/wvn.12223

Khanna, R., & Yen, T. (2014). Computerized physician order entry: Promise, perils, and experience. *The Neurohospitalist, 4*(1), 26–33. http://doi.org/10.1177/1941874413495701

Kumar, S., Merchant, S., & Reynolds, R. (2013). Tele-ICU: Efficacy and cost-effectiveness of remotely managing critical care. *Perspectives in Health Information Management.* Retrieved from http://perspectives.ahima.org/tele-icu-efficacy-and-cost-effectiveness-of-remotely-managing-critical-care/

Melnyk, B. M. (2004). Integrating levels of evidence into clinical decision-making. *Pediatric Nursing, 30*(4), 323–326.

Melnyk, B. M., & Fineout-Overholt, E. (2011). *Evidence based practice in nursing & healthcare. A guide to best practice.* Philadelphia, PA: Wolters Kluwer/Lippincott Williams & Wilkins.

National Institute of Nursing Research. (n.d.). *History.* Retrieved August 3, 2017, from https://www.ninr.nih.gov/aboutninr/history

OpenClinical. (n.d.). *DSS success factors.* Retrieved July 31, 2017, from http://www.openclinical.org/dss-SuccessFactors.html

Polit, D. F., & Beck, C. T. (2014). *Essentials of nursing research: Appraising evidence for nursing practice* (8th ed.). Philadelphia, PA: Wolters Kluwer/Lippincott Williams & Wilkins.

Thompson, C., Cullum, N., McCaughan, D., Sheldon, T., & Raynor, P. (2004). Nurses, information use, and clinical decision making: The real world potential for evidence based decisions in nursing. *Evidence Based Nursing, 7*(3), 68–72.

University of North Carolina. (2017). *Using evidenced based nursing in practice.* Retrieved August 3, 2017, from http://guides.lib.unc.edu/ebn_practice

Index